Advances in Bioactivation Research

Biotechnology: Pharmaceutical Aspects

Advances in Bioactivation Research

Adnan A. Elfarra
Schools of Veterinary Medicine and Pharmacy
Center for Molecular and Environmental Toxicology
University of Wisconsin-Madison

Springer

AAPS PRESS

Editor
Adnan A. Elfarra
Schools of Veterinary Medicine and Pharmacy
Center for Molecular and Environmental Toxicology
University of Wisconsin-Madison
elfarra@svm.vetmed.wisc.edu

ISBN: 978-0-387-77299-8 e-ISBN: 978-0-387-77300-1
DOI 10.1007/978-0-387-77300-1

Library of Congress Control Number: 2008934609

Printed on acid-free paper

springer.com

Contents

Part II Tissue-Specific Features and Risk Assessment Applications

Preface

I have always been interested in chemistry and biology. My undergraduate, graduate, and postdoctoral trainings in pharmacy, medicinal chemistry and pharmacology, respectively, have strengthened this interest and led me to realize that significant advances in medicine have frequently been realized because of research at the chemistry–biology interface. I am hoping that this comprehensive volume on recent advances in bioactivation research will stimulate pharmacologists, medicinal chemists, pharmaceutical scientists, and graduate students in these fields and related areas to consider and use bioactivation research when they explore and chart new frontiers in drug design and drug development and when they consider ways to reduce the side effects of existing drugs by making prodrugs. As for the toxicologists and environmental health scientists, I hope this volume will help them generate the knowledge needed to understand better mechanisms of toxicity to improve human risk assessments and intervention methods after occupational or environmental exposure to various hazardous chemicals.

Adnan A. Elfarra, Ph.D.

Part I

General Concepts and Basic Mechanisms

1

Metabolic Concerns in Drug Design

Jeffrey P. Jones
Department of Chemistry, Washington State University, Pullman, WA 99164, USA
e-mail: jpj@wsu.edu

Keywords: Cytochrome P450 · Aldehyde Oxidase · Drug–Drug Interactions · Mechanism-based · Virtual Screening · ADMET · Regioselectivity

1.1. Introduction

Due to recent technological innovations, such as genomics, combinatorial chemistry, and high-throughput screening, the identification of disease targets and of compounds that are active against these targets ("leads") can now be carried out efficiently. With the acceleration of these early steps of the drug discovery process, the last step of lead optimization has become the new "bottleneck" that is responsible for a substantial portion of the estimated $800 million and the approximately 14 years that it takes to get a new drug to market (Dimasi 2001; Lehmann Brothers 2001).

Lead optimization aims to maximize a compound's ADMET (absorption, distribution, metabolism, excretion, toxicity) properties while at the same time maintaining its potency and selectivity for the target. A variety of approaches have been developed to expedite lead optimization. These approaches include in vitro ADMET screens with increased throughput and quick in vivo assays early in the discovery process. However, these lead optimization strategies still require multiple cycles of compound design, synthesis, and screening. They are cumbersome and often fail to predict the in vivo human condition. The net result is that many compounds with poor ADMET profiles are progressing from early discovery to the pre-development threshold where they fail as drugs. Pfizer reports that only one out of every 12 compounds that enter its development pipeline successfully emerges as a commercial drug (Milne 2000). An estimated 21–35% of these compound failures result from toxicity (Prentis, Lis and Walker 1988).

A.A. Elfarra (ed.), *Advances in Bioactivation Research*, DOI: 10.1007/978-0-387-77300-1_1,

Beyond the development phase, ADMET problems can surface once a drug is launched and used by a broad and diverse patient population. They manifest themselves as overt toxicity problems in specific patient populations or as drug–drug interaction reactions in patients who take multiple drugs. A recent study suggests that 6.7% of hospitalized patients suffer serious adverse drug reactions, defined as those resulting in further hospitalization or causing disability or death (Lazarou, Pomeranz and Corey 1998). In a single year, adverse drug reactions may cause 75 000—135 000 deaths in the US, making such reactions the sixth leading cause of death. Overall, in the US, ADMET liabilities are estimated to account for a significant portion of the $136 billion yearly cost of drug-related morbidity and mortality (Jankel, McMillan and Martin 1994).

Obviously, new technologies are needed to expedite the development and decision-making process at this stage of drug development. One approach is to complement existing experimental approaches with computational models that permit the virtual screening of up to thousands of compounds. Such models promise to dramatically reduce the requirement for repeated physical synthesis and screening of the compounds and thus to expedite drug development and to reduce costs. They also permit the evaluation and optimization of multiple ADMET properties in a more parallel fashion and at an earlier stage of the drug discovery process than is supported by current screening methodologies. Application of these models during drug development would thus lead to the design of compounds with not just "adequate" but "optimal" ADMET properties that are expected to have a greater chance of development success and to lead to better medicines.

1.2. Overview of Computational Modeling of ADMET

Computational models for the cytochrome P450 enzymes are some of the most useful for the characterization and optimization of drug candidates, due to the almost universal importance of the P450 enzymes in drug development programs. The important features of predictive models are (1) regioselectivity (or site of metabolism), (2) substrate affinity, and (3) metabolic rates.

Predicting the site of metabolism is of fundamental importance in the process of compound redesign (Zamora, Afzelius and Cruciani 2003; Zhou et al. 2006). A metabolically labile compound with a single-site major metabolite can be improved by altering the reactivity of that site. As described below, influencing rates of metabolism by decreasing the reactivity of a site can be complicated by P450 enzyme's ability to produce multiple metabolites from a given substrate. Even with this caveat, compound redesign remains one of the single most important uses of metabolic models. In addition, the ability to predict the fractional importance of a given metabolite allows the medicinal chemist to put pro-toxins in the molecule if they are predicted to be a very minor metabolite. Predicting regioselectivity therefore provides important information for the chemist on how to redesign a molecule to have a longer half-life, or to avoid toxicity.

The affinity of a compound for a given metabolic enzyme is an important feature in determining the compound's metabolic profile. In general, a compound with high affinity for an enzyme will be a substrate for that enzyme, although some compounds that have very high affinity are not good substrates (He et al. 1999). Since almost all drug metabolism occurs at subsaturating (first order) drug concentrations in vivo, the observed rate of metabolism is proportional to affinity. In addition, since all substrates are competitive inhibitors the binding affinity of a molecule to a metabolic enzyme determines its potential to inhibit that enzyme and results in drug–drug interactions (Rao et al. 2000). Since the normal therapeutic concentrations of drugs are about 0.1–10 μM, drugs that bind to important metabolic enzymes with less than 10-μM affinities have the potential to inhibit the metabolism of other drugs and cause drug interactions (Rettie and Jones 2005).

Predicting overall rate of clearance of a compound is the most useful and problematic aspect of predictive metabolism. Metabolic rates impact bioavailability and overall clearance of drugs. An ideal drug has an oral bioavailability and a clearance that allows for dosing once a day. Drugs with high first pass metabolism will soon lose market share to newer drugs with more ideal pharmacokinetics. To predict metabolic rates, the affinity, free fractions of drug, and the maximum turnover rate of the metabolic enzyme must be predicted. For the P450 enzymes the maximum turnover is dependent on the ability of the substrate to start the catalytic cycle by initiating the reduction of P450 by P450 reductase, the amount of hydrogen peroxide produced, and the activation energy of substrate oxidation by the active-oxygen species (Cpd I) process relative to reduction of Cpd I to water (Figure 1.1).

While P450 enzymes are arguably the single most important enzyme family, to understand the metabolism of a drug and the potential for toxicity, the drug's total metabolic profile must be considered. Recently a number of models have been made for predicting glucoronide formation

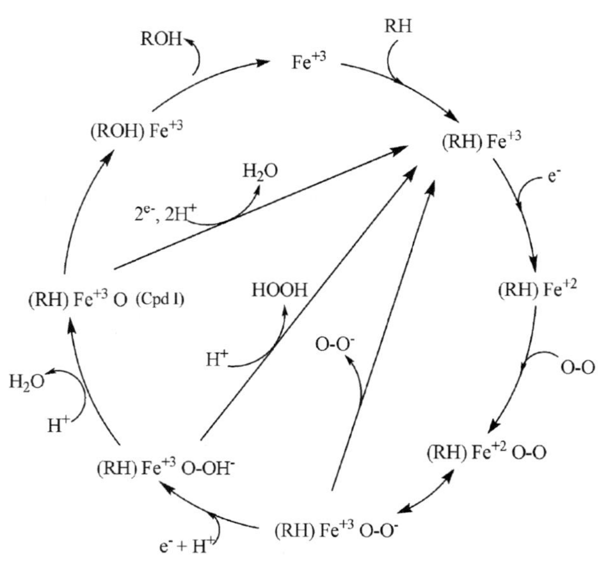

Figure 1.1 The catalytic cycle of P450 enzymes.

(Sorich et al. 2003). To effectively predict ADMET properties in whole animals, methods for predicting the enzymes, including all phase I and phase II enzymes, will be required. Furthermore, as a new generation of drugs are produced that have good (low rates and binding affinities) metabolic profiles with regard to the P450 enzymes, other metabolic enzymes will become more important. At present the efforts to reduce cytochrome P450 metabolic lability have increased the number of azaheterocyclic structures tested for their potential as new drug entities (Obach 2004; Obach et al. 2004; Obach and Walsky 2005). Replacing a carbon in an aromatic ring with a nitrogen decreases the electron density in the aromatic ring carbons thereby decreasing P450-mediated aromatic oxidation. These electron-deficient carbons then become susceptible to nucleophilic attack by aldehyde oxidase (AO). The recent attention given by Pfizer to this enzyme attests to AO's growing significance. Given that the discovery process takes over 10 years in general, we can expect to see a significant increase in the number of drugs metabolized by this enzyme over the next decade.

1.3. Predicting Inhibition/Affinities: Drug–Drug Interactions and Drug Design

1.3.1. Cytochrome P450 Inhibition

The vast majority of drug compounds interact with the cytochrome P450 (CYP)-containing microsomal enzyme system. In most cases, the interactions are detoxifying in that they result in more polar molecules that have greater water solubility and are more susceptible to elimination from the body, or further phase II metabolism. However, metabolism by P450 enzymes can also "bioactivate" a compound by introducing into the compound highly reactive and toxic functionalities (toxicophores) (Park et al. 2005). For example, the oxidation of acetaminophen by CYP2E1 and CYP3A4 produces a reactive quinone imine (Streeter et al. 1984). At large doses, the phase II metabolism pathways that would normally remove this reactive metabolite can become saturated and the metabolite accumulates, leading to hepatic toxicity (Mitchell et al. 1974). Bioactivation by P450 will be discussed later in this chapter.

In addition to reactive intermediate formation, P450-mediated metabolism can also lead to toxicity via P450 enzyme inhibition. Inhibition of P450 enzymes can affect the metabolism of co-administered drugs and thus lead to adverse drug–drug interactions. Posicor (mibefradil), for example, was used to control hypertension and angina. However, Posicor is a potent P450 inhibitor and interferes with the metabolism of other drugs commonly prescribed for high blood pressure. It was the potential for these drug–drug interactions that caused Posicor to be withdrawn from the market in June 1998, only a year after its launch (Krayenbuhl et al. 1999).The most important phase I enzymes are the family of cytochrome P450 enzymes (or CYPs), of which there are approximately 60 enzymes in humans (Nelson et al. 1996). The P450s are heme-containing monooxygenase enzymes. Half of all drugs are metabolized in part by the P450s and 30% of all drugs are metabolized primarily by P450s (Gonzalez 1992). P450 enzymes catalyze a number of reactions, including aliphatic hydroxylations, hydrogen-atom abstractions, aromatic oxidations, and metabolism at carbonyl groups or at heteroatoms (Jones, Mysinger and Korzekwa 2002).

Over 99% of the oxidative metabolism of drugs by humans is mediated by just six P450 isozymes (CYP1A2, CYP2C9, CYP2C19, CYP2D6, CYP2E1, and CYP3A4), and CYP3A4, CYP2D6, and CYP2C9 alone mediate over 90% of human drug oxidation (Li and Jurima-Romet 1997). While CYP1A2 is not a major drug-metabolizing enzyme it tends to metabolize relatively planer structures, giving rise to such reactive intermediates as epoxides, phenols, and conjugated electrophiles. Therefore, it may have a larger role in P450-mediated toxicities.

Drug–drug interactions causing toxicity is often the result of P450 enzyme inhibition. These inhibitory drug–drug interactions can arise from three different mechanisms, which need to be addressed by separate computational approaches. Competitive reversible inhibition is a result of either simple competition for binding to the enzyme active site or reversible coordination with the prosthetic heme of the enzyme (type II binding) (Ortiz de Montellano 1995). Irreversible inhibition occurs after compound oxidation. Most irreversible inhibitors covalently modify the protein or the prosthetic heme of the enzyme such that the enzyme activity is irreversibly destroyed in a process called suicide inhibition or mechanism-based inactivation. Metabolic intermediate complex (MI complex) inhibitors form a species that complexes to the prosthetic heme of the P450 enzyme (Sharma, Roberts and Hollenberg 1996). A form of inhibition called "time-dependent inactivation" is due to suicide inhibition and MI complex formation, reducing the concentration of active P450 available over time. Bioreactive intermediates are similar to suicide inhibitors in that they require metabolic activation to a reactive species that can covalently interact with macromolecules. However, they are different from time-dependent inactivators in that metabolites produced are less reactive and diffuse from the P450 active site and modify other cellular components (Fisher, et al. 1993). Through damage to the cellular macromolecules, normal cellular functions are disrupted and result in toxicities.

Some caveats may play an important role in interpreting results from computational models for predicting drug–drug interactions resulting from high affinity that have not been addressed extensively in the literature are as follows:

1. *Allosteric concerns* – For a number of P450 enzymes atypical kinetics is observed, as a result of multiple substrates binding in the same active site. (It is also possible that allosteric activation may also occur from binding to a site remote from the active site.) This has obvious implication for predicting binding affinity, since each substrate may have multiple Ki values, and inhibition constant may depend on the substrate used. For example, Rock and coworkers have recently found that when different fluorescent probes are used as substrates, different Ki values are found for the same inhibitor (Hummel et al. 2006). To date no good models have been made to predict multiple binding sites, and the data for building such a model are difficult to obtain. However, most atypical kinetics is observed

at high substrate concentrations, and perhaps models that only consider a single site are the most appropriate for predicting drug–drug interactions (Jones 2004). One practical aspect of data collection, that in part stems from these issues, is that more general models will be built from datasets constructed with the use of multiple substrates to determine inhibition constants (Kumar et al. 2006). Recently a computational method has been published for screening 2C9 substrates for the potential for allosteric activation (Locuson et al. 2007).

2. *Metabolically activated inhibitors* – Predicting metabolites that will bind very tightly to the heme (MI complexes), and suicide inactivation that destroys enzyme activity, requires not only a binding model but a model that predicts the amount of the reactive intermediate that causes inhibition. At times the MI complex is formed only after multiple oxidations, increasing the problems associated with predicting the event. Given the problems associated with predicting rates of P450-mediated reactions (see below), the only way to address this issue at this time is to use regioselectivity predictions, and include them in the models. This will work for closely related compounds that form similar amounts of hydrogen peroxide and water, but will fail for substrates that have different coupling of NADPH consumption to product formation.

3. Type II binding of substrates is another problem that needs to be addressed for the accurate prediction of affinity and rates of metabolism. In general, some of the tightest competitive inhibitors of cytochrome P450 enzymes are compounds that can coordinate a nitrogen to the iron of the heme. Inhibition by type II binding had been used clinically in compounds such as ketoconazole, but these compounds have a strong potential for inhibiting P450 enzyme in a nonspecific way. For example, the antifungal agent and type II binder fluconazole have been shown to be a teratogen; presumably, this is a result of inhibiting steroid biosynthesis in the developing fetus (Lopez-Rangel and Van Allen 2005). Most models for affinity assume a common binding mode. Since type II binding compounds which coordinate to heme bind differently than normal competitive inhibitors they should not be included in any model that assumes a specific binding orientation.

Even with these caveats a number of good models exist for predicting binding affinity (Hudelson and Jones 2006; Mao et al. 2006; Yamashita et al. 2006; Jensen et al. 2007; Korhonen et al. 2007) and a number of recent reviews discuss these models in detail (Ekins, Berbaum and Harrison 2003; Rettie and Jones 2005; Arimoto 2006). Both three-dimensional (3D) and 2D quantitative structure–activity relationships (QSARs) have been made for the important metabolic enzymes, except P4502E1. The 2D models have the advantage of being easy to use, and do not require alignment of the molecules. The 3D models have the advantage of providing information about what interactions are important in binding, and are more useful in drug redesign to decrease binding affinity. In general most of the models are able to predict Ki values with errors of about 1 log unit. The models for 3A4 are the hardest to construct and give the worst predictions. This is mostly a result of the prevalence of allosteric binding of substrates and inhibitors of this enzyme. Since no modeling method gives outstanding predictive capability, using multiple models and looking for a consensus gives the best results (O'Brien and de Groot 2005).

1.3.2. Predicting Metabolites: Efficient Redesign and Avoiding Bioactivation Pathways

The cytochrome P450 enzyme family metabolizes an amazing diversity of substrates as dictated by both electronic features and binding features. First, the active sites can accommodate a diverse set of substrates, most likely with nonspecific binding interactions (Higgins et al. 2001; Dowers and Jones 2006). Second, the oxidant used by the enzyme is very reactive and can oxidize a wide variety of functional groups. This combination of weak nonspecific binding interactions and a strong oxidant, results in both broad substrate selectivity and broad regioselectivity. One method for predicting the site of metabolism of P450-mediated reactions is to combine the reactivity of each potential site of metabolism (electronic effects) with any relevant accessibility effects (binding).

Experiments indicate that reaction energetics is independent of enzyme structure and that reactivity plays a major role in the regioselectivity of substrate oxidation (Jones, Rettie and Trager 1990; Karki et al. 1995; Manchester et al. 1997; Higgins et al. 1998). For example, the tendency for oxidation of a certain functional group generally follows the relative stability of the intermediate radicals that are formed – for example, N-dealkylation>O-dealkylation>2 carbon oxidation > 1 carbon oxidation. In support of this view, several studies have shown that strong correlations between regioselectivity can be developed using rather simple quantum chemical models that do not take into account the protein structure (Jones, Mysinger and Korzekwa 2002; Singh et al. 2003). These results are in contrast to results of kinetic experiments which show that a step prior to substrate oxidation (electron transfer) is the rate-limiting step in the catalytic cycle (Figure 1.1). The main reason that quantum chemical methods can predict regioselectivity is that a competition exists between a number of different positions in the molecule for the reactive-oxygen species. If two potential sites can approach the reactive-oxygen species the site with the lowest activation energy will be oxidized to a greater extent. This was first observed for molecules in which deuterium replaced hydrogen at the site of oxidation. Deuterium increases the activation energy by about 1 kcal mol^{-1} and alters regioselectivity. This is known as isotopically sensitive branching, or metabolic switching (Jones et al. 1986; Miwa and Lu 1987).

The kinetics of branched pathways was first described by Trager and coworkers (Jones et al. 1986) while the phenomenon was observed earlier by Lu and coworkers (Miwa, Walsh and Lu 1984). It was observed that if octane was substituted in the C1 position with deuterium then less 1-octanol was produced and more 2- and 3-octanol were formed, while the overall amount of product at all three positions remained unchanged. Another example of branching as a result of deuterium substitution is the oxidation of norcamphor by P450cam when it is substituted with deuterium (Atkins and Sligar 1987). In this case a smaller amount of over product from norcamphor is observed than if it has hydrogens, even though the rate-limiting step is not norcamphor hydroxylation. Atkins and Sligar found that the isotope effect was observed because of branching to the alternate product water (the third decoupling pathway in Figure 1.1).

Branching to water is most likely not an important pathway for compounds with very reactive position of oxidation, since this pathway appears to occur at a rate that is comparable to benzylic oxidation. However, for high-activation-energy reactions like aliphatic hydroxylation it can be a major branched pathway. This is most likely the reason why activation energies can be used to predict the rates of halogenated hydrocarbons, and these compounds' ability to modify proteins after bioactivation as described below (Harris et al. 1992; Yin, Jones and Anders 1995; Yin, Anders and Jones 1996). In short, for high-activation-energy metabolic processes, such as aliphatic hydroxylation, water formation provides an alternate faster pathway that unmasks reactivity differences. For compounds with moderate or low activation energies water formation will be a minor pathway and will not unmask rates of reaction (Higgins et al. 1998). For these types of oxidations an alternate metabolite of comparable activation energy must be available for oxidation (Higgins et al. 2001). In this case the major determinant in predicting regioselectivity is the ability of the two sites of oxidation to approach the active-oxygen species and to rapidly interchange at a rate faster than oxidation (Higgins et al. 2001). Fortunately, most drug molecules have a plethora of sites that can be oxidized as shown for simvastatin in Figure 1.2. For this molecule 19 different sites can be oxidized by P450. If all the sites can rapidly interchange and approach the active-oxygen species the most prevalent metabolites can be predicted by relatively simple quantum mechanical calculations to determine the activation energy for oxidation as described below.

Branching also has another important feature, in that it allows for the measurement of the difference in activation energies for different metabolic pathways. When two enzyme–substrate (ES) complexes rapidly interchange, the product ratios reflect the differences in activation energies as described by the Curtin–Hammett postulate (Seeman 1983). This method has been used to calibrate electronic models for aliphatic and aromatic oxidation (Higgins et al. 2001; Jones, Mysinger and Korzekwa 2002).

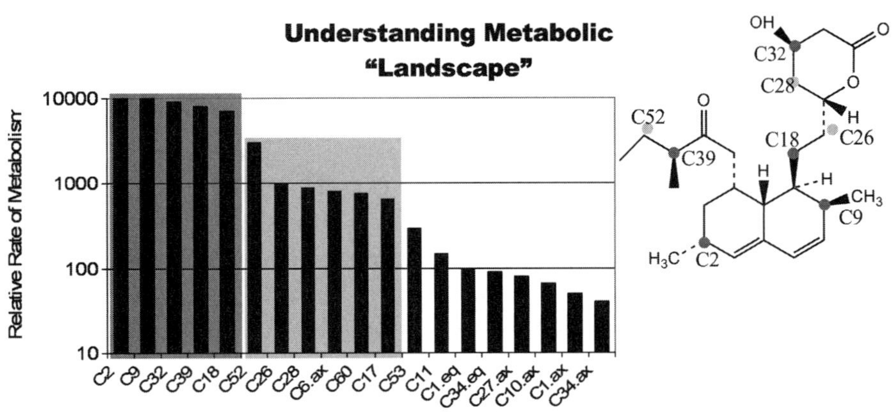

Figure 1.2 The potential sites of oxidation of simvastatin, and the predicted ease of oxidation of each site. The *dark-shaded* region contains the positions that are easily oxidized. Moderately stable sites are *lightly shaded.*

The first attempt at understanding the role of electronic effects for a series of reactions was published in 1990 by Korzekwa (Korzekwa, Jones and Gillette 1990). While limited in computational power relative to today's standards, semiempirical AM1 calculations were used to look at the barrier heights for a series of reactions modeling hydrogen-atom abstraction from carbons attached to different functional groups. The activation energies reproduced the generally accepted reactivity of functional groups with N-dealkylation having a lower barrier than O-dealkylation, and aliphatic hydroxylation having the highest barriers. A linear free energy relationship (Eq. 1) was established that allowed for the rapid prediction of activation energies from ground-state calculations:

$$\Delta H_{\mathrm{act.}} = 2.60 + 0.22(\Delta H)_{\mathrm{R}} + 2.38(\mathrm{IP}_{\mathrm{rad}}), \qquad (1.1)$$

where $(\Delta H)_R$ is the AM1 heat of reaction with *p*-nitrosophenoxy radical, and IP_{rad} is the ionization potential of the radical product. The activation energy for each position in a molecule is calculated by obtaining the energy and ionization potential of each radical. Aromatic oxidation is modeled by the energy of the tetrahedral intermediate.

The activation energies from this model were first applied to predicting the LD50 values for a series of nitriles (Grogan et al. 1992). In this case toxicity arises from oxidation adjacent to the nitrile group which releases cyanide (Figure 1.3). It was assumed that oxidation at any other position would not result in death. While none of these molecules were drug-like this was one of the first models to rationally predict toxicity based on a mechanism, and it illustrates how regioselectivity models can be used in drug design when a potential toxicophore is needed for pharmacological activity.

Another early application of the AM1 method was for the prediction of metabolism of halogenated hydrocarbons used as anesthetics, and in compressors for refrigeration. The in vivo metabolism of four halohydrocarbons was determined in rats and compared with the predicted enthalpy of activation using the AM1 model for P450-mediated reactivity (Harris et al. 1992) and a strong correlation was observed (r^2 = 0.955).

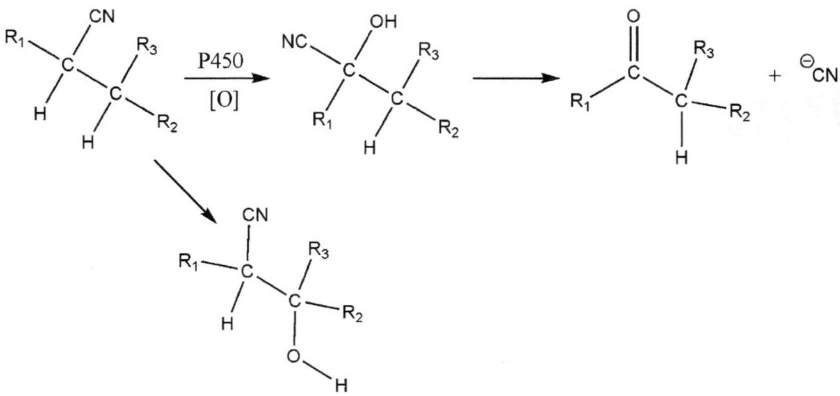

Figure 1.3 The two pathways that lead to either cyanide release and death or a stable metabolic product.

Furthermore, the amount of protein adducts as estimated by immunoblots also showed a rank-order correlation. This work was extended for the prediction of regioselectivity in HCFC-141 and HCFC-131 (Yin et al. 1995; Yin, Anders and Jones 1996), and for the rates of metabolism of six halogenated hydrocarbons in microsomes and purified human 2E1 to again give very strong correlations between rates and activation energies (Yin, Jones and Anders 1995). Our ability to predict rates in this case is a result of the overall slow rate of reaction for hydrocarbon oxidations. Since, as mentioned above, water formation is a branched pathway from Cpd I and is favored over hydrocarbon oxidation, as the activation energy for the hydrocarbon is increased the amount of water formed increases and the amount of product decreases. Another important feature is that these are structurally related compounds that most likely bind with similar affinities, and have similar abilities to start the catalytic cycle. Finally, these simple AM1 methods have been used to predict the relative rate of activation of water contaminants to help in understanding the potential mutagenicity of halogenated hydrocarbons in drinking water (Tornero-Velez et al. 2004).

Since not all reactions mediated by P450 enzyme involve hydrogen-atom abstraction, other models are required for aromatic hydroxylation, epoxidation of alkenes, N-oxidation, and sulfoxidation. Simple AM1 models for aromatic hydroxylation have been developed by us and integrated with the aliphatic models (Jones, Mysinger and Korzekwa 2002). For these models we used methoxy radical and correlated the enthalpy of reaction for tetrahedral intermediate formation to the activation energy for the process. Experimental data was than used to calibrate the activation energies for aromatic oxidation with those for aliphatic oxidation. If this calibration was not done, aromatic oxidation is predicted to be the major metabolite for all compounds with an aromatic ring. Experimentally, aromatic oxidation is very similar in activation energy to benzylic oxidation. Problems with these models occur when a compound has multiple fused aromatic rings. In this case it is possible to predict if aromatic hydroxylation will occur, but the absolute regioselectivity is dictated by steric concerns, and the stability of any epoxides that are formed (Dowers et al. 2004b).

N-oxides and *S*-oxides are also formed by P450-mediated reaction. Heterocyclic *N*-oxides are relatively easily formed with relative reactivities being close to aliphatic epoxide formation. However, while this is a relatively facile reaction, substituents ortho to the nitrogen in the ring will significantly hinder this reaction (Dowers et al. 2004). Sulfoxidation is another very facile reaction that electronically is favored over N-dealkylation by about 1–2 kcal mol^{-1} (Volz, Rock and Jones 2002). In general sulfur oxidation will be a major route of metabolism unless the sulfur is made electron deficient, or is sterically hindered.

When these simple AM1-based computational methods are applied to drugs that are substrates for P450 3A4 they are very successful at predicting regioselectivity. The literature was reviewed for compounds that had reported major metabolites for 3A4 metabolism in vitro. For some compounds a number of metabolites were reported. The AM1 model for hydrogen-atom abstraction (Korzekwa, Jones and Gillette 1990), or where appropriate the newer model for aromatic hydroxylation (Jones, Mysinger and Korzekwa 2002) for predicting activation energy was then applied to each aliphatic or aromatic site of potential oxidation in the drug. Out of the 82 compounds presented in Figure 1.4 all the reported metabolites were correctly predicted for 62 of them. For the remaining compounds at least one of the reported metabolites was reported to be among the top three for 13 drugs. In most of these cases a number of positions are predicted to have very similar activation energies. Only 7 drugs did not have the major metabolite in the top three predicted sites. For most of these molecules the low-activation-energy positions are sterically hindered. Thus, a simple fast model predicts the site of metabolism with about 75% accuracy.

Given that most of these molecules are very complex and have a number of sites of metabolism the high level of predictability is unexpected. To illustrate this, the predictions for a simvastatin will be evaluated. Simvastatin is shown in Figure 1.2, and has 19 possible positions of metabolism. Of the 19 possible metabolic positions the top 5 are predicted to have similar relative rates of metabolism based on activation energy, with the highest metabolic rates predicted to be at the C2 position which is the observed major site of metabolism (Prueksaritanont et al. 1997). Hydrogen-atom abstraction from the C2 position produces an allylic radical, which is stabilized by resonance. A very similar activation energy is predicted for the C9 position which is also allylic and three other positions in the molecule. From the predicted relative rates the effect of having similar activation energies becomes apparent with the first three sites having some differences in activation energy but having very little difference in predicted rate. In terms of drug design this means that at least the first three sites, and reasonably the five easiest sites of oxidation, would need to be altered to have a meaningful change in the clearance of simvastatin. It should be noted that these are relative rates and can be used for redesign since other factors that affect rates, such as affinity, the ability to start the catalytic cycle by initial electron transfer, and the amount of

All Observed Sites Among Top Three Electronically Activated

Adinazolam	Cyclobenzaprine	Haloperidol	Oxybutynin	Terbinafine
Alfentanil	Delavirdine	Imipramine	Pimobendan	Terbuthylazine
Amitriptyline	Dextromethorphan	LAAM	Pimozide	Testosterone
Atrazine	Diazepam	Lidocaine	Pranidipine	Tolterodine
Azelastine	Diclofenac	Lilopristone	Progesterone	Toremifene
Beta-arteether	Diltiazem	Lovastatin	Propafenone	Trazodone
Buprenorphine	Ebastine	Meloxicam	Ropinirole	Triazolam
Citalopram	Erythromycin	Methadone	Ropivacaine	Trimethadione
Clomipramine	Estrone	Midazolam	Salicylate	Verapamil
Clozapine	Etoposide	Mifepristone	Sertraline	Zaleplon
Cocaine	Felodipine	Nifedipine	Simvastatin	
Codeine	Fentanyl	Nitrendipine	Tamoxifen	
CQA	Halofantrine	Onapristone	Teniposide	

At Least One Site Among Top Three

Ametryne	Granisetron	Nevirapine	Ritonavir	Zopiclone
Budesonide	H259-31	Omeprazole	Terbutryne	
Clarithromycin	MK-639	Rifabutin	Terfenadine	

Figure 1.4 The prediction success and failure of a simple AM1 electronic model for regioselectivity.

hydrogen peroxide release, are the same since it is an intramolecular competition (Porter, Branchflower and Trager 1977). However, the rate of metabolism of simvastatin cannot be compared with other molecules using this method. The site(s) of metabolism for five other compounds plus simvastatin are given in Figure 1.5. In general, the major sites of metabolism are activated by nitrogen. Cocaine, propafenone, trimethadione, and diazepam all are oxidized adjacent to a nitrogen. This is a result of the lone pair of electron decreasing the activation energy for hydrogen abstraction. For simvastatin, diazepam, and meloxicam the site of metabolism is adjacent to a double bond and hydrogen-atom abstraction is stabilized by resonance. Overall, when two sites of metabolism are predicted to have the same probability of oxidation, the less-hindered site is the site of metabolism.

While this model has been shown to work for 3A4 and for 2E1, it unlikely to work for substrates for 2D6 and 2C9 since both these enzymes orient the substrate in the active site. It can even be shown that for 3A4 the hydrophobic nature of the active site biases orientation, and an increase in predictability can be obtained by biasing reactivity toward hydrophobic portions of the molecule.

This method of modeling uses the accepted mechanism for oxidation of a carbon–hydrogen bond, and for aromatic hydroxylation. Hydrogen-atom abstraction is used to model dealkylation reactions and aliphatic oxidation, assuming the Groves hydrogen-atom abstraction rebound mechanism (Groves et al. 1978) shown in Figure 1.6. Aromatic oxidation is modeled by the formation of a tetrahedral intermediate and is independent of whether the tetrahedral intermediate collapses to an epoxide or rearranges to give phenol directly (Jones, Mysinger and Korzekwa 2002). It is also assumed that all P450 enzymes have similar energetics with respect to the active-oxygen species, and that only a single such

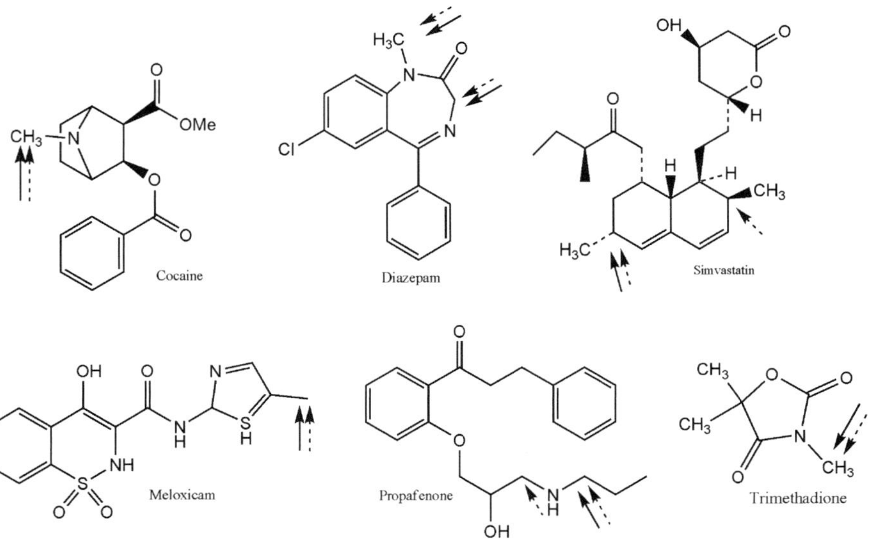

Figure 1.5 The observed (*solid arrow*) and predicted (*dotted arrow*) sites of metabolism of selected drugs from Figure 1.4.

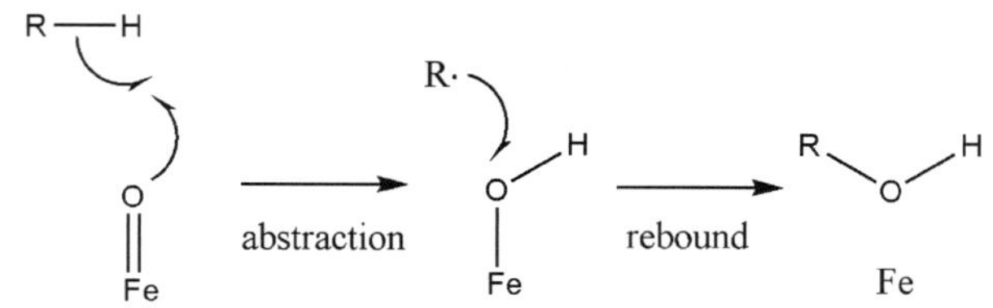

Figure 1.6 Groves hydrogen abstraction rebound mechanism.

reactive-oxygen species exists. This is consistent with a number of studies that have concluded that the transition states as reflected by isotope effects are almost identical for different P450 enzymes for hydrogen-atom abstraction reactions (Higgins et al. 1998; Higgins et al. 2001). One caveat to this finding is that recently a number of reactions have been attributed to the iron-hydroperoxy species known as Compound 0 (Vaz and Coon 1987; Coon and Vaz 1988; Vaz, Roberts and Coon 1990; Volz, Rock and Jones 2002; Chandrasena et al. 2004; Cryle and De Voss 2006). Most of this work is dependent on increases in rates of a given reaction or changes in product ratios for mutation of a threonine in the I-helix involved in proton transfer to the Compound 0 to from Cpd I (Figure 1.7). The threonine mutant was first made by Imai et al., in 1989 and according to electron paramagnetic resonance (EPR) studies this mutant increases the steady-state concentration of Compound 0 (Denisov, Makris and Sligar 2001).

Given that the rate-limiting step is prior to Compound 0 formation, low steady-state level of Compound 0 would be expected for each enzyme. It is not clear if each enzyme would catalyze the breakdown of Compound 0 with similar rates, and small differences in rates would have relatively large differences in the steady-state concentration of this species. Considering that this rate is dependent upon proton delivery to the oxygen distal to the iron, difference in tertiary structure that alters the flow of protons might vary to a large extent. Furthermore, the substrate also can play a role in the lifetime of Compound 0 (French et al. 2001; Davydov et al. 2005) since it may alter the ability of the enzyme to deliver a proton to the distal oxygen and instead lead to proximal protonation and hydrogen peroxide release (Figure 1.7b). Thus, any reaction dependent on Compound 0 may be expected to behave very differently for different P450 enzymes and possibly will have different branching ratios with different substrates. Reactions that may be mediated in part by Compound 0 include epoxidation (Vaz,

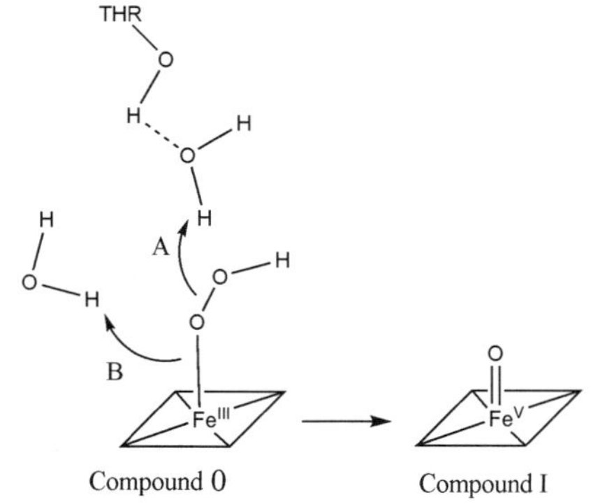

Figure 1.7 **(a)** Proton transfer to give Compound I. **(b)** Proton transfer to release hydrogen peroxide.

McGinnity and Coon 1998; Jin et al. 2003; Jin, Bryson and Dawson 2004), sulfoxidation (Volz, Rock and Jones 2002; Cryle and De Voss 2006), aliphatic oxidation of cyclopropanes (Newcomb, Hollenberg and Coon 2003; Chandrasena et al. 2004), ipso-substitution of substitutes phenols (i.e., aromatic carbon that has a substituent) (Vatsis and Coon 2002), reaction with acetylenes to generate reactive-oxygen species (Blobaum et al. 2004), deformylation of aldehydes (Vaz et al. 1996), N-dealkylation, and aromatic hydroxylation (Hutzler et al. 2003; Keizers et al. 2005). The enzymes involved include the mammalian enzymes 2D6, 2E1, 2B4, 101, 102, and the potential for multiple reactive species has been reviewed recently (Newcomb, Hollenberg and Coon 2003; Jin, Bryson and Dawson 2004).

The main tool that has been used to probe for multiple oxidants is mutation of the threonine residue that is conserved in most P450 enzymes and responsible for coordinating proton delivery from a water molecule to the distal oxygen of the iron-hydroperoxy species (Figure 1.7a). By far the most convincing of these studies report an increase or no change in the amount of product formed when the mutant that slows Cpd I formation is used, implying that oxidation does not come from Cpd I. For example, the T268A mutant of P450BM3 results in a decrease in fatty acid oxidation, but no change in the rate or stereochemistry of oxidation of thiafatty acids (Cryle and De Voss 2006). This provides strong evidence that sulfoxidation occurs from Compound 0. Supporting this conclusion is the fact that sulfoxidation has been found to come from a different oxidant than N-dealkylation of dimethylanilines (Volz, Rock and Jones 2002). Another compelling study used the T309A mutant of P4502D6 and found that the rates of aliphatic N-dealkylation of dextromethorphan and 3,4-methylenedioxymethylamphetamine and aromatic hydroxylation of bufuralol were increased while O-dealkylation of these substrates was decreased. Finally, for the T303A mutant of P4502E1 the rates of epoxide formation were found to increase for styrene, cyclohexene, *cis*-2-butene, and *trans*-2-butene but not for oxidation at the allylic position (Vaz, McGinnity and Coon 1998). Finally, ipso-substitution of a number of phenols is increased with this 2E1 mutant (Vatsis and Coon 2002). The simplest interpretation of these results is that the iron-hydroperoxy species is responsible for the reactions that increase in rate (sulfoxidation, aliphatic N-demethylation, epoxidation, and ipso-substitution), and that Cpd I is responsible for the reactions that decrease in rate (O-dealkylation, aliphatic hydroxylation, and allylic hydroxylation).

In contrast to the findings with the mutants, a number of these same types of reactions have been shown to come from a common reactive-oxygen intermediate (Higgins et al. 2001), and for N-dealkylation of *N*,*N*-dimethylanilines the reactive species has been shown to be Cpd I (Dowers et al. 2004). Aromatic oxidation, N-oxide formation, and O-dealkylation have also been shown to come from a common intermediate (Dowers and Jones 2006). Interestingly, when the O-dealkylation and N-dealkylation reactivity of dextromethorphan are explored by the T309A mutant of 2D6, O-dealkylation is assigned to Cpd I and N-dealkylation to Compound 0 (Hutzler et al. 2003; Keizers et al. 2005). This leads to a situation where most reaction types (N-dealkylation, aromatic oxidation, etc.) catalyzed by P450 may result from either Compound 0 or Cpd I, with O-dealkylation, straight-chain aliphatic compounds, and N-oxidation of heterocyclic amines being the only reactions unanimously identified as only coming from Cpd I.

Theory has been used to look at the potential for the iron-hydroperoxo species to mediate different P450 reactions. The results have been stated rather unambiguously by Kamachi et al. (2003) when they used density functional methods "... to look at whether or not the iron(III)-hydroperoxo species can participate in olefin epoxidation with the iron(IV)-oxo species (Cpd I). The answer is negative." Shaik and coworkers have also looked at the reactivity of the iron(III)-hydroperoxo species (Compound 0) and found that in comparison to Cpd I oxidation the barrier heights are at least 23 kcal mol^{-1} higher for Compound 0 than Cpd I (Ogliaro et al. 2002) and concluded that the iron-hydroperoxo species cannot be a second oxidant. However in a more recent work Shaik and coworkers have stated that in the absence of any Cpd I formation, Compound 0 may act as an oxidant (Hirao, Kumar and Shaik 2006). Specifically they looked at the T252A mutant of P450cam and concluded that hydroxylation of 5-methylenenylcamphor could possibly occur from Compound 0 if no Cpd I is present with a barrier height only 6 kcal mol^{-1} higher than Cpd I.

Surrogate oxygen donors are molecules that can donate oxygen to the resting heme to generate Cpd I directly without having Compound 0 as an intermediate. Obviously, given the concern about whether Compound 0 or Compound 1 is the active oxidant in P450, a molecule that will only form Cpd I would be highly desirable. The major caveat is that the surrogate generated Cpd I must have the same reactivity as the native Cpd I. Three surrogates, cumene hydroperoxide, iodosobenzene, (Guengerich, Yun and MacDonald 1996) and the *N*-oxide of *N,N*-dimethylaniline (Dowers et al. 2004) have been used to measure the kinetic isotope effects for *N,N*-dimethylaniline dealkylation. Of these three oxygen donors only the *N*-oxide of *N,N*-dimethylaniline gave the same isotope effect as the native enzyme system. Both cumene hydroperoxide and iodosobenzene gave significantly larger isotope effects indicating a change in mechanism. However, while this might make the *N*-oxide of *N,N*-dimethylaniline seem like the best surrogate oxygen donor, it has never been reported to oxidize any substrate other then *N,N*-dimethylaniline. While iodosobenzene supports a number of P450-mediated reactions, besides giving different isotope effects, it often gives different ratios of products (Berg, Ingelman-Sundberg and Gustafsson 1979; Chandrasena et al. 2004), and causes heme degradation at a rate that exceeds the rate of oxidation (Macdonald et al. 1989). Cumene hydroperoxide also seems to give large isotope effects for N-demethylation of amitriptyline (Hutzler et al. 2003) and to give different product ratios for bufuralol (Keizers et al. 2005) and indole (Li et al. 2005). Thus, at this time it would appear that no good oxygen surrogate is available for Cpd I-mediated reactions.

An alternate possibility for a second oxidant that has been put forth by Shaik and coworker is that spin-selective reactivity may be responsible for the experimental observations that require multiple oxidants (Shaik et al. 2005). Density functional theory (DFT) predicts that multiple spin states of Cpd I exist with very small differences in their energetics. Thus, high-spin Cpd I has a lower barrier for sulfoxidation than low-spin Cpd I (Sharma et al. 2003), while the low-spin state is responsible for hydrogen-atom abstractions. Very small changes in structure around the heme lead to changes in the energetic ordering of the spin states. Thus, a mutant that changes threonine to alanine, which would change the environment above the heme, may change the spin reaction manifold and alter reactivity (Watanabe 2001; Shaik et al. 2005). Recently, spin-selective reactivity has been proposed to be the reason why iodosobenzene has a different reactivity than the native P450 system (Cho et al. 2007). When iodosobenzene donates oxygen to the heme it initially forms a high-spin Cpd I that in theoretical calculations gives large isotope effects consistent with experiment.

Thus, a contrasting view of the potential for predicting metabolites arises from the work published on the mechanism, which appears very complex, and the application of relatively simple models mentioned above to predicting the actual regioselectivity of the metabolism of drugs. Understanding these different mechanistic possibilities, and when they come into play, should increase our predictive capabilities.

An extension of the models developed in the early 1990s has recently been reported by Olsen et al., in which the simple AM1 calculations were extended to more rigorous DFT methods and the transition states for building the model used a heme model instead of a simpler radical (Olsen et al. 2006). These studies confirmed that AM1 model for predicting activation energies works rather well at predicting the more computationally demanding DFT full-heme activation energies. This study also found that different functional groups could just be grouped into primary aliphatic, secondary aliphatic, aromatic, dealkylation with sulfur or oxygen adjacent, and N-dealkylation and used to predict reactivity with high accuracy. Finally these authors combined site accessibility and reactivity to make predictions for progesterone and dextromethorphan.

An automated approach has recently been developed into a commercial program, Metasite. The main advantage of this program over the methods mentioned above is that the system is automated and different steric accessibility parameters have been developed for CYP1A2, CYP2C9, CYP2C19, CYP2D6, and CYP3A4 based on crystal structure and homology models. This method uses GRID (a computer program to define 3D space) flexible interaction fields to estimate if the reactive atom is accessible and a reactivity parameter based on ab initio methods, which are then used to define reactive fragments: when a significantly different fragment is encountered an AM1 calculation is used (Cruciani et al. 2005). For 3A4 the predictive capacity is about 78% for 340 compounds, very close to the 75% reported above for the AM1 model alone.

The Metasite program has recently been evaluated for statin metabolism (Caron, Ermondi and Testa 2007). This effort assessed the regioselectivity of metabolism of seven statins by 3A4 and 2C9, and they found an overall success rate that was very similar to the original report of about 77%. In a separate study that compared Metasite and a docking methodology in predicting metabolites of 227 known 3A4 substrates, Metasite was found to be the best method, predicting 78% of the major metabolites versus 57% for the docking methods (Zhou et al. 2006). Thus, consistent predictions of the major metabolite with electronic methods alone or with crystal structure corrections for accessibility have yet to consistently exceed the 80% success rate.

The complex mechanistic issues mentioned above may be the reason for this limit in predictive capability. Another possibility has recently been presented by Shaik and coworkers who hypothesized that the activation energy was not the only variable that needed to be accounted for in predicting regioselectivity, and that the regioselectivity ratio also reflected the overall energy of the products as calculated in the active site (Cohen et al. 2006). Therefore, products that interact with the heme strongly are not formed to as high an extent as those that interact weakly.

1.3.3. Predicting Rates of P450-Mediated Reactions

As described above we have successfully predicted the rates of reaction of very poor substrates using our simple AM1 model (Yin, Jones and Anders 1995; Tornero-Velez et al. 2004). Our ability to make these rate predictions is a result of a number of features of these reactions that are not general. Therefore, in general it is not possible to use activation energy, and the parameters associated with predicting regioselectivity, to predict rates. The following four features of the reaction must be very similar or known to make rate predictions:

1. *Affinity of the substrate for the enzyme* – Since metabolism usually occurs at subsaturating concentrations of substrate, the higher the affinity of the substrate to the enzyme, the faster the rate of metabolism.
2. *Peroxide formation* – In addition to the decoupling pathway to form water, the peroxy or superoxy intermediates can also dissociate to decouple the enzymatic cycle (Figure 1.1). The degree of peroxy decoupling is probably a whole-molecule property and is dependent on whether Compound 0 is protonated on the proximal or distal oxygen (Figure 1.7). If all other features are identical, the substrate that makes the least amount of peroxide will be metabolized the fastest.
3. *Composite site lability* – Composite site lability is the fraction of maximum velocity based on all activation energy values in the molecule. This is essentially a fractional velocity calculated for the substrate oxidation step that is determined by the relative importance of water formation. For compounds with easily oxidized sites, such as N-dealkylation and epoxidation pathways, this value approaches 1. In other words, if one site is made more difficult the overall flux to give product remains the same since a number of products come from low-energy pathways. For compounds that are very stable, such as halogenated hydrocarbon oxidation, the log of this value is proportional to activation energy. The scale of this parameter is compressed in the reactive region since water formation cannot compete with the metabolism of labile sites, while very stable compounds will branch to water, giving the perception that less product is being formed, since water is not normally counted as product.
4. *Reduction rates* – The rate-limiting steps in the catalytic cycle of the P450s is enzyme reduction, and substrate interactions in the active site can influence the rate of reduction. A very significant influence on

reduction rate occurs when the substrate can complex with the heme within the active site, called type II binding. Although this results in an increased affinity to the active site, the rate of metabolism is decreased because a large fraction of the heme can no longer be reduced and bind oxygen. Conversely, compounds that bind directly above the heme and excluded water increase the rate of reduction and are metabolized at an overall higher rate.

In the case of the halogenated hydrocarbons the compounds are all very similar in structure, and it is likely that they have similar affinity for CYP2E1. They also have similar size, which most likely gives similar branching to peroxide. The composite site liability is low, leading to high amount of water formation which gives a constant branched pathway to unmask differences in reactivity. It is not clear what factors alter the reduction rates of CYP2E1, but from the results all the substrates must give rather similar amounts of reduction.

For drug-like molecules these four features will rarely be the same. For example, the compounds we tested for regioselectivity that are given in Figure 1.4 for the most part have very different structures and are known to have different K_i and K_M values which would lead to differences in the binding affinity, reduction rates, and peroxide formation. Most drugs contain functional groups that have relatively high reactivity, such as alkyl group attached to nitrogen and oxygen. These highly reactive groups make the electronic component less important since the maximum rate is not determined by oxidation rate, but rather by other features. Thus, when one considers the flux of metabolism the electronic component becomes less important when the drug has a very reactive group. While affinity can be modeled reasonably well, model for peroxide formation and reduction rates are much less straightforward. Overall, predicting rates is one of the most important, but as yet generally unattainable goal in ADMET prediction.

1.4. Summary

Predictive models are important tools for increasing the efficiency of drug development. Lead generation and optimization is best accomplished by the consideration of multiple parameters, including properties involved in ADMET processes. Predictive ADMET models allow for consideration of these properties prior to synthesis and therefore for incorporation of these properties into compound design and redesign. The emphasis of the work described here has been on the development and application of predictive models for cytochrome P450 enzymes but more global models need to be developed that include other important metabolic enzymes. The models available now predict regioselectivity, or site of metabolism, and affinity. Additionally, concepts and relationships from these models can be incorporated into models of the rate of metabolism for a series of compounds, although this has not been routinely done. ADMET models can be used to design compounds with more optimal metabolic characteristics, including low rates of metabolism, decreased potential for drug–drug interactions, and decreased likelihood of metabolically mediated toxicity. Ultimately, the goal is to apply predictive tools to help decrease the huge attrition in drug discovery and development, and to help design better medicines.

Acknowledgments. This work was supported in part by ES009122 and GM 32165.

References

Arimoto, R. 2006. Computational models for predicting interactions with cytochrome p450 enzyme. Curr. Top. Med. Chem. 6:1609–1618.

Atkins, W. M., and Sligar, S. G. 1987. Metabolic switching in cytochrome P-450cam: Deuterium isotope effects on regiospecificity and the monooxygenase/oxidase ratio. J. Am. Chem. Soc. 109:3754–3760.

Berg, A., Ingelman-Sundberg, M., and Gustafsson, J. A. 1979. Purification and characterization of cytochrome P-450 meg. J. Biol. Chem. 254(12):5264–5271.

Blobaum, A. L., Kent, U. M., Alworth, W. L., and Hollenberg, P. F. 2004. Novel reversible inactivation of cytochrome P450 2E1 T303A by tert-butyl acetylene: the role of threonine 303 in proton delivery to the active site of cytochrome P450 2E1. J. Pharmacol. Exp. Ther. 310(1):281–290.

Caron, G., Ermondi G., and Testa, B. 2007. Predicting the oxidative metabolism of statins: An application of the MetaSite (R) algorithm. Pharm. Res. 24(3):480–501.

Chandrasena, R. E. P., Vatsis, K. P., Coon, M. J., Hollenberg, P. F., and Newcomb, M. 2004. Hydroxylation by the hydroperoxy-iron species in cytochrome P450 enzymes. J. Am. Chem. Soc. 126(1):115–126.

Cho, K. Y., Moreau, Y., Kumar, D., Rock, D. A., Jones, J. P., and Shaik, S. 2007. Formation of the active species of cytochrome P450 by using iodosylbenzene: A case for spin-selective reactivity. Chemistry: A European Journal: Published Online.

Cohen, S., Kozuch, S., Hazan, C., and Shaik, S. 2006. Does substrate oxidation determine the regioselectivity of cyclohexene and propene oxidation by cytochrome P450? J. Am. Chem. Soc. 128:11028–11029.

Coon, M. J., and Vaz, A. D. 1988. Role of cytochrome P-450 in hydrocarbon formation from xenobiotic and lipid hydroperoxides. Prog. Clin. Biol. Res. 274:497–507.

Cruciani, G., Carosati, E., De Boeck, B., Ethirajulu, K., Mackie, C., Howe, T., and Vianello, R. 2005. MetaSite: Understanding metabolism in human cytochromes from the perspective of the chemist. J. Med. Chem. 48:6970–6979.

Cryle, M. J., and De Voss, J. J. 2006. Is the ferric hydroperoxy species responsible for sulfur oxidation in cytochrome P450s. Angewandte Chemie-International Edition 45: 8221–8223.

Davydov, R., Perera, R., Jin, S. X., Yang, T. C., Bryson, T. A., Sono, M., Dawson J. H., and Hoffman, B. M. 2005. Substrate modulation of the properties and reactivity of the oxy-ferrous and hydroperoxo-ferric intermediates of cytochrome P450cam as shown by cryoreduction-EPR/ENDOR spectroscopy. J. Am. Chem. Soc. 127:1403–1413.

Denisov, I. G., Makris, T. M., and Sligar, S. G. 2001. Cryotrapped reaction intermediates of cytochrome p450 studied by radiolytic reduction with phosphorus-32. J. Biol. Chem. 276:11648–11652.

Dimasi, J. A. 2001. New drug development in the United States from 1963 to 1999. Clin. Pharmacol. Ther. 69:286–296.

Dowers, T. S., and Jones, J. P. 2006. Kinetic isotope effects implicate a single oxidant for cytochrome P450-mediated O-dealkylation, N-oxygenation, and aromatic hydroxylation of 6-methoxyquinoline. Drug Metab. Dispos. 34:1288–1290.

Dowers, T. S., Rock, D. A., Rock, D. A., and Jones, J. P. 2004a. Kinetic isotope effects implicate the iron-oxene as the sole oxidant in P450-catalyzed N-dealkylation. J. Am. Chem. Soc. 126:8868–8869.

Dowers, T. S., Rock, D. A., Rock, D. A., Perkins, B. N. S., and Jones, J. P. 2004b. An analysis of the regioselectivity of aromatic hydroxylation and N-oxygenation by cytochrome P450 enzymes. Drug Metab. Dispos. 32:328–332.

Ekins, S., Berbaum, J., and Harrison, R. K. 2003. Generation and validation of rapid computational filters for CYP2D6 and CYP3A4. Drug Metab. Dispos. 31:1077–1080.

Fisher, R., Brendel, K., and Hanzlik, R. P. 1993. Correlation of metabolism, covalent binding and toxicity for a series of bromobenzene derivatives using rat liver slices in vitro. Chem. Biol. Interact. 88:191–198.

French, K. J., Strickler, M. D., Rock, D. A., Rock, D. A., Bennett, G. A., Wahlstrom, J. L., Goldstein, B. M., and Jones, J. P. 2001. Benign synthesis of 2-ethylhexanoic acid by cytochrome P450cam: Enzymatic, crystallographic, and theoretical studies. Biochemistry 40:9532–9538.

Gonzalez, F. J. 1992. Human cytochrome P450: problems and prospects. TiPs Reviews 13:346–352.

Grogan, J., DeVito, S. C., Pearlman, R. S., and Korzekwa, K. R. 1992. Modeling cyanide release from nitriles: Prediction of cytochrome P450 mediated acute nitrile toxicity. Chem. Res. Toxicol. 5:548–552.

Groves, J. T., McClusky, G. A., White, R. E., and Coon, M. J. 1978. Aliphatic hydroxylation by highly purified liver microsomal cytochrome P450. Evidence for a carbon radical intermediate. Biochem. Biophys. Res. Commun. 81:154–160.

Guengerich, F. P., Yun C., and MacDonald, T. L. 1996. Evidence for a 1-electron oxidation mechanism in N-dealkylation of *N,N*-dialkylanilines by cytochrome P450 2B1. J. Biol. Chem. 271:27321–27329.

Harris, J. W., Jones, J. P., Martin, J. L., LaRosa, A. C., Olson, M. J., Pohl, L. R., and Anders, M. W. 1992. Pentahaloethane-based chlorofluorocarbon substitutes and halothane: Correlation of in vivo hepatic protein-trifluoroacetylation and urinary trifluoroacetic acid excretion with calculated enthalpies of activation. Chem. Res. Toxicol. 5:720–725.

He, M., Korzekwa, K. R., Jones, J. P., Rettie, A. E., and Trager, W. F. 1999. Structural forms of phenprocoumon and warfarin that are metabolized at the active site of CYP2C9. Arch. Biochem. Biophys. 372:16–28.

Higgins, L., Bennett, G. A., Shimoji, M., and Jones, J. P. 1998. Evaluation of cytochrome P450 mechanism and kinetics using kinetic deuterium isotope effects. Biochemistry 37:7039–7046.

Higgins, L., Korzekwa, K. R., Rao, S., Shou, M., and Jones, J. P. 2001. An assessment of the reaction energetics for cytochrome P450-mediated reactions. Arch. Biochem. Biophys. 385:220–230.

Hirao, H., Kumar, D., and Shaik, S. 2006. On the identity and reactivity patterns of the "second oxidant" of the T252A mutant of cytochrome P450(cam) in the oxidation of 5-methylenenylcamphor. J. Inorg. Biochem. 100:2054–2068.

Hudelson, M. G., and Jones, J. P. 2006. Line-walking method for predicting the inhibition of P450 drug metabolism. J. Med. Chem. 49:4367–4373.

Hummel, M. A., Tracy, T. S., Hutzler, J. M., Wahlstrom, J. L., Zhou Y., and Rock, D. A. 2006. Influence of fluorescent probe size and cytochrome b5 on drug–drug interactions in CYP2C9. J. Biomol. Screen. 11:303–309.

Hutzler, J. M., Powers, F. J., Wynalda, M. A., and Wienkers, L. C. 2003. Effect of carbonate anion on cytochrome P450 2D6-mediated metabolism in vitro: the potential role of multiple oxygenating species. Arch. Biochem. Biophys. 417:165–175.

Jankel, C. A., McMillan, J. A., and Martin, B. C. 1994. Effect of drug interactions on outcomes of patients receiving warfarin or theophylline. Am. J. Hosp. Pharm. 51:661–666.

Jensen, B. F., Vind, C., Padkjaer, S. B., Brockhoff, P. B., and Refsgaard, H. H. 2007. In silico prediction of cytochrome P450 2D6 and 3A4 inhibition using Gaussian kernel weighted k-nearest neighbor and extended connectivity fingerprints, including structural fragment analysis of inhibitors versus noninhibitors. J. Med. Chem. 50:501–511.

Jin, S., Makris, T. M., Bryson, T. A., Sligar, S. G., and Dawson, J. H. 2003. Epoxidation of olefins by hydroperoxo-ferric cytochrome P450. J. Am. Chem. Soc. 125:3406–3407.

Jin, S. X., Bryson, T. A., and Dawson, J. H. 2004. Hydroperoxoferric heme intermediate as a second electrophilic oxidant in cytochrome P450-catalyzed reactions. J. Biol. Inorg. Chem. 9:644–653.

Jones, J. P. 2004. Metabolic menages a trois: what does it mean for drug design? Drug Discov. Today **9**:592–592.

Jones, J. P., Korzekwa, K. R., Rettie, A. E., and Trager, W. F. 1986. Isotopically sensitive branching and its effect on the observed intramolecular isotope effects in cytochrome P450 catalyzed reactions: a new method for the estimation of intrinsic isotope effects. J. Am. Chem. Soc. 108:7074–7078.

Jones, J. P., Mysinger, M., and Korzekwa, K. R. 2002. Computational models for cytochrome P450: a predictive electronic model for aromatic oxidation and hydrogen atom abstraction. Drug Metab. Dispos. 30:7–12.

Jones, J. P., Rettie, A. E., and Trager, W. F. 1990. Intrinsic isotope effects suggest that the reaction coordinate symmetry for the cytochrome P450 catalyzed hydroxylation of octane is isozyme independent. J. Med. Chem. 33:1242–1246.

Kamachi, T., Shiota, Y., Ohta, T., and Yoshizawa, K. 2003. Does the hydroperoxo species of cytochrome P450 participate in olefin epoxidation with the main oxidant, Cpd I? Criticism from density functional theory calculations. Bull. Chem. Soc. Jpn. 76:721–732.

Karki, S., Dinnocenzo, J. P., Jones, J. P., and Korzekwa, K. R. 1995. Mechanism of oxidative amine dealkylation of substituted *N,N*-dimethylanilines by cytochrome P-450 – application of isotope effect profiles. J. Am. Chem. Soc. 117:3657–3664.

Keizers, P. H. J., Schraven, L. H. M., de Graaf, C., Hidestrand, M., Ingelman-Sundberg, M., van Dijk, B. R., Vermeulen, N. P. E., and Commandeur, J. N. M. 2005. Role of the conserved threonine 309 in mechanism of oxidation by cytochrome P450 2D6. Biochem. Biophys. Res. Commun. 338:1065–1074.

Korhonen, L. E., Turpeinen, M., Rahnasto, M., Wittekindt, C., Poso, A., Pelkonen, O., Raunio, H., and Juvonen, R. O. 2007. New potent and selective cytochrome P450 2B6 (CYP2B6) inhibitors based on three-dimensional quantitative structure–activity relationship (3D-QSAR) analysis. Br. J. Pharmacol. 150:932–42.

Korzekwa, K. R., Jones, J. P., and Gillette, J. R. 1990. Theoretical studies on cytochrome P-450 mediated hydroxylation: A predictive model for hydrogen atom abstractions. J. Am. Chem. Soc. 112:7042–7046.

Krayenbuhl, J. C., Vozeh, S., Kondo-Oestreicher, M., and Dayer, P. 1999. Drug–drug interactions of new active substances: mibefradil example. Eur. J. Clin. Pharmacol. 55:559–565.

Kumar, V., Wahlstrom, J. L., Rock, D. A., Warren, C. J., Gorman, L. A., and Tracy, T. S. 2006. CYP2C9 inhibition: impact of probe selection and pharmacogenetics on in vitro inhibition profiles. Drug Metab. Dispos. 34:1966–1975.

Lazarou, J., Pomeranz, B. H., and Corey, P. N. 1998. Incidence of adverse drug reactions in hospitalized patients: a meta-analysis of prospective studies. JAMA 279:1200–1205.

Lehmann Brothers, R. 2001. The Fruits of Genomics. p. 26.

Li, Q. S., Ogawa, J., Schmid, R. D., and Shimizu, S. 2005. Indole hydroxylation by bacterial cytochrome P450 BM-3 and modulation of activity by cumene hydroperoxide. Biosci. Biotechnol. Biochem. 69:293–300.

Li, A. P., and Jurima-Romet, M. 1997. Overview: pharmacokinetic drug–drug interactions. Adv. Pharmacol. 43:1–6.

Locuson, C. W., Gannett, P. M., Ayscue, R., and Tracy, T. S. 2007. Use of simple docking methods to screen a virtual library for heteroactivators of cytochrome P450 2C9. J. Med. Chem. 50:1158–65.

Lopez-Rangel, E., and Van Allen, M. I. 2005. Prenatal exposure to fluconazole: an identifiable dysmorphic phenotype. Birth Defects Res. A Clin. Mol. Teratol. 73:919–23.

Macdonald, T. L., Gutheim, W. G., Martin, R. B., and Guengerich, F. P. 1989. Oxidation of substituted *N,N*-dimethylanilines by cytochrome P-450: estimation of the effective oxidation–reduction potential of cytochrome P-450. Biochemistry 28:2071–2077.

Manchester, J. I., Dinnocenzo, J. P., Higgins, L. A., and Jones, J. P. 1997. A new mechanistic probe for cytochrome P450 – an application of isotope effect profiles. J. Am. Chem. Soc. 119:5069–5070.

Mao, B., Gozalbes, R., Barbosa, F., Migeon, J., Merrick, S., Kamm, K., Wong, E., Costales, C., Shi, W., Wu, C., and Froloff, N. 2006. QSAR modeling of in vitro inhibition of cytochrome P450 3A4. J. Chem. Inf. Model. 46:2125–2134.

Milne, G. 2000. New Drug Development in U.S. Pfizer J.

Mitchell, J. R., Thorgeirsson, S. S., Potter, W. Z., Jollow, D. J., and Keiser H. 1974. Acetaminophen-induced hepatic injury: protective role of glutathione in man and rationale for therapy. Clin. Pharmacol. Ther. 16:676–684.

Miwa, G. T., Walsh, J. S., and Lu, A. Y. 1984. Kinetic isotope effects on cytochrome P450-catalyzed reactions: the oxidative O-dealkylation of 7-ethoxycoumarin. J. Biol. Chem. 259:3000–3004.

Miwa, G. T., and Lu, A. Y. H. 1987. Kinetic isotope effects and 'metabolic switching' in cytochrome P450-catalyzed reactions. BioEssays 7:215–219.

Nelson, D. R., Koymans, L., Kamataki, T., Stegeman, J. J., Feyereisen, R., Waxman, D. J., Waterman, M. R., Gotoh, O., Coon, M. J., Estabrook, R. W., Gunsalus, I. C., and Nebert, D. W. 1996. P450 superfamily: update on new sequences, gene mapping, accession numbers and nomenclature. Pharmacogenetics 6:1–42.

Newcomb, M., Hollenberg, P. F., and Coon, M. J. 2003. Multiple mechanisms and multiple oxidants in P450-catalyzed hydroxylations. Arch. Biochem. Biophys. 409:72–79.

Obach, R. S. 2004. Potent inhibition of human liver aldehyde oxidase by raloxifene. Drug Metab. Dispos. 32:89–97.

Obach, R. S., Huynh, P., Allen, M. C., and Beedham, C. 2004. Human liver aldehyde oxidase: inhibition by 239 drugs. J. Clin. Pharmacol. 44:7–19.

Obach, R. S., and Walsky, R. L. 2005. Drugs that inhibit oxidation reactions catalyzed by aldehyde oxidase do not inhibit the reductive metabolism of ziprasidone to its major metabolite, *S*-methyldihydroziprasidone: an in vitro study. J. Clin. Psychopharmacol. 25:605–608.

O'Brien, S. E., and de Groot, M. J. 2005. Greater than the sum of its parts: combining models for useful ADMET prediction. J. Med. Chem. 48:1287–91.

Ogliaro, F., de Visser, S. P., Cohen, S., Sharma, P. K., and Shaik, S. 2002. Searching for the second oxidant in the catalytic cycle of cytochrome P450: a theoretical investigation of the iron(III)-hydroperoxo species and its epoxidation pathways. J. Am. Chem. Soc. 124:2806–2817.

Olsen, L., Rydberg, P., Rod, T. H., and Ryde, U. 2006. Prediction of activation energies for hydrogen abstraction by cytochrome P450. J. Med. Chem. 49:6489–6499.

Ortiz de Montellano, P. R. 1995. Cytochrome P450:Structure, Mechanism, and Biochemistry. New York: Plenum.

Park, K., Williams, D. P., Naisbitt, D. J., Kitteringham, N. R., and Pirmohamed, M. 2005. Investigation of toxic metabolites during drug development. Toxicol. Appl. Pharmacol. 207(2 Suppl):425–434.

Porter, W. R., Branchflower, R. V., and Trager, W. F. 1977. A kinetic method for the determination of multiple forms of microsomal cytochrome P-450. Biochem. Pharmacol. 26:549–550.

Prentis, R. A., Lis, Y., and Walker, S. R. 1988. Pharmaceutical innovation by the seven UK-owned pharmaceutical companies (1964–1985). Br. J. Clin. Pharmacol. 25:387–396.

Prueksaritanont, T., Gorham, L. M., Ma, B., Liu, L., Yu, X., Zhao, J. J., Slaughter, D. E., Arison, B. H., and Vyas, K. P. 1997. In vitro metabolism of simvastatin in humans [SBT]identification of metabolizing enzymes and effect of the drug on hepatic P450s. Drug Metab. Dispos. 25:1191–1199.

Rao, S., Aoyama, R., Schrag, M., Trager, W. F., Rettie, A., and Jones, J. P. 2000. A refined 3-dimensional QSAR of cytochrome P450 2C9: computational predictions of drug interactions. J. Med. Chem. 43:2789–2796.

Rettie, A. E., and Jones, J. P. 2005. Clinical and toxicological relevance of CYP2C9: Drug–drug interactions and pharmacogenetics. Ann. Rev. Pharmacol. Toxicol. 45:477–494.

Seeman, J. I. 1983. Effect of conformational changes on reactivity in organic chemistry. Evaluations, applications, and extensions of Curtin–Hammett/Winstein–Holness kinetics. Chem. Rev. 83:83–134.

Shaik, S., Kumar, D., de Visser, S. P., Altun, A., and Thiel, W. 2005. Theoretical perspective on the structure and mechanism of cytochrome P450 enzymes. Chem. Rev. 105: 2279–2328.

Sharma, P. K., De Visser, S. P., and Shaik, S. 2003. Can a single oxidant with two spin states masquerade as two different oxidants? A study of the sulfoxidation mechanism by cytochrome p450. J. Am. Chem. Soc. 125:8698–8699.

Sharma, U., Roberts, E. S., and Hollenberg, P. F. 1996. Formation of a metabolic intermediate complex of cytochrome P4502B1 by clorgyline. Drug Metab. Dispos. 24:1247–1253.

Singh, S. B., Shen, L. Q., Walker, M. J., and Sheridan, R. P. 2003. A model for predicting likely sites of CYP3A4-mediated metabolism on drug-like molecules. J. Med. Chem. 46:1330–1336.

Sorich, M. J., Miners, J. O., McKinnon, R. A., Winkler, D. A., Burden, F. R., and Smith. P. A. 2003. Comparison of linear and nonlinear classification algorithms for the prediction of drug and chemical metabolism by human UDP-glucuronosyltransferase isoforms. J. Chem. Inf. Comput. Sci. 43:2019–2024.

Streeter, A. J., Dahlin, D. C., Nelson, S. D., and Baillie, T. A. 1984. The covalent binding of acetaminophen to protein. Evidence for cysteine residues as major sites of arylation in vitro. Chem. Biol. Interact. 48:349–66.

Tornero-Velez, R., Ross, M. K., Granville, C., Laskey, J., Jones, J. P., DeMarini, D. M., and Evans, M. V. 2004. Metabolism and mutagenicity of source water contaminants 1,3-dichloropropane and 2,2-dichloropropane. Drug Metab. Dispos. 32:123–131.

Vatsis, K. P., and Coon, M. J. 2002. Ipso-substitution by cytochrome P450 with conversion of p-hydroxybenzene derivatives to hydroquinone: evidence for hydroperoxo-iron as the active oxygen species. Arch. Biochem. Biophys. 397:119–129.

Vaz, A. D., Pernecky, S. J., Raner, G. M., and Coon, M. J. 1996. Peroxo-iron and oxenoid-iron species as alternative oxygenating agents in cytochrome P450-catalyzed reactions: switching by threonine-302 to alanine mutagenesis of cytochrome P450 2B4. Proc. Natl. Acad. Sci. USA 93:4644–4648.

Vaz, A. D., and Coon, M. J. 1987. Hydrocarbon formation in the reductive cleavage of hydroperoxides by cytochrome P-450. Proc. Natl. Acad. Sci. USA 84:1172–1176.

Vaz, A. D. N., McGinnity, D. F., and Coon, M. J. 1998. Epoxidation of olefins by cytochrome P450: Evidence from site-specific mutagenesis for hydroperoxo-iron as an electrophilic oxidant. Proc. Natl. Acad. Sci. USA 95:3555–3560.

Vaz, A. D., Roberts, E. S., and Coon, M. J. 1990. Reductive beta-scission of the hydroperoxides of fatty acids and xenobiotics: role of alcohol-inducible cytochrome P-450. Proc. Natl. Acad. Sci. USA 87:5499–5503.

Volz, T. J., Rock, D. A., and Jones, J. P. 2002. Evidence for two different active oxygen species in cytochrome p450 BM3 mediated sulfoxidation and N-dealkylation reactions. J. Am. Chem. Soc. 124:9724–9725.

Watanabe, Y. 2001. Alternatives to the oxoferryl porphyrin cation radical as the proposed reactive intermediate of cytochrome P450: two-electron oxidized Fe(III) porphyrin derivatives. J. Biol. Inorg. Chem. 6:846–856.

Yamashita, F., Fujiwara, S., Wanchana, S., and Hashida, M. 2006. Quantitative structure/activity relationship modelling of pharmacokinetic properties using genetic algorithm-combined partial least squares method. J. Drug Target. 14:496–504.

Yin, H., Anders, M. W., Korzekwa, K. R., Higgins, L., Thummel, K. E., Kharasch, E. D., and Jones, J. P. 1995. Designing safer chemicals: predicting the rates of metabolism of halogenated alkanes. Proc. Nat. Acad. Sci. USA 92:11076–11080.

Yin, H. Q., Anders, M. W., and Jones, J. P. 1996. Metabolism Of 1,2-dichloro-1-fluoroethane and 1-fluoro-1,2,2-trichloroethane – electronic factors govern the regioselectivity of cytochrome P450-dependent oxidation. Chem. Res. Toxicol. 9:50–57.

Yin, H. Q., Jones, J. P., and Anders, M. W. 1995. Metabolism of 1-fluoro-1,1,2-trichloroethane, 1,2-dichloro-1,1-difluoroethane, and 1,1,1-trifluoro-2-chloroethane. Chem. Res. Toxicol. 8:262–268.

Zamora, I., Afzelius, L., and Cruciani, G. 2003. Predicting drug metabolism: A site of metabolism prediction tool applied to the cytochrome P4502C9. J. Med. Chem. 46:2313–2324.

Zhou, D. S., Afzelius, L., Grimm, S. W., Andersson, T. B., Zauhar, R. J., and Zamora, I. 2006. Comparison of methods for the prediction of the metabolic sites for CYP3A4-mediated metabolic reactions. Drug Metab. Dispos. 34: 976–983.

2

Role of Bioactivation in Idiosyncratic Drug Toxicity: Structure–Toxicity Relationships

Amit S. Kalgutkar

Pharmacokinetics, Dynamics and Metabolism Department, Pfizer Global Research & Development, Groton, CT06340, USA

e-mail: amit.kalgutkar@pfizer.com

Keywords: Bioactivation · Idiosyncratic · Reactive Metabolite · P450 · Liver · Drug · Hepatotoxicity · Glutathione · DNA

2.1. Adverse Drug Reactions

Adverse drug reactions (ADRs) continue to be a significant contributor to overall attrition statistics in the pharmaceutical industry. ADRs pose a significant health problem since they contribute to patient morbidity and mortality and represent one of the most common causes for pharmaceutical product recalls and black-box warning labels. Of a total of 548 drugs approved in the period from 1975 to 1999, 45 drugs (8.2%) acquired one or more black-box warnings and 16 (2.9%) were withdrawn from the market (Lasser et al. 2002). An estimated 100 000 fatalities annually are attributed to ADRs making it the fourth to sixth leading cause of death in the United States (Lazarou, Pomeranz and Corey 1998). Therefore, increased emphasis has been placed on the identification of indicators of ADRs in preclinical species and humans as early as possible in the overall discovery/development process.

Adverse drug reactions can be classified into two categories namely type A and type B reactions. Type A or augmented reactions account for approximately 80% of all ADRs and are predictable from the known primary or secondary pharmacology of the drug. They show simple dose–response relationships and, therefore, can be usually avoided by dose reduction and are rarely life-threatening. Type A ADRs can be routinely identified in preclinical toxicological investigations. Typical examples of type A ADRs include the risk of hypotension with antihypertensives and hemorrhage with anticoagulants. Currently, risk assessment of overall toxicity in the clinic is usually based on the safety margin of the drug candidate, which is often the ratio of the no observable adverse effect

A.A. Elfarra (ed.), *Advances in Bioactivation Research*, DOI: 10.1007/978-0-387-77300-1_2,

level (NOAEL) in the most sensitive preclinical species and the anticipated efficacious dose/systemic exposure in humans. A combination of clinical signs and histopathological evaluations serve as standard paradigm for identification of organ toxicity in animals, and the risk assessment is then extrapolated to humans. If an adverse event is observed in laboratory animals at systemic drug exposures near those anticipated for clinical efficacy, the drug is generally abandoned from further development. This traditional approach for organ toxicity risk assessment has poor predictability for type B reactions (Olson et al. 2000), since these reactions are not related to the known pharmacology of the drug, and although they are dose-dependent in susceptible individuals, they can occur at any dose within the usual therapeutic range. Although less common than type A reactions, type B reactions can be serious and may be life-threatening. Type B reactions are extremely host-dependent, usually rare, and therefore referred to as idiosyncratic ADRs (IADRs). Furthermore, there are no general animal models that can predict the occurrence of IADRs in humans. Idiosyncratic ADRs can be just as idiosyncratic in animals as they are in humans and furthermore it is rare for animals to show all of the biochemical, clinical, and morphological features characteristic of IADRs in humans. This is not surprising considering that many of the manifestations of idiosyncratic reactions to the same drug can be different in different humans. Comprehensive reviews on this subject have recently appeared in the literature (Roth et al. 2003; Shenton, Chen and Uetrecht 2004).

Given the low frequency of occurrence of type B reactions and lack of available animal models, large clinical trials, exposing perhaps up to 10 000 patients to a new therapeutic agent prior to registration, may not suffice in detecting IADRs reliably. An additional complication is that IADRs usually manifest as overt or symptomatic disease and can occur with intermediate (1–8 weeks) or long (1 year) periods of latency. Drugs can adversely affect almost any organ in the body; however, potentially life-threatening IADRs noted for several drugs include hepatotoxicity, severe cutaneous reactions, anaphylaxis, and blood dyscrasias. Among these, drug-induced liver toxicity is the most common cause for the withdrawal of a drug from the market and it accounts for approximately one-half of the cases of acute liver failure and mimics all forms of acute and chronic liver disease (Gunawan and Kaplowitz 2004). An estimated 1400 drugs have been implicated in causing liver damage in greater than one occasion (Biour et al. 2000). Manifestations of liver injury range from mild, asymptomatic changes in serum transaminases, which occur at high frequency with a number of drugs, to fulminant hepatic failure, which although rare is potentially life-threatening and may necessitate a liver transplant.

2.2. Link Between Drug Metabolism and Type B ADRs

One of the liver's main physiological roles is the metabolism of drugs into hydrophilic metabolites (via a combination of oxidative, reductive, and hydrolytic phase I and conjugating phase II pathways) in order to facilitate their elimination. Considering that the liver is exposed to high concentrations of drugs/metabolites after oral administration, it is not altogether surprising that the organ is often a target for drug-induced toxicity. In most cases hepatic metabolism results in the loss of biological activity of the parent drug, and such metabolic reactions are therefore regarded as detoxification pathways. However, depending on the structural features present in some drugs, the same metabolic events on occasion can generate chemically reactive and toxic metabolites. The concept of drug metabolism to chemically reactive species that covalently modify critical protein components leading to some form of toxicity has its basis in the field of carcinogenicity (Fieser 1938; Miller and Miller 1947), which proposed the carcinogenic and hepatotoxic activity of polycyclic aromatic hydrocarbons and aminoazo dyes to arise from their bioactivation to reactive metabolites. Extension of these concepts to human drug-induced hepatotoxicity was provided from studies in the 1970s on the covalent binding to hepatic tissue by structurally diverse drugs including acetaminophen (Cohen et al. 1997). Based on these collective findings gathered over the last 50 years, biotransformation of relatively inert organic compounds to reactive electrophilic intermediates including free radicals, commonly referred to as metabolic activation or bioactivation, has been speculated to contribute toward certain drug-induced toxicities, including hepatotoxicity, cutaneous ADRs, and blood dyscrasias (Kaplowitz 2004). Inadequate detoxification of reactive metabolites is thought to represent a pathogenic mechanism for tissue necrosis, carcinogenicity, teratogenicity, and immune-mediated toxicity (Figure 2.1; Kaplowitz 2004).

Drug-metabolizing enzymes have evolved to process a plethora of structurally diverse xenobiotics, which are encountered by the organism. These enzymes, however, cannot distinguish between xenobiotics that are bioactivated to reactive metabolites and those that are not. Whether bioactivation will occur for any given molecule will depend on two key factors: (1) does the molecule possess a functionality and/or architecture that is susceptible to bioactivation and (2) is there an alternative (higher affinity but innocuous) route of metabolism within the molecule that minimizes the potential bioactivation of the "suspect" chemical motif within that molecule. Most bioactivation reactions in the liver involve either oxidation or reduction and can often

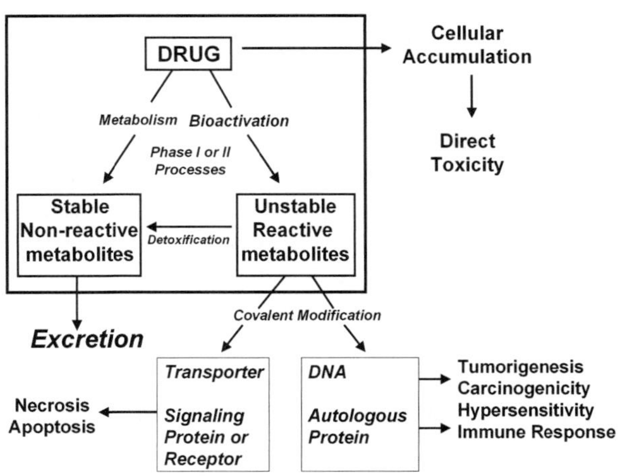

Figure 2.1 Proposed role of bioactivation in drug toxicity.

be attributed mainly to the action of cytochrome P450 enzymes. In several cases, cytosolic enzymes, such as aldehyde oxidase or alcohol dehydrogenases, have also been noted to participate in the catalysis of bioactivation pathways. Conjugative pathways including glucuronidation and sulfation are also known to transform latent functional groups into electrophilic intermediates. In some cases, bioactivation can involve a single enzymatic reaction, whereas in other cases, multiple enzymatic and/or chemical steps are involved in the production of the ultimate toxin. Besides the liver, neutrophils and monocytes can metabolize drugs to reactive metabolites, especially those drugs that have nitrogen or sulfur in a low oxidation state. The major system involved in this oxidation is the combination of NADPH oxidase and myeloperoxidase (MPO), which generates hypochlorous acid. In such cases, the dominant toxicity will be agranulocytosis and/or aplastic anemia, not hepatotoxicity.

While the detection of a bioactivation process in vitro is relatively straightforward, the downstream consequences of this process as it relates to toxicity remain poorly understood, although, two hypotheses have been proposed to explain the phenomenon. Foremost amongst them is the hapten hypothesis that proposes covalent modification of proteins by a reactive metabolite leading to a "foreign" protein that, in some cases, translates to an immune-mediated adverse reaction. Failure to downregulate potentially deleterious immune responses due to a "foreign" macromolecule may cause ADRs in susceptible patients (Matzinger 2002). For example, sulfonamides such as sulfamethoxazole cause a variety of ADRs including fever, skin rashes, hepatitis, nephritis, and blood dyscrasias, many of which are idiosyncratic in nature. The identification of drug-specific T cells in systemic circulation and blister fluid of susceptible population provides convincing evidence that adverse events associated with sulfamethoxazole require activation of the host's immune system (Hess et al. 1999). In the case of sulfamethoxazole, the immune activation is thought to involve a P450-catalyzed bioactivation of the aniline group to a reactive nitroso metabolite capable of covalently binding to cellular constituents (Hess et al. 1999). The danger hypothesis, which aims to account for the idiosyncratic nature of ADRs in patients, further expands on the hapten hypothesis. In this proposal, drug–macromolecule conjugates lead to cell damage, which in turn generates a "danger signal" that ultimately can result in antibody- or cytotoxic T-cell-mediated responses (Uetrecht 1999). The variability in incidence of such a response in patients is thought to be due to high interindividual differences in the competing processes of cell damage, repair, and host cell defense.

Since the initial hypothesis that covalent binding of acetaminophen to "critical" hepatic proteins may be associated with its hepatotoxic effects, there has been a plethora of publications on the identification of susceptible protein targets (Pumford and Halmes 1997). However, few have attempted to distinguish "critical" from "noncritical" proteins. With acetaminophen, more than 30 hepatic proteins form conjugates with acetaminophen after a toxic overdose of the drug to rodent species (Hinson et al. 2004; Park et al. 2005). The concomitant inactivation of multiple proteins during this process suggests that failure in the cellular machinery is a consequence of multiple parallel events rather than a simple cascade or signaling mechanism. Overall, the complex nature of these events severely limits our ability to predict whether in vitro bioactivation and accompanying covalent binding of a potential drug candidate to hepatic tissue(s) will or will not ultimately translate in some form of toxicity in animals or for that matter in humans. Even if the drug candidate fails to cause organ toxicity in preclinical species, there is always some concern that the bioactivation observed in human hepatic tissue may have the potential to elicit idiosyncratic immune-mediated ADRs in the susceptible population.

2.3. Assays to Monitor Reactive Metabolites in Drug Discovery

Formation of reactive metabolites has received considerable attention and several in vitro assays have been established to monitor and address this phenomenon. Reactive electrophilic metabolites are generally short-lived (with the possible exception of some acyl glucuronides) and are not usually detectable in circulation. Their intracellular formation can be inferred from conjugates derived from reaction with endogenous nucleophiles. Their formation may be modulated by enzyme induction and/or inhibition, and gene deletion in mammals. However, none of these experimental approaches are directly applicable to humans. Consequently, human exposure to chemically reactive metabolites in the liver and in the general circulation is impossible to quantify. Given the inability to predict whether bioactivation phenomenon detected in vitro will ultimately lead to toxicity in the clinic, a general strategy adopted by many within the pharmaceutical community involves the assessment of reactive metabolite formation as early as possible in the selection of drug candidates, with the goal of eliminating or minimizing the formation of reactive species by rational structural modification of lead chemical matter.

2.3.1. Covalent Binding

Availability of a radiolabeled compound allows a quantitative assessment of the amount of covalent binding either in vitro (e.g., liver microsomes, cytosol, or S-9 fractions) or in tissue or blood/plasma obtained from preclinical in vivo studies. Some companies have adopted a limit of 50 pM mg^{-1} liver microsomal protein as the cutoff for further development (Evans et al 2004; Evans and Baillie 2005). This limit is based on the commonly observed amount of covalent binding detected in the livers of animals receiving a prototypic hepatotoxin (e.g., acetaminophen, bromobenzene, furosemide, or 4-ipomeanol), which is associated with overt hepatoxicity (about 1000 pM mg^{-1} microsomal protein) and a 20-fold safety margin. However, it should be noted that the 50 pM mg^{-1} microsomal protein is not a hard cutoff. The rigor with which teams adhere to this limit depends on multiple factors such as the therapeutic area, the duration of therapy (acute versus chronic), the target population, first in class or best in class and, of course, the anticipated human pharmacokinetics and dose. Covalent binding studies can be performed in vivo as well. Either tissue or blood/plasma can be examined for the degree of covalent binding. However, covalent binding may require multiple dosing to establish the true impact of the compound. Reactive metabolites formed after the first dose may be efficiently trapped by nucleophiles such as glutathione (GSH) and eliminated from the body (e.g., via the bile). Once GSH is depleted, the extent of covalent binding with cellular or circulating proteins may increase rapidly, which could result in an ADR. The advantage of covalent binding studies is that they directly measure covalent binding of reactive metabolites to macromolecules, which could cause an adverse immunological response or direct organ toxicity. Nevertheless, no information is available about the nature of the covalently modified proteins. Furthermore, since many drugs display a degree of covalent modification of proteins, but only a fraction thereof cause toxicity, a direct link with a toxicological endpoint is not guaranteed. Indeed, the mechanism of action of some drugs (e.g., aspirin, finasteride, clopidogrel, and omeprazole) involves covalent binding to the target. For finasteride the binding specifically involves 5α-reductase and, therefore, no toxicity due to off-target covalent binding is observed. An added disadvantage of this approach is that covalent binding experiments are laborious. Finally, radiolabeled material is not routinely available in early drug discovery at most pharmaceutical companies.

2.3.2. Reactive Metabolite Characterization as Stable Sulfydryl, Amino, and/or Cyano Conjugates

Methodology to elucidate the structure(s) of reactive metabolites typically involves in vitro "trapping" experiments conducted using liver microsomes, cytosol, or S-9 fractions supplemented with NADPH and appropriate nucleophilic trapping agents including thiols (e.g., naturally occurring tripeptide and soft nucleophile GSH and its ethyl ester derivative or *N*-acetylcysteine), amines (e.g., *N*-acetyllysine, semicarbazide, and methoxylamine), or cyanide anion; analysis of the resulting metabolites by liquid chromatography-tandem mass spectrometry (LC-MS/MS) is employed to detect and characterize stable conjugates with the exogenously added nucleophile. Elucidation of the structure of these adducts can provide indirect information on the structure of the electrophilic species, thereby providing insight into the bioactivation mechanism and hence a rationale on which to base subsequent chemical intervention strategies. These trapping agents also serve as surrogate markers of covalent binding of the electrophile to microsomal protein. GSH adducts can be analyzed by LC-MS/MS using either the full-scan mode or constant neutral loss scanning for 129 Da (glutamyl moiety) to detect GSH-related conjugates (Baillie and Davis 1993; Soglia et al. 2004). Hard electrophiles (e.g., electrophilic carbonyl compounds) will preferentially react with hard nucleophiles including amines (e.g., semicarbazide and methoxylamine), amino acids (e.g., lysine), and DNA bases (e.g., guanine and cytosine) (Zhang et al. 1996; Dalvie et al. 2002) affording the corresponding Schiff base, which can be further stabilized by the addition of reducing agents (e.g., sodium borohydride or sodium cyanoborohydride) to generate the more stable amine conjugates. Typical in vitro conditions require the addition of 5 mM of amine trapping agent to the microsomal mixture followed by LC-MS/MS analysis for the formation of stable imine conjugates as indicated in the case of furan ring opening to reactive β-dicarbonyl metabolites (Zhang et al. 1996). The cyanide anion is a "hard" nucleophile that can be used to trap iminium species. Gorrod et al. (1991) have developed a simple screening method that detects reactive iminium intermediates via reaction with [^{14}C]-cyanide. Extent of radiolabeled cyanide incorporation in test compounds that are suspected of forming reactive iminium intermediates is normalized with reference to a standard compound (e.g., S-nicotine). Utilizing this methodology, iminium ion formation has been assessed for several structurally diverse cyclic tertiary amines (Gorrod and Aislaitner 1994).

2.3.3. Enzyme Inactivation Studies

In some instances, P450-mediated oxidative bioactivation of drugs to reactive intermediates leads to irreversible inactivation of the P450 enzyme by the reactive species prior to its release from the active site (Murray 1997). Because metabolic activation precludes enzyme inactivation, these drugs fall into the category of mechanism-based inactivators. The mechanism-based inactivation of P450 enzymes may result from irreversible alkylation of an active-site amino acid or the heme prosthetic group or a combination of both. In general, heme alkylation invariably inactivates P450, whereas amino acid alkylation may result in loss of catalytic activity. Inactivation of P450 enzymes often translates into clinically relevant drug–drug interactions as well as immune-mediated IADRs, which can be potentially deleterious. The ability of drug candidates to inactivate P450 function is typically screened for in an industry setting.

2.3.4. Metabolite Identification

A thorough understanding of metabolic pathways and the biochemical mechanisms by which metabolites are generated can provide insight to the potential of a compound to yield a reactive species. Both in vitro and in vivo approaches can and should be performed to gain a detailed understanding of the biotransformation pathways that a drug candidate may undergo. Often times, stable downstream metabolites derived from non-enzymatic processing of electrophilic intermediates provide important clues on the generation of reactive metabolites (e.g., the detection of carboxylic acid metabolite in the metabolism of terminal alkynes provides evidence for the generation of a reactive ketene intermediate). The possibility that metabolism occurs at an alternate site and not on the structural alert itself, can also be assessed in these studies. In the absence of an alternate chemical series, this information may be critical toward nominating a candidate containing a structural alert for clinical development.

2.4. Strategies to Abrogate Reactive Metabolite Formation: Structure–Activity Relationship Studies

The propensity of a drug candidate to undergo bioactivation to reactive intermediates, usually electrophiles, is a function of the chemistry that ensues following metabolism. Information to qualify certain functional groups as structural alerts (Figure 2.2) has been inferred from myriad

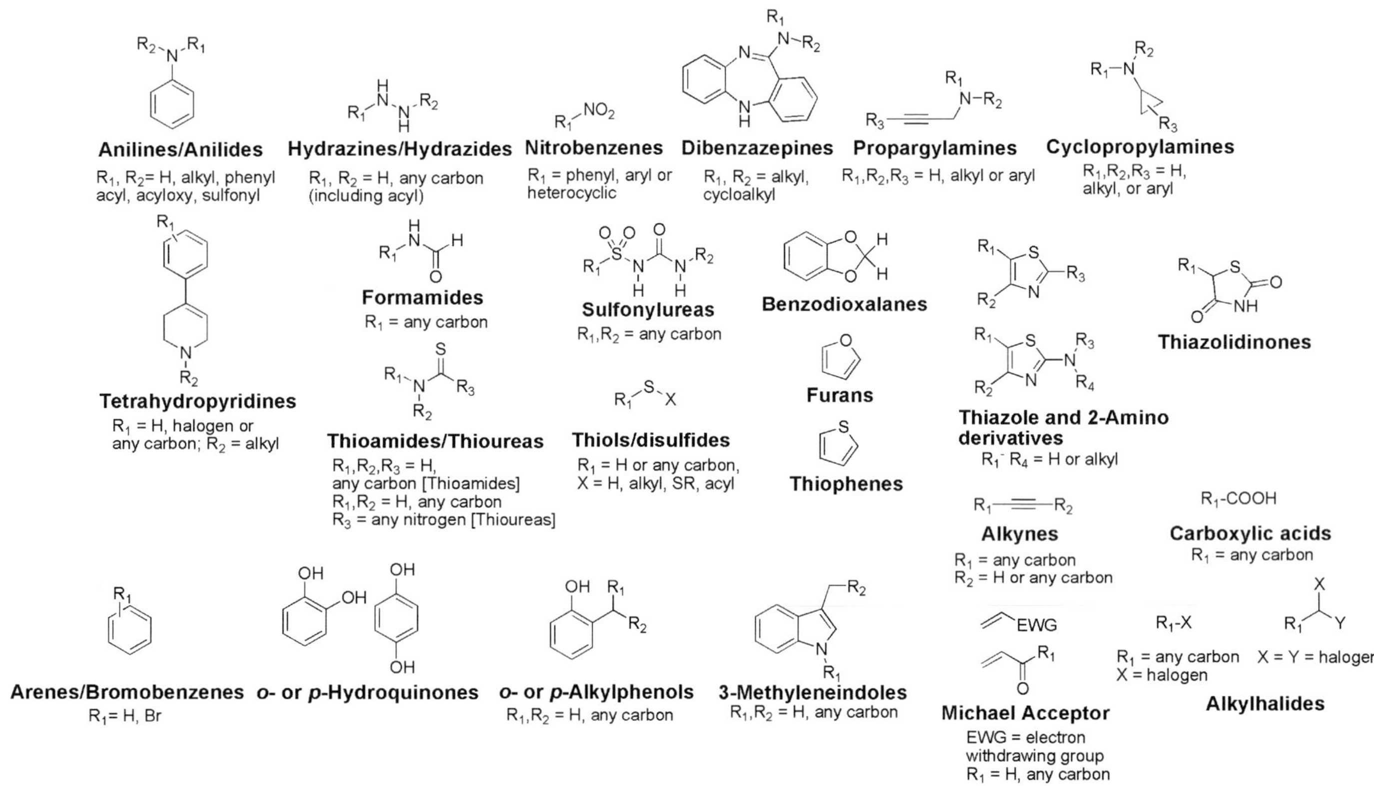

Figure 2.2 A comprehensive list of organic functional groups susceptible to bioactivation.

examples of protoxins containing these motifs, which upon bioactivation affords reactive metabolites. A comprehensive review that summarizes the existing bioactivation pathways for these functional groups has been recently published (Kalgutkar et al. 2005a). The scope of this concept can be further expanded to include numerous drugs that contain putative structural alerts and are associated with some form of toxicity. Indeed, for many such drugs reactive metabolites formation has been demonstrated and serves to provide a circumstantial link between bioactivation and toxicity. Figure 2.3 provides a glimpse of drugs that have been withdrawn due to toxicity and are also prone to bioactivation. For an exhaustive review on this subject, the reader is advised to refer to the article by Kalgutkar and Soglia (2005).

Numerous examples documenting the elimination of bioactivation liabilities via chemical manipulations have been presented in the literature. In several cases, elimination of bioactivation liability in prototype drugs has also resulted in the elimination of toxicity in the successor agent. It is noteworthy to point out that structural alterations which successfully eliminate the propensity of new chemical leads to undergo bioactivation may also confer a detrimental effect on the desired pharmacological

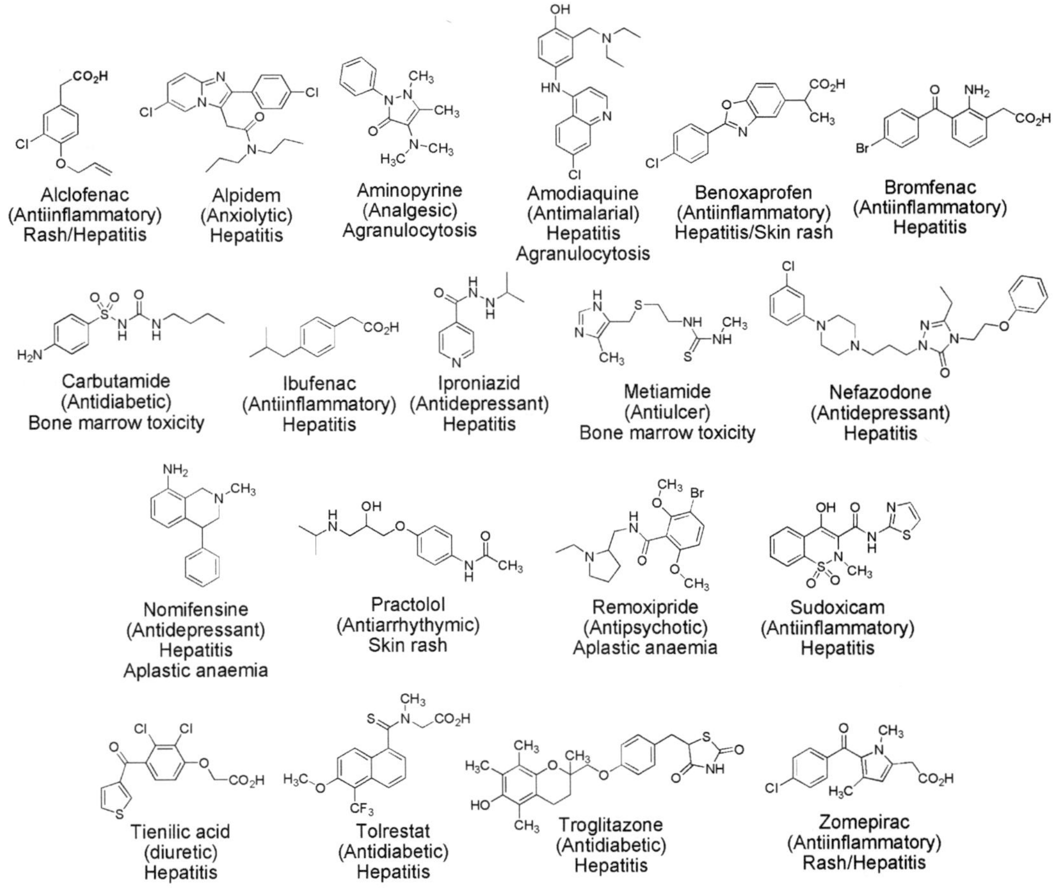

Figure 2.3 Examples of drugs susceptible to bioactivation, which have been withdrawn due to ADRs.

(possible changes in agonist/antagonist behavior and/or subtype selectivity for target receptor or enzyme) and pharmacokinetic attributes of the chemical matter. Therefore, chemical intervention strategies toward the elimination of bioactivation phenomenon are often an iterative process, the success of which is heavily dependent on a close working relationship between medicinal chemists, pharmacologists, and metabolism scientists.

2.4.1. Removal of Structural Alerts

There are several strategies that medicinal chemists can utilize toward elimination of bioactivation potential of lead chemical matter. Foremost amongst which is a strategy involving direct replacement of the potential structural alert with substituents that are generally resistant to metabolism or with groups that undergo biotransformation to nonreactive metabolites. Circumstantial evidence, whereupon removal of structural alerts in prototype therapeutic agents translates into a markedly improved safety profile is illustrated in Figure 2.4. Removal of the aniline substituents in the antiarrhythmic agent procainamide and the antidiabetic agent carbutamide, which are known to be associated with bone marrow toxicity (carbutamide has been withdrawn from the market due to life-threatening bone marrow toxicity), results in flecainide and tolbutamide, respectively, that are devoid of the IADRs observed with the prototype drugs. Likewise, the bone marrow toxicity associated with the prototype H2 receptor antagonist metiamide that led to its withdrawal has not been observed with cimetidine. A key structural difference between the two compounds is the replacement of the thiourea substituent in metiamide that is subject to bioactivation with nonreactive guanidine functionality in cimetidine.

Structure–bioactivation relationships on clozapine and its analogs have been examined (Liegeois et al. 1995, 1999). Replacing the nitrogen that connects the two aryl rings on clozapine with oxygen or sulfur results in marketed drugs loxapine and quetiapine, respectively, that do not undergo peroxidase-mediated bioactivation to the reactive iminium species in neutrophils – a metabolic fate, which has been speculated to contribute toward clozapine-induced agranulocytosis (Figure 2.4) (Uetrecht 1994; Liegeois et al. 1999). Despite administration at doses comparable to clozapine, cases of agranulocytosis with quetiapine and loxapine are extremely rare.

An additional example wherein reactive metabolite formation can be eliminated by direct replacement of the offending motifs is evident in structure–toxicity studies on the antimalarial agent amodiaquine, which has been withdrawn from prophylactic use due to cases of hepatotoxicity and agranulocytosis. Tingle et al. (1995) have shown that exchanging the C'4-phenolic OH group in the antimalarial drug amodiaquine with a fluorine results in a compound that does not undergo the obligatory peroxidase-mediated two-electron oxidation process on the 4-aminophenol motif to the corresponding electrophilic quinone-imine as discernible with the parent compound (see Figure 2.4). It is interesting to note that incorporation of steric bulk around the C'4-phenolic OH group as means to prevent oxidation, however, is not successful in the case of amodiaquine as indicated with the analogous antimalarials pyronaridine and cycloquine that are equally susceptible to bioactivation as the parent drug (Naisbitt et al. 1998).

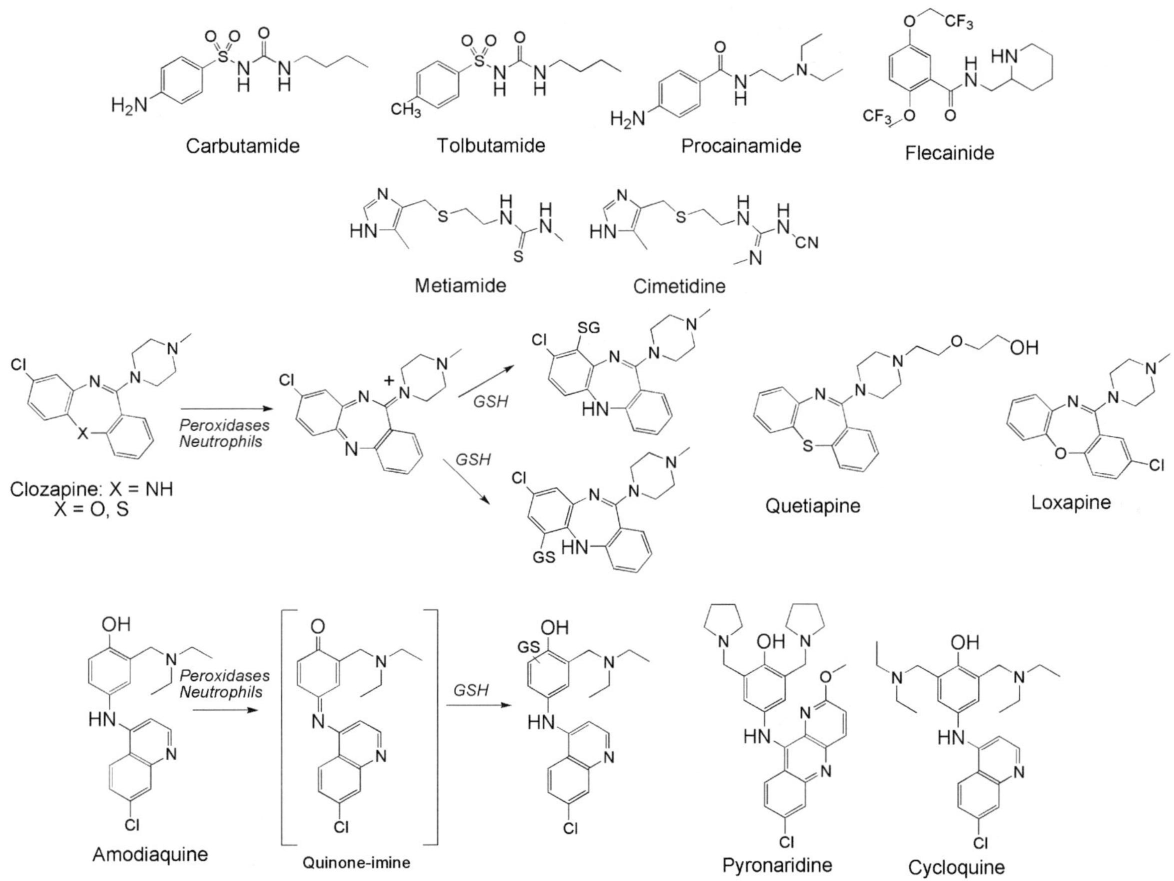

Figure 2.4 Circumstantial evidence linking chemical structure to IADRs: removal of structural alerts.

2.4.2. Blocking Sites of Bioactivation

An alternate approach involves blocking the site of initial metabolism that precludes bioactivation. The strategy is particularly effective in eliminating reactive metabolite formation in instances when bioactivation occurs in a stepwise fashion via an enzymatic or nonenzymatic processing (oxidative, elimination, or rearrangement) of the initially formed latent metabolite(s). In this scenario, neighboring functional groups can participate in the process of sequential metabolic or nonmetabolic steps leading to reactive metabolite formation (e.g., oxidative metabolism of phenol to ortho- or para-hydroquinone followed by further oxidation to the corresponding quinones). An example of successful implementation of this approach to prevent reactive metabolite formation is evident from structure–bioactivation studies conducted on a novel potassium channel opener (Compound **1**) (see Figure 2.5) to elucidate the mechanism of bioactivation resulting in potent mechanism-based inactivation of P4503A4 (Wu et al. 2003). Saturation of the cinnamoyl double bond (compound **2**) or insertion of fluorine on the phenyl ring in the cinnamoyl portion of **1** to afford **3** did not abolish P450 inactivation, whereas replacement of the morpholine ring with a hydrogen atom to afford **4** or substitution of the hydrogen ortho to the morpholine ring with a fluorine atom to yield **5** were successful methods toward eliminating P4503A4 inactivation by **1**. The lack of P450 inactivation by **5** is consistent with a bioactivation pathway involving the initial aromatic hydroxylation ortho to the morpholine ring (or para to the benzylamine methine). Further two-electron oxidation of this initial metabolite by P450 can result in the formation of the reactive quinone-imine or quinone-methide intermediates. The potential formation of either reactive intermediates can be avoided by the introduction of the fluorine atom. In the present example, Compound **5** not only is devoid of P450 inactivation liability but it also retains the pharmacological and pharmacokinetic properties of the prototype Compound **1**.

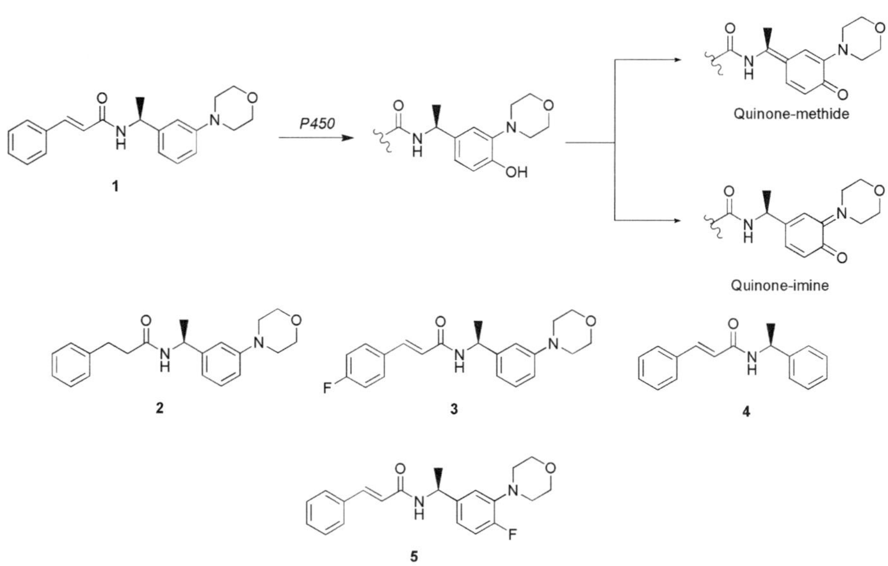

Figure 2.5 Strategies to abrogate reactive metabolite formation: blocking sites of bioactivation.

2.4.3. Introduction of Alternate Metabolic Soft Spots

Apart from strategies that focus on replacement of structural alerts or blocking metabolic sites that preclude bioactivation, chemists can also introduce metabolic soft spots elsewhere on the pharmacophore to divert metabolism. An example of this concept is evident with nifidepine, a well-tolerated drug, despite containing the nitroaromatic structural alert (Figure 2.6). The major metabolic pathways of nifedipine identified in humans are restricted to biotransformations on the available soft spots including oxidation of the 1,4-dihydropyridine ring, hydrolysis of both the methyl ester groups, and/or hydroxylation of the methyl substituent followed by lactonization (Bocker and Guengerich 1986; Guengerich, Peterson and Bocker 1988). There is no evidence for formation of metabolites derived from reductive metabolism of the nitro group in humans.

Additional examples that highlight the success of this strategy are displayed in Figures 2.6 and 2.7. Toxicity associated with platelet aggregation inhibitor ticlopidine has been linked to the P450 or MPO-catalyzed bioactivation of its thiophene ring to reactive *S*-oxides or *S*-chloride intermediates that covalently bind to hepatic proteins and neutrophils, respectively (Figure 2.6; Liu and Uetrecht 2000). In the case of structurally similar drug clopidogrel, introduction of the additional methyl ester group results in a metabolic shift such that ester hydrolysis to the inactive carboxylic acid metabolite constitutes the principal metabolic fate (>85% in circulation) of this drug (Figure 2.6; Reist et al. 2000). Of much interest in this context is the observation that clopidogrel by itself is inactive and requires biotransformation to produce inhibition of platelet aggregation in vivo. Recently, Pereillo et al. (2002) have identified a thiophene ring scission product as the active metabolite of clopidogrel. The formation of this active carboxylic acid metabolite presumably occurs via a P450-catalyzed oxidation of the thiophene ring in clopidogrel to yield a 2-oxothiophene metabolite, hydrolytic cleavage of which generates the active component (see Figure 2.6). Whether the formation of electrophilic intermediates during the oxidative metabolism of the thiophene ring in clopidogrel occurs, remains unknown. Finally, it is important to note that the daily dose of clopidogrel (75 mg) is approximately sixfold lower than that of ticlopidine (500 mg) and this feature may play a key role in the markedly improved safety profile of clopidogrel.

The anxiolytic agent alpidem was withdrawn from the market within the first year of its commercial release due to severe hepatotoxicity that led to fatalities or required immediate liver transplantation. In contrast, the structural analog zolpidem does not possess the hepatotoxic liability associated with its predecessor. Although the reason(s) for this discrepancy remains unclear, it is interesting to note that the chloro-imidazopyridine ring in alpidem is subject to P450 bioactivation leading to the formation of a reactive epoxide that reacts with GSH to yield sulfydryl conjugates (see Figure 2.6), which have been detected in humans (Durand et al. 1992). A key structural difference in the two drugs is the replacement of the two chlorine atoms in alpidem with two metabolically labile methyl groups in zolpidem. Indeed, the primary biotransformation pathways of zolpidem in humans is restricted to the oxidative metabolism of both methyl groups to the corresponding alcohol

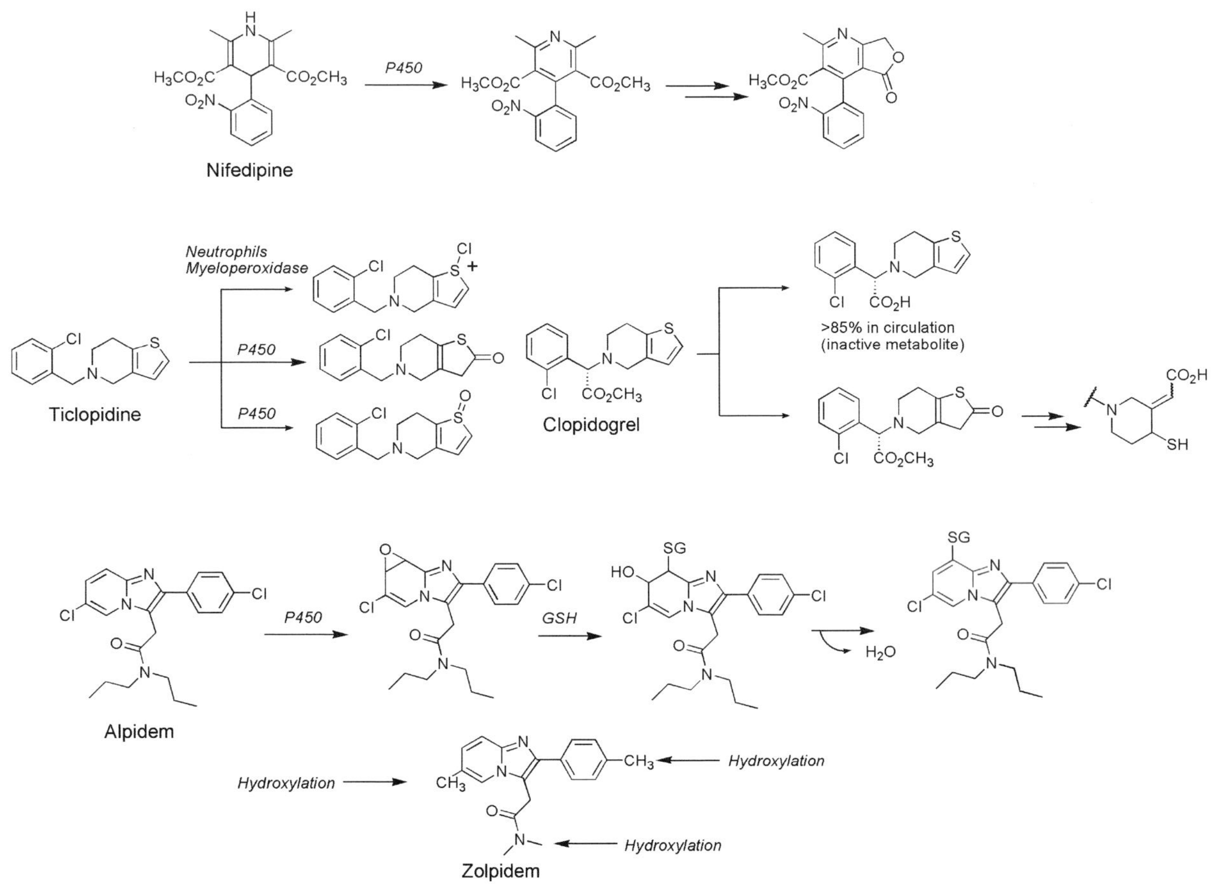

Figure 2.6 Strategies to abrogate reactive metabolite formation: introducing alternate metabolic soft spots.

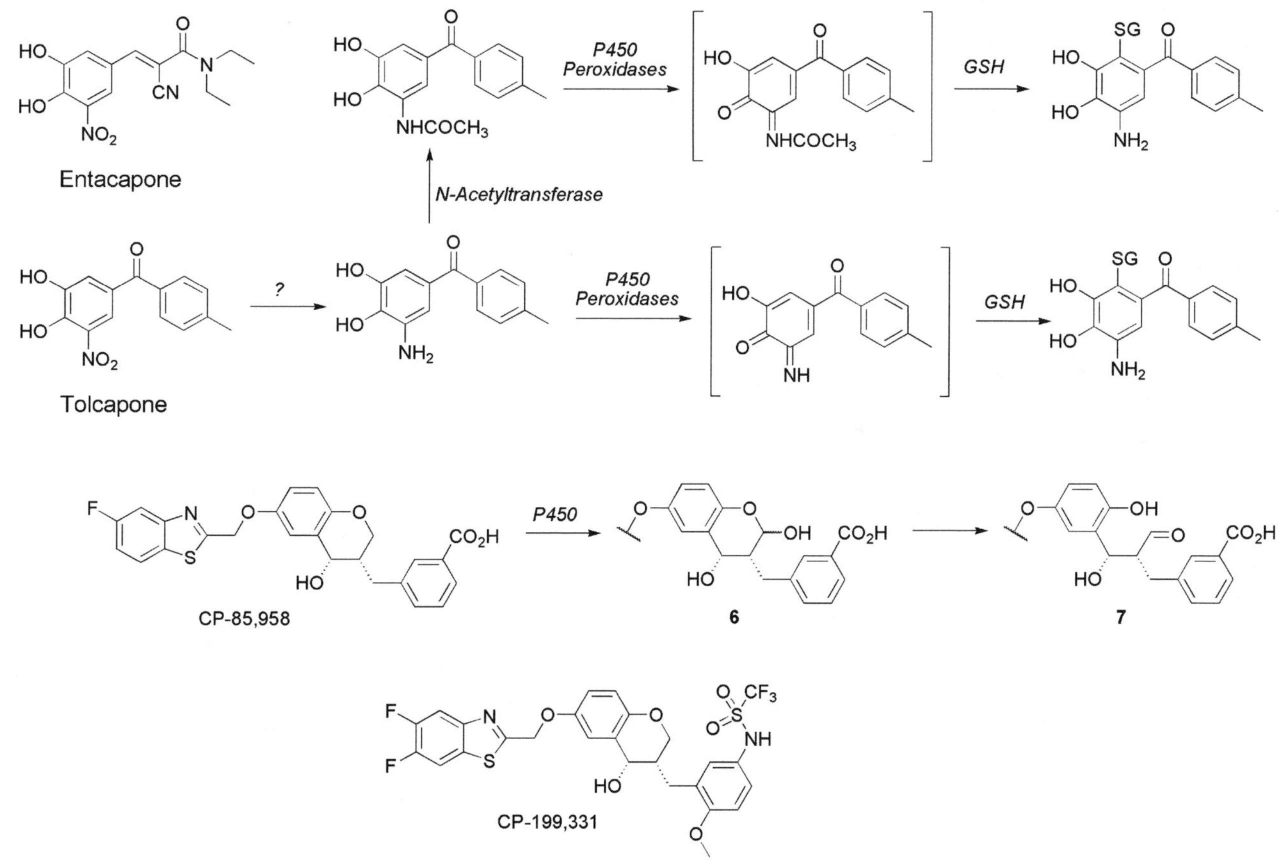

Figure 2.7 Additional examples where presence of alternate metabolic spots eliminates bioactivation.

and carboxylic acid metabolites and no sulfydryl conjugates of zolpidem have been observed in humans (Durand et al. 1992). Furthermore, alpidem also exhibits potent inhibition of mitochondrial respiration and also depletes GSH in primary hepatocyte cultures, phenomena that are not observed with zolpidem even at high concentrations (Berson et al. 2001). Finally, as observed with clopidogrel and ticlopidine, the daily dose of zolpidem (5–10 mg QD) is significantly lower than that of alpidem (50–200 mg), a feature that may represent an additional and perhaps a more important mitigating factor.

The two catechol-*O*-methyltransferase inhibitors tolcapone and entacapone used for the treatment of Parkinson's disease also provide important illustrations of the effectiveness of this strategy. The use of tolcapone has been associated with a number of problems, including abnormalities in liver function tests and three cases of fatal hepatotoxicity. These problems have led to the drug being withdrawn from the market in some countries and the introduction of a black-box warning and intensive monitoring requirements in the United States. These ADRs, however, do not occur with the use of the structurally related drug entacapone despite administration at doses similar to tolcapone (200–1000 mg QD). Both tolcapone and entacapone are extensively metabolized in humans; a significant portion of tolcapone biotransformation proceeds via reduction of the nitrobenzene group to the aniline derivative, which is then transformed to the corresponding anilide by *N*-acetyltransferase (Jorga et al. 1999). Smith et al. (2003) have shown that both the aniline and the anilide metabolites of tolcapone undergo facile two-electron oxidation to the corresponding quinone-imine metabolites that are trapped with GSH (Figure 2.7). In contrast, no reduction of the nitrobenzene group in entacapone (see Figure 2.7) has been observed in humans and its principal clearance pathway involves N-deethylation of the tertiary amide substituent, isomerization of the active E-isomer to the inactive Z-isomer, followed by glucuronidation of the catechol motif (Wikberg et al. 1993).

A final example is provided with the two cysteinyl leukotriene antagonists CP-85958 and CP-199331 (see Figure 2.7). The clinical development of CP-85958 was discontinued due to unacceptable hepatotoxicity in monkeys (Chambers et al. 1999). Examination of monkey bile samples after dosing with CP-85958 revealed the presence of significant quantities of the corresponding lactol metabolite **6**, presumably generated from a P450-mediated hydroxylation α to the oxygen atom in the chromanol ring. Considering that the toxicity in the monkey may be mediated by the lactol derivative by ring opening to a potentially reactive hydroxyaldehyde intermediate **7**, which can bind to biomacromolecules, an obvious backup strategy was to eliminate this metabolic liability. Numerous structure–activity studies were conducted to prevent hydroxylation of the chromanol ring and efforts included blocking the site of hydroxylation or introducing substituents prone to metabolism at an alternate site in the molecule. Replacement of the benzoic acid portion in CP-85958 that was resistant to oxidative metabolism, with the more labile 4-methoxyphenyl-methanesulfonamide led to the discovery of CP-199331 that not only demonstrated enhanced efficacy against asthma in preclinical models, but also was devoid of hepatotoxic events in the monkey (Chambers et al. 1999). Metabolism studies in primate and human hepatocytes indicated that the principal route of metabolism of CP-199331 involved O-demethylation of the labile anisole group followed by glucuronidation of the corresponding phenol; no hydroxylation on the chromanol ring in CP-199331 was discernible in the primate and human (Kuperman et al. 2001).

2.4.4. Modulation of Biochemical Reactivity via Steric Hindrance

Strategies incorporating substituents either directly on the structural alert or in its immediate vicinity to provide steric hindrance and/or modulate its electronic properties to minimize bioactivation have also been implemented. The success of the former methodology toward the elimination of biochemical reactivity is illustrated with carboxylic acid analogs, which form reactive acyl glucuronides. Idiosyncratic ADRs associated with many carboxylic acid-containing drugs have been attributed to the covalent modification of essential proteins by the corresponding acyl glucuronide metabolites. The covalent binding may occur via two different pathways (Figure 2.8). The first is a transacylation mechanism, where a nucleophilic amino acid on a protein attacks the carbonyl group of the primary acyl glucuronide leading to the formation of an acylated protein and free glucuronic acid. The second is a mechanism of Schiff base formation where condensation occurs between the aldehyde group of a rearranged acyl glucuronide with a lysine residue or an amine group of the N-terminus, leading to the formation of a glycated protein. The formation of the

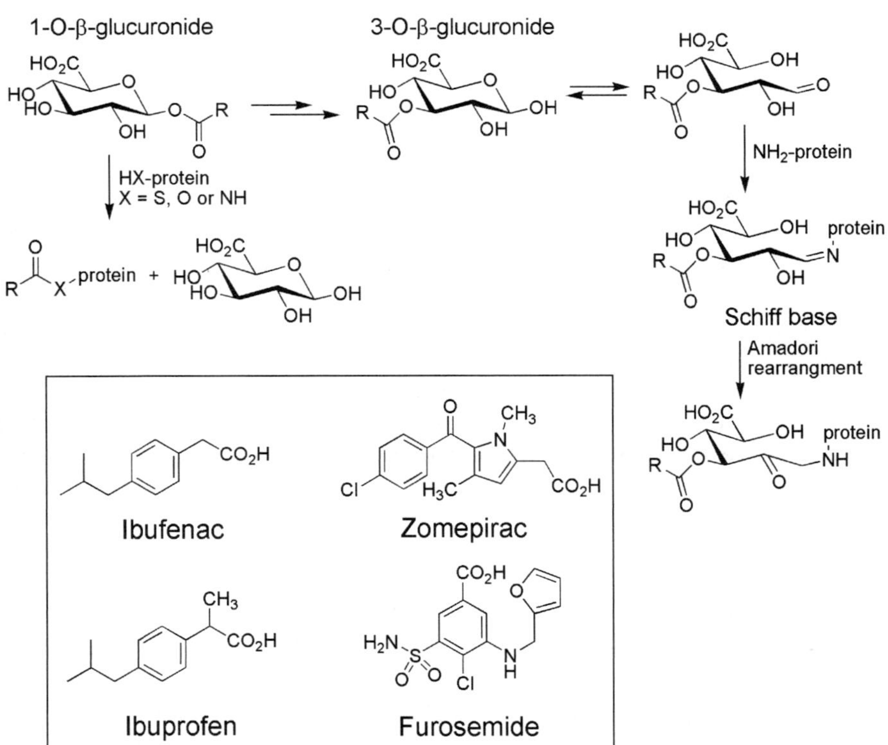

Figure 2.8 Strategies to diminish biochemical reactivity of electrophiles via introducing steric hindrance.

iminium species is reversible but may be followed by an Amadori rearrangement of the imino sugar to the more stable 1-amino-2-keto product (Ding et al. 1993). A structural relationship between acyl glucuronide degradation to the Schiff base and covalent binding has also been proposed (Benet et al. 1993). Acyl glucuronides of acetic acid derivatives such as the NSAIDs ibufenac, tolmetin, and zomepirac, all of which have been withdrawn due to toxicity, exhibit the highest level of rearrangement and covalent binding, whereas mono-α-substituted acetic acids (2-substituted propionic acids) such as ibuprofen, considered to be the safest nonsteroidal anti-inflammatory drug (NSAID) exhibit intermediate level of acyl glucuronide rearrangement and covalent binding (Bolze et al. 2002; Wang et al. 2004). In contrast, benzoic acid derivatives (e.g., furosemide) indicate the least amount of rearrangement and covalent binding. Overall, these observations imply that inherent electronic and steric properties must modulate the rate of acyl glucuronide rearrangement. For example, resonance stabilization of the carboxylic acid group by the aromatic ring in benzoic acids could be the reason for the lowest extent of acyl glucuronide rearrangement, whereas 2-substituted propionic acid derivatives could display a slower rearrangement rate than the corresponding acetic acid analogs due to the steric hindrance provided by the α-methyl substituent. In this aspect, it is noteworthy to point out that while ibuprofen is considered to be the safest NSAID in the market, its close-in analogue ibufenac was withdrawn due to severe hepatotoxicity. The only structural difference between the two drugs is the presence of the α-methyl substituent in ibuprofen, which presumably slows the rearrangement of the glucuronide (Castillo and Smith 1995).

2.4.5. Modulation of Biochemical Reactivity via Changes in the Electronic Properties

Bioactivation of the alkylhalide substituents in inhaled anesthetics to extremely reactive acylating agents is usually due to the availability of an extractable hydrogen atom on the halogenated alkyl carbon. In susceptible patients, halothane, isoflurane, and desflurane can produce severe hepatic injury by an immune response directed against reactive acyl halides covalently bound to hepatic proteins (Satoh et al. 1989). However, the relative incidence of hepatotoxicity due to these agents appears to directly correlate with the extent of their conversion to acyl halides by P450, which in turn may be governed by the leaving group ability of the respective substituents within these drugs. As is seen in Figure 2.9, halothane, which exhibits the greatest incidence of hepatotoxicity in the clinic, undergoes the most conversion to reactive acyl chloride, a feature that can be attributed to the presence of bromide substituent, which is a good leaving group. In contrast, isofluorane and desfluorane also undergo oxidative metabolism resulting in the formation of reactive acyl halides, but the degree to which these anesthetics are bioactivated is significantly lower than halothane (Njoko et al. 1997). Thus, the lower yield of acyl halide formation with isofluorane may be traced back to changes in the electronic environment that reduce overall affinity toward metabolism or to the relatively poor leaving group ability of the difluoromethoxy group compared to the bromide.

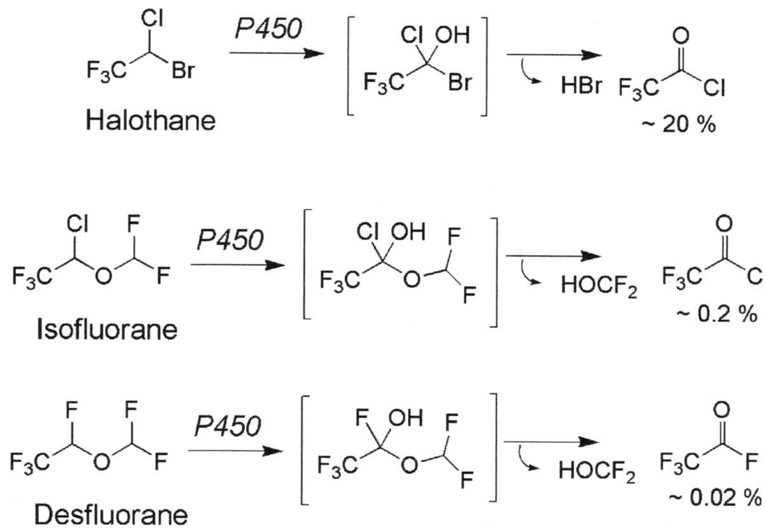

Figure 2.9 Strategies to diminish biochemical reactivity of electrophiles via modulation of electronic properties.

2.5. Factors That Mitigate IADR Risks Associated with Drug Candidates Containing Structural Alerts

There are several other variables that will impact whether the presence of a putative structural alert in a drug candidate will eventually manifest in unanticipated toxicity. First of all, the susceptibility of a functional group to metabolic activation needs to be clearly understood, since there are several examples of commercially successful drugs, which do not exhibit toxicity despite containing structural alerts (Figure 2.10). In many such cases, the structural alert is not involved in metabolism and the primary clearance mechanism normally proceeds via metabolism at an alternate site or by nonmetabolic processes. In other instances, bioactivation may be discernible in standard in vitro systems such as liver microsomes, but the principal clearance mechanism in vivo may involve an altogether different and perhaps more facile metabolic pathway yielding nonreactive metabolites. For example, the two phenolic groups in the selective estrogen receptor modulator raloxifene undergo P4503A4-catalyzed bioactivation in human liver microsomes generating electrophilic quinonoid intermediates (Chen et al. 2002); however, in vivo, glucuronidation of the same phenolic groups in the gut and liver constitutes the principal clearance pathway of raloxifene in humans (Figure 2.10; Kemp, Fan and Stevens 2002). Thus, the likelihood of raloxifene bioactivation in vivo may be in question when compared with the phase II conjugation process, a feature that may provide an explanation for the rare occurrence of ADRs, despite administration at moderately high daily doses of 60 mg QD. When encountered with the challenge of progressing a drug candidate associated with reactive metabolite formation, due consideration also must be given to the intended therapeutic area (e.g., a major unmet medical need or a

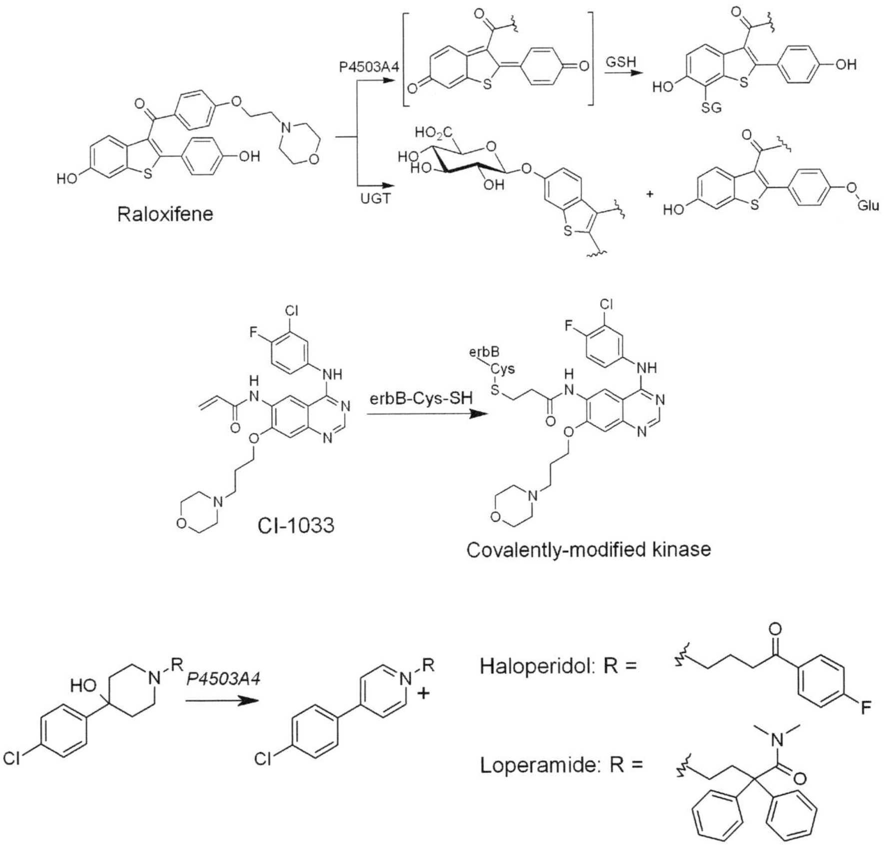

Figure 2.10 Balancing bioactivation with variables such as therapeutic benefits, regimen, and alternate clearance mechanisms.

life-threatening disease) and usage (acute versus chronic therapy). For example, CI-1033 is an intrinsically electrophilic compound but has shown significant promise in the treatment of breast and other cancers. CI-1033 irreversibly inhibits all four members of the erbB receptor tyrosine kinase family via a chemical reaction of its α,β-unsaturated acrylamide group with a cysteine residue (Figure 2.10) in the ATP-binding pocket in these enzymes (Allen et al. 2003).

Drugs used in a chronic setting appear to be more prone to ADRs than those used in an acute setting. Because toxicity is evident only after few weeks of administration, agents that are administered for 2 weeks or less are rarely associated with bioactivation-related toxicities. This is illustrated with the widely used antidiarrheal agent loperamide that is rarely associated with ADRs, especially, tardive dyskinesia and Parkinsonism, despite its structural similarity to haloperidol and despite its P4503A4-catalyzed metabolism to a potentially neurotoxic pyridinium intermediate (Figure 2.10; Kalgutkar and Nguyen 2004). Plausible reason(s) for the lack of neurotoxic complications associated with loperamide use relative to haloperidol include (1) opiate activity that is restricted to the gastrointestinal tract, (2) therapy that usually last for a few days versus haloperidol use in a chronic setting, and (3) the findings that loperamide and its positively charged pyridinium metabolite, but not haloperidol, are p-glycoprotein substrates and are denied access to the central nervous system (CNS), where they can potentially damage critical neurons.

Finally, the efficacious dose of the drug candidate may be pivotal as a factor mitigating the risk of toxicity. Type B ADRs are often referred to as dose-independent, but this certainly does not appear to be the case. For instance, the risk of hydralazine-induced lupus is dose-dependent, with a significant increase in frequency at doses >200 mg QD (Cameron and Ramsay 1984). Furthermore, there are no examples of drugs that are dosed below 10 mg day^{-1} that cause IADRs. There are many examples of two structurally related drugs that possess a common structural alert prone to bioactivation, but the one administered at the lower dose is much safer than the one given at a higher dose (Figure 2.11) (e.g., the alpidem/zolpidem and the ticlopidine/clopidogrel comparisons, previously mentioned). Olanzapine forms the same reactive iminium species that is presumably thought to be responsible for clozapine-induced agranulocytosis (Gardner et al. 1998), yet occurrence of agranulocytosis with olanzapine is extremely rare. A major difference between the two drugs is the dose; clozapine is administered at doses exceeding several 100 mg QD, whereas the recommended daily dose of olanzapine is 10 mg QD.

Additional examples of potential low therapeutic dose as a mitigating factor for ADRs are depicted with tadalafil, a PDE5 inhibitor for the treatment of erectile dysfunction, the antidepressant paroxetine, the hypnotic quazepam, the antihypertensive prazosin, and the estrogen ethinylestradiol. The benzodioxalane group in tadalafil is bioactivated by P450 to the corresponding reactive catechol metabolite, a process that also results in the mechanism-based inactivation of P4503A4 activity in vitro (Ring et al. 2005). However, there are no reports of ADRs (especially

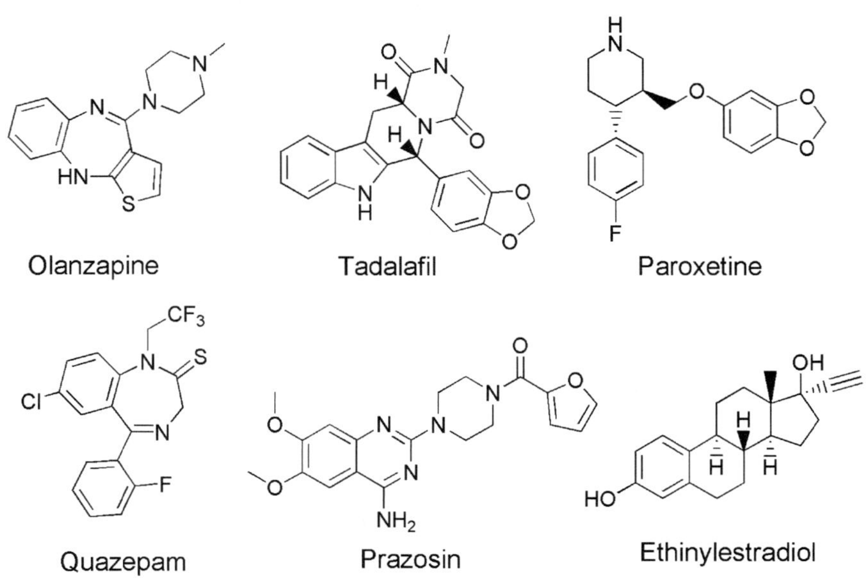

Figure 2.11 Examples of low-dose drugs devoid of IADRs despite forming reactive intermediates.

hepatotoxicity) associated with tadalafil use at the recommended dose of 10–20 mg QD and, furthermore, tadalafil also does not produce significant changes in the clearance of drugs metabolized by P4503A4 (Ring et al. 2005). In a similar fashion, paroxetine undergoes a P4502D6-catalyzed scission of its benzodioxalane group to the reactive catechol metabolite, which is known to partition between further oxidation to reactive *O*-quinone [Dr. Chandra Prakash, Pfizer Global Research & Development, unpublished observations] or undergo O-methylation catalyzed by catechol-*O*-methyltransferase (Haddock et al. 1989). Cleavage of the benzodioxalane group in paroxetine also results in the mechanism-based inactivation of P4502D6 (Bertelsen et al. 2003). Despite these liabilities, ADRs including hepatotoxicity associated with paroxetine use are extremely rare (Carvajal et al. 2002), a feature that may be linked to a moderately low dose of 20–50 mg day^{-1} and/or to the immediate detoxification of the catechol metabolite by O-methylation.

S-oxidation of the thioamide substituent in quazepam followed by hydrolysis of the potentially electrophilic S-oxide intermediate to the corresponding amide constitutes the rate-limiting step in the metabolism of the drug in humans (Kato et al. 2003), yet there are no reports of potentially life-threatening toxicity linked to the use of this agent, which is administered at a daily dose of 15 mg. Likewise, there are no adverse findings with the use of the antihypertensive agent prazosin at the recommended daily dose of 1 mg, despite the presence of the furan and the dimethoxybenzene rings in its structure (Jaillon 1980). Finally, ethinylestradiol, the major estrogenic component of many oral contraceptives, undergoes bioactivation at two different regions within its architecture (oxidation of the phenol and the acetylenic substituents to the corresponding catechol and ketene intermediates) that results in suicide inactivation of P4503A4 and a high degree of covalent binding to hepatic tissue (Lin, Kent and Hollenberg 2002), but does not elicit a toxicological response in the clinic. The extremely low oral dose of 0.035 mg must represent a significant mitigating factor.

2.6. Exploring Biochemical Mechanisms of Toxicity Other Than (or in Addition to) Bioactivation

There are cases where mechanisms other than (or in addition to) bioactivation can result in a toxicological outcome as was discussed earlier with the alpidem/zolpidem case. A second example is the bioactivation and formation of glutathione adducts for the nontricyclic antidepressant nefazodone. Severe hepatotoxicity resulting in death or the need for a liver transplant has been reported for nefazodone (Choi 2003) and the incidence (29 cases of hepatic injury per 100,000 patient years) far exceeds that associated with other antidepressants on the market (generally less than 4 cases of hepatic injury per 100 000 patient years). Recently, nefazodone was voluntarily withdrawn from the market. Following incubation of nefazodone with human liver microsomes and recombinant P4503A4 fortified with GSH, a GSH adduct associated with the 3-chlorophenyl piperazine moiety (Figure 2.12) was detected (Kalgutkar et al. 2005b). The authors suggested that formation of this GSH adduct was mediated via

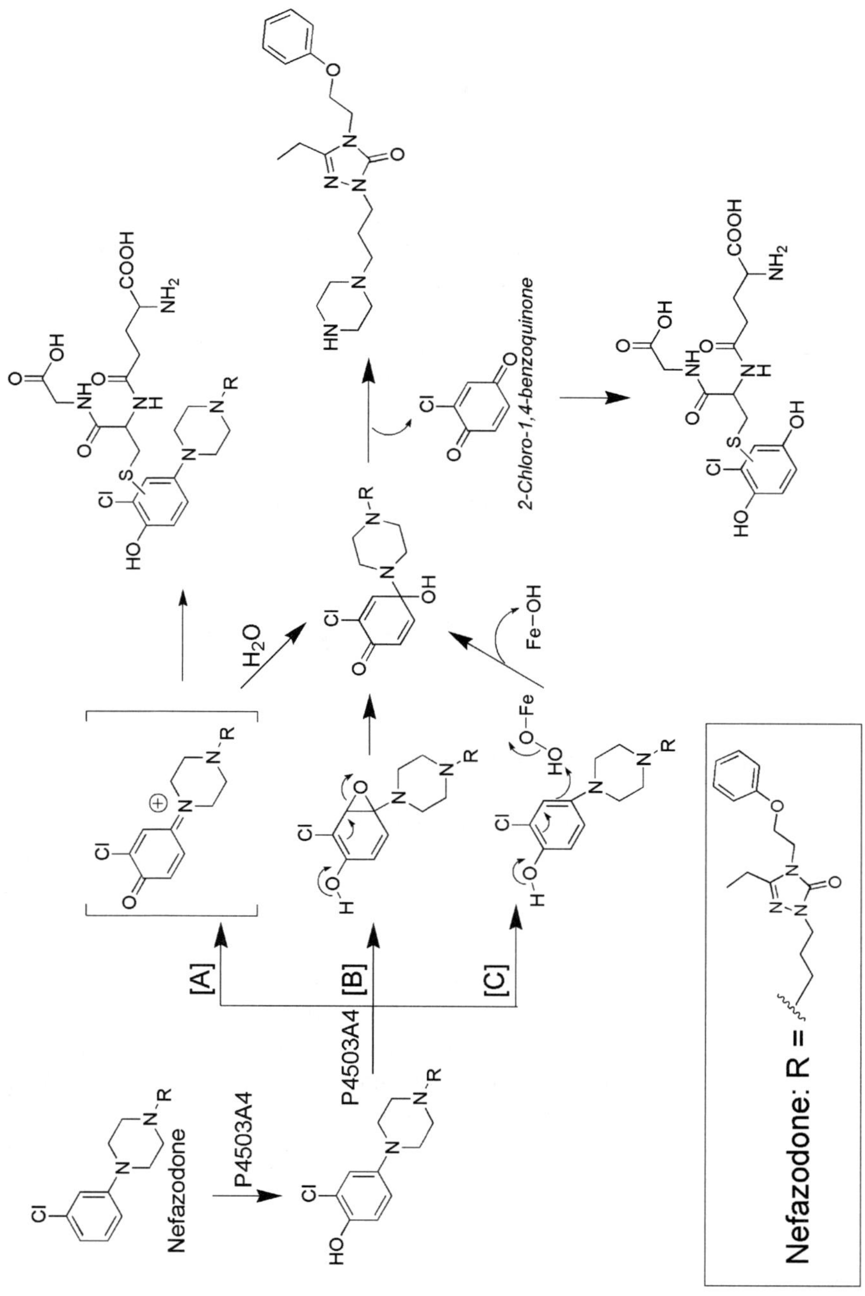

Figure 2.12 Bioactivation pathways of the nontricyclic antidepressant agent nefazodone.

para-hydroxylation of the chlorophenyl ring followed by two-electron oxidation to the reactive quinone-imine (Figure 2.12, pathway A). A novel N-dearylated metabolite was detected as well and it was speculated that its formation should be accompanied by release of 2-chloro-1,4-benzoquinone. Indirect evidence for release of 2-chloro-1,4-benzoquinone was obtained via trapping of this intermediate with GSH (Figure 2.12, pathways B and C) and detection of the adduct by LC-MS/MS. Although these data point to a potential liability for nefazodone, it must be emphasized that an unambiguous link between the formation of reactive metabolites and the observed hepatotoxicity has not been established. Moreover, recent evidence suggests that the parent compound itself is responsible for the clinical hepatotoxicity (Kostrubsky et al. 2006). In vitro and in vivo studies were performed, which indicate that nefazodone inhibits the human bile salt export pump (BSEP) in the liver. Interestingly, the structurally related drug and anxiolytic agent buspirone, which is not associated with overt hepatoxicity, does not form GSH adduct(s) (Kalgutkar et al. 2005b) and is not a BSEP inhibitor (Kostrubsky et al. 2006). In vivo rat studies showed an increase in serum bile acids following administration of nefazodone, but not for buspirone. In vitro hepatocyte studies in the presence of 1-aminobenzotriazole (ABT), a nonspecific mechanism-based inhibitor of P450 enzymes, increased the cytotoxicity. ABT inhibited the hydroxylation of nefazodone, which is the first step in formation of GSH adducts. These two observations together suggest that the metabolic bioactivation is not the mechanism responsible for nefazodone toxicity. This example highlights the difficulty associated with finding the root mechanistic cause for toxicity.

2.7. Concluding Remarks

There can be little debate on the value of predicting potential adverse events associated with drug candidates as early as possible in the overall discovery/development process, since safety-related issues continue to significantly contribute to overall attrition statistics in the pharmaceutical industry. In an increasing number of cases, a broader understanding of the molecular basis for idiosyncratic pathomechanisms has aided to replace a vague perception of a class effect with a sharper picture of an individual molecular peculiarity. A low-risk strategy in drug discovery could potentially preclude the use of structural alerts susceptible to bioactivation altogether, but this is likely to limit a detailed exploration of SAR around a chemical series of interest. Thus, a proactive approach between medicinal chemists, pharmacologists, and metabolism scientists in establishing detailed pharmacological SAR alongside screening for bioactivation potential is more appropriate and balanced especially in the lead optimization stage. If the chemical matter is susceptible to bioactivation, then efforts to minimize metabolic activation by iterative chemical interventions should be considered. If an alternate structural series that does not form reactive metabolites is available, then this series could be progressed as a suitable replacement for further optimization of pharmacology and/or absorption, distribution, metabolism, and excretion (ADME) properties. The potential for toxicity of a new drug candidate depends on a variety of factors including its overall disposition (extent of metabolism via bioactivation pathway relative to latent metabolic or nonmetabolic fate), daily dose (20 mg or less), therapeutic regimen (acute versus chronic), and the intended target population; factors that need to be taken into consideration when making a final decision to develop a drug candidate that is bioprocessed to reactive intermediates. Likewise, appropriate consideration needs to be given for drug candidates for potential treatment options for unmet and urgent medical needs. Despite decades of research in the arena of bioactivation and toxicity, accurate prediction of the toxicity potential of a drug candidate susceptible to bioactivation remains elusive. Future advances in the areas of immunology, genetics, and proteomics will hopefully provide a coherent relationship between covalent modification of biomacromolecules by reactive metabolites and a toxicity outcome. Toxicogenomics also represents a powerful new tool that may show gene and protein changes earlier and at treatment levels below the limits of detection of traditional measures of toxicity. Finally, considering that the meaning of the term "idiosyncrasy" literally translates to a characteristic belonging to, and distinguishing, an individual, the "one-size-fits-all" paradigm in drug discovery/development may need to be examined in greater detail.

References

Allen, L. F., Eiseman, I. A., Fry, D. W., and Lenehan, P. F. 2003. CI-1033, an irreversible pan-erbB receptor inhibitor and its potential application for the treatment of breast cancer. Semin. Oncol. 30:65–78.

Baillie, T. A., and Davis, M. R. 1993. Mass spectrometry in the analysis of glutathione conjugates. Biol. Mass Spectrom. 22:319–325.

Benet, L. Z., Spahn-Langguth, H., Iwakawa, S., Volland, C., Mizuma, T., Mayer, S., Mutschler, E., and Lin, E. T. 1993. Predictability of the covalent binding of acidic drugs in man. Life Sci. 53:141–146.

Berson, A., Descatoire, V., Sutton, A., Fau, D., Maulny, B., Vadrot, N., Feldmann, G., Berthon, B., Tordjmann, T., and Pessayre, D. 2001. Toxicity of alpidem, a peripheral benzodiazepine receptor ligand, but not zolpidem, in rat hepatocytes: role of mitochondrial permeability transition and metabolic activation. J. Pharmacol. Exp. Ther. 299:793–800.

Bertelsen, K. M., Venkatakrishnan, K., Von Moltke, L .L., Obach, R. S., and Greenblatt, D. J. 2003. Apparent mechanism-based inhibition of human CYP2D6 in vitro by paroxetine: comparison with fluoxetine and quinidine. Drug Metab. Dispos. 31:289–293.

Biour, M., Poupon, R., Grange, J. D., and Chazouilleres, O. 2000. Drug-induced hepatotoxicity. The 13th updated edition of the bibliographic database of drug-related liver injuries and responsible drugs. Gastroenterol. Clin. Biol. 24:1052–1091.

Bocker, R. H., and Guengerich, F. P. 1986. Oxidation of 4-aryl- and 4-alkyl-substituted 2,6-dimethyl-3,5-bis(alkoxycarbonyl)-1,4-dihydropyridines by human liver microsomes and immunochemical evidence for the involvement of a form of cytochrome P-450. J. Med. Chem. 29:1596–1603.

Bolze, S., Bromet, N., Gay-Feutry, C., Massiere, F., Boulieu, F., and Hulot, T. 2002. Development of an in vitro screening model for the biosynthesis of acyl glucuronide metabolites and the assessment of their reactivity toward human serum albumin. Drug Metab. Dispos. 30:404–413.

Cameron, H. A., and Ramsay, L. E. 1984. The lupus syndrome induced by hydralazine: a common complication with low dose treatment. Br. Med. J. 289:410–412.

Carvajal, G. P., Garcia, D., Sanchez, S. A., Velasco, M. A., Rueda, D., and Lucena, M. I. 2002. Hepatotoxicity associated with the new antidepressants. J. Clin. Psychiatry 63:135–137.

Castillo, M., and Smith, P. C. 1995. Disposition and reactivity of ibuprofen and ibufenac acyl glucuronides in vivo in the rhesus monkey and in vitro with human serum albumin. Drug Metab. Dispos. 23:566–572.

Chambers, R. J., Marfat, A., Antognoli, G. W., Cheng, J. B., Damon, D. B., Kuperman, A. V., Liston, T. C., Mebus, C., Pillar, J. S., Shirley, J. T., and Watson, J. W. 1999. Discovery of CP-199330 and CP-199331: two potent and orally efficacious cysteinyl LT1 receptor antagonists devoid of liver toxicity. Bioorg. Med. Chem. Lett. 9:2773–2778.

Chen, Q., Ngui, J. S., Doss, G. A., Wang, R. W., Cai, X., DiNinno, F. P., Blizzard, T. A., Stearns, R. A., Evans, D. C., Baillie, T. A., and Tang, W. 2002. Cytochrome P450 3A4-mediated bioactivation of raloxifene: irrever-sible enzyme inhibition and thiol adduct formation. Chem. Res. Toxicol. 15:907–914.

Choi, S. 2003. Nefazodone (Serzone) withdrawn because of hepatotoxicity. Can. Med. Assoc. J. 169:1187.

Cohen, S. D., Pumford, N. R., Khairallah, E. A., Boekelheide, K., Pohl, L. R., Amouzadeh, H. R., and Hinson, J. A. 1997. Selective protein covalent binding and target organ toxicity. Toxicol. Appl. Pharmacol. 143:1–12.

Dalvie, D. K., Kalgutkar, A. S., Khojasteh-Bakht, S. C., Obach, R. S., and O'Donnell, J. P. 2002. Biotransformation reactions of five-membered aromatic heterocyclic rings. Chem. Res. Toxicol. 15:269–299.

Ding, A., Ojingwa, J. C., McDonagh, A. F., Burlingame, A. L., and Benet, L. Z. 1993. Evidence for covalent binding of acyl glucuronides to serum albumin via an imine mechanism as revealed by tandem mass spectrometry. Proc. Natl. Acad. Sci. U.S.A. 90:3797–3801.

Durand, A., Thenot, J. P., Bianchetti, G., Morselli, P. L. 1992. Comparative pharmacokinetic profile of two imidazopyridine drugs: zolpidem and alpidem. Drug Metab. Rev. 24:239–266.

Evans, D. C., and Baillie, T. A. 2005. Minimizing the potential for metabolic activation as an integral part of drug design. Curr. Opin. Drug Discov. Dev. 8:44–50.

Evans, D. C., Watt, A. P., Nicoll-Griffith, D. A., and Baillie, T. A. 2004. Drug–protein adducts: an industry perspective on minimizing the potential for drug bioactivation in drug discovery and development. Chem. Res. Toxicol. 17:3–16.

Fieser, L. F. 1938. Carcinogenic activity, structure, and chemical reactivity of polynuclear aromatic hydrocarbons. Am. J. Cancer 34:37–124.

Gardner, I., Zahid, N., Maccrimmon, D., and Uetrecht, J. P. 1998. A comparison of the oxidation of clozapine and olanzapine to reactive metabolites and the toxicity of these metabolites to human leukocytes. Mol. Pharmacol. 53:991–998.

Gorrod, J. W., and Aislaitner, G. 1994. The metabolism of alicyclic amines to reactive iminium ion intermediates. Eur. J. Drug Metab. Pharmacokinet. 19:209–217.

Gorrod, J. W., Whittlesea, C. M., and Lam, S. P. 1991. Trapping of reactive intermediates by incorporation of 14C-sodium cyanide during microsomal oxidation. Adv. Exp. Med. Biol. 283:657–664.

Guengerich, F. P., Peterson, L. A., and Bocker, R. H. 1988. Cytochrome P-450-catalyzed hydroxylation and carboxylic acid ester cleavage of Hantzsch pyridine esters. J. Biol. Chem. 263:8176–8183.

Gunawan, B., and Kaplowitz, N. 2004. Clinical perspectives on xenobiotic-induced hepatotoxicity. Drug Metab. Rev. 36:301–312.

Haddock, R. E., Johnson, A. M., Langley, P. F., Nelson, D. R., Pope, J. A., Thomas, D. R., and Woods, F. R. 1989. Metabolic pathway of paroxetine in animals and man and the comparative pharmacological properties of its metabolites. Acta Psychiatr. Scand. Suppl. 350:24–26.

Hess, D. A., Sisson, M. E., Suria, H., Wijsman, J., Puvanesasingham, R., Madrenas, J., and Rieder, M. J. 1999. Cytotoxicity of sulfonamide reactive metabolites: apoptosis and selective toxicity of CD8(+) cells by the hydroxylamine of sulfamethoxazole. FASEB J. 13:1688–1698.

Hinson, J. A., Reid, A. B., McCullough, S. S., and James, L. P. 2004. Acetaminophen-induced hepatotoxicity: role of metabolic activation, reactive oxygen/nitrogen species, and mitochondrial permeability transition. Drug Metab. Rev. 36:805–822.

Jaillon, P. 1980. Clinical pharmacokinetics of prazosin. Clin. Pharmacokinet. 5:365–376.

Jorga, K., Fotteler, B., Heizmann, P., and Gasser, R. 1999. Metabolism and excretion of tolcapone, a novel inhibitor of catechol-*O*-methyltransferase. Br. J. Clin. Pharmacol. 48:513–520.

Kalgutkar, A. S., Gardner, I., Obach, R. S., Shaffer, C. L., Callegari, E., Henne, K. R., Mutlib, A. E., Dalvie, D. K., Lee, J. S., Nakai, Y., O'Donnell, J. P., Boer, J., and Harriman, S. P. 2005a. A comprehensive listing of bioactivation pathways of organic functional groups. Curr. Drug Metab. 6:121–225.

Kalgutkar, A. S., and Nguyen, H. T. 2004. Identification of an *N*-methyl-4-phenylpyridinium-like metabolite of the antidiarrheal agent loperamide in human liver microsomes: underlying reason(s) for the lack of neurotoxicity despite the bioactivation event. Drug Metab. Dispos. 32:943–952.

Kalgutkar, A. S., and Soglia, J. R. 2005. Minimizing the potential for metabolic activation in drug discovery. Exp. Opin. Drug Metab. Toxicol. 1:91–142.

Kalgutkar, A. S., Vaz, A. D., Lame, M. E., Henne, K. R., Soglia, J., Zhao, S. X., Abramov, Y. A., Lombardo, F., Collin, C., Hendsch, Z. S., and Hop, C. E. 2005b. Bioactivation of the nontricyclic antidepressant nefazodone to a reactive quinone-imine species in human liver microsomes and recombinant cytochrome P450 3A4. Drug Metab. Dispos. 33:243–253.

Kaplowitz, N. 2004. Drug-induced liver injury. Clin. Infect. Dis. 38:S44–S48.

Kato, K., Yasui-furukori, N., Fukasawa, T., Aoshima, T., Suzuki, A., Kanno, M., and Otani, K. 2003. Effects of itraconazole on the plasma kinetics of quazepam and its two active metabolites after a single oral dose of the drug. Ther. Drug Monit. 25:473–477.

Kemp, D. C., Fan, P. W., and Stevens, J. C. 2002. Characterization of raloxifene glucuronidation in vitro: contribution of intestinal metabolism to presystemic clearance. Drug Metab. Dispos. 30:694–700.

Kostrubsky, S. E., Strom, S. C., Kalgutkar, A. S., Kulkarni, S., Atherton, J., Mireles, R., Feng, B., Kubik, R., Hanson, J., Urda, E., and Mutlib, A. E. 2006. Inhibition of hepatobiliary transport as a predictive method for clinical hepatotoxicity of nefazodone. Toxicol. Sci. 90:451–459.

Kuperman, A. V., Kalgutkar, A. S., Marfat, A., Chambers, R. J., and Liston, T. E. 2001. Pharmacokinetics and metabolism of a cysteinyl leukotriene-1 receptor antagonist from the heterocyclic chromanol series in rats: in vitro–in vivo correlation, gender-related differences, isoform identification, and comparison with metabolism in human hepatic tissue. Drug Metab. Dispos. 29:1403–1409.

Lasser, K. E., Allen, P. D., Woolhandler, S. J., Himmelstein, D. U., Wolfe, S. M., and Bor, D. H. 2002. Timing of new black box warnings and withdrawals for prescription medications. J. Am. Med. Assoc. 287:2215–2220.

Lazarou, J., Pomeranz, B. H., and Corey, P. N. 1998. Incidence of adverse drug reactions in hospitalized patients: a meta-analysis of prospective studies. J. Am. Med. Assoc. 279:1200–1205.

Liegeois, J. F., Bruhwyler, J., Petit, C., Damas, J., DeLarge, J., Geczy, J., Kauffmann, J. M., Lamy, M., Meltzer, H., and Mouithys-Mickalad, A. 1999. Oxidation sensitivity may be a useful tool for the detection of the hematotoxic potential

of newly developed molecules: application to antipsychotic drugs. Arch. Biochem. Biophys. 370:126–137.
Liegeois, J. F., Rogister, F., DeLarge, J., Pincemail, J. 1995. Peroxidase-catalysed oxidation of different dibenzazepine derivatives. Arch. Pharm. (Weinheim) 328:109–112.
Lin, H. L., Kent, U. M., and Hollenberg, P. F. 2002. Mechanism-based inactivation of cytochrome P450 3A4 by 17 alpha-ethynylestradiol: evidence for heme destruction and covalent binding to protein. J. Pharmacol. Exp. Ther. 301:160–167.
Liu, Z. C., and Uetrecht, J. P. 2000. Metabolism of ticlopidine by activated neutrophils: implications for ticlopidine-induced agranulocytosis. Drug Metab. Dispos. 28:726–730.
Matzinger, P. 2002. The danger model: a renewed sense of self. Science 296:301–305.
Miller, E. C., and Miller, J. A. 1947. The presence and significance of bound aminoazo dyes in the livers of rats fed p-dimethylaminoazobenzene. Cancer Res. 7:468–480.
Murray, M. 1997. Drug-mediated inactivation of cytochrome P450. Clin. Exp. Pharmacol. Physiol. 24:465–470.
Naisbitt, D. J., Williams, D. P., O'Neill, P. M., Maggs, J. L., Willock, D. J., Pirmohamed, M., and Park, B. K. 1998. Metabolism-dependent neutrophil cytotoxicity of amodiaquine: a comparison with pyronaridine and related antimalarial drugs. Chem. Res. Toxicol. 11:1586–1595.
Njoko, D., Laster, M. J., Gong, D. H., Eger, E. I. II., Reed, G. F., and Martin, J. L. 1997. Biotransformation of halothane, enflurane, isoflurane, and desflurane to trifluoroacetylated liver proteins: association between protein acylation and hepatic injury. Anesth. Analg. 84:173–178.
Olson, H., Betton, G., Robinson, D., Thomas, K., Monro, A., Kolaja, G., Lilly, P., Sanders, J., Sipes, G., Bracken, W., Dorato, M., Van Deun, K., Smith, P., Berger, B., Heller, A. 2000. Concordance of the toxicity of pharmaceuticals in humans and in animals. Regul. Toxicol. Pharmacol. 32:56–67.
Park, B. K., Kitteringham, N. R., Maggs, J. L., Pirmohamed, M., and Williams, D. P. 2005. The role of metabolic activation in drug-induced hepatotoxicity. Annu. Rev. Pharmacol. Toxicol. 45:177–202.
Pereillo, J. M., Maftouh, M., Andrieu, A., Uzabiaga, M. F., Fedeli, O., Savi, P., Pascal, M., Herbert, J. M., Maffrand, J. P., and Picard, C. 2002. Structure and stereochemistry of the active metabolite of clopidogrel Drug Metab. Dispos. 30:1288–1295.
Pumford, N. R., and Halmes, N. C. 1997. Protein targets of xenobiotic reactive intermediates. Ann. Rev. Pharmacol. Toxicol. 37:91–117.
Reist, M., Roy-De Vos, M., Montseny, J. P., Mayer, J. P., Carrupt, P. A., Berger, Y., and Testa, B. 2000. Very slow chiral inversion of clopidogrel in rats: a pharmacokinetic and mechanistic investigation. Drug Metab. Dispos. 28:1405–1410.
Ring, B. J., Patterson, B. E., Mitchell, M. I., Vandenbranden, M., Gillespie, J., Bedding, A. W., Jewell, H., Payne, C. D., Forgue, S. T., Eckstein, J., Wrighton, S. A., and Phillips, D. L. 2005. Effect of tadalafil on cytochrome P450 3A4-mediated clearance: studies in vitro and in vivo. Clin. Pharmacol. Ther. 77:63–75.
Roth, R. A., Luyendyk, J. P., Maddox, J. F., and Ganey, P. E. 2003. Inflammation and drug idiosyncrasy – is there a connection? J. Pharmacol. Exp. Ther. 307:1–8.
Satoh, H., Martin, B. M., Schulick, A. H., Christ, D. D., Kenna, J. G., and Pohl, L. R. 1989. Human anti-endoplasmic reticulum antibodies in sera of patients with halothane-induced hepatitis are directed against a trifluoroacetylated carboxylesterase. Proc. Natl. Acad. Sci. U.S.A. 86:322–326.
Shenton, J. M., Chen, J., and Uetrecht, J. P. 2004. Animal models of idiosyncratic drug reactions. Chem. Biol. Interact. 150:53–73.

Smith, K. S., Smith, P. L., Heady, T. N., Trugman, J. M., Harman, W. D., and MacDonald, T. L. 2003. In vitro metabolism of tolcapone to reactive intermediates: relevance to tolcapone liver toxicity. Chem. Res. Toxicol. 16:123–128.

Soglia, J. R., Harriman, S. P., Zhao, S., Barberia, J., Cole, M. J., Boyd, J. G., and Contillo, L. G. 2004. The development of a higher throughput reactive intermediate screening assay incorporating micro-bore liquid chromatography-micro-electrospray ionization-tandem mass spectrometry and glutathione ethyl ester as a trapping agent. J. Pharm. Biomed. Anal. 36:105–116.

Tingle, M. D., Jewell, H., Maggs, J. L., O'Neill, P. M., and Park, B. K. 1995. The bioactivation of amodiaquine by human polymorphonuclear leucocytes in vitro: chemical mechanisms and the effects of fluorine substitution. Biochem. Pharmacol. 50:1113–1119.

Uetrecht, J. P. 1994. Metabolism of drugs by leukocytes. Drug Metabol. Drug Interact. 11:259–282.

Uetrecht, J. P. 1999. New concepts in immunology relevant to idiosyncratic drug reactions: the "danger hypothesis" and innate immune system. Chem. Res. Toxicol. 12:387–395.

Wang, J., Davis, M., Li, F., Azam, F., Scatina, J., and Talaat, R. 2004. A novel approach for predicting acyl glucuronide reactivity via Schiff base formation: development of rapidly formed peptide adducts for LC/MS/MS measurements. Chem. Res. Toxicol. 17:1206–1216.

Wikberg, T., Vuorela, A., Ottoila, P., and Taskinen, J. 1993. Identification of major metabolites of the catechol-*O*-methyltransferase inhibitor entacapone in rats and humans. Drug Metab. Dispos. 21:81–92.

Wu, Y. J., Davis, C. D., Dworetzky, S., Fitzpatrick, W. C., Harden, D., He, H., Knox, R. J., Newton, A. E., Philip, T., Polson, C., Sivarao, D. V., Sun, L. Q., Tertyshnikova, S., Weaver, D., Yeola, S., Zoeckler, M., and Sinz, M. W. 2003. Fluorine substitution can block CYP3A4 metabolism-dependent inhibition: identification of (S)-*N*-[1-(4-fluoro-3- morpholin-4-ylphenyl)ethyl]-3-(4-fluorophenyl)acrylamide as an orally bioavailable KCNQ2 opener devoid of CYP3A4 metabolism-dependent inhibition. J. Med. Chem. 46:3778–3781.

Zhang, K. E., Naue, J. A., Arison, B., and Vyas, K. P. 1996. Microsomal metabolism of the 5-lipoxygenase inhibitor L-739010: evidence for furan bioactivation. Chem. Res Toxicol. 9:547–554.

3

Michael Addition–Elimination Reactions: Roles in Toxicity and Potential New Therapeutic Applications

Adnan A. Elfarra and Renee J. Krause
Department of Comparative Biosciences, Division of Pharmaceutical Sciences, and Center for Molecular and Environmental Toxicology, University of Wisconsin, Madison, Wisconsin, USA
e-mail: elfarra@svm.vetmed.wisc.edu

Keywords: GSH Conjugation · GSH S-Transferases · FMOs, P450s · Cysteine S-Conjugates · Trichloroethylene · Tetrachloroethylene · Protein Adducts and Cross-Links · DCVC, DCVC Sulfoxide · TCVC · TCVC Sulfoxide · Thiopurines · Prodrugs · Cancer Chemotherapy

3.1. Introduction

Activated olefins of the type XCH = CHY, where Y is an electron-withdrawing group and X is a good leaving group, can undergo nucleophilic vinylic substitution reactions by a single-step or a multistep addition–elimination mechanism, depending on the chemical structure of the olefin and the reaction conditions. While nucleophilic vinylic substitution reactions have been extensively characterized and described in the chemical literature (Koch and Kielbania 1970; Kahn and Hehre 1986; Hackett et al. 1990; Rappoport 1992; Galli, Gentili and Rappoport 1994), only recently have these reactions been recognized to occur at physiological conditions and have been implicated in biological activity. The purpose of this chapter is to review recent experimental evidence that documents occurrence of Michael addition–elimination reactions in intact mammalian cells, both in vitro and in vivo. Evidence implicating these reactions in the mechanisms of nephrotoxicity and renal carcinogenicity of the halogenated hydrocarbons, trichloroethylene, and tetrachloroethylene will also be discussed. Finally, adaptation of Michael addition–elimination reactions to design new anticancer prodrugs that can undergo bioactivation by biological thiols, such as glutathione (GSH) and glutathione S-transferases (GST), to release the cytoxic drug 6-mercaptopurine (6-MP) or 6-thioguanine (6-TG) will also be described. Furthermore, data demonstrating the

A.A. Elfarra (ed.), *Advances in Bioactivation Research*, DOI: 10.1007/978-0-387-77300-1_3,

effectiveness of this prodrug approach in increasing the efficacy of 6-MP and 6-TG against tumor cells while decreasing the known side-effects of these drugs on the bone marrow and small intestine will be reviewed.

3.2. Formation of Michael Acceptors During Metabolism of Halogenated Hydrocarbons

The nephrotoxicity and renal carcinogencity of the halogenated hydrocarbons trichloroethylene and tetrachloroethylene have long been associated with the GSH-conjugation pathway and the formation of the corresponding cysteine S-conjugates, namely, *S*-(1,2-dichlorovinyl)-L-cysteine (DCVC) and *S*-(1,2,2-trichlorovinyl)-L-cysteine (TCVC), respectively (Figure 3.1). While DCVC and TCVC can undergo bioactivation by cysteine conjugate β-lyases (Elfarra and Anders 1984; Elfarra 2005; Anders 2007; also see Chapter 12 of this volume), oxidation of the sulfur moiety of DCVC by recombinant rabbit and human flavin-containing monooxygenase 3 (FMO3) to form the Michael acceptor, DCVC sulfoxide (DCVCS; Figure 3.1) has recently been demonstrated to represent an alternative bioactivation mechanism (Ripp et al. 1997; Krause, Lash and Elfarra 2003). Two high-performance liquid chromatography (HPLC) peaks, corresponding to the two DCVCS diastereomers were detected upon incubation of DCVC with rabbit liver microsomes in the presence of NADPH, with the late eluting peak (diastereomer II) constituting greater than 95% of the total DCVCS peak areas. Because the microsomal activity was inhibited by methimazole, a known FMO inhibitor, whereas inclusion of superoxide dismutase, catalase, 1-benzylimidazole, a cytochrome P450 inhibitor, or solubilization of the microsomes with emulgen 911 did not inhibit the S-oxidase activity, FMO3 was implicated as the primary catalyst of DCVC oxidation in rabbit liver microsomes (Ripp et al. 1997).

Oxidation of the sulfur moiety of TCVC by recombinant rabbit FMO3, rat and rabbit liver microsomes, and rat kidney microsomes to form the Michael acceptor TCVC sulfoxide (TCVCS) has also been demonstrated (Ripp et al. 1997; Elfarra and Krause 2007) with rat and rabbit liver

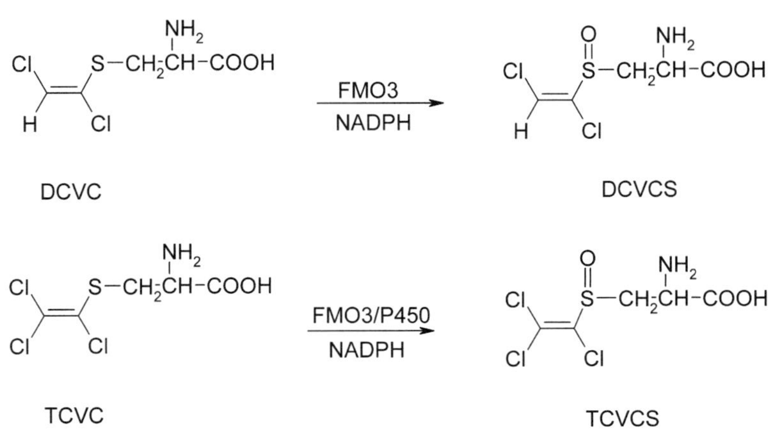

Figure 3.1 Metabolism of the cysteine S-conjugates, DCVC and TCVC, to their corresponding sulfoxides.

microsomes exhibiting a fivefold higher activity than rat kidney microsomes. In distinction from the DCVC S-oxidase activity which was mediated solely by FMO3, the TCVC S-oxidase activity was mediated by both FMOs and cytochrome P450s (Ripp et al. 1997; Elfarra and Krause 2007). Collectively, these results suggest that *S*-vinyl cysteine *S*-conjugates undergo enzymatic oxidation to yield reactive vinyl sulfoxides (Michael acceptors), and that depending upon the chemical structure of the substrate FMOs and/or P450s may be involved in these metabolic reactions.

3.3. Stabilities and Chemical Reactivities of DCVCS and TCVCS

Both DCVCS and TCVCS react readily with cellular thiols to yield multiple products (Sausen and Elfarra 1991; Ripp et al. 1997; Barshteyn and Elfarra 2007). The half-life of DCVCS when incubated with 3.3 equivalents of GSH in phosphate buffer at pH 7.4 and 37°C was only 1.2 min, whereas the half-life of TCVCS under similar incubation conditions was approximately 20 min (Figure 3.2). Both of the DCVCS diastereomeric peaks disappeared at the same time upon the addition of GSH indicating similar reactivities for the DCVCS diastereomers toward GSH. When *N*-acetyl-L-cysteine (NAC) was used as the nucleophile instead of GSH, the half-lives of the two DCVCS diastereomers were 13.8 and 9.4 min and these half-lives decreased upon increasing the incubation pH (Table 3.1), possibly due to a higher amount of the NAC sulfhydryl group being present in the deprotonated state, which is more favorable for nucleophilic attack.

One of the products formed from the reaction of DCVCS and GSH has been characterized as the GSH monoadduct, *S*-[1-chloro-2-(*S*-glutathionyl)vinyl]-L-sulfoxide (Figure 3.3), a product formed by the Michael addition of GSH to DCVCS followed by the loss of HCl (Sausen and Elfarra 1991). Interestingly, this GSH-DCVCS monoadduct was detectable within 1 h in the bile of rats given DCVCS (230 μmol kg^{-1}). Because

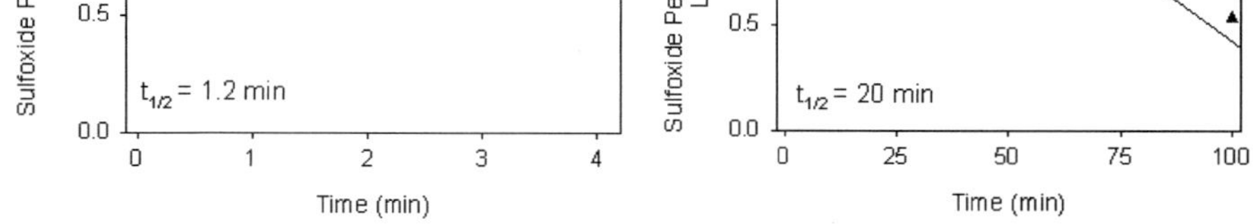

Figure 3.2 Stability of DCVCS (3 mM) and TCVCS (3 mM) in the presence of GSH (10 mM) at physiological conditions (phosphate buffer pH 7.4, 37°C). Data were taken from Ripp et al. (1997).

Table 3.1 Half-lives ($t\frac{1}{2}$) of DCVCS (3 mM) diastereomers when incubated at 37°C in the presence of *N*-acetyl-L-cysteine (10 mM) at various pHs.

pH	Diastereomer I $t\frac{1}{2}$ (min)	Diastereomer II $t\frac{1}{2}$ (min)
7.4	13.8	9.4
9.0	8.3	5.5

Data taken from Barshteyn and Elfarra (2007).

the DCVCS treatment also reduced hepatic and renal nonprotein thiol concentrations at 1 h to 74% and 27% of that in control rats, respectively, these results suggest formation of DCVCS–GSH adducts represents a major pathway for DCVCS metabolism in liver and kidney cells. Consistent with these results, treatment of human proximal tubular cells with DCVCS caused significant depletion of cellular GSH (Lash et al. 2003). Treatment of rats with TCVCS (230 μmol kg^{-1}) did not alter nonprotein thiol concentrations in the liver, but decreased nonprotein thiol concentrations in the kidney by nearly 50% compared with saline-treated rats (Elfarra and Krause 2007). The greater selectivity of TCVCS toward nonprotein thiols in the kidney in comparison with DCVCS could be explained by the slower reactivity of TCVCS, allowing more time for TCVCS to be actively transported and concentrated in kidney cells.

Three monoadducts [two diastereomers of *S*-[1-chloro-2-(*N*-acetyl-L-cystein-*S*-yl)vinyl]-L-cysteine (monoadducts I and II) and *S*-[2-chloro-2-(*N*-acetyl-L-cystein-*S*-yl]-cysteine sulfoxide (monoadduct III)] and one diadduct [*S*-[2,2-(*N*-acetyl-L-cystein-*S*-yl)vinyl]-L-cysteine sulfoxide (diadduct I)] (Figure 3.4) have recently been characterized from the reaction of DCVCS (3 mM) with NAC (10 mM) at physiological conditions (pH 7.4 and 37°C) (Barshteyn and Elfarra 2007). Monoadducts I and II were likely formed by Michael addition of NAC to the terminal vinylic carbon of the two DCVCS diastereomers followed by a *trans*-elimination of HCl (the highly acidic proton on the carbon adjacent to the sulfoxide moiety and the chlorine atom on the terminal carbon, Figure 3.4). While monoadduct III could be formed from the initial Michael addition product after a less favorable loss of HCl (the proton on the terminal carbon and the chlorine atom on the carbon adjacent to the sulfoxide moiety, Figure 3.4), stability studies with monoadduct II in the presence of NAC provided evidence for rearrangement of monoadduct II to monoadduct III through the formation of cyclic chloronium ion (Figure 3.5) as an alternative mechanism for the

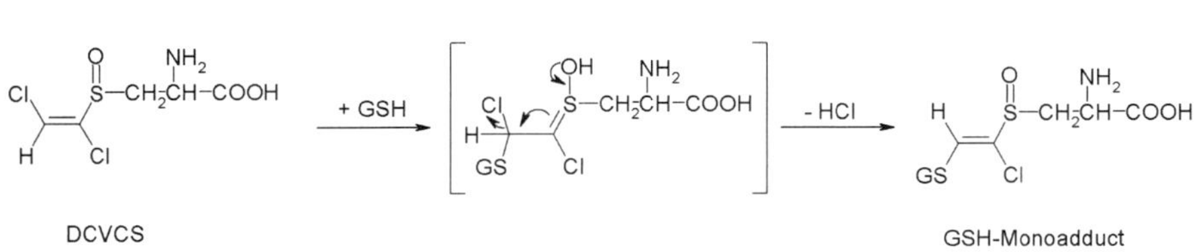

Figure 3.3 The reaction of DCVCS with GSH to form a GSH-monoadduct.

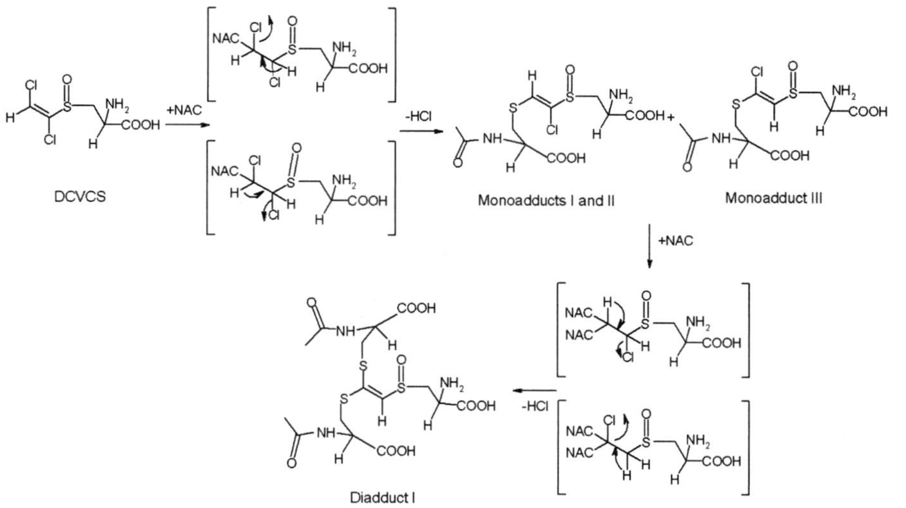

Figure 3.4 Proposed mechanism for the formation of monoadducts I, II, and III and diadduct I from the reaction of DCVCS with *N*-acetyl-L-cysteine (NAC).

formation of monoadduct III. Because incubations of monoadduct I, II, or III with NAC resulted in the formation of diadduct I, all three monoadducts are likely to contribute to the formation of diadduct I, as shown in Figure 3.4. The formation of all adducts was rapid and time-dependent (with relative ratios of 29%, 31%, 12%, and 24% for monoadducts I, II, and III, and diadduct I, respectively), providing strong evidence that DCVCS could modify protein thiols and act as a protein crosslinking agent. Recently, multiple DCVS-globin monoadducts and crosslinks

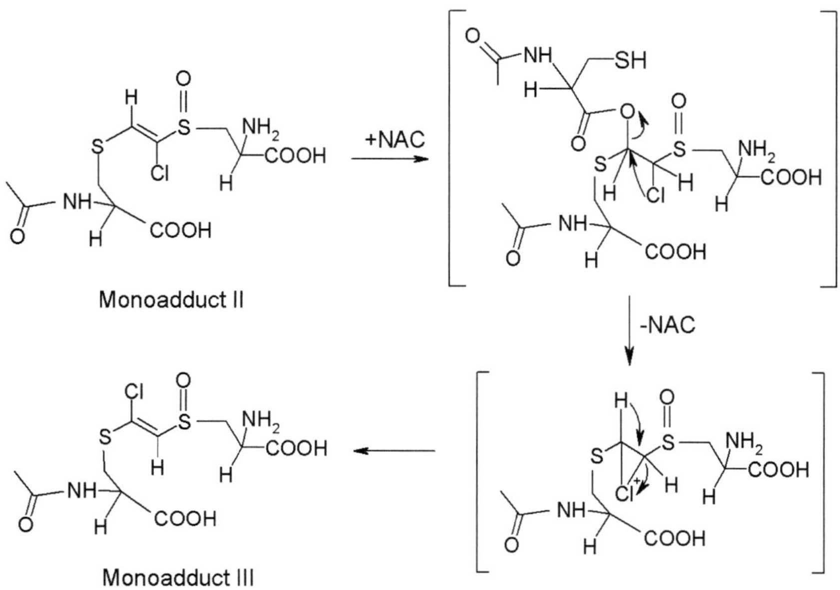

Figure 3.5 Proposed mechanism for the formation of monoadduct III from monoadduct II.

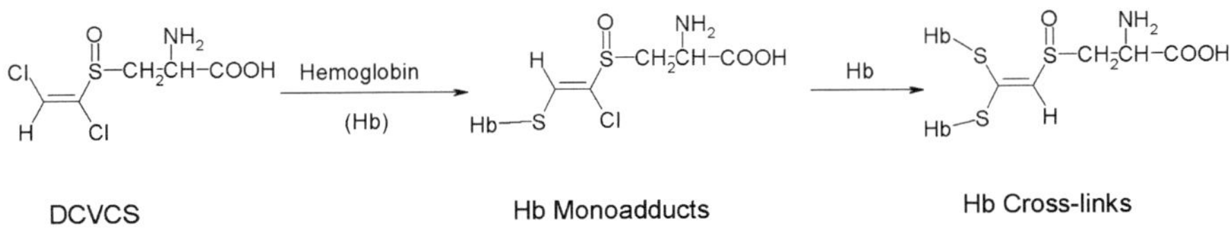

Figure 3.6 Reaction of DCVCS with hemoglobin to form monoadducts and cross-links.

(Figure 3.6) have been detected by sodium dodecyl sulfate polyacrylamide gel electrophoresis (SDS-PAGE) and mass spectrometry after both incubations of DCVCS (0.9–450 μM) with rat erythrocytes and subsequent to treatment of rats with DCVCS (Barshteyn and Elfarra 2008).

3.4. Nephrotoxicity of DCVCS and TCVCS

In vivo studies in rats have shown DCVCS and TCVCS to be much more potent nephrotoxicants than DCVC and TCVC, respectively (Lash et al. 1994; Elfarra and Krause 2007). A dose of 230 μmol kg^{-1} DCVCS caused anuria, severe proximal tubular necrosis, and a nearly eightfold increase in blood urea nitrogen (BUN), whereas an equimolar dose of DCVC failed to cause nephrotoxicity (Figure 3.7). Treatment of rats with TCVCS caused a

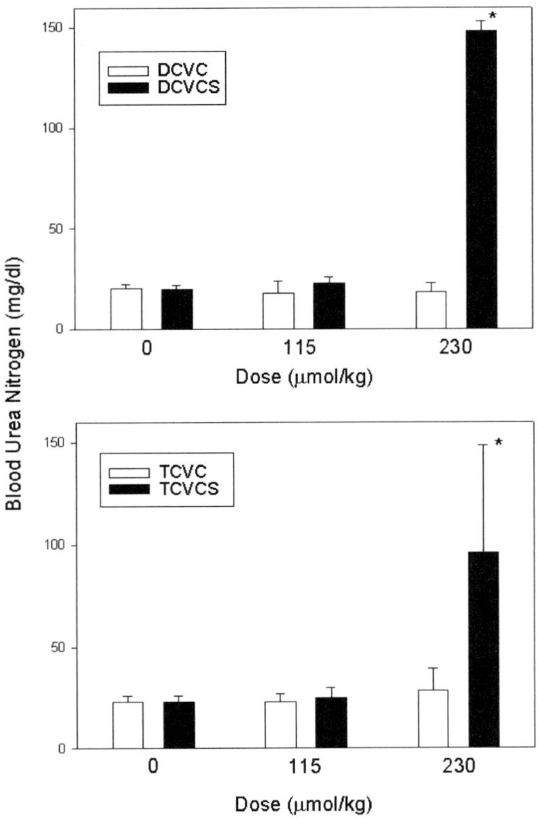

Figure 3.7 Blood urea nitrogen levels 24 h after male Sprague–Dawley rats were treated with DCVC, DCVCS, TCVC, and TCVCS.

nearly threefold increase in BUN (Figure 3.7) and severe tubular necrosis, whereas rats given the equimolar dose of TCVC failed to increase BUN and only exhibited mild-to-moderate acute tubular necrosis. Because pretreatment of rats with aminooxyacetic acid, a selective cysteine conjugate β-lyase inhibitor, enhanced TCVC toxicity, these results suggest TCVCS may play a prominent role in TCVC-induced nephrotoxicity. With DCVC, the aminooxyacetic acid pretreatment provided partial protection against DCVC-induced nephrotoxicity, suggesting a role for both cysteine conjugate β-lyase and FMO3 in the nephrotoxicity of DCVC. Because recombinant human FMO3 has recently been shown to convert DCVC to DCVCS (Krause, Lash and Elfarra 2003), and as little as 10 μM DCVCS has been shown to decrease the cellular ATP concentration by approximately 60% and induce apoptosis in primary cultures of human renal proximal tubular cells (Lash et al. 2003), DCVC and TCVC could be oxidized in human tissues to yield DCVCS and TCVCS, respectively, which could then contribute to DCVC and TCVC toxicity in human cells. As discussed above, the high reactivities and cross-linking abilities of DCVCS and TCVCS toward protein thiols are likely to play roles in their high nephrotoxic potency.

3.5. Addition–Elimination Reactions and the Bioactivation of Anticancer Thiopurine Prodrugs

In an effort to develop new thiopurine produgs, we characterized the metabolism of *cis*-3-(9*H*-purin-6-ylthio)acrylic acid (*cis*-PTA; Figure 3.8), *cis*-6-(2-acetylvinylthio)purine (*cis*-AVTP), and *trans*-6-(2-acetylvinyl)guanine (*trans*-AVTG), potential prodrugs of the chemotherapeutic drugs 6-MP and 6-TG targeting tumors with upregulated GSH levels (Gunnarsdottir and Elfarra 1999; Gunnarsdottir, Rucki and Elfarra 2002; Gunnarsdottir et al. 2002; Gunnarsdottir and Elfarra 2003). These prodrugs were envisioned to act as Michael acceptors and undergo GSH-mediated addition–elimination reactions (Figure 3.9) to yield 6-MP and 6-TG. In vitro results showed high reactivity of *cis*-AVTP and *trans*-AVTG toward

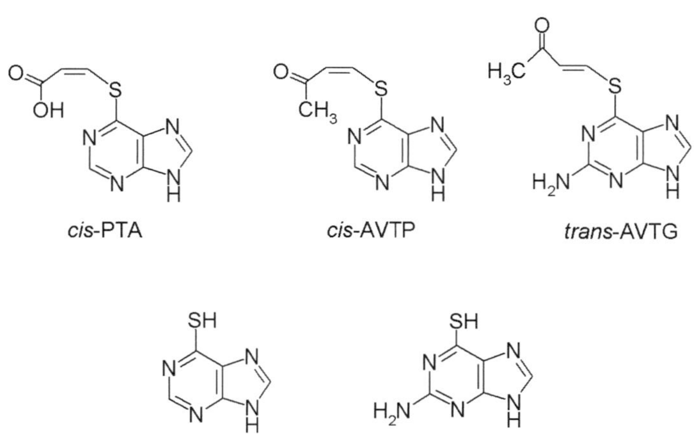

Figure 3.8 Structures of three potential Michael acceptors envisioned to be prodrugs of 6-MP or 6-TG.

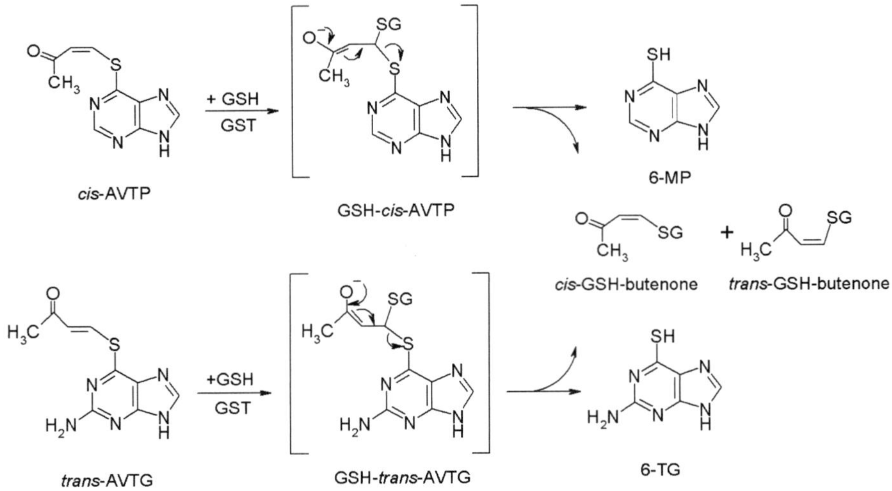

Figure 3.9 GSH-dependent metabolism of *cis*-AVTP and *trans*-AVTG to their corresponding thiopurines.

GSH and production of 6-MP and 6-TG at high rates, whereas the rates of conversion of *cis*-PTA to 6-MP was very slow possibly due to ionization of the carboxylic acid moiety of *cis*-PTA at physiological pH which decreased the reactivity toward GSH. The primary GSH conjugates, *cis*- and *trans*-4-glutathionylbuten-2-one, formed from the reaction of *cis*-AVTP or *trans*-AVTG with GSH, can react with a second molecule of GSH to form a di-GSH-conjugate, 4-(bis-glutathionyl)butan-2-one (Figure 3.10).

Cellular uptake and metabolism of *trans*-AVTG in the two human renal carcinoma cell lines A-498 and ACHN, which were initially used as models, were rapid and associated with depletion of intracellular GSH. Pretreatment of the cells with diethyl maleate decreased the formation of 6-TG from *trans*-AVTG consistent with the role of GSH in the generation of 6-TG (Gunnarsdottir, Rucki and Elfarra 2002). Interestingly, the prodrug delivered more 6-TG to the cells than did 6-TG itself. While both *cis*-AVTP and *trans*-AVTG can react nonenzymatically with GSH, the rates of these reactions can be enhanced significantly by glutathione transferases (Eklund et al. 2007). Among 13 examined human glutathione

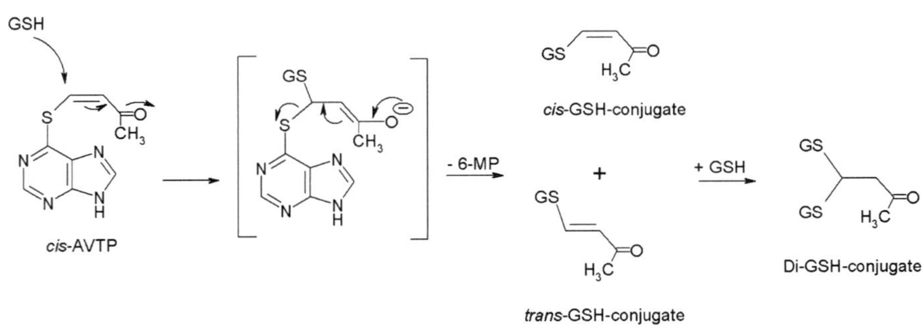

Figure 3.10 Proposed mechanism for the formation of the mono- and di-glutathionyl conjugates of butanone derived from *cis*-AVTP.

transferases, GST M1-1 and GST A4-4 were the most efficient catalysts with *trans*-AVTG, whereas GST M1-1 and GST M2-2 exhibited the highest activity with *cis*-AVTP. Thus, tumors expressing high levels of GST M1-1 or GST A4-4 may be particularly sensitive to chemotherapy with *cis*-AVTP or *trans*-AVTG.

Mice treated with the prodrugs excreted in urine a lower fraction of the administered dose as 6-MP or 6-TG and its further metabolites than did mice treated with equivalent 6-TG doses (Gunnarsdottir et al. 2002). No unchanged prodrug was detected in urine of mice given *cis*-AVTP or *trans*-AVTG. Interestingly, distinct patterns of tissue metabolites were observed after treatments of mice with *cis*-AVTP, *trans*-AVTG, and 6-TG, and a higher liver/plasma metabolite ratio was observed after *trans*-AVTG treatment than after *cis*-AVTP or 6-TG treatments, which exhibited similar liver/plasma ratios (Gunnarsdottir and Elfarra 2003). The distinct patterns of tissue metabolites observed after the different treatments suggest the prodrugs might exhibit tissue selectivity as chemotherapeutic agents, and may explain the decreased intestinal and bone marrow toxicity observed with the prodrugs in comparison with 6-TG (Gunnarsdottir, Rucki and Elfarra 2002; Gunnarsdottir et al. 2002).

3.6. *cis*-AVTP and *trans*-AVTG are More Cytotoxic in Tumor Cells Than 6-MP or 6-TG

The cytotoxicities of *cis*-AVTP and *trans*-AVTG were evaluated in the anticancer screening program of the National Cancer Institute using more than 50 cell lines derived from bone marrow, skin, central nervous system (CNS), lung, colon, ovary, breast, prostate, and kidney, and the results were compared with the cytotoxicities of 6-MP and 6-TG obtained in the same screen (Gunnarsdottir and Elfarra 2004). The results showed that the prodrugs had enhanced cytotoxicity compared with their parent thiopurines (Table 3.2), consistent with previous findings in the human renal cell carcinoma cell lines ACHN and A-498 (Gunnarsdottir, Rucki and Elfarra 2002). Interestingly, *cis*-AVTP was more effective against renal cancer cells

Table 3.2 The median TGI[a], GI_{50}, and LC_{50} values obtained for 6-TG, 6-MP, *cis*-AVTP, and *trans*-AVTG in the National Cancer Institute anticancer screen.

Cytotoxicity parameter	6-TG	6-MP	*cis*-AVTP	*trans*-AVTG
TGI	44.8[b]	>100	4.6	12.9
GI_{50}	1.1	4.0	0.6	1.0
LC_{50}	>100	>100	38.6	76.2

[a]TGI refers to the drug concentration required to inhibit tumor cell growth.
GI_{50} refers to the drug concentration that reduces tumor cell growth by 50% compared with untreated controls.
LC_{50} refers to the drug concentration required to decrease tumor cell numbers by 50% compared with untreated controls.
[b]All values are given in micromolar concentration (μM).
Data were taken from Gunnarsdottir and Elfarra (2004).

than *trans*-AVTG, whereas the latter was more effective against ovarian cancer cells, and both prodrugs exhibited high growth-inhibitory activities in leukemic cells and melanoma cells.

3.7. *cis*-AVTP and *trans*-AVTG Exhibited Reduced In Vivo Toxicity Than 6-TG

In vivo studies in mice have shown less bone marrow toxicity associated with the administration of *cis*-AVTP and *trans*-AVTG compared with 6-TG. The prodrugs caused no reduction of circulating white blood cells, whereas mice treated with equimolar or 60% lower doses of 6-TG demonstrated significant leucopenia (Gunnarsdottir, Rucki and Elfarra 2002). Mice given multiple doses of 6-TG and, to a lesser extent *trans*-AVTG but not *cis*-AVTP, exhibited increased myeloid:erythroid (M:E) ratios in bone marrow (Table 3.3; Gunnarsdottir et al. 2002). The increased M:E ratio likely results from severe erythroid hypoplasia rather than granulocytic hyperplasia in bone marrow because erythroid cells were virtually absent from bone marrow, and there was no evidence of tissue inflammation with sequestered leukocytes. Intestinal epithelial crypt cell apoptosis was also more extensive in mice given 6-TG than in those treated with *trans*-AVTG. Mice given *cis*-AVTP had little intestinal apoptosis. No liver or kidney lesions were detected after mice were treated with *cis*-AVTP or *trans*-AVTG, but mild increases in the activities of the hepatocellular leakage enzymes, alaninine aminotransferase and aspartate aminotransferase, were observed in mice treated with *trans*-AVTG. Furthermore, inflammation was not detected in any of the tissues examined. Collectively, these results suggest that the thiopurine prodrugs exhibit less in vivo toxicity than 6-TG and provide justification for future investigations into the efficacy of the prodrugs against tumors in vivo.

Table 3.3 Myeloid:erythroid (M:E) ratio in the bone marrow of CD-1 heterozygous nude male mice treated with vehicle alone (control), *cis*-AVTP, *trans*-AVTG, or 6-TG.

		M:E ratio (mean)[a]	
Prodrug	**Dose (μmol kg^{-1})**	**One cycle[b]**	**Two cycles**
Control		1.7:1	1.6:1
cis-AVTP	8.5	ND[c]	1.4:1
	21.25	1.8:1	1.8:1
trans-AVTG	8.5	ND	3.2:1
	21.25	6.6:1	5.7:1
6-TG	8.5	ND	11.8:1
	21.25	44.8:1	86.5:1

[a]All values are the means of results obtained with four animals.
[b]One cycle consisted of a once daily i.p. injection for 3 consecutive days whereas two cycles consisted of once daily i.p. injections for 3 consecutive days, repeated again 5 days later.
[c]ND – Not done.
Data were taken from Gunnarsdottir et al. (2002).

3.8. Conclusions

The preceeding discussion demonstrates that olefins of the general structure XCH = CHY, where X is a good leaving group (e.g., a halogen or a thiopurine moiety) and Y is an electron-withdrawing group (e.g. a sulfoxide or a ketone moiety), can undergo thiol-mediated addition–elimination reactions in mammalian cells and may result in the formation of protein crosslinks. While the thiol-mediated addition–elimination reactions of DCVCS and TCVCS were associated with severe renal toxicity, the reactions of *cis*-AVTP and *trans*-AVTG with thiols were associated with enhanced cytotoxicities in tumor cell lines and caused less systemic toxicity than 6-TG in mice in vivo. Based on these results, similar addition–elimination reactions may play a role in the toxicity of other cysteine S-conjugates of halogenated olefins after metabolism to their corresponding sulfoxides. Other activated olefins, where X is a drug moiety that, similar to the thiopurines, can act as a leaving group may also be synthesized for evaluation as prodrugs. In this regard, it should be recognized that the rates of the addition–elimination reactions are likely to vary depending on the exact chemical structure of the activated olefin, as demonstrated above among DCVCS and TCVCS or among *cis*-PTA and *cis*-AVTP, and these rates are likely to be important determinants of biological activity.

Acknowledgements. Research conducted in our laboratory was made possible primarily by Grant DK 44295 from the National Institute of Diabetes and Digestive and Kidney Diseases.

References

Anders, M. W. 2007. Chemical toxicology of reactive intermediates formed by the glutathione-dependent bioactivation of halogen-containing compounds. Chem. Res. Toxicol. 21:145–159.

Barshteyn, N., and Elfarra, A. A. 2007. Formation of three *N*-acteyl-L-cysteine monoadducts and one diadduct by the reaction of *S*-(1,2-dichlorovinyl)-L-cysteine sulfoxide with *N*-acetyl- L-cysteine at physiological conditions: chemical mechanisms and toxicological implications. Chem. Res. Toxicol. 20:1563–1569.

Barshteyn, N., and Elfarra, A. A. 2008. Detection of multiple globin mono-adducts and cross-links after exposure of rat erythrocytes to *S*-(1,2-dichlorovinyl)-L-cysteine sulfoxide both in vitro and in vivo. Toxicol. Sci. 102:77.

Eklund, B. I., Gunnarsdottir, S., Elfarra, A. A., and Mannervik, B. 2007. Human glutathione transferases catalyzing the bioactivation of anticancer thiopurine prodrugs. Biochem. Pharmacol. 73:1829–1841.

Elfarra, A. A. 2005. Renal cytochrome P450s and flavin-containing monooxygenases: potential roles in metabolism and toxicity of 1,3-butadiene, trichloroethylene, and tetrachloroethylene. In Methods in Pharmacology and Toxicology, Drug Metabolism and Transport: Molecular Methods and Mechanisms. Lash, L., ed., pp.1–18. Totowa: Humana Press Inc.

Elfarra, A. A., and Anders, M. W. 1984. Renal processing of glutathione conjugates: role in nephrotoxicity. Biochem. Pharmacol. 33:3729–3732.

Elfarra, A. A., and Krause, R. J. 2007. *S*-(1,2,2-trichlorovinyl)-L-cysteine sulfoxide, a reactive metabolite of *S*-(1,2,2-trichlorovinyl)-L-cysteine formed in rat liver and kidney microsomes, is a potent nephrotoxicant. J. Pharmacol. Exp. Ther. 321:1–7.

Galli, C., Gentili, P., and Rappoport, Z. 1994. Competition of mechanisms in nucleophilic substitution of vinyl halides. An unequivocal example of the vinylic $S_{RN}1$ route. J. Org. Chem. 59:6786–6795.

Gunnarsdottir, S., and Elfarra, A. A. 1999. Glutathionine-dependent metabolism of cis-(9H-purin-6-ylthio) acrylic acid to yield the chemotherapeutic drug 6-mercaptopurine: evidence for two distinct mechanisms in rats. J. Pharmacol. Exp. Ther. 290: 950–957.

Gunnarsdottir, S., and Elfarra, A. A. 2003. Distinct tissue distribution of metabolites of the novel glutathione-activated thiopurine prodrugs *cis*-6-(2-acetylvinylthio)purine and *trans*-6-(2-acetylvinylthio)guanine and 6-thioguanine in the mouse. Drug Metab. Dispos. 31:718–726.

Gunnarsdottir, S., and Elfarra, A. A. 2004. Cytotoxicity of the novel glutathione-activated thiopurine prodrugs *cis*-AVTP [*cis*-6-(2-acetylvinylthio)-purine] and *trans*-AVTG [*trans*-6-(2-acetylvinylthio)guanine]: results from the National Cancer Institute's anticancer drug screen. Drug Metab. Dispos. 32:321–327.

Gunnarsdottir, S., Rucki, M., and Elfarra, A. A. 2002. Novel glutathione-dependent thiopurine prodrugs: evidence for enhanced cytotoxicity in tumor cells and for decreased bone marrow toxicity in mice. J. Pharmacol. Exp. Ther. 301:77–86.

Gunnarsdottir, S., Rucki, M., Phillips, L. A., Young, K. M., and Elfarra, A. A. 2002. The glutathione-activated thiopurine prodrugs *trans*-6-(2-acetylvinylthio)guanine and *cis*-6-(2-acetylvinylthio)purine cause less in vivo toxicity than 6-thioguanine after single- and multiple-dose regimens. Mol. Cancer Ther. 1:1211–1220.

Hackett, A. G., Kotyk, J. J., Fujiwara, H., and Logusch, E. W. 1990. Identification of a unique glutathione conjugate of trichloroacrolein using heteronuclear multiple quantum coherence ^{13}C nuclear magnetic resonance spectroscopy. J. Am. Chem. Soc. 112:3669–3671.

Kahn, S. D., and Hehre, W. J. 1986. Modeling chemical reactivity. 3. Stereochemistry of Michael additions of vinyl sulfoxides. J. Am. Chem. Soc. 108:7399–7400.

Koch, H. F., and Kielbania, A. J. 1970. Nucleophilic reactions of fluoroolefins. Evidence for a carbanion intermediate in vinyl and allyl displacement reactions. J. Am. Chem. Soc. 92:729–730.

Krause, R. J., Lash, L. H., and Elfarra, A. A. 2003. Human kidney flavin-containing monooxygenases and their potential roles in cysteine S-conjugate metabolism and nephrotoxicity. J. Pharmacol. Exp. Ther. 304:185–191.

Lash, L. H., Putt, D. A., Hueni, S. E., Krause, R. J., and Elfarra, A. A. 2003. Roles of necrosis, apoptosis, and mitochondrial dysfunction in *S*-(1,2-dichlorovinyl)-L-cysteine sulfoxide-induced cytotoxicity in primary cultures of human renal proximal tubular cells. J. Pharmacol. Exp. Ther. 305:1163–1172.

Lash, L. H., Sausen, P. J., Duescher, R. J., Cooley, A. J., and Elfarra, A. A. 1994. Roles of cysteine conjugate β-lyase and *S*-oxidase in nephrotoxicity: studies with *S*-(1,2-dichlorovinyl)-L-cysteine and *S*-(1,2-dichlorovinyl)-L-cysteine sulfoxide. J. Pharmacol. Exp. Ther. 269:374–383.

Rappoport, Z. 1992. The rapid steps in nucleophilic vinylic "addition–elimination" substitution. Recent developments. Acc. Chem. Res. 25:474–479.

Ripp, S. L., Overby, L. H., Philpot, R. M., and Elfarra, A. A. 1997. Oxidation of cysteine S-conjugates by rabbit liver microsomes and cDNA-expressed flavin-containing monooxygenases: studies with *S*-(1,2-dichlorovinyl)-L-cysteine, *S*-(1,2,2-trichlorovinyl)-L-cysteine, *S*-allyl-L-cysteine, and *S*-benzyl-L-cysteine. Mol. Pharmacol. 51:507–515.

Sausen, P. J., and Elfarra, A. A. 1991. Reactivity of cysteine S-conjugate sulfoxides: formation of *S*-[1-chloro-2-(*S*-glutathionyl)vinyl]-L-cysteine sulfoxide by the reaction of *S*-(1,2-dichlorovinyl)-L-cysteine sulfoxide with glutathione. Chem. Res. Toxicol. 4:655–660.

4

Induction of Drug-Metabolizing Enzymes: Contrasting Roles in Detoxification and Bioactivation of Drugs and Xenobiotics

Sharon L. Ripp

Department of Pharmacokinetics, Dynamics and Metabolism, Pfizer Global Research & Development, Groton, CT 06340, USA

e-mail: sharon.l.ripp@pfizer.com

Keywords: PXR · CAR · AhR · FXR · CYPs · Phase I Metabolism · Phase II Metabolism

4.1. Introduction

Enzyme induction, in the context of this chapter, is a process by which expression of certain drug-metabolizing enzymes and/or transporters is increased by drug or xenobiotic exposure. In recent years, there have been marked advances in the understanding of mechanisms of enzyme induction and more facile means of measuring gene expression changes. These advances have led to increased awareness of the ability of drugs and xenobiotics to cause enzyme induction, with increasing need to identify and manage risks associated with this process. Enzyme induction is generally considered a means to detoxify xenobiotics by increasing their clearance. When considering medicines, enzyme induction can result in drug–drug interactions and/or loss of efficacy by causing decreased exposure to coadministered medications. However, there is also a concern that enzyme induction can be more than a detoxification route or drug–drug interaction problem, in that it could lead to increased generation of toxic and/or reactive metabolites and increased toxicity. The purpose of this chapter is to examine enzyme induction and consider the evidence for its role in detoxification versus bioactivation of drugs and xenobiotics. A brief introduction to enzyme induction and mechanisms is included.

A.A. Elfarra (ed.), *Advances in Bioactivation Research*, DOI: 10.1007/978-0-387-77300-1_4,

4.2. Enzyme Induction

The primary mechanism by which drugs or xenobiotics can cause enzyme induction is by way of activation of gene transcription. Most commonly, a drug or xenobiotic is considered an inducer if it activates a nuclear receptor, thereby causing increased expression of that receptor's target genes. The nuclear receptors that have the broadest ligand selectivity and are most commonly involved in activation of transcription of drug-metabolizing enzymes and transporters are the aryl hydrocarbon receptor (AhR), pregnane X receptor (PXR), and constitutive androstane receptor (CAR). There are additional nuclear receptors that are activated by a narrower range of compounds, and are involved in activation of transcription of a more limited set of target genes; these are farnesyl X receptor (FXR), liver X receptor (LXR), and peroxisome proliferator-activated receptors (PPARs). Additional mechanisms of enzyme induction that are relevant to drug-metabolizing enzymes and transporters are the activation of the Nrf2 transcription factor by redox active agents and the induction of cytochrome P450 2E1 by substrate stabilization of the protein. The target genes for these various receptors that are of interest to the study of drug metabolism include various phase I metabolizing enzymes (e.g., cytochrome P450 s (CYPs)) as well as phase II conjugating enzymes (e.g., glutathione S-transferases (GSTs), uridine diphosphate glucuronosyl transferases (UGTs), and sulfotransferases (SULTs)). Target genes can also include numerous uptake or efflux transporters, for example, organic anion transporting peptide (OATP) and multidrug resistance proteins (MDR1, MRP2). Each of the receptor pathways involved in the different enzyme induction processes will be reviewed in more detail below, and are summarized in Table 4.1.

Table 4.1 Pathways for induction of human drug-metabolizing enzymes and transporters.

Induction pathway	Activators/ligand examples	Target gene examples
AhR	TCDD, benzo[a]pyrene, 3-methylcholanthrene, indole[3,2-b]carbazole, other polychlorinated biphenyls and polycyclic aromatic hydrocarbons	ALDH3A1, CYP1A1, CYP1A2, CYP1B1, CYP2S1, GSTA1, NQO1, UGT1A6
PXR	Rifampicin, phenobarbital, hyperforin, phenytoin, carbamazepine, nifedipine, clotrimazole, lovastatin	ALAS, ALDH1A4, CYP2A6, CYP2B6, CYP2C8, CYP2C9, CYP3A4, GSTA2, MDR1, MRP2, MRP3, OATP2, UGT1A1, UGT1A6
CAR	Phenobarbital, CITCO	ALAS, ALDH1A4, CYP2A6, CYP2B6, CYP2C8, CYP2C9, CYP3A4, GSTA2, SULT1A1, UGT1A1, UGT1A6
Nrf2	tBHQ, sulforaphane, oltipraz	GCS, GSTs, HO-1, NQO1
Protein and/or mRNA stabilization	Ethanol, acetone, ketone bodies	CYP2E1

4.3. Overview of Enzyme Induction Pathways

4.3.1. Aryl Hydrocarbon Receptor (Aromatic Hydrocarbon/CYP1 Inducers)

The induction of CYP1 enzymes through AhR activation has been arguably the most actively studied pathway in the enzyme induction research field. The study of aryl hydrocarbon/CYP1A pathway has progressed from the initial identification of the association of the AhR locus with aryl hydrocarbon hydroxylase activity, to the purification and identification of the AhR, to the development of AhR knockout mice and realization of this receptor's roles in a myriad of physiological responses (Nebert and Gelboin 1968; Niwa et al. 1975; Poland, Glover and Kende et al. 1976; Fernandez-Salguero et al. 1995). Despite the fact that this has been an active area of research for nearly 40 years, new functions and roles for the AhR are still being uncovered. The AhR is known to be involved not only in induction of xenobiotic-metabolizing enzymes, but also in cell cycle regulation (both apoptosis and proliferation), and plays a role in numerous physiological pathways, including liver and immune system development and vascular remodeling (Marlowe and Puga 2005; Rifkind 2006).

The AhR is a ligand-activated transcription factor of the basic helix-loop-helix/Per-Arnt-Sim (bHLH-PAS) family. The understanding of the mechanism of activation of the AhR continues to evolve; a current model for the mechanism of ligand activation of AhR is summarized as follows (Figure 4.1; reviewed in Riddick et al. 2003). In the unliganded, inactive

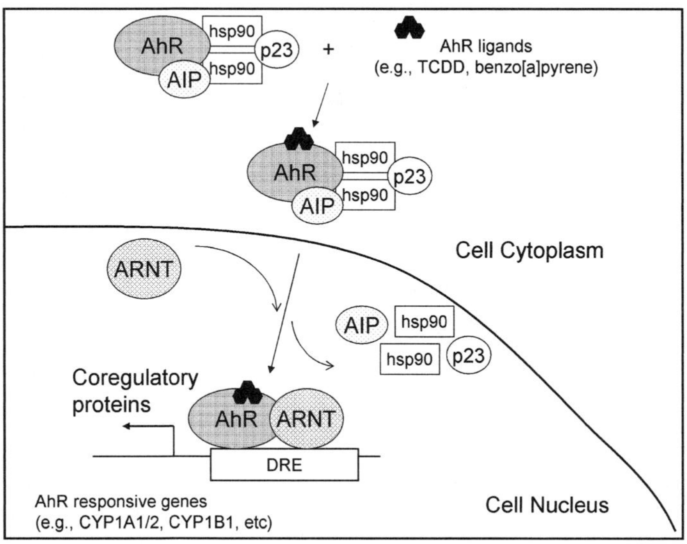

Figure 4.1 Regulation of gene transcription by AhR. In the absence of activating ligand, AhR is retained in the cytoplasm in a complex with various heat shock proteins/chaperones. Upon ligand binding and activation, the AhR translocates to the nucleus where it forms a heterodimer with ARNT. The AhR/ARNT heterodimer binds to specific DNA sequences in the 5′-regulatory region of responsive genes, and interacts with general transcription factors and coregulatory proteins, resulting in the modulation of gene transcription.

state, AhR resides in the cytoplasm, in complex with a dimer of heat shock protein 90, the cochaperone p23, and an immunophilin-related protein called AhR-interacting protein (AIP, a.k.a. ARA9 or XAP2). Upon ligand activation, AhR dissociates from this complex and translocates to the nucleus where it forms a heterodimer with AhR nuclear translocator (ARNT). The AhR/ARNT heterodimers bind to DNA sequences in the 5′-regulatory regions of target genes, and interact with various coactivator, corepressor, and/or general trancription factor proteins to positively or negatively regulate gene transcription (Hankinson 2005). The DNA sequences that bind AhR/ARNT are known as dioxin-responsive elements (DREs), or alternatively as xenobiotic-responsive elements (XREs). Target genes include numerous drug- and xenobiotic-metabolizing enzymes (Table4.1), the most intensively studied of which are members of the CYP1 family. In fact, one of the originally identified bioactivation pathways, metabolism of benzo[a]pyrene to the carcinogenic diol epoxide, is mediated by CYP1A isozymes, and inducible by AhR ligands. Ligand activators of AhR include planar aromatic compounds such as 2,3,7,8-tetrachlorodibenzo-*p*-dioxin (TCDD), polychlorinated biphenyls (PCBs), benzo[a]pyrene, 3-methylcholanthrene, as well as dietary chemicals such as tryptophan and indole derivatives (e.g., indole[2,3-b]carbazole; Denison and Nagy 2003). In addition, the dietary component common in red wine, resveratrol, has been shown to be an antagonist of the AhR (Ciolino, Daschner and Yeh 1998). There is also evidence for endogenous compounds activating the AhR; for example, it was recently reported that AhR in endothelial cells can be activated by modified low-density lipoprotein (LDL), providing a potential explanation for the vascular defects in AhR-null mice (McMillan and Bradfield 2007).

Since AhR is involved in so many cellular processes, it is reasonable to think that ligand activators of AhR could have profound effects on an organism. Indeed, TCDD, a very potent AhR ligand, produces a plethora of biological effects including chloracne, tumor promotion, and thymic atrophy (Nebert 1989). TCDD is also somewhat unusual as a member of the class of AhR activators in that it is not a substrate for the drug-metabolizing enzymes induced by AhR. However, with other AhR ligands, some of the potentially toxic sequelae of AhR activation are offset by the detoxification reactions catalyzed by the AhR-responsive drug-metabolizing enzymes. These contrasting effects will be discussed further in Section 4.5.1.

4.3.2. Pregnane X Receptor (CYP3A Inducers)

The nuclear receptor PXR (NR1I2) was first identified in 1998 as the ligand-activated transcription factor mediating CYP3A induction by steroids (Bertilsson et al. 1998; Blumberg et al. 1998; Kliewer et al. 1998).[1] The identification of the role of PXR marked a major advance in understanding of the mechanisms behind CYP3A induction, and paved the way for a

---

[1] PXR, or pregnane X receptor, is also known as the pregnane activated receptor (PAR) or the steroid and xenobiotic receptor (SXR). The majority of recent literature uses the name PXR, and hence this convention is followed herein.

flurry of subsequent research into the role of CYP3A induction in detoxification, drug–drug interactions, and bioactivation.

Pregnane X receptor belongs to the nuclear receptor superfamily of ligand-activated transcription factors that includes vitamin D receptor (VDR; NR1I1), the CAR (NR1I3), PPAR (NR1C), and others (Germain et al. 2006). Members of this NR1 subfamily of nuclear receptors typically function as heterodimers with the retinoid X receptor (RXR; NR2B1). In the unactivated state, the PXR/RXR heterodimers are thought to be retained in the cytoplasm, bound to heat shock proteins and/or various chaperone proteins (Squires, Sueyoshi and Negishi 2004). Upon ligand binding, PXR/RXR translocates to the nucleus, binds DNA in the 5′-regulatory region of target genes, and interacts with various coregulatory proteins thereby effecting gene transcription (Figure 4.2; reviewed in Stanley et al. 2006).

Genes regulated by PXR code for a wide array of proteins involved in transport and metabolism of drugs and endogenous compounds. Perhaps the most widely recognized PXR target gene is CYP3A4. Since CYP3A4 is involved in the metabolism of an estimated 50% of all marketed drugs, increases in CYP3A4 expression by PXR activation can have profound effects on the clearance of drug substrates and results in drug–drug interactions. Conversely, increased CYP3A4 can be a protective mechanism

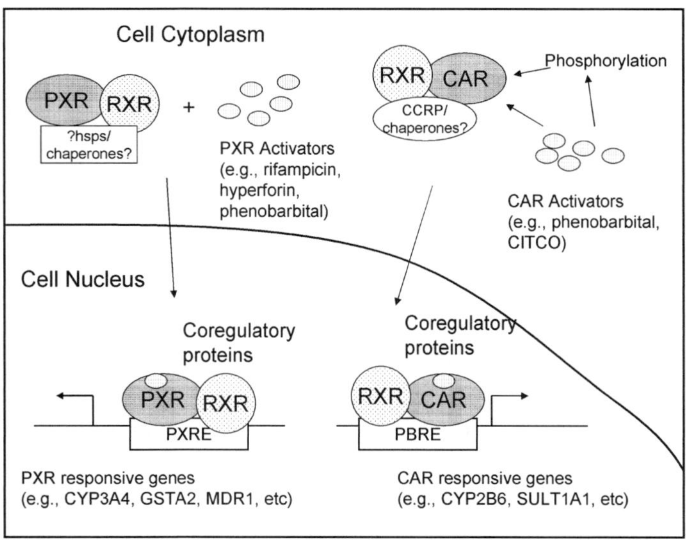

Figure 4.2 Regulation of gene transcription by PXR or CAR. Under basal conditions the PXR/RXR or CAR/RXR heterodimers are thought to be retained in the cytoplasm, likely bound to heat shock proteins and/or other chaperones – for example, the cytosolic CAR retention protein (CCRP). Upon ligand binding, and/or activation by phosphorylation, the PXR/RXR or CAR/RXR heterodimers translocate to the nucleus where they bind specific DNA sequences in the 5′-regulatory region of responsive genes. Gene transcription is modulated by interactions of the heterodimeric complexes with coregulatory proteins, including TIF2, SRC-1, SMRT, and/or NCoR. For a more comprehensive review of these factors, refer to Stanley et al. (2006).

whereby potentially toxic xenobiotic or endogenous compounds are cleared more quickly. CYP3A4 is only one of many PXR target genes that also include numerous other CYPs, GSTA2, MDR1, MRP2, OATP2, and UGT1A6 (Table 4.1). Therefore, activation of PXR is thought to be primarily a protective response whereby uptake, metabolism, and efflux of potentially toxic compounds are increased.

Activators of PXR include natural and synthetic steroids and steroid metabolites such as corticosterone, dexamethasone, and dehydroepiandrosterone, and numerous pharmaceutical and nutriceutical agents such as rifampicin, nifedipine, lovastatin, clotrimazole, and hyperforin (Blumberg et al. 1998; Kliewer et al. 1998; Lehmann et al. 1998). Very few antagonists of PXR have been identified to date. The natural product-derived drug known as ecteinascidin 743 (ET-743) blocks activation of PXR with IC_{50} values in the nanomolar range (Synold, Dussault and Forman 2001). A recent report shows that the isothiocyanate compound sulforaphane is an antagonist of human PXR, and can inhibit both basal and inducible expression of CYP3A4, with IC_{50} values in the micromolar range (Zhou et al. 2007). Interestingly, ketoconazole, a molecule well known for its ability to competitively inhibit CYP3A4, also can antagonize the activity of PXR and other nuclear receptors (Huang et al. 2007). Ketoconazole apparently acts by disrupting the interaction between the nuclear receptor and the coactivator protein, steroid receptor coactivator 1 (SRC-1).

In contrast to classical nuclear hormone receptors such as estrogen receptor (ER) and glucocorticoid receptor (GR), steroid activators of PXR exhibit low affinity, with EC_{50} values in the low micromolar range rather than the low nanomolar range typical of classical hormone receptors. Therefore, it appears that PXR is responsive to supraphysiological concentrations of steroids and metabolites, which is consistent with the assertion that PXR acts as a sensor, responding to potentially toxic concentrations of xenobiotics and endogenous compounds by initiating a protective gene expression response.

4.3.3. Constitutive Androstane Receptor (Phenobarbital-Like Inducers)

Although induction of CYP2B genes by phenobarbital treatment had been known for many years, the fact that this induction was mediated via a nuclear receptor, now known as the CAR), was not realized until 1998 (Honkakoski et al. 1998). The challenge in identifying CAR was due in part to the fact the phenobarbital inductive effect on CYP2B genes was observed in vivo and in primary hepatocytes, but was not reproduced in continuously cultured cell lines. Subsequently, it was discovered that in vivo and in primary hepatocytes, CAR is sequestered in the cytoplasm, and translocates to the nucleus upon ligand binding or upon phosphorylation (Kawamoto et al. 1999). Like the closely related receptor PXR, CAR exists as a heterodimer with RXR (Figure 4.2). Once in the nucleus, the CAR/RXR heterodimer is constitutively active; therefore, the translocation event is essentially a receptor activation event. The apparent lack of active CAR in cultured cell lines was due to the fact that CAR was already located in the nucleus under basal conditions, and hence was constitutively active (Kobayashi et al. 2003).

The first compounds identified that interact with CAR were actually the inverse agonists androstanol and androstenol (Forman et al. 1998). These compounds are termed inverse agonists in that they bind to CAR, but rather than activate the receptor, they deactivate its constitutive activity. Subsequently, it was discovered that regular agonist ligands also exist for CAR, for example 1,4-*bis*[2-(3,5-dichloropyridyloxy)] benzene (TCPOBOP)(mouse CAR; Tzameli et al., 2000) and (6-(4-chlorophenyl)imidazo[2,1-b](1,3)-thiazole-5-carbaldehyde-*O*-(3,4-dichlorobenzyl)oxime) (CITCO) (human CAR; Maglich et al. 2003). CAR can also be activated in a ligand-independent manner. Phenobarbital, the prototypical inducer of CYP2B6 (Cyp2b10 in mice), does not appear to be a ligand for CAR, but rather activates the receptor via activation of receptor phosphorylation (Kawamoto et al. 1999; Rencurel et al. 2006). In addition, nutritional and metabolic stresses, such as fasting and caloric restriction, can activate CAR (Maglich et al. 2004), and this apparently occurs through receptor phosphorylation activated by cAMP/protein kinase A (Ding et al. 2006).

Soon after the discovery that CAR was involved in the phenobarbital-mediated induction of CYP2B enzymes, it became clear that CAR, like PXR, mediated the induction of numerous additional drug-metabolizing enzymes, including phase II enzymes and transporters, such as GSTA2, UGT1A1, and MDR1 (Maglich et al. 2002; Maglich et al. 2003). In addition, it was recognized that many of the ligands that activate CAR can also activate PXR, although the inverse is not necessarily true, since CAR has a smaller ligand-binding pocket and narrower ligand selectivity than PXR. There is also overlap in the target genes of these two receptors; for example, both CAR and PXR can activate transcription of CYP3A4, CYP2B6, and UGT1A6 (Moore et al. 2000; Maglich et al. 2002; Wei et al. 2002). Therefore, it appears that both CAR and PXR are part of a protective response to xenobiotic exposure – regulating genes involved in uptake, metabolism, and excretion of potentially toxic substances.

4.3.4. Other Nuclear Receptors: FXR (Bile Acids), LXR (Sterols), PPAR (Fibrates), VDR (Vitamin D)

Additional members of the NR1 subfamily of nuclear receptors, namely FXR, LXRα, PPAR, and VDR are also involved in regulation of CYPs and/or transporters. However, these receptors differ from CAR and PXR in that they are predominantly involved in metabolism and homeostasis of endogenous compounds. These receptors also do not exhibit the broad ligand selectivity seen with PXR or CAR, but rather have a more specific set of ligands. For example, FXR is activated by natural bile acids, which results in repression of the expression of CYP7A1, the enzyme catalyzing the rate-limiting step in the conversion of cholesterol to bile acids (Makishima et al. 1999; Parks et al. 1999; Masubuchi 2006). LXRα is activated by oxidized cholesterol metabolites (oxysterols), and when activated causes increased expression of cholesterol-metabolizing enzymes, including CYP7A1 (Peet et al. 1998). VDR binds 1,25-dihydroxy-vitamin

D_3 (calcitriol) with high affinity, and regulates genes involved in calcium and phosphate homeostasis (Reschly and Krasowski 2006). Activated VDR has also been shown to increase expression of CYP3A4 in intestinal cell lines and in primary human hepatocytes (Thummel et al. 2001; Drocourt et al. 2002). Although VDR has a very limited ligand selectivity compared to PXR and CAR, it can be activated by high concentrations of the potentially toxic secondary bile acid LCA, resulting in increased clearance of this compound from the liver (Makishima et al. 2002). Although VDR activation can result in increased expression of several CYPs, the relative importance of this pathway for CYP induction is currently unclear since VDR has a very limited set of ligands relative to PXR and CAR.

The PPARα (NR1C1) was originally identified as the receptor activated by compounds known to cause peroxisome proliferation in rodents (Issemann and Green 1990). Two additional PPAR family members – PPARγ (NR1C3) and PPARδ (NR1C2, also called PPARβ) – were subsequently identified. The PPARs are ligand-activated transcription factors, specifically involved in fatty acid and lipid metabolism and homeostasis. The PPARs are activated by endogenous compounds (e.g., fatty acids, leukotriene B4 (PPARα), and prostaglandin J2 (PPARγ)) and by drugs (e.g., fibrates (PPARα) and thiazolidinediones (PPARγ)). However, with the exception of these latter two classes of drugs that are specifically targeted toward these receptors, PPARs are not generally activated by drugs and xenobiotics, and do not induce typical drug-metabolizing enzymes and transporters. Since FXR, LXR, PPAR, and VDR are not typically involved in detoxification or bioactivation of drugs and xenobiotics, they will not be discussed any further.

4.3.5. Nrf2/Keap1 (ARE Inducers)

The induction of phase II enzymes such as GSTs, UGTs, NAD[P]H:quinone oxidoreductase (NQO1), and gamma-glutamylcysteine synthetase (GCS) in response to antioxidants and chemopreventive chemicals is mediated by the transcription factor known as nuclear factor erythroid 2-related factor 2 (Nrf2) (Kobayashi and Yamamoto 2006). The Nrf2 pathway differs significantly from the typically ligand-activated transcription factors discussed above. The Nrf2 is not a member of the nuclear receptor superfamily, but rather belongs to the cap ‘n’ collar subfamily of the basic region leucine zipper transcription factors. The Nrf2 heterodimerizes with a member of the small Maf transcription factor family to bind DNA sequences known as antioxidant response elements (AREs)[2] in the 5′-flanking regions of target genes (Venugopal and Jaiswal 1996; Itoh et al. 1997).

Activators of the Nrf2 pathway include antioxidants (tert-butylhydroquinone), chemopreventive agents (sulforaphane and oltipraz), electrophiles, and oxidative stress. These inducers are not ligands for Nrf2, but rather activate the transcription factor indirectly via protein stabilization.

[2] AREs are also known as electrophile responsive elements, or EpREs.

Much research has focused on this unique mechanism of activation of the Nrf2/ARE pathway, and the reader is referred to several good reviews on the subject (Nguyen, Yang and Pickett 2004; Kobayashi and Yamamoto 2006; Zhang 2006). A summary of the current understanding is that under basal conditions, most of the cellular Nrf2 is retained in the cytoplasm, bound to a protein known as Keap1, which serves to target Nrf2 for degradation via the ubiquitin-dependent proteasome pathway (Figure 4.3). The Keap1 protein contains an unusually large number of cysteine residues, which are thought to act as redox sensors for the Keap1/Nrf2 complex. Upon treatment with ARE inducers and/or under conditions of oxidative stress, one or more cysteine residues of Keap1 becomes modified, thereby disrupting the interactions with Nrf2 (Itoh et al. 1999). There is evidence that some inducers and/or their reactive metabolites directly modify specific cysteine residues in Keap1 (Dinkova-Kostova et al. 2002; Zhang and Hannink 2003). The disruption of the interactions between Keap1 and Nrf2 result in stabilization of Nrf2 protein. Stabilized Nrf2 can translocate to the nucleus, where it forms a heterodimer with a

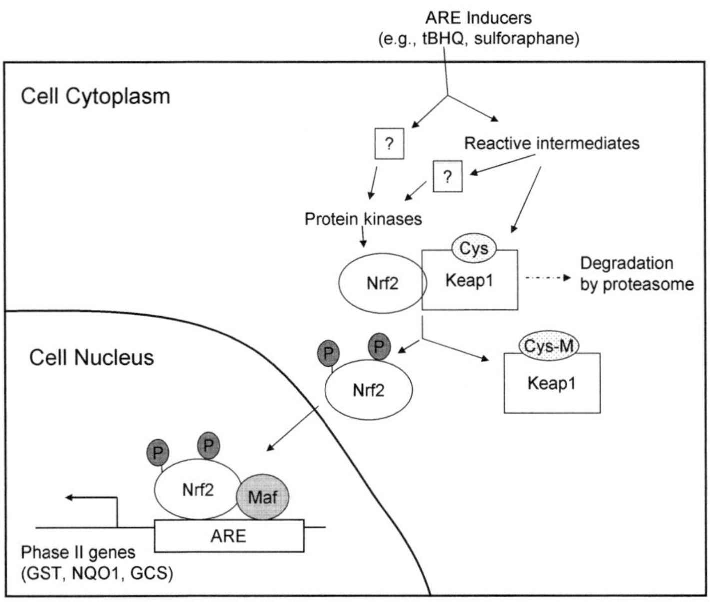

Figure 4.3 Regulation of Nrf2–Keap1 by ARE inducers. Schematic representation of factors involved in activation of ARE-mediated gene expression by ARE inducers. Under basal conditions, most cellular Nrf2 is thought to be bound to Keap1, which keeps Nrf2 in the inactive state and enhances its degradation. Treatment with ARE inducers causes the release of Nrf2 from Keap1, by activation of Nrf2 phosphorylation and/or by modification of cysteine residue(s) on Keap1. Disruption of the Nrf2/Keap1 interaction results in stabilization of Nrf2, translocation to the nucleus, heterodimerization with a small Maf protein, and activation of gene transcription. Note that recent evidence indicates that the Nrf2/Keap1 complex may shuttle between cytoplasm and nucleus. Cys indicates one of several cysteine residues thought to be involved in regulation of Keap1. Cys-M, modified cysteine residue; P, phosphorylated Ser, Thr, or Tyr residue. Figure adapted from Nguyen et al. (2004) with permission from Elsevier.

small Maf protein, and binds to ARE sequences, thereby activating transcription of target genes. In addition, phosphorylation of Nrf2 plays a role in its stabilization and translocation to the nucleus. Several different protein kinases have been shown to be involved in phosphorylation of Nrf2, including PKC, PERK, and MAP kinase family members (Yu et al. 1999; Huang, Nguyen and Pickett 2000; Cullinan et al. 2003). The exact mechanisms of how ARE inducers activate these kinases to phosphorylate Nrf2 are not clear at this time.

In summary, it appears that compounds known as ARE inducers activate Nrf2-mediated transcriptional activation indirectly via protein stabilization and enhanced translocation to the nucleus. The stabilization and translocation of Nrf2 can be achieved by disruption of interactions with Keap1 and/or phosphorylation. Activation of the Nrf2/ARE pathway initiates a general cytoprotective response that allows cells to better defend against electrophiles and oxidative stress, as described in Section 4.5.3.

4.3.6. Ethanol-Type Induction (CYP2E1 Inducers)

The induction of CYP2E1 by ethanol is unusual in that it involves stabilization of protein rather than ligand activation of a receptor/transcription factor (reviewed in Gonzalez 2007). To date, CYP2E1 is the only CYP isozyme known to be regulated in this manner. The role of substrate stabilization of CYP2E1 was shown in elegant studies using in vivo labeling of CYP2E1 in rats. The degradation of the enzyme was found to be biphasic, with half-lives of approximately 7 hours and 32 hours for the two phases (Song et al. 1989). In rats treated with CYP2E1 inducers, the rapid half-life component was missing, and only the longer half-life component remained. This suggested that the presence of substrate shifted the protein to the longer half-life form, thereby explaining the increase in microsomal CYP2E1 content.

There is also evidence that CYP2E1 can be induced by way of mRNA stabilization. This observation was made in diabetic rats, in which levels of CYP2E1 mRNA and protein were increased, but gene transcription was not increased (Song et al. 1987). Subsequent studies have shown that this induction can be reversed by treatment with insulin, and a nucleotide sequence in the 5′-region of the mRNA that mediates this reversal has recently been identified (Truong et al. 2005). That insulin is involved in regulation of CYP2E1 is consistent with the postulated role of CYP2E1 in a secondary pathway of gluconeogenesis (Koop and Casazza 1985). For a more detailed discussion of the mechanisms of CYP2E1 induction, the reader is referred to the Chapter 6.

Drugs and xenobiotic inducers of CYP2E1 are typically low molecular weight and are substrates for CYP2E1, for example, ethanol, acetone, pyrazole, and isoniazid. A notable example of consequences of this induction is the increased CYP2E1-mediated metabolism of acetaminophen to *N*-acetyl-*p*-benzoquinone-imine (NAPQI), which represents a bioactivation reaction. The consequences of CYP2E1 induction with respect to acetaminophen metabolism will be discussed in more detail in Section 4.5.4

4.4. Techniques in Enzyme Induction Research

The understanding of the pathways involved in enzyme induction, the target genes, and the effect of induction on physiological and toxicological events has advanced significantly in the last decade. The enzyme induction field has benefited from technological advances in receptor binding and coactivator assays, gene expression arrays, and in improved transgenic mouse models. The needs of pharmaceutical companies to screen new compounds for enzyme induction potential has led to the development of numerous higher-throughput cell assays. This section is devoted to a survey of various technical approaches to the study of enzyme induction and is intended to briefly cover both classical techniques (e.g., CYP activity assays in treated hepatocytes) and newer technologies (e.g., transgenic mice models), and discuss the impact that these techniques have had on research in enzyme induction.

4.4.1. Measuring Induction Potential of New Chemical Entities

Researchers involved in the discovery and development of new chemical entities, such as pharmaceuticals and food additives, need to know whether a given compound has the potential to induce drug-metabolizing enzymes. This is important, as enzyme induction can increase a compound's own metabolism (termed "autoinduction") and/or the metabolism of other substrates. For example, drugs that induce levels of CYP3A4, an enzyme involved in metabolism of numerous pharmaceutical agents, can cause drug–drug interactions by causing increased clearance of coadministered drugs. Therefore, the ability of a new chemical entity to bind and/or activate PXR, as well as AhR and CAR, is often assessed early in the discovery process, and hence numerous test systems have been developed for measuring induction potential. Since there are considerable species differences in the ability of compounds to activate the different pathways, in vivo studies in preclinical species (rats, mice) are not typically used for this testing. Rather, numerous in vitro assays using human-derived reagents are used, as described below.

4.4.1.1. Primary Cultures of Human Hepatocytes

The classic technique for measuring the ability of a compound to induce drug-metabolizing enzymes is by short-term culture and treatment of primary human hepatocytes, followed by measurement of CYP levels. Typically, cells are isolated from livers by collagenase perfusion, then plated and cultured for 2–3 days prior to addition of the compound of interest (LeCluyse et al. 2000). Cells are generally exposed to the compound for an additional 3 days, followed by measurement of CYP levels. Cytochrome P450 levels can be determined by enzyme activity measurements using isoform-selective probe substrates – for example, testosterone 6β-hydroxylation to measure CYP3A4, and/or measurement of mRNA levels. In some cases, immunoquantitation of protein levels is also done. The benefits of primary human hepatocyte cultures are that they contain the native receptors and enzymes of interest in induction studies. They also have metabolic capabilities similar to the intact liver. Some drawbacks of this technique are that human liver specimens are not easily obtained, and isolation of hepatocytes can yield cells of variable quality. The development of cryopreservation techniques has improved the availability of primary human hepatocytes, but many cryopreserved cells are not plateable and therefore cannot be maintained in culture. There is also significant interdonor variability in basal and inducible CYP levels in different hepatocyte preparations, making it more difficult to compare activities across experiments and across laboratories. Also, due to hepatocyte availability constraints, the method is low throughput. Due to some of these limitations, numerous additional in vitro assays have been developed to assess enzyme induction potential, as discussed below.

4.4.1.2. Reporter Gene Assays

Reporter gene assays using cultured cell lines have proven to be a relatively facile and widely used tool to study individual induction pathways. Continuously cultured cell lines, for example, HepG2, Huh7, etc., are typically transfected with an expression plasmid encoding a nuclear receptor (e.g., PXR) and a reporter gene plasmid. The reporter gene plasmid contains part of the 5′-regulatory region of a target gene (e.g., CYP3A4) connected to the coding portion of a "reporter" gene, typically luciferase or chloramphenicol acetyl transferase (CAT), due to the ease of detection of their enzymatic activities. When the transfected cells are treated with inducers, expression of the reporter gene is measured. Reporter gene systems offer advantages over primary hepatocyte cultures in terms of availability, cost, ease of culture, and potential for high-throughput applications. A limitation of the reporter gene system is that generally only a limited portion of the 5′-regulatory region of the target gene of interest is used, such that the gene expression response may not translate to the full response that would be observed in vivo or in primary hepatocytes. Also, typically the transient transfection of a receptor plasmid results in overexpression of that receptor, which may result in a different magnitude of response relative to the primary hepatocyte assay. The continuously cultured cell lines also lack expression of some of the liver-specific proteins, and hence have a more dedifferentiated phenotype compared to primary hepatocytes (Castell et al. 2006). Despite these limitations, the reporter gene system has been very useful in identifying the potential of compounds to cause induction.

Pregnane X receptor has been particularly amenable to reporter gene methodologies, and there is a good correlation between activation of PXR/CYP3A4 induction in reporter gene assays and activation of PXR/CYP3A4 induction in primary hepatocytes (Luo et al. 2002; Sinz et al. 2006). Activation of AhR/CYP1A induction is also readily observed in reporter gene assays, and generally does not require the transfection of AhR expression plasmids, since cell lines typically express AhR at adequate basal levels (Ciolino, Daschner and Yeh 1998). On the other hand, reporter gene assays have not worked as well for detecting activators of CAR (Honkakoski et al. 1998). Apparently, when CAR is overexpressed in cultured cell lines, much of it localizes in the nucleus where it is constitutively active, and hence further ligand-dependent activation of CAR above the background of constitutive activity is difficult to detect. One system that has been successfully used for detecting CAR activators is the use of CAR-transfected cells treated with androstenol. Androstenol is an inverse agonist that blocks the constitutive activity of CAR, thereby allowing CAR activation to be detected above background (Sueyoshi et al. 1999).

4.4.1.3. Immortalized Hepatocytes and Minimally Derived Hepatocyte Lines

The desire to combine the ease, reproducibility, and throughput of reporter gene assays with the ability to measure native receptor and target gene expression as in primary hepatocytes has led to the development of both immortalized and minimally derived hepatocyte lines. The term "immortalized hepatocytes" refers to cells that originated from primary human hepatocytes that have been transformed and are capable of growing in culture. The term minimally derived hepatocytes refers to cell lines, originally derived from hepatoma cells, that have not been extensively passaged. Both immortalized hepatocytes and minimally derived hepatocytes retain a more differentiated phenotype relative to cell lines that have been extensively cultured. The Fa2N4 immortalized hepatocytes have been used successfully to measure induction via PXR and AhR pathways (Mills et al. 2004; Ripp et al. 2006). The Fa2N4 cells are derived from primary human hepatocytes that had been transformed with SV40 large T antigen. When the cells are cultured in the absence of serum, they maintain a differentiated phenotype like that of primary hepatocytes. They express various nuclear receptors, transporters, and CYPs, although the basal enzyme activity is lower than that of primary hepatocytes (Mills et al. 2004). Fa2N4 cells offer advantages over reporter gene assays in that they do not require transfection or overexpression of nuclear receptors and reporter genes, but rather they rely on native human receptors and target gene expression. In addition, the Fa2N4 cells offer advantages over primary human hepatocytes in terms of availability and reproducibility.

The HepaRG cell line represents a minimally derived cell line that can be continuously maintained, but can also be cultured in such a way as to develop a more differentiated, hepatocyte-like morphology (Guillouzo et al. 2007). When cultured in the presence of 2% dimethyl sulfoxide (DMSO) for 30days, the cells express CYPs (with the exception of CYP2D6), transporters, and other liver-specific proteins at levels near those of primary hepatocytes (Aninat et al. 2006). The cells also show inducibilty of CYP1A and CYP3A, although the CYP3A effect needs to be done under non-DMSO culture conditions in order to observe inducibility (Aninat et al. 2006).

4.4.1.4. Ligand-Binding or Coactivator Recruitment Assays

Activation of nuclear receptors by new chemical entities can be a result of direct ligand binding to a nuclear receptor, or due to indirect modification of the receptor, for example, via phosphorylation. It is useful to know the mechanisms of receptor activation, and whether a compound is actually a ligand for a receptor. There are several different methods for assessing this, including scintillation proximity assay (SPA), fluorescence resonance electron transfer assay (FRET), or coactivator-dependent receptor ligand assay (CARLA) (Krey et al. 1997; Jones et al. 2000; Kliewer, Goodwin and Willson 2002). In a SPA, the receptor is expressed and immobilized on scintillant-containing beads, which are then incubated with radiolabeled compound. When compound is bound to receptor, the scintillant is activated and can be readily measured. Binding affinity of unlabeled compounds can be determined in the same system, by measuring concentrations required to compete with a high-affinity radiolabeled ligand. The CARLA experiments are useful when no radiolabeled ligand for a receptor is available. The CARLA assay measures the protein–protein interactions between SRC-1 and the receptor of interest, which happens only if the receptor has been ligand activated (Krey et al. 1997). Similarly, the ligand-induced interaction of a nuclear receptor with SRC-1 can be measured by FRET assay, by using fluorophore-labeled proteins (Moore et al. 2000). These ligand-binding assay techniques offer insight into how a compound activates a receptor, whether direct or indirect, as well as the relative affinity of that compound for the receptor.

4.4.1.5. In Silico Models

There is interest, particularly within the pharmaceutical industry, in the use of in silico tools to predict induction potential, thereby enabling the design of compounds that avoid interaction with nuclear receptors. Researchers have used a combination of crystal structures, site-directed mutagenesis studies, and pharmacophore models to better understand the ligand-binding sites of PXR and CAR (reviewed in Poso and Honkakoski 2006). Despite the considerable effort that has been put into the development of in silico prediction tools, the ability to predict PXR and CAR activation remains elusive. The large size and flexibility of the PXR-binding pocket makes development of a robust in silico model more of a challenge. The situation with CAR is even more complex. Although CAR has a smaller binding pocket with less flexibility, the subtle structural changes that determine whether ligands of CAR are activators or inhibitors is still being defined. Despite the challenges, the promise of in silico prediction tools drives continued research and effort in this area.

4.4.2. Use of Gene Arrays to Find Novel Target Genes and Elucidate Wider Role of Nuclear Receptor Activation

The study of nuclear receptor biology and target gene regulation has been greatly facilitated by the ability to broadly profile gene expression (mRNA) changes through the use of gene expression arrays. Arrays are available that allow simultaneous profiling of anywhere from a few dozen to thousands of genes. Some arrays are enriched in genes coding for drug-metabolizing enzymes and transporters, while others are enriched in genes important in pharmacological or toxicological pathways. In addition, several companies offer the ability to make customized gene arrays. The basic technique for a gene expression array experiment involves isolating RNA from control and treated cells or tissues, reverse transcription and labeling of the RNA using fluorescence or biotin systems, hybridization to the gene array, and detection and analysis of the hybridized products through specialized instrumentation and software. More specific technical aspects of gene expression arrays will not be addressed here, but the reader is referred to the literature cited in the examples that follow, as well as array manufacturers' websites.

Gene expression arrays have been used for two primary purposes related to enzyme induction: to profile gene expression changes caused by chemical treatment and/or to profile gene expression changes induced by lack or overexpression of a nuclear receptor. For example, the pleiotropic effects of rifampicin on hepatic gene expression have been assessed by microarray analysis of primary human hepatocytes treated with rifampicin, emphasizing the breadth of changes in drug-metabolizing enzymes and transporters upon rifampicin treatment (Rae et al. 2001). Similarly, the gene expression array analysis has helped to elucidate the broad physiological and toxicological responses to TCDD treatment (Hanlon et al. 2005). Gene expression array analysis is also useful in characterizing gene expression changes in receptor knockout mice. For example, the role of CAR in the pleiotropic hepatic effects of phenobarbital treatment was studied using gene expression profiling in CAR knockout and wild-type mice (Ueda et al. 2002). This study was one of the first to show that gene regulation by CAR extended beyond drug metabolism, and included genes involved in energy metabolism. In addition, this work suggested that the effects of phenobarbital treatment had both CAR-dependent and CAR-independent aspects. Rosenfeld et al. compared global gene expression changes between wild-type and PXR knockout mice, as well as mice expressing a constitutively activated form of human PXR (Rosenfeld et al. 2003). This study confirmed the PXR dependence of known target genes such as Cyp3a11 and Cyp2b10, and revealed additional target genes that were induced (e.g., carboxylesterases) or suppressed (e.g., Cyp4a10) in the activated hPXR transgenic mice. The above examples represent only a small fraction of the studies that have employed gene expression array analysis to aid in our understanding of enzyme induction and the diversity of target genes and pathways affected by nuclear receptor activation.

4.4.3. Use of Transgenic and Knockout Mice in Induction Rresearch

Transgenic and knockout mouse models have contributed greatly to the understanding of the role of nuclear receptors in modulation of gene expression and in vivo response to chemical stress. One key use of knockout mouse models has been to clarify the role of a given receptor in enzyme induction as a result of inducer treatment. For example, the generation of the first CAR knockout mouse was key to understanding phenobarbital induction (Wei et al. 2000). Prior to this mouse model, CAR had been hypothesized to be the mediator of phenobarbital induction of CYP2B genes; however, data from expression studies in cultured cell lines yielded conflicting results. The role of CAR was unambiguously confirmed with the generation of the CAR knockout mouse. Cyp2b10 was strongly upregulated by phenobarbital and TCPOBOP in wild-type, but not in CAR knockout mice (Wei et al. 2000). Transgenic mice have also been useful in translating interspecies differences in receptor ligand selectivity exhibited by PXR and CAR. For example, mice that express a human form of PXR show Cyp3a induction in response to the human PXR agonist rifampicin, but not in response to the mouse PXR agonist PCN (Xie et al. 2000; Ma et al. 2007). Similarly transgenic mice expressing hCAR have been generated, and demonstrate responsiveness to hCAR activators (Zhang et al. 2002; Huang et al. 2005). Researchers have also generated mice that express a constitutively activated form of human PXR, in order to assess consequences of receptor activation without confounding effects of chemical treatment (Xie et al. 2000).

There are numerous examples that demonstrate the importance of transgenic mouse models in understanding the role of nuclear receptors/enzyme induction pathways in the toxicity of chemical treatments. For example, PXR knockout mice are more susceptible to hepatotoxicity caused by lithocholic acid, and are resistant to the hepatoprotective effects of PCN treatment, supporting the hypothesis that PXR is critical for detoxification of potentially toxic bile acids (Staudinger et al. 2001; see Section 4.5.2). The Nrf2 knockout mice are more sensitive to numerous toxicants than wild-type mice and are resistant to the chemopreventive effects of oltipraz – data that support a prominent role for Nrf2 in detoxification (Chan Han and Kan 2001; Ramos-Gomez et al. 2001; see Section 4.5.3).

Genetically modified mouse models have also been useful in assessing the roles of nuclear receptors in normal physiology. For example, AhR knockout mice exhibited decreased viability, defects in liver and immune function, and additional abnormalities (Fernandez-Salguero et al., 1995; Rifkind 2006). These knockout mice studies revealed that AhR function extended beyond xenobiotic sensing/enzyme induction, to that of a key transcription factor involved in numerous physiological processes.

4.5. Consequences of Enzyme Induction – Examples of Detoxification and/or Bioactivation

Enzyme induction is widely believed to be part of an adaptive response to potentially toxic insult such as exposure to environmental contaminants (e.g., TCDD, PAHs), drugs (e.g., acetaminophen, phenytoin), or excess concentrations of endogenous chemicals (e.g., excess bile acids or bilirubin). However, it is also recognized that in some cases enzyme induction can result in bioactivation to more toxic substances. Whether enzyme induction represents a bioactivation or detoxification pathway can be quite complex and dependent on many different factors. The following are well-studied examples of enzyme induction that aim to illustrate some of these factors and complexity. In some cases, the examples reflect a clear detoxification role for enzyme induction, while in others there are elements of both detoxification and bioactivation.

4.5.1. Consequences of AhR Activation

The activation of AhR is known to produce a multitude of gene expression changes that include induction of drug-metabolizing enzymes, most notably, CYPs 1A1, 1A2, and 1B1. Whether this induction represents a detoxification pathway or a bioactivation pathway has been a matter of discussion for many years (Conney 1967; Parkinson and Hurwitz 1991;

Ioannides and Parke 1993; Nebert et al. 2004). As early as the 1950 s it was recognized that treatment with various polycyclic aromatic hydrocarbons (PAHs) resulted in induction of drug-metabolizing enzymes, although at this time the existence of AhR and CYPs was not known (Brown, Miller and Miller 1954). These early studies revealed that enzyme induction led to increased metabolism; this induction was viewed as an adaptive and predominantly protective response to chemical exposure (Conney 1967). Indeed, numerous studies showed that PAH-mediated enzyme induction reduced chemical carcinogenesis (reviewed in Conney 1967; Parkinson and Hurwitz 1991). The 1960 s brought the identification of cytochrome P450 s and the recognition that the enzymes induced by PAH treatment were of this cytochrome P450 monooxygenase class (Omura and Sato 1962; Sladek and Mannering 1966). At the same time, there was increasing recognition that these enzymes were also involved in the bioactivation of procarcinogens; for example, CYP1A1 catalyzes the first step in metabolism of benzo[a]pyrene to the carcinogenic diol-epoxide, and CYP1A2 catalyzes the N-hydroxylation of 2-acetylaminofluorene to a carcinogenic metabolite (Miller, Miller and Hartmann 1961; Sims et al. 1974). Increasingly, the ability of a chemical or drug to cause induction of CYP1 enzymes was viewed as an indicator of likely toxicity and carcinogenicity of that compound (reviewed in Ioannides and Parke 1993). This illustrates the seemingly contradictory effects of CYP1 induction – on the one hand increasing bioactivation of toxins/carcinogens, and on the other hand decreasing carcinogenicity in vivo.

The development of knockout mice has helped to clarify the roles of AhR and the CYP1 enzymes in these various bioactivation and detoxification pathways. Surprisingly, Cyp1a1-null and Cyp1a2-null mice showed increased sensitivity to benzo[a]pyrene and 4-aminobiphenyl toxicities, respectively (Tsuneoka et al. 2003; Uno et al. 2004), suggesting that in vivo, these enzymes provide a protective response to these chemical toxins. An interesting example of the complex nature of the in vitro versus in vivo response to CYP1 induction is that of the role of CYP1 enzymes in bone marrow toxicity. CYP1B1, which is constitutively expressed in numerous tissues including bone marrow, is required for bioactivation of PAHs and subsequent bone marrow toxicity (Heidel et al. 2000; Galvan et al. 2003). However, induction of CYP1A1 in the liver ameliorates PAH-induced bone marrow toxicity (Galvan et al. 2003). Therefore, although CYP1B1 induction results in increased toxicity to bone marrow cells in vitro, these effects can be offset in vivo due to increased metabolism in the liver. Another example of the complexity around in vivo effects of CYP1 induction involve the observation of increased formation of DNA and protein adducts in AhR-null mice and in Cyp1a1-null mice treated orally with benzo[a]pyrene (Sagredo et al. 2006; Uno et al. 2006). This observation, along with the aforementioned increased toxicity of oral benzo[a]pyrene treatment in Cyp1a1-null mice (Uno et al. 2004), is in contrast to an observed decrease in skin tumorigenesis in AhR-null mice by topically administered benzo[a]pyrene (Shimizu et al. 2000). These data again support the notion that increased Cyp1a1 metabolism in the liver (e.g., after oral benzo[a]pyrene treatment) can offset the potential bioactivation reactions in extrahepatic tissues such as skin.

Therefore, several possibilities emerge for the explanation of the contradictory effects of CYP1 induction (reviewed in Nebert et al. 2004; Rifkind 2006). Bioactivation and detoxification may be dependent upon constitutive versus inducible CYP expression in different tissues, and the relative contributions of major clearing organs (liver and intestine, after oral administration), versus metabolism to bioactive species in target tissues (skin, bone marrow, and thymus). Also, while CYP1-mediated metabolism might represent an initial bioactivation reaction, whether the ultimate product is toxic likely depends on other factors, such as how tightly coupled the phase I product is to detoxifying phase II enzymes. Taken together, what is emerging from these years of research is that CYP1 induction via AhR activation likely represents part of an adaptive response to toxic insult, and that this induction response represents neither solely a bioactivation pathway nor solely a detoxification pathway, but rather a pleiotropic response that has components of each. Whether bioactivation or detoxification is the predominant in vivo outcome of CYP1 induction cannot necessarily be predicted from in vitro experiments, due to the complexities around compound-specific metabolism, tissue-specific expression of various CYPs, and the interplay between these factors.

4.5.2. Enzyme Induction in Detoxification of Supraphysiological Concentrations of Endogenous Compounds

Endogenous chemicals such as bilirubin and bile acids serve essential roles in mammalian physiology, yet excess levels of these compounds can also result in pathophysiological conditions. Bilirubin is a natural breakdown product of heme, and is normally metabolized and excreted in the bile. However, impairments in the heme metabolic pathways can result in increased serum bilirubin, which if high enough can enter central nervous system (CNS) tissues and cause neurotoxicities including encephalopathy. Bile acids serve important roles in aiding absorption of lipids and fat-soluble vitamins and serve to aid solubilization of lipids and cholesterol metabolites for excretion in the bile. However, at supraphysiological concentrations, bile acids are toxic to cells and hence impairments in bile acid metabolism and/or excretion can lead to hepatotoxicity. Cholestasis, or the impairment or cessation of bile flow, leads to buildup of bile acids and subsequent liver damage.

The prototypical inducers rifampicin and phenobarbital have been used empirically for many years to treat cholestasis (Javor et al. 1973; Hoensch et al. 1985). However, it was not until relatively recently that the roles of nuclear receptor activation and enzyme induction were elucidated as part of the mechanism underlying this treatment. In 2001, seminal studies were published that demonstrated the importance of the nuclear receptor PXR in metabolism of potentially toxic bile acids (Staudinger et al. 2001). This work showed that treatment of mice with PCN resulted in increased expression of Oatp2 and Cyp3a11, and decreased expression of Cyp7a1. These gene expression changes would result in increased hepatic uptake and metabolism of bile acids, and decreased formation of bile acids from cholesterol. Moreover, it was shown that PXR is activated by supraphysiological concentrations of bile acids. By comparing wild-type and

PXR-null mice, the effects on gene expression were confirmed to be PXR-dependent, and PCN was shown to protect from lithocholic acid-mediated hepatotoxicity in a PXR-dependent manner (Staudinger et al. 2001). These authors therefore proposed that PXR serves as a sensor of lithocholic acid and mediates gene expression changes to reduce concentrations of the potentially toxic bile acids, and hence protects against liver toxicity. Further studies utilizing both PXR-null and hPXR transgenic mice confirmed the results of Staudinger et al., and also showed that expression of a constitutively active hPXR protected mice from lithocholic acid-induced liver injury (Xie et al. 2001). Subsequent investigations have also demonstrated a critical role for PXR in the response to excess cholesterol and cholesterol metabolites (Sonoda et al. 2005). When fed a diet rich in cholesterol and cholic acid, PXR-null mice exhibited hepatorenal failure, whereas the same diet was well-tolerated in wild-type mice. Taken together, these studies exemplify that in addition to responding to and enhancing detoxification of drugs and xenobiotics, PXR also plays a key role in detoxification of endogenous metabolic intermediates.

A role for nuclear receptor activation and enzyme induction in detoxification of endogenous compounds is not limited to PXR. The related receptor CAR has been shown to be involved in the induction of metabolic enzymes involved in the conjugation and excretion of bilirubin (Huang et al. 2003). The potent mouse CAR agonist TCPOBOP induced hepatic expression of known components of the bilirubin clearance pathway – UGT1A1, MRP2, SLC21A6, GSTA1, and GSTA2 – in wild-type but not CAR-null mice. In addition, wild-type mice respond to hyperbilirubinemia by increasing bilirubin clearance, whereas CAR-null mice were deficient in this important protective response (Huang et al. 2003). These valuable studies now provide mechanistic insight into phenobarbital therapy for hyperbilirubinemia, a treatment that has been used for many years, but had previously been mechanistically not well understood.

More recently, there is evidence that PXR activation has protective effects beyond that of induction of proteins involved in metabolism/excretion. Recent evidence demonstrates that PXR activation affects expression of numerous genes involved in cell cycle and repair, such as growth arrest and DNA damage-inducible 45β (Gadd45β) and suppression of tumorigenicity 5 (St5) (Guzelian et al. 2006). These data support the notion that activation of PXR initiates a protective response that extends beyond metabolism.

4.5.3. ARE Inducers and Nrf2 Pathway in Detoxification and Chemoprevention

One of the quintessential examples of the critical role of induction of drug-metabolizing enzymes in detoxification is that of the antioxidant-responsive Nrf2 pathway. Compounds that induce this pathway include chemopreventive agents, antioxidants, and reactive-oxygen species (ROS), for example, sulforaphane, tBHQ, and H_2O_2. Activation of the antioxidant response via the transcription factor Nrf2 results in increased expression of a plethora of cytoprotective factors, including phase II drug-metabolizing enzymes (GSTs, NQO1), epoxide hydrolase, glutathione synthetic enzymes, heat shock proteins, NADPH-regenerating enzymes, and enzymes involved in the ubiquitin-mediated degradation pathway (Thimmulappa et al. 2002; Kwak et al. 2003).

The importance of the Nrf2 pathway to the detoxification response is exemplified in studies using Nrf2 knockout mice. These mice have lower basal expression and lack of inducibility of key phase II enzymes, resulting in increased sensitivity to toxins and carcinogens. For example, Nrf2-null mice are more sensitive to benz(a)pyrene-induced gastric neoplasia and *N*-nitrosobutyl(4-hydroxybutyl)amine-induced bladder carcinoma (Ramos-Gomez et al. 2001; Iida et al. 2004). Not only are the Nrf2-null mice more sensitive to carcinogenic agents, but the chemoprotective effects of ARE inducers, such as oltipraz, are lost in these mice. Nrf2-null mice are also more sensitive to acute toxin treatment and oxidative stressors, such as acetaminophen, cigarette smoke, and hyperoxia (Chan, Han and Kan 2001; Enomoto et al. 2001; Cho et al. 2002; Rangasamy et al. 2004). Very recent studies have demonstrated a protective role for Nrf2 in the presence of elevated levels of ROS due to CYP2E1 (Gong and Cederbaum 2006). These studies showed that induction of CYP2E1 by ethanol treatment resulted in increased Nrf2. This appeared to be part of a protective response; blocking Nrf2 resulted in increased ROS and decreased glutathione in cells overexpressing CYP2E1. Taken together, it is clear that the activation of ARE-containing genes through Nrf2 is a critical cytoprotective mechanism that results in detoxification of numerous ROS- and electrophile-producing compounds.

4.5.4. Consequences of Enzyme Induction on the Bioactivation of Acetaminophen

Acetaminophen is a classic example of a compound that is bioactivated by CYP metabolism to form a reactive metabolite capable of causing toxicity. Much research has focused on the mechanisms of acetaminophen bioactivation and toxicity, particularly hepatotoxicity, and the reader is referred to several excellent reviews on this topic (James, Mayeux and Hinson 2003; Hinson et al. 2004; Park et al. 2005). It is within the scope of this chapter to discuss enzyme induction and acetaminophen bioactivation, and review recent evidence pointing to roles for multiple induction processes.

Acetaminophen is a widely used over-the-counter analgesic drug that is metabolized by a combination of sulfation, glucuronidation, and CYP-mediated oxidation (Figure 4.4). The sulfation and glucuronidation reactions are considered detoxification pathways, and result in excretion of conjugated acetaminophen (James, Mayeux and Hinson 2003). The CYP oxidation pathway yields the reactive metabolite NAPQI, and hence is considered a bioactivation pathway (Dahlin et al. 1984). At therapeutic concentrations of acetaminophen, most metabolism is thought to occur through the phase II (conjugation) routes; however, at high acetaminophen concentrations, these conjugation pathways can become saturated and cofactors depleted, sending more compound through the CYP oxidation pathway (Park et al. 2005).

The metabolism of acetaminophen to NAPQI can be catalyzed by CYP2E1, CYP1A2, and CYP3A4 (Raucy et al. 1989; Thummel et al.

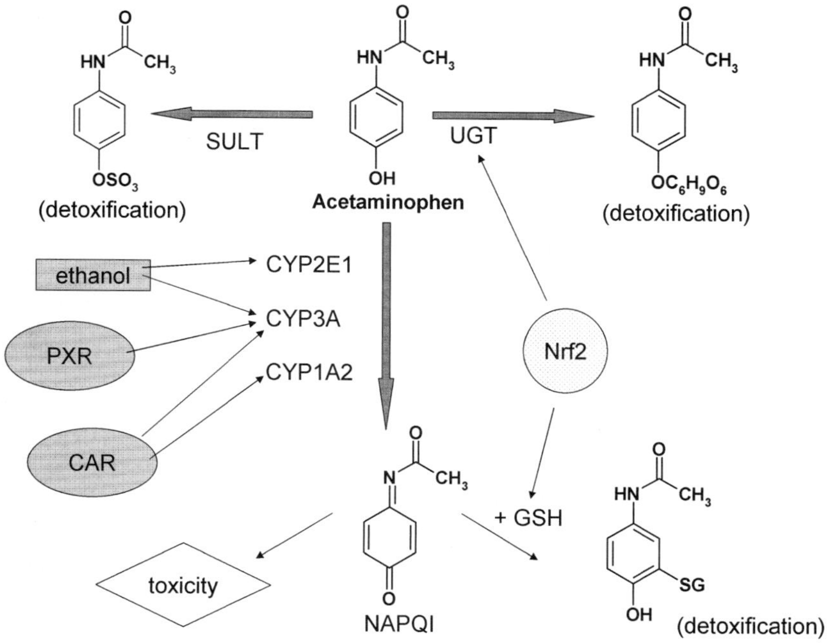

Figure 4.4 Potential effects of enzyme induction pathways on acetaminophen bioactivation and detoxification. Acetaminophen is metabolized by sulfation, glucuronidation, and CYP oxidation. The sulfation and glucuronidation pathways are considered detoxification routes, while the CYP oxidation pathway generates NAPQI, a reactive and toxic species. Ethanol has been shown to enhance the toxicity of acetaminophen in rodents and humans, presumably through CYP2E1 and/or CYP3A induction, resulting in increased NAPQI formation. Activation of CAR or PXR has been shown to enhance acetaminophen toxicity in rodent studies, likely by way of CYP3A induction. Studies in Nrf2-null mice suggest that activation of Nrf2 ameliorates acetaminophen toxicity, presumably by increasing glutathione conjugation of NAPQI, and/or by induction of UGT and SULT activity leading to increased conjugation of acetaminophen.

1993). Therefore, any compound that induces one or more of these CYPs could theoretically enhance the toxicity of acetaminophen. Indeed, there is strong evidence that treatment with ethanol enhances the hepatotoxicity of acetaminophen (Teschke, Stutz and Strohmeyer 1979; McClain et al. 1980). This effect is thought to be due to CYP2E1 induction, but recent evidence suggests that ethanol can also induce CYP3A forms, which could also contribute to the enhanced toxicity effect (Kostrubsky et al. 1997). PCN, a PXR activator and inducer of CYP3A in rodents, also potentiates the hepatotoxic effect of acetaminophen in mice, and is thought to be due to PXR-dependent induction of Cyp3a-mediated bioactivation (Guo et al. 2004). Phenobarbital and TCPOBOP treatments also enhance the hepatotoxicity of acetaminophen in mice (Mitchell et al. 1973; Zhang et al. 2002). Studies in knockout mice demonstrated that this effect was CAR-dependent and apparently involved Cyp1a2 and Cyp3a11, but not Cyp2e1 modulation by CAR (Zhang et al. 2002).

There is also evidence in the literature to suggest that some induction pathways can ameliorate the toxicity of acetaminophen. Since the reactive species NAPQI can be detoxified by conjugation with glutathione (Albano et al. 1985), inducers that affect GST activity or glutathione synthesis could affect acetaminophen-mediated toxicity. Indeed, mice that are deficient in Nrf2, a transcription factor involved in regulation of glutathione biosynthetic enzymes, as well as some UGTs and GSTs (see Section 4.3.5), are much more sensitive to acetaminophen hepatotoxicity than wild-type mice (Chan et al. 2001; Enomoto et al. 2001). This suggests the possibility that ARE-type inducers, which activate Nrf2, could have a protective effect against acetaminophen toxicity.

The studies outlined above clearly support the notion that induction of CYP2E1, CYP1A2, and/or CYP3A results in increased hepatotoxicity of acetaminophen in rodents, and that activation of the Nrf2 pathway could ameliorate this toxicity. However, how each of these induction pathways may or may not contribute to acetaminophen toxicity in humans is less clear. There is ample evidence that alcohol consumption can enhance the hepatotoxicity of acetaminophen in humans (McClain et al. 1980; Zimmerman and Maddrey 1995), but the importance of the other induction pathways (PXR, CAR, and Nrf2) in bioactivation or detoxification of acetaminophen in humans remains to be demonstrated.

4.5.5. Consequences of CYP3A Induction by Troglitazone

Troglitazone is an example of a compound for which enzyme induction has been implicated as a causal factor in the development of hepatotoxicity (Kassahun et al. 2001). Troglitazone was the first of the thiazolidinedione class of PPARγ agonists, and was used as an insulin-sensitizing agent for the treatment of type 2 diabetes. Troglitazone was associated with rare instances of severe liver injury, and was withdrawn from the market in 2000. Since that time, there have been numerous studies aimed at identifying the cause of the liver injury associated with troglitazone. Since it is beyond the scope of this chapter to examine all potential mechanisms of troglitazone hepatotoxicity, the reader is referred to several reviews on the topic (Smith 2003; Chojkier 2005; Hastings 2006; Masubuchi 2006). It is within the scope of this chapter to examine the role of enzyme induction in troglitazone hepatotoxicity, and to review available evidence both for and against a role for enzyme induction in bioactivation and hepatotoxicity of troglitazone.

Troglitazone was first suspected of being a CYP3A inducer based on increases in 6β-hydroxy cortisol/cortisol ratios in clinical studies (Koup, Anderson and Loi 1998), and was later found to cause drug–drug interaction with other CYP3A substrates (Loi et al. 1999). Troglitazone was then identified as a CYP3A inducer using primary human hepatocytes (Ramachandran et al. 1999). Further studies using primary human hepatocytes revealed that not only troglitazone, but also the structurally related compounds rosiglitazone and pioglitazone were capable of inducing CYP3A in primary hepatocytes (Sahi et al. 2003), and activating PXR in cell culture (Sinz et al. 2006). While all three thiazolidinediones induce CYP3A in vitro, only troglitazone caused CYP3A induction in vivo. It appears that the three thiazolidinediones have similar potency against PXR, and cause similar degree of upregulation of CYP3A protein in vitro (Sahi et al. 2003; Ripp et al. 2006). The fact that only troglitazone causes induction in vivo is readily explained by the difference in dose and exposure among the three compounds. Troglitazone was used clinically at doses ranging from 200 mg to 600 mg per day, whereas pioglitazone and rosiglitazone are given at doses of 15–45 mg and 2–8 mg per day, respectively. The free plasma levels that would be expected to correlate with drug available for binding and activating PXR are much higher for troglitazone than for the other two thiazolidinediones. Note that troglitazone is often referred to as a "potent inducer," compared to rosiglitazone and pioglitazone; however, this is actually a misstatement in that the pharmacological potency of all three compounds for PXR is similar, it is instead the in vivo exposures that differ (Smith et al. 2007).

In humans, troglitazone is metabolized by sulfation, glucuronidation, and CYP oxidation, the latter pathway leading to formation of a quinone metabolite (Loi et al. 1999; Smith 2003; Figure 4.5). The sulfate conjugate (M1) and the quinone metabolite (M3) are the most abundant circulating metabolites in humans, and are present at levels greater than or equal to levels of the parent (Loi et al. 1999). Troglitazone is metabolized in human liver microsomes to M3, and a number of additional reactive metabolites that can be trapped by glutathione (Kassahun et al. 2001). Metabolism to M3 can be catalyzed by a number of different CYP isoforms, with CYP3A4 and CYP2C8 isoforms thought to be the predominant ones (Yamazaki et al. 1999). Several investigators have hypothesized that the ability of troglitazone to induce its own metabolism to reactive metabolites is one of the factors contributing to the idiosyncratic hepatotoxicity incidence with this compound (Kassahun et al. 2001; Hastings 2006). Although this is a reasonable hypothesis, it does not appear to be supported by available data. Perhaps the most compelling evidence against this hypothesis is that in humans, troglitazone does not appear to induce

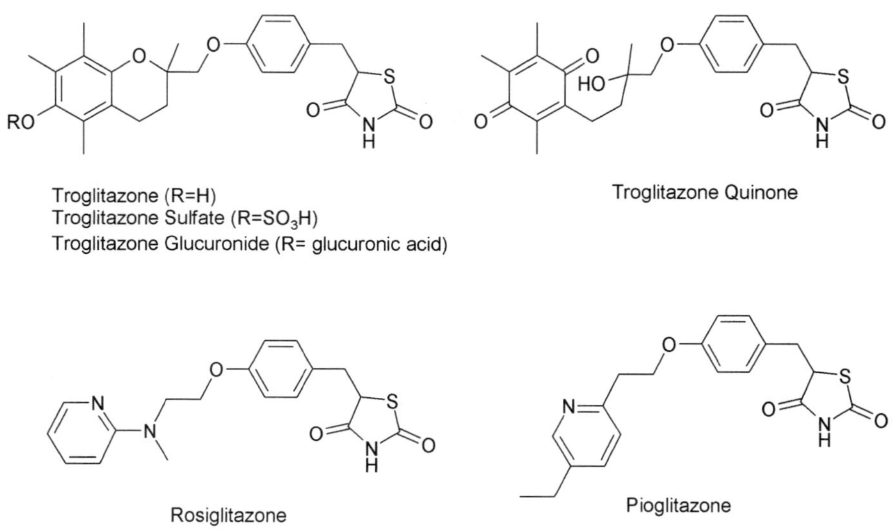

Figure 4.5 Structures of troglitazone and metabolites, rosiglitazone, and pioglitazone.

its own metabolism. If induction contributed to increased metabolism and generation of reactive metabolites in humans, then upon multiple doses steady-state levels of troglitazone should decrease, and levels of metabolites should increase. However, steady-state exposures of troglitazone M1 and M3 were similar after single-dose or multiple-dose administration (Loi et al. 1999). Therefore, even though troglitazone treatment was shown to cause CYP3A4 induction in vivo using prototypical substrates, it does not appear to induce its own metabolism. One possible explanation for this is that M3 formation in vivo is catalyzed by a CYP form other than CYP3A4.

A study by Tettey et al. (2001) specifically examined the toxicity of the quinone metabolite of troglitazone in both rat and human hepatocytes, and found that the quinone metabolite was actually less cytotoxic than the parent troglitazone in both systems. In addition, induction of CYP3A in rat hepatocytes resulted in increased formation of glutathione adducts, but produced only a marginal, but not statistically significant, increase in the toxicity of troglitazone (Tettey et al. 2001). Hewitt et al. examined the correlation between expression of drug-metabolizing activities and cytotoxicity of troglitazone in human hepatocytes, and found that there was no link between increased metabolic activity and increased toxicity. In fact, hepatocytes with higher levels of CYP3A and glucuronidation activities showed less sensitivity to troglitazone cytotoxicity (Hewitt et al. 2002).

Taken together, the currently available data suggest that enzyme induction does not contribute to the hepatotoxicity of troglitazone. There are other proposed mechanisms for the hepatotoxicity of troglitazone for which the data are more convincing, including inhibition of hepatic transporters resulting in accumulation of bile acids and bilirubin, and/or initiation of mitochondrial injury (Smith 2003; Hastings 2006; Masubuchi 2006).

4.5.6. Enhancement of Cocaine Bioactivation by Phenobarbital-Like Inducers

It has been known for sometime that the hepatotoxicity of cocaine is enhanced by phenobarbital pretreatment, both in vitro and in vivo (Boelsterli and Goldlin 1991). Several investigators have studied the relationship between induction and cocaine hepatotoxicity and the findings provide a nice illustration of the complexity of induction as a detoxification versus a bioactivation event (Boelsterli and Goldlin 1991; Bornheim 1998; Wei et al. 2000). In rats, cocaine is metabolized by CYP2B1 to the N-demethylated metabolite. Induction of CYP2B1 by phenobarbital enhances metabolism and hepatotoxicity, both in vitro and in vivo, and inhibition of CYP2B1 acts conversely (Boelsterli et al. 1992). However, in mice and humans, metabolism of cocaine is mediated by CYP3A and CYP2B forms (Pasanen et al. 1995). In mouse studies, phenobarbital pretreatment induces both CYP3A and CYP2B forms, and enhances cocaine hepatotoxicity. However, dexamethasone pretreatment also induces CYP3A and CYP2B forms to a similar extent as phenobarbital, yet dexamethasone does not potentiate hepatotoxicity (Bornheim 1998).

One plausible explanation for these seemingly conflicting results is that dexamethasone induces liver esterases in addition to CYP3A and CYP2B, resulting in rapid conversion of cocaine to a nonhepatotoxic metabolite. Phenobarbital induction does not show this marked induction of liver esterase activity (Bornheim 1998). This cocaine hepatotoxicity example illustrates the importance of recognizing that typical enzyme inducers increase expression of numerous target genes, and therefore multiple clearance mechanisms need to be considered when deciding whether activation of a given induction pathway will produce overall increase or decrease in bioactivation.

4.6. Conclusions

Ever since the 1950s, and the initial observations that exposure to certain chemicals could increase the activity of drug-metabolizing enzymes, understanding of the mechanisms and consequences of enzyme induction has advanced considerably. The identification of ligand-activated transcription factors, AhR, PXR, CAR, and others, have enabled the facile identification of compounds that activate the various enzyme induction pathways. Advances in gene expression techniques have enabled the identification of target genes and pathways, and the development of transgenic and knockout mouse lines have helped clarify the role of different receptors and enzymes in these pathways. The physiological consequences of enzyme induction remain an area of much interest and debate. Enzyme induction can be considered an adaptive response to chemical exposure that enhances clearance and detoxification, or a maladaptive response leading to bioactivation and enhanced toxicity. Whether the consequences of enzyme induction by any particular compound is on balance a detoxification event versus a bioactivation event cannot necessarily be predicted by in vitro assays, since these are typically focused on only a subset of affected pathways. Predicting outcome requires an understanding of all affected pathways, and their tissue-specific and compound-specific considerations. Therefore enzyme induction is sure to continue to be the subject of many more years of engaging research.

References

Albano, E., Rundgren, M., Harvison, P. J., Nelson, S. D., and Moldeus, P. 1985. Mechanisms of *N*-acetyl-*p*-benzoquinone imine cytotoxicity. Mol. Pharmacol. 28:306–311.

Aninat, C., Piton, A., Glaise, D., Le Charpentier, T., Langouet, S., Morel, F., Guguen-Guillouzo, C., and Guillouzo, A. 2006. Expression Of cytochromes P450, conjugating enzymes and nuclear receptors in human hepatoma HepaRG cells. Drug Metab. Dispos. 34:75–83.

Bertilsson, G., Heidrich, J., Svensson, K., Asman, M., Jendeberg, L., Sydow-Backman, M., Ohlsson, R., Postlind, H., Blomquist, P., and Berkenstam, A. 1998. Identification of a human nuclear receptor defines a new signaling pathway for CYP3A induction. Proc. Natl. Acad. Sci. USA 95:12208–12213.

Blumberg, B., Sabbagh Jr., W., Juguilon, H., Bolado Jr., J., van Meter, C. M., Ong, E. S., and Evans, R. M. 1998. SXR, a novel steroid and xenobiotic-sensing nuclear receptor. Genes Dev. 12:3195–3205.

Boelsterli, U. A., and Goldlin, C. 1991. Biomechanisms of cocaine-induced hepatocyte injury mediated by the formation of reactive metabolites. Arch. of Toxicol. 65:351–360.

Boelsterli, U. A., Lanzotti, A., Goldlin, C., and Oertle, M. 1992. Identification of cytochrome P-450IIB1 as a cocaine-bioactivating isoform in rat hepatic microsomes and in cultured rat hepatocytes. Drug Metab. Dispos. 20:96–101.

Bornheim, L. 1998. Effect of cytochrome P450 inducers on cocaine-mediated hepatotoxicity. Toxicol. Appl. Pharmacol. 150:158–165.

Brown, R. R., Miller, J. A., and Miller, E. C. 1954. The metabolism of methylated aminoazo dyes. IV. Dietary factors enhancing demethylation in vitro. J. Biol. Chem. 209:211–222.

Castell, J. V., Jover, R., Martinez-Jimenez, C. P., and Gomez-Lechon, M. 2006. Hepatocyte cell lines: their use, scope and limitations in drug metabolism studies. Expert Opin. Drug Metab. Toxicol. 2:183–212.

Chan, K., Han, X.-D., and Kan, Y. W. 2001. An important function of Nrf2 in combating oxidative stress: Detoxification of acetaminophen. Proc. Natl. Acad. Sci. USA 98:4611–4616.

Cho, H.-Y., Jedlicka, A. E., Reddy, S. P. M., Kensler, T. W., Yamamoto, M., Zhang, L.-Y., and Kleeberger, S. R. 2002. Role of NRF2 in protection against hyperoxic lung injury in mice. Am. J. Respir. Cell Mol. Biol. 26:175–182.

Chojkier, M. 2005. Troglitazone and liver injury: In search of answers. Hepatology 41:237–246.

Ciolino, H. P., Daschner, P. J., and Yeh, G. C. 1998. Resveratrol inhibits transcription of CYP1A1 in vitro by preventing activation of the aryl hydrocarbon receptor. Cancer Res. 58:5707–5712.

Conney, A. H. 1967. Pharmacological implications of microsomal enzyme induction. Pharmacol. Rev. 19:317–366.

Cullinan, S. B., Zhang, D., Hannink, M., Arvisais, E., Kaufman, R. J., and Diehl, J. A. 2003. Nrf2 is a direct PERK substrate and effector of PERK-dependent cell survival. Mol. Cell. Biol. 23:7198–7209.

Dahlin, D. C., Miwa, G. T., Lu, A. Y. H., and Nelson, S. D. 1984. *N*-acetyl-*p*-benzoquinone imine: A cytochrome P450-mediated oxidation product of acetaminophen. Proc. Natl. Acad. Sci. USA 81:1327–1331.

Denison, M. S., and Nagy, S. R. 2003. Activation of the aryl hydrocarbon receptor by structurally diverse exogenous and endogenous chemicals. Ann. Rev. Pharmacol. Toxicol. 43:309–334.

Ding, X., Lichti, K., Kim, I., Gonzalez, F. J., and Staudinger, J. L. 2006. Regulation of constitutive androstane receptor and its target genes by fasting, cAMP, hepatocyte nuclear factor {alpha}, and the coactivator peroxisome proliferator-activated receptor {gamma} coactivator-1{alpha}. J. Biol. Chem. 281:26540–26551.

Dinkova-Kostova, A. T., Holtzclaw, W. D., Cole, R. N., Itoh, K., Wakabayashi, N., Katoh, Y., Yamamoto, M., and Talalay, P. 2002. Direct evidence that sulfhydryl groups of Keap1 are the sensors regulating induction of phase 2 enzymes that protect against carcinogens and oxidants. Proc. Natl. Acad. Sci. USA 99:11908–11913.

Drocourt, L., Ourlin, J.-C., Pascussi, J.-M., Maurel, P., and Vilarem, M.-J. 2002. Expression of CYP3A4, CYP2B6, and CYP2C9 is regulated by the vitamin D receptor pathway in primary human hepatocytes. J. Biol. Chem. 277:25125–25132.

Enomoto, A., Itoh, K., Nagayoshi, E., Haruta, J., Kimura, T., O'Connor, T., Harada, T., and Yamamoto, M. 2001. High sensitivity of Nrf2 knockout mice to acetaminophen hepatotoxicity associated with decreased expression of ARE-regulated drug metabolizing enzymes and antioxidant genes. Toxicol. Sci. 59:169–177.

Fernandez-Salguero, P., Pineau, T., Hilbert, D. M., McPhail, T., Lee, S. S., Kimura, S., Nebert, D. W., Rudikoff, S., Ward, J. M., and Gonzalez, F. J. 1995. Immune system impairment and hepatic fibrosis in mice lacking the dioxin-binding Ah receptor. Science 268:722–726.

Forman, B. M., Tzameli, I., Choi, H.-S., Chen, J., Simha. D., Seol, W., Evans, R. M., and Moore, D. D. 1998. Androstane metabolites bind to and deactivate the nuclear receptor CAR-[beta]. Nature 395:612–615.

Galvan, N., Jaskula-Sztul, R., MacWilliams, P. S., Czuprynski, C. J., and Jefcoate, C. R. 2003. Bone marrow cytotoxicity of benzo[a]pyrene is dependent on CYP1B1 but is diminished by Ah receptor-mediated induction of CYP1A1 in liver. Toxicol. Appl. Pharmacol. 193:84–96.

Germain, P., Staels, B., Dacquet, C., Spedding, M., and Laudet, V. 2006. Overview of nomenclature of nuclear receptors. Pharmacol. Rev. 58:685–704.

Gong, P., and Cederbaum, A. I. 2006. Nrf2 is increased by CYP2E1 in rodent liver and HepG2 cells and protects against oxidative stress caused by CYP2E1. Hepatology 43:144–153.

Gonzalez, F. J. 2007. CYP2E1. Drug Metab. Dispos. 35:1–8.

Guillouzo, A., Corlu, A., Aninat, C., Glaise, D., Morel, F., and Guguen-Guillouzo, C. 2007. The human hepatoma HepaRG cells: A highly differentiated model for studies of liver metabolism and toxicity of xenobiotics. Chem.-Biol. Interact. 168:66–73.

Guo, G. L., Moffit, J. S., Nicol, C. J., Ward, J. M., Aleksunes, L. A., Slitt, A. L., Kliewer, S. A., Manautou, J. E., and Gonzalez, F. J. 2004. Enhanced acetaminophen toxicity by activation of the pregnane X receptor. Toxicol. Sci. 82:374–380.

Guzelian, J., Barwick, J. L., Hunter, L., Phang, T. L., Quattrochi, L. C., and Guzelian, P. S. 2006. Identification of genes controlled by the pregnane X receptor by microarray analysis of mRNAs from pregnenolone 16{alpha}-carbonitrile-treated rats. Toxicol. Sci. 94:379–387.

Hankinson, O. 2005. Role of coactivators in transcriptional activation by the aryl hydrocarbon receptor. Arch. Biochem. Biophys. 433:379–386.

Hanlon, P. R., Zheng, W., Ko, A. Y., and Jefcoate, C. R. 2005. Identification of novel TCDD-regulated genes by microarray analysis. Toxicol. Appl. Pharmacol. 202:215–228.

Hastings, K. L. 2006. The use of hepatotoxic signals to predict the safety of peroxisome proliferator-activated receptor agonists. Expert Opinion on Drug Metab. Toxicol. 2:489–492.

Heidel, S. M., MacWilliams, P. S., Baird, W. M., Dashwood, W. M., Buters, J. T. M., Gonzalez, F. J., Larsen, M. C., Czuprynski, C. J., and Jefcoate, C. R. 2000. Cytochrome P4501B1 mediates induction of bone marrow cytotoxicity and preleukemia cells in mice treated with 7,12-dimethylbenz[a]anthracene. Cancer Res. 60:3454–3460.

Hewitt, N. J., Lloyd, S., Hayden, M., Butler, R., Sakai, Y., Springer, R., Fackett, A., and Li, A P. 2002. Correlation between troglitazone cytotoxicity and drug metabolic enzyme activities in cryopreserved human hepatocytes. Chem. Biol. Interact. 142:73–82.

Hinson, J. A., Reid, A. B., McCullough, S. S., and James, L. P. 2004. Acetaminophen-induced hepatotoxicity: Role of metabolic activation, reactive oxygen/

nitrogen species, and mitochondrial permeability transition. Drug Metab. Rev. 36:805–822.

Hoensch, H. P., Balzer, K., Dylewizc, P., Kirch, W., Goebell, H., and Ohnhaus, E. E. 1985. Effect of rifampicin treatment on hepatic drug metabolism and serum bile acids in patients with primary biliary cirrhosis. Eur. J. Clin. Pharmacol. 28:475–477.

Honkakoski, P., Zelko, I., Sueyoshi, T., and Negishi, M. 1998. The nuclear orphan receptor CAR-retinoid X receptor heterodimer activates the phenobarbital-responsive enhancer module of the CYP2B gene. Mol. Cell. Biol. 18:5652–5658.

Huang, H. C., Nguyen, T., and Pickett, C. B. 2000. Regulation of the antioxidant response element by protein kinase C-mediated phosphorylation of NF-E2-related factor 2. Proc. Natl. Acad. Sci. USA 97:12475–12480.

Huang, W., Zhang, J., Chua, S. S., Qatanani, M., Han, Y., Granata, R., and Moore, D. D. 2003. Induction of bilirubin clearance by the constitutive androstane receptor (CAR). Proc. Natl. Acad. Sci. USA 100:4156–4161.

Huang, W., Zhang, J., Washington, M., Liu, J., Parant, J. M., Lozano, G., and Moore, D. D. 2005 Xenobiotic stress induces hepatomegaly and liver tumors via the nuclear receptor constitutive androstane receptor. Mol. Endocrinol. 19:1646–1653.

Huang, H., Wang, H., Sinz, M., Zoeckler, M., Staudinger, J., Redinbo, M. R., Teotico, D. G., Locker, J., Kalpana, G. V., and Mani, S. 2007. Inhibition of drug metabolism by blocking the activation of nuclear receptors by ketoconazole. Oncogene 26:258–268.

Iida, K., Itoh, K., Kumagai, Y., Oyasu, R., Hattori, K., Kawai, K., Shimazui, T., Akaza, H., and Yamamoto, M. 2004. Nrf2 is essential for the chemopreventive efficacy of oltipraz against urinary bladder carcinogenesis. Cancer Res. 64:6424–6431.

Ioannides, C., and Parke, D. V. 1993. Induction of cytochrome P4501 as an indicator of potential chemical carcinogenesis. Drug Metab. Rev. 25:485–501.

Issemann, I., and Green S. 1990. Activation of a member of the steroid hormone receptor superfamily by peroxisome proliferators. Nature 347:645–650.

Itoh, K., Chiba,T., Takahashi, S., Ishii, T., Igarashi, K., Katoh, Y., Oyake, T., Hayashi, N., Satoh, K., Hatayama, I., Yamamoto, M., and Nabeshima, Y.-I. 1997. An Nrf2/small Maf heterodimer mediates the induction of phase II detoxifying enzyme genes through antioxidant response elements. Biochem. Biophys. Res. Commun. 236:313–322.

Itoh, K., Wakabayashi, N., Katoh, Y., Ishii, T., Igarashi, K., Engel, J. D., and Yamamoto, M. 1999. Keap1 represses nuclear activation of antioxidant responsive elements by Nrf2 through binding to the amino-terminal Neh2 domain. Genes Dev. 13:76–86.

James, L. P., Mayeux, P. R., and Hinson, J. A. 2003. Acetaminophen-induced hepatotoxicity. Drug Metab. Dispos. 31:1499–1506.

Javor, T., Gogl, A., Horvath, T., and Tenyi, I. 1973. Effects of phenobarbital treatment on biliary excretion in man. Drug Metab. Dispos. 1:424–427.

Jones, S. A., Moore, L. B., Shenk, J. L., Wisely, G. B., Hamilton, G. A., McKee, D. D., Tomkinson, N. C. O., LeCluyse, E. L., Lambert, M. H., Willson, T. M., Kliewer, S. A., and Moore, J. T. 2000. The pregnane X receptor: A promiscuous xenobiotic receptor that has diverged during evolution. Mol. Endocrinol. 14:27–39.

Kassahun, K., Pearson, P. G., Tang, W., McIntosh, I., Leung, K., Elmore, C., Dean, D., Wang, R., Doss, G., and Baillie, T. A. 2001. Studies on the metabolism of troglitazone to reactive intermediates in vitro and in vivo. Evidence for novel

biotransformation pathways involving quinone methide formation and thiazolidinedione ring scission. Chem. Res. Toxicol. 14:62–70.
Kawamoto, T., Sueyoshi, T., Zelko, I., Moore, R., Washburn, K., and Negishi, M. 1999. Phenobarbital-responsive nuclear tanslocation of the receptor CAR in induction of the CYP2B gene. Mol. Cell. Biol. 19:6318–6322.
Kliewer, S. A., Goodwin, B., and Willson, T. M. 2002. The nuclear pregnane X receptor: A key regulator of xenobiotic metabolism. Endocr. Rev. 23:687–702.
Kliewer, S. A., Moore, J. T., Wade, L., Staudinger, J. L., Watson, M. A., Jones, S. A., McKee, D. D., Oliver, B. B., Willson, T. M., Zetterstrom, R. H., Perlmann, T., and Lehmann, J. M. 1998. An orphan nuclear receptor activated by pregnanes defines a novel steroid signaling pathway. Cell 92:73–82.
Kobayashi, K., Sueyoshi, T., Inoue, K., Moore, R., and Negishi, M. 2003. Cytoplasmic accumulation of the nuclear receptor CAR by a tetratricopeptide repeat protein in HepG2 cells. Mol. Pharmacol. 64:1069–1075.
Kobayashi, M., and Yamamoto, M. 2006. Nrf2-Keap1 regulation of cellular defense mechanisms against electrophiles and reactive oxygen species. Adv. Enzyme Regulation 46:113–140.
Koop, D. R., and Casazza, J. P. 1985. Identification of ethanol-inducible P-450 isozyme 3a as the acetone and acetol monooxygenase of rabbit microsomes. J. Biol. Chem. 260:13607–13612.
Kostrubsky, V. E., Szakacs, J. G., Jeffery, E. H., Wood, S. G., Bement, W. J., Wrighton, S. A., Sinclair, P. R., and Sinclair, J. F. 1997. Role of CYP3A in ethanol-mediated increases in acetaminophen hepatotoxicity. Toxicol. Appl. Pharmacol. 143:315–323.
Koup, J. R., Anderson, G. D., and Loi, C. M. 1998. Effect of troglitazone on urinary excretion of 6beta-hydroxycortisol. J. Clin. Pharmacol. 38:815–818.
Krey, G., Braissant, O., L'Horset, F., Kalkhoven, E., Perroud, M., Parker, M. G., and Wahli, W. 1997. Fatty acids, eicosanoids, and hypolipidemic agents identified as ligands of peroxisome proliferator-activated receptors by coactivator-dependent receptor ligand assay. Mol. Endocrinol. 11:779–791.
Kwak, M.-K., Wakabayashi, N., Itoh, K., Motohashi, H., Yamamoto, M., and Kensler, T. W. 2003. Modulation of gene expression by cancer chemopreventive dithiolethiones through the Keap1–Nrf2 pathway. Identification of novel gene clusters for cell survival. J. Biol. Chem. 278:8135–8145.
LeClusye, E., Madan, A., Hamilton, G., Carroll, K., DeHaan, R., and Parkinson, A. 2000. Expression and regulation of cytochrome P450 enzymes in primary cultures of human hepatocytes. J. Biochem. Mol. Toxicol. 14:177–188.
Lehmann, J. M., McKee, D. D., Watson, M. A., Willson, T. M., Moore, J. T., and Kliewer, S. A. 1998. The human orphan nuclear receptor PXR is activated by compounds that regulate CYP3A4 gene expression and cause drug interactions. J. Clin. Invest. 102:1016–1023.
Loi, C. M., Young, M., Randinitis, E., Vassos, A. B., and Koup, J. R. 1999. Clinical pharmacokinetics of troglitazone. Clin. Pharmacokinet. 37:91–104.
Luo, G., Cunningham, M., Kim, S., Burn, T., Lin, J., Sinz, M., Hamilton, G., Rizzo, C., Jolley, S., Gilbert, D., Downey, A., Mudra, D., Graham, R., Carroll, K., Xie, J., Madan, A., Parkinson, A., Christ, D., Selling, B., LeCluyse, E., and Gan, L.-S. 2002. CYP3A4 induction by drugs: Correlation between a pregnane X receptor reporter gene assay and CYP3A4 expression in human hepatocytes. Drug Metab. Dispos. 30:795–804.
Ma, X., Shah, Y., Cheung, C., Guo, G. L., Feigenbaum, L., Krausz, K. W., Idle, J. R., and Gonzalez, F. J. 2007. The pregnane X receptor gene-humanized mouse: A model for investigating drug–drug interactions mediated by cytochromes P450 3A. Drug Metab. Dispos. 35:194–200.

Maglich, J. M., Parks, D. J., Moore, L. B., Collins, J. L., Goodwin, B., Billin, A. N., Stoltz, C. A., Kliewer, S. A., Lambert, M. H., Willson, T. M., and Moore, J. T. 2003. Identification of a novel human constitutive androstane receptor (CAR) agonist and its use in the identification of CAR target genes. J. Biol. Chem. 278:17277–17283.
Maglich, J. M., Stoltz, C. M., Goodwin, B., Hawkins-Brown, D., Moore, J. T., and Kliewer, S. A. 2002. Nuclear pregnane X receptor and constitutive androstane receptor regulate overlapping but distinct sets of genes involved in xenobiotic detoxification. Mol. Pharmacol. 62:638–646.
Maglich, J. M., Watson, J., McMillen, P. J., Goodwin, B., Willson, T. M., and Moore, J. T. 2004. The nuclear receptor CAR is a regulator of thyroid hormone metabolism during caloric restriction. J. Biol. Chem. 279:19832–19838.
Makishima, M., Lu, T. T., Xie, W., Whitfield, G. K., Domoto, H., Evans, R. M., Haussler, M. R., and Mangelsdorf, D. J. 2002. Vitamin D receptor as an intestinal bile acid sensor. Science 296:1313–1316.
Makishima, M., Okamoto, A. Y., Repa, J. J., Tu, H., Learned, R. M., Luk, A., Hull, M. V., Lustig, K. D., Mangelsdorf, D. J., and Shan, B. 1999. Identification of a nuclear receptor for bile acids. Science 284:1362–1365.
Marlowe, J. L., and Puga, A. 2005. Aryl hydrocarbon receptor, cell cycle regulation, toxicity, and tumorigenesis. J. Cell. Biochem. 96:1174–1184.
Masubuchi, Y. 2006. Metabolic and nonmetabolic factors determining troglitazone hepatotoxicity: A review. Drug Metab. Pharmacokinet. 21:347–356.
McClain, C. J., Kromhout, J. P., Peterson, F. J., and Holtzman, J. L. 1980. Potentiation of acetaminophen hepatotoxicity by alcohol. JAMA 244:251–253.
McMillan, B. J., and Bradfield, C. A. 2007. The aryl hydrocarbon receptor is activated by modified low-density lipoprotein. Proc. Natl. Acad. Sci. USA 104:1412–1417.
Miller, E. C., Miller, J. A., and Hartmann, H. A. 1961. *N*-hydroxy-2-acetylaminofluorene: a metabolite of 2-acetylaminofluorene with increased carcinogenic activity in the rat. Cancer Res. 21:815–824.
Mills, J. B., Rose, K. A., Sadagopan, N., Sahi, J., and de Morais, S. M. F. 2004. Induction of drug metabolism enzymes and MDR1 using a novel human hepatocyte cell line. J. Pharmacol. Exp. Ther. 309:303–309.
Mitchell, J. R., Jollow, D. J., Potter, W. Z., Davis, D. C., Gillette, J. R., and Brodie, B. B. 1973. Acetaminophen-induced hepatic necrosis. I. Role of drug metabolism. J. Pharmacol. Exp. Ther. 187:185–194.
Moore, L. B., Parks, D. J., Jones, S. A., Bledsoe, R. K., Consler, T. G., Stimmel, J. B., Goodwin, B., Liddle, C., Blanchard, S. G., Willson, T. M., Collins, J. L., and Kliewer, S. A. 2000. Orphan nuclear receptors constitutive androstane receptor and pregnane X receptor share xenobiotic and steroid ligands. J. Biol. Chem. 275:15122–15127.
Nebert, D. W. 1989. The Ah locus: Genetic differences in toxicity, cancer, mutation, and birth defects. Crit. Rev. Toxicol. 20:153–174.
Nebert, D. W., Dalton, T. P., Okey, A. B., and Gonzalez, F. J. 2004. Role of aryl hydrocarbon receptor-mediated induction of the CYP1 enzymes in environmental toxicity and cancer. J. Biol. Chem. 279:23847–23850.
Nguyen, T., Yang, C. S., and Pickett, C. B. 2004. The pathways and molecular mechanisms regulating Nrf2 activation in response to chemical stress. Free Rad. Biol. Med. 37:433–441.
Niwa, A., Kumaki, K., Nebert, D.W., and Poland, A. P. 1975. Genetic expression of aryl hydrocarbon hydroxylase activity in the mouse. Distinction between the "responsive" homozygote and heterozygote at the Ah locus. Arch. Biochem. Biophys. 166:559–564.
Omura, T., and Sato, R. 1962. A new cytochrome in liver microsomes. J. Biol. Chem. 237:PC1375–1376.

Park, B. K., Kitteringham, N. R., Maggs, J. L., Pirmohamed, M., and Williams, D. P. 2005. The role of metabolic activation in drug-induced hepatotoxicity. Ann. Rev. Pharmacol. Toxicol. 45:177–202.

Parkinson, A., and Hurwitz, A. 1991. Omeprazole and the induction of human cytochrome P-450: a response to concerns about potential adverse effects. Gastroenterology 100:1157–1164.

Parks, D. J., Blanchard, S. G., Bledsoe, R. K., Chandra, G., Consler, T. G., Kliewer, S. A., Stimmel, J. B., Willson, T. M., Zavacki, A. M., Moore, D. D., and Lehmann, J. M. 1999. Bile acids: Natural ligands for an orphan nuclear receptor. Science 284:1365–1368.

Pasanen, M., Pellinen, P., Stenback, F., Juvonen, R. O., Raunio, H., and Pelkonen, O. 1995. The role of CYP enzymes in cocaine-induced liver damage. Arch. Toxicol. 69:287–290.

Peet, D. J., Turley, S. D., Ma, W., Janowski, B. A., Lobaccaro, J.-M. A., Hammer, R. E., and Mangelsdorf, D. J. 1998. Cholesterol and bile acid metabolism are impaired in mice lacking the nuclear oxysterol receptor LXR[alpha]. Cell 93:693–704.

Poland, A., Glover, E., and Kende, E.S. 1976. Stereospecific, high affinity binding of 2,3,7,8-tetrachlorodibenzo-p-doxin by hepatic cytosol. Evidence that the binding species is receptor for induction of aryl hydrocarbon hydroxylase. J. Biol. Chem. 251:4936–4946.

Poso, A., and Honkakoski, P. 2006. Ligand recognition by drug-activated nuclear receptors PXR and CAR: structural, site-directed mutagenesis and molecular modeling studies. Mini-Rev. Med. Chem. 6:937–943.

Rae, J. M., Johnson, M. D., Lippman, M. E., and Flockhart, D. A. 2001. Rifampin is a selective, pleiotropic inducer of drug metabolism genes in human hepatocytes: Studies with cDNA and oligonucleotide expression arrays. J. Pharmacol. Exp. Ther. 299:849–857.

Ramachandran, V., Kostrubsky, V. E., Komoroski, B. J., Zhang, S., Dorko, K., Esplen, J. E., Strom, S. C., and Venkataramanan, R. 1999. Troglitazone increases cytochrome P-450 3A protein and activity in primary cultures of human hepatocytes. Drug Metab. Dispos. 27:1194–1199.

Ramos-Gomez, M., Kwak, M.-K., Dolan, P. M., Itoh, K., Yamamoto, M., Talalay, P., and Kensler, T. W. 2001. Sensitivity to carcinogenesis is increased and chemoprotective efficacy of enzyme inducers is lost in nrf2 transcription factor-deficient mice. Proc. Natl. Acad. Sci. USA 98:3410–3415.

Rangasamy, T., Cho, C. Y., Thimmulappa, R. K., Zhen, L., Srisuma, S. S., Kensler, T. W., Yamamoto, M., Petrache, I., Tuder, R. M., and Biswal, S. 2004. Genetic ablation of Nrf2 enhances susceptibility to cigarette smoke-induced emphysema in mice. J. Clin. Invest. 114:1248–1259.

Raucy, J. L., Lasker, J. M., Lieber, C. S., and Black, M. 1989. Acetaminophen activation by human liver cytochromes P450IIE1 and P450IA2. Arch. Biochem. Biophys 271:270–283.

Rencurel, F., Foretz, M., Kaufmann, M. R., Stroka, D., Looser, R., Leclerc, I., da Silva Xavier, G., Rutter, G. A., Viollet, B., and Meyer, U. A. 2006. Stimulation of AMP-activated protein kinase is essential for the induction of drug metabolizing enzymes by phenobarbital in human and mouse liver. Mol. Pharmacol. 70:1925–1934.

Reschly, E. J., and Krasowski, M. D. 2006. Evolution and function of the NR1I nuclear hormone receptor subfamily (VDR, PXR, and CAR) with respect to metabolism of xenobiotics and endogenous compounds. Curr. Drug Metab. 7:349–365.

Riddick, D. S., Lee, C., Bhathena, A., and Timsit, Y. E. 2003. The 2001Veylien Henderson Award of the Society of Toxicology of Canada. Positive and negative

transcriptional regulation of cytochromes P450 by polycyclic aromatic hydrocarbons. Can. J. Physiol. Pharmacol. 81:59–77.
Rifkind, A. B. 2006. CYP1A in TCDD toxicity and in physiology – with particular reference to CYP dependent arachidonic acid metabolism and other endogenous substrates. Drug Metab. Rev. 38:291–335.
Ripp, S. L., Mills, J. B., Fahmi, O. A., Trevena, K. A., Liras, J. L., Maurer, T. S., and de Morais, S. M. 2006. Use of immortalized human hepatocytes to predict the magnitude of clinical drug–drug interactions caused by CYP3A4 induction. Drug Metab. Dispos. 34:1742–1748.
Rosenfeld, J. M., Vargas, R, Jr., Xie, W., and Evans, R. M 2003. Genetic profiling defines the xenobiotic gene network controlled by the nuclear receptor pregnane X receptor. Mol Endocrinol 17:1268–1282.
Sagredo, C., Ovrebo, S., Haugen, A., Fujii-Kuriyama, Y., Baera, R., Botnen, I. V., and Mollerup, S. 2006. Quantitative analysis of benzo[a]pyrene biotransformation and adduct formation in Ahr knockout mice. Toxicol. Lett. 167:173–182.
Sahi, J., Black, C. B., Hamilton, G. A., Zheng, X., Jolley, S., Rose, K. A., Gilbert, D., LeCluyse, E. L., and Sinz, M. W. 2003. Comparative effects of thiazolidinediones on in vitro P450 enzyme induction and inhibition. Drug Metab. Dispos. 31:439–446.
Shimizu, Y., Nakatsuru, Y., Ichinose, M., Takahashi, Y., Kume, H., Mimura, J., Fujii-Kuriyama, Y., and Ishikawa, T. 2000. Benzo[a]pyrene carcinogenicity is lost in mice lacking the aryl hydrocarbon receptor. Proc. Natl. Acad. Sci. USA 97:779–782.
Sims, P., Grover, P. L., Swaisland, A., Pal, K., and Hewer, A. 1974. Metabolic activation of benzo(a)pyrene proceeds by a diol-epoxide. Nature 252:326–328.
Sinz, M. W., Kim, S., Zhu, Z., Chen, T., Anthony, M., Dickinson, K., and Rodrigues, A. D. 2006. Evaluation of 170 xenobiotics as transactivators of human pregnane X receptor (hPXR) and correlation to known CYP3A4 drug interactions. Curr. Drug Metab. 7:375–388.
Sladek, N. E., and Mannering, G. J. 1966. Evidence for a new P-450hemoprotein in hepatic microsomes from methylcholanthrene treated rats. Biochem. Biophys. Res. Commun. 24:668–674.
Smith, M. T. 2003. Mechanisms of troglitazone hepatotoxicity. Chem. Res. Toxicol. 16:679–687.
Smith, D. A., Dickins, M., Fahmi, O. A,, Iwasaki, K., Lee, C., Obach, R. S., Padbury, G., de Morais, S. M., Ripp, S. L., Stevens, J., Voorman, R., and Youdim, K. 2007. The time to move cytochrome P450 induction into mainstream pharmacology is long overdue. Drug Metab. Dispos. 35:697–698.
Song, B.J., Matsunaga, T., Harwick, J.P., Park, S.S., Veech, R.L., Yang, C.S., Gelboin, H.V., and Gonzalez, F.G. 1987. Stabilization of cytochrome P450j messenger ribonucleic acid in the diabetic rat. Mol. Endocrinol. 1:542–547.
Song, B. J., Veech, R. L., Park, S. S., Gelboin, H. V., and Gonzalez, F. J. 1989. Induction of rat hepatic *N*-nitrosodimethylamine demethylase by acetone is due to protein stabilization. J. Biol. Chem. 264:3568–3572.
Sonoda, J., Chong, L. W., Downes, M., Barish, G. D., Coulter, S., Liddle, C., Lee, C.-H., and Evans, R. M. 2005. Pregnane X receptor prevents hepatorenal toxicity from cholesterol metabolites. Proc. Natl. Acad. Sci. USA 102:2198–2203.
Squires, E. J., Sueyoshi, T., and Negishi, M. 2004. Cytoplasmic localization of pregnane X receptor and ligand-dependent nuclear translocation in mouse liver. J. Biol. Chem. 279:49307–49314.
Stanley, L. A, Horsburgh, B. C., Ross, J., Scheer, N., and Wolf, C. R. 2006. PXR and CAR: Nuclear receptors which play a pivotal role in drug disposition and chemical toxicity. Drug Metab. Rev. 38:515–597.

Staudinger, J. L., Goodwin, B., Jones, S. A., Hawkins-Brown, D., MacKenzie, K. I., LaTour, A., Liu, Y., Klaassen, C. D., Brown, K. K., Reinhard, J., Willson, T. M., Koller, B. H., and Kliewer, S. A. 2001. The nuclear receptor PXR is a lithocholic acid sensor that protects against liver toxicity. Proc. Natl. Acad. Sci. USA 98:3369–3374.

Sueyoshi, T., Kawamoto, T., Zelko, I., Honkakoski, P., and Negishi, M. 1999. The repressed nuclear receptor CAR responds to phenobarbital in activating the human CYP2B6 gene. J. Biol. Chem. 274:6043–6046.

Synold, T. W., Dussault, I., and Forman, B. M. 2001. The orphan nuclear receptor SXR coordinately regulates drug metabolism and efflux. Nat. Med. 7:584–590.

Teschke, R., Stutz, G., and Strohmeyer, G. 1979. Increased paracetamol-induced hepatotoxicity after chronic alcohol consumption. Biochem. Biophys. Res. Commun. 91:368–374.

Tettey, J. N., Maggs, J. L., Rapeport, W. G., Pirmohamed, M., and Park, B. K. 2001. Enzyme-induction dependent bioactivation of troglitazone and troglitazone quinone in vivo. Chem. Res. Toxicol. 14:965–974.

Thimmulappa, R. K., Mai, K. H., Srisuma, S., Kensler, T. W., Yamamoto, M., and Biswal, S. 2002. Identification of Nrf2-regulated genes induced by the chemopreventive agent sulforaphane by oligonucleotide microarray. Cancer Res. 62:5196–5203.

Thummel, K. E., Brimer, C., Yasuda, K., Thottassery, J., Senn, T., Lin, Y., Ishizuka, H., Kharasch, E., Schuetz, J., and Schuetz, E. 2001. Transcriptional control of intestinal cytochrome P-4503A by 1alpha,25-dihydroxy vitamin D3. Mol. Pharmacol. 60:1399–1406.

Thummel, K. E., Lee, C. A., Kunze, K. L,, Nelson, S. D., and Slattery, J. T. 1993. Oxidation of acetaminophen to *N*-acetyl-*p*-aminobenzoquinone imine by human CYP3A4. Biochem. Pharmacol. 45:1563–1569.

Truong, N.T., Moncion, S., Barouki, R., Beaune, P., and de Waziers, I. 2005. Regulatory sequence responsible for insulin destabilization of cytochrome P450 2B1 (CYP2B1) mRNA. Biochem. J. 388:227–235.

Tsuneoka, Y., Dalton, T. P., Miller, M. L., Clay, C. D., Shertzer, H. G., Talaska, G., Medvedovic, M., and Nebert, D. W. 2003. 4-Aminobiphenyl-induced liver and urinary bladder DNA adduct formation in Cyp1a2(–/–) and Cyp1a2(+/+) mice. J. Natl. Cancer Inst. 95:1227–1237.

Tzameli, I., Pissios, P., Schuetz, E. G., and Moore, D. D. 2000. The xenobiotic compound 1,4- *bis*[2-(3,5-dichloropyridyloxy)]benzene is an agonist ligand for the nuclear receptor CAR. Mol. Cell. Biol. 20:2951–2958.

Ueda, A., Hamadeh, H. K., Webb, H. K., Yamamoto, Y., Sueyoshi, T., Afshari, C. A., Lehmann, J. M., and Negishi, M. 2002. Diverse roles of the nuclear orphan receptor CAR in regulating hepatic genes in response to phenobarbital. Mol. Pharmacol. 61:1–6.

Uno, S., Dalton, T. P., Derkenne, S., Curran, C. P., Miller, M. L., Shertzer, H. G., and Nebert, D. W. 2004. Oral exposure to benzo[a]pyrene in the mouse: Detoxication by inducible cytochrome P450 is more important than metabolic activation. Mol. Pharmacol. 65:1225–1237.

Uno, S., Dalton, T. P., Dragin, N., Curran, C. P., Derkenne, S., Miller, M. L., Shertzer, H. G., Gonzalez, F. J., and Nebert, D. W. 2006. Oral benzo[a]pyrene in Cyp1 knockout mouse lines: CYP1A1 important in detoxication, CYP1B1 metabolism required for immune damage independent of total-body burden and clearance rate. Mol. Pharmacol. 69:1103–1114.

Venugopal, R., and Jaiswal Anil, K. 1996. Nrf1 and Nrf2 positively and c-Fos and Fra1 negatively regulate the human antioxidant response element-mediated expression of NAD(P)H:quinone oxidoreductase1 gene. Proc. Natl. Acad. Sci. USA 93:14960–14965.

Wei, P., Zhang, J., Dowhan, D. H., Han, Y., and Moore, D. D. 2002. Specific and overlapping functions of the nuclear hormone receptors CAR and PXR in xenobiotic response. Pharmacogenomics J. 2:117–126.

Wei, P., Zhang, J., Egan-Hafley, M., Liang, S., and Moore, D. D. 2000. The nuclear receptor CAR mediates specific xenobiotic induction of drug metabolism. Nature 407:920–923.

Xie, W., Barwick, J. L., Downes, M., Blumberg, B., Simon, C. M., Nelson, M. C., Neuschwander-Tetri, B. A., Brunt, E. M., Guzelian, P. S., and Evans, R. M. 2000. Humanized xenobiotic response in mice expressing nuclear receptor SXR. Nature 406:435–439.

Xie, W., Radominska-Pandya, A., Shi, Y., Simon, C. M., Nelson, M. C., Ong, E. S., Waxman, D. J., and Evans, R. M. 2001. An essential role for nuclear receptors SXR/PXR in detoxification of cholestatic bile acids. Proc. Natl. Acad. Sci. USA 98:3375–3380.

Yamazaki, H., Shibata, A., Suzuki, M., Nakajima, M., Shimada, N., Guengerich, F. P., and Yokoi, T. 1999. Oxidation of troglitazone to a quinone-type metabolite catalyzed by cytochrome P-450 2C8 and P-450 3A4 in human liver microsomes. Drug Metab. Dispos. 27:1260–1266.

Yu, R., Lei, W., Mandlekar, S., Weber, M. J., Der, C. J., Wu, J., and Kong, A. N. T. 1999. Role of a mitogen-activated protein kinase pathway in the induction of phase II detoxifying enzymes by chemicals. J. Biol. Chem. 274:27545–27552.

Zhang, D. D. 2006. Mechanistic studies of the Nrf2–Keap1 signaling pathway. Drug Metab. Rev. 38:769–789.

Zhang, D. D., and Hannink, M. 2003. Distinct cysteine residues in Keap1 are required for Keap1-dependent ubiquitination of Nrf2 and for stabilization of Nrf2 by chemopreventive agents and oxidative stress. Mol. Cell. Biol. 23:8137–8151.

Zhang, J., Huang, W., Chua, S. S., Wei, P., and Moore, D. D. 2002. Modulation of acetaminophen-induced hepatotoxicity by the xenobiotic receptor CAR. Science 298:422–424.

Zhou, C., Poulton, E.-J., Grun, F., Bammler, T. K., Blumberg, B., Thummel, K. E., and Eaton, D. L. 2007 The dietary isothiocyanate sulforaphane is an antagonist of the human steroid and xenobiotic nuclear receptor. Mol Pharmacol 71:220–229.

Zimmerman, H. J., and Maddrey, W. C. 1995 Acetaminophen (paracetamol) hepatotoxicity with regular intake of alcohol: Analysis of instances of therapeutic misadventure. Hepatology 22:767–773.

5

Mechanism-Based Inactivation of Cytochrome P450 2A and 2B Enzymes

Sharon E. Murphy and Linda B. von Weymarn
University of Minnesota Cancer Center, Minneapolis, MN 55455, USA
e-mail: murph062@umn.edu

Keywords: Cytochrome P450 · P450 · CYP2A6 · CYP2B6 · CYP2B1 · Nicotine · Isothiocyanates · 8-Methoxypsoralen · Ethynylestradiol

5.1. Introduction

Inhibition of cytochrome P450 enzymes (P450s) contributes significantly to drug–drug interactions (Wienkers and Heath 2005) and recently it has been suggested that mechanism-based inactivation may play a greater role in these interactions than previously recognized (Zhang and Wong 2005). Mechanism-based inactivation of P450s may also be caused by exposure to compounds present in tobacco and food. This inactivation may result in an increase in the toxicity of drugs or other xenobiotics. Alternatively, mechanism-based inactivators (MBIs) may have a positive affect; for example, inactivation of the enzymes that catalyze the metabolic activation of procarcinogens. Mechanism-based inactivators of all human hepatic drug-metabolizing P450 enzymes have been identified (Table 5.1): the majority of these inactivate P450 3A4, the major human drug-metabolizing enzyme. In this chapter we will focus our discussion on the mechanism-based inactivation of two less abundant and less well-studied hepatic enzymes, P450 2B6 and P450 2A6. In addition, some recent studies on the mechanism-based inactivation of P450 2A13, an enzyme believed to play a role in the metabolic activation of the tobacco-specific lung carcinogen, 4-(methylnitrosamino)-1-(3-pyridyl)-1-butanone (NNK), will be discussed.

A.A. Elfarra (ed.), *Advances in Bioactivation Research*, DOI: 10.1007/978-0-387-77300-1_5,

Table 5.1 Human mechanism-based inactivators.

P450	MBI		References
1A1/1A2	Carbamazepine	1A2 in HLM	Masubuchi et al. (2001)
	Clorgyline	1A2	Polasek et al. (2006)
	Coriandrin	1A1 (purified)	Cai et al. (1996)
	Dihydralazine	HLM, B-lymphoblastoid microsomes	Masubuchi and Horie (1999)
	Furafylline	1A2 in HLM	Kunze and Trager (1993)
	Oltipraz	*E.coli* membranes	Langouet et al. (2000)
	Rhapontigenin	1A1 (bacterial membrane)	Chun et al. (2001)
	trans-Resveratrol	1A2 (Supersomes), HLM	Chang, Chen and Lee (2001)
	Zileuton	1A2 in HLM	Lu et al. (2003)
2A6/2A13	Benzylisothiocyanate (BITC)	2A6 and 2A13 (purified from *E. coli*)	von Weymarn, Chun and Hollenberg (2006b)
	(R)-(+)-Menthofuran	HLM, 2A6 purified from *E. coli*	Khojasteh-Bakht et al. (1998)
	8-Methoxysporalen (8-MOP)	2A6 and 2A13 (purified from *E. coli*)	von Weymarn et al. (2005) Koenigs et al. (1997)
	Nicotine	2A6 and 2A13 (purified from *E. coli*)	von Weymarn, Brown and Murphy (2006a)
	Phenethylisothiocyanate (PEITC)	2A6 and 2A13 (purified from *E. coli*)	von Weymarn, Chun and Hollenberg (2006b)
2B6	Bergamottin	Purified from *E. coli*	Tassaneeyakul et al. (2000)
	Clopidogrel	2B6 Superosomes, HLM	Richter et al. (2004)
	N-(3,5-dichloro-4-pyridyl)-4-methoxy-3-(prop-2-ynyloxy)benzamide	2B6 Superosomes	Fan et al. (2003)
	Efavirenz and 8-hydroxyefavirenz	Purified from *E. coli*	Bumpus, Kent and Hollenberg (2006)
	17α-Ethynylestradiol	Purified from *E. coli*	Kent et al. (2002b)
	Glabridine	Purified from *E. coli*	Kent et al. (2002a)
	Phencyclidine	Purified from *E. coli*	Jushchyshyn, Kent and Hollenberg (2003)
	2-Phenyl-2-(1-piperidinyl)propane	Purified from *E. coli*	Chun et al. (2000)
	n-Propylxanthate	Purified from *E. coli*	Kent, Yanev and Hollenberg (1999)
	Ticlopidine	2B6 Superosomes, HLM	Richter et al. (2004)
	Tamoxifen	Purified from *E. coli*	Sridar et al. (2002)
	N,N′,N″-triethylenethiophosphoramide tTEPA	Purified from *E. coli*	Harleton et al. (2004) Richter et al. (2005)
2C8	Amiodarone Fluoxetine Isoniazid Nortriptyline Phenelzine Verapamil	*E. c*oli membranes	Polasek et al. (2004)

2C9	Silybin	Purified from *E. coli*	Sridar et al. (2004)
	Suprofen	Recombinant 2C9	O′Donnell et al. (2003)
	Tienilic acid	Yeast microsomes	Jean et al. (1996)
2C19	Phenelzine	*E. coli* membranes, HLM	Polasek et al. (2006)
	Ticlopidine	Yeast microsomes	Ha-Duong et al. (2001)
2D6	5-fluoro-2-[4-[(2-phenyl-1H-imidazol-5-yl)methyl]-1-piperazinyl]pyrimidine	Superosomes, HLM	Palamanda et al. (2001)
	Paroxetine	HLM	Bertelsen et al. (2003)
2E1	Trichloroethylene	*E. coli* membranes	Cai and Guengerich (2001)
3A4	Amiodarone		Ohyama et al. (2000)
	Ampenprenavir	Superosomes, HLM	Ernest, Hall and Jones (2005)
	Bergamottin	HLM	Tassaneeyakul et al. (2000)
	Clarithromycin	Superosomes	Mayhew, Jones and Hall (2000)
	Delavirdine	β-lymphoblast microsomes, HLM	Voorman et al. (1998)
	N-desmethyl dilitiazem	Superosomes	Mayhew, Jones and Hall (2000)
	Diclofenac	β-lymphoblast microsomes, HLM	Masubuchi, Ose and Horie (2002)
	Dihydralazine	HLM, B-lymphoblastoid microsomes	Masubuchi and Horie (1999)
	6′,7′-Dihydroxybergamottin	HLM, Purified from *E. coli*	Tassaneeyakul et al. (2000) Schmiedlin-Ren et al. (1997)
	Dilitiazem	Superosomes	Mayhew, Jones and Hall (2000)
	Erythromycin	β-lymphoblast microsomes, HLM	Kanamitsu et al. (2000)
	17α-Ethynylestradiol	Purified from *E. coli*	Lin, Kent and Hollenberg (2002)
	Fluoxetine	Superosomes	Mayhew, Jones and Hall (2000)
	Gestodene	HLM, purified from *E. coli*	Guengerich (1990)
	4-Ipomeanol		Alvarez-Diez and Zheng (2004)
	Irinotecan	Superosomes	Hanioka et al. (2002)
	Limonin	HLM	Iwata et al. (2005)
	Lopinavir	Superosomes, HLM	Ernest, Hall and Jones (2005)
	Mibefradil	HLM	Prueksaritanont et al. (1999)
	Midazolam	Purified from *E. coli*	Khan et al. (2002)
	Mifepristone	Purified from *E. coli*	He, Woolf and Hollenberg (1999)
	Nelfinavir	Superosomes, HLM	Ernest, Hall and Jones (2005)

(*Continued*)

Table 5.1 (*Continued*).

P450	MBI		References
	Nicardipine	HLM, Baculovirus microsomes	Ma, Prueksaritanont and Lin (2000)
	Nor-Verapamil	HLM, Superosomes	Wang, Jones and Hall (2004)
	Phenelzine	*E. coli* membranes, HLM	Polasek et al. (2006)
	Raloxifene	HLM, superosomes	Chen et al. (2002)
	Resveratrol	Baculovirus microsomes	Chan and Delucchi (2000)
	Ritonavir	Superosomes, HLM	Ernest, Hall and Jones (2005)
	Rutaecarpine	HLM	Iwata et al. (2005)
	Saquinavir	Superosomes, HLM	Ernest, Hall and Jones (2005)
	Silybin	Purified from *E.Coli*	Sridar et al. (2004)
	Tamoxifen	HLM, superosomes	Zhao et al. (2002)
	Verapamil	HLM, Superosomes	Wang, Jones and Hall (2004)
	Zafirlukast	Superosomes, HLM	Kassahun et al. (2005)

The mechanism-based inactivators included in this table meet at least two of the criteria for mechanism-based inactivation. The kinetics of inactivation is reported, whenever possible, and in addition at least irreversibility or mechanism of inactivation is also assessed.

5.2. Characterization of Mechanism-Based Inactivation

An enzyme inactivator is any compound that causes the irreversible or quasi-irreversible loss of enzymatic activity. The definition of a mechanism-based or suicide inactivator is more specific. Pratt and Kranz defined an MBI simply as an enzyme inactivator that requires the mechanism of the target enzyme (Krantz 1992; Pratt 1992). The definition that will be used in this chapter is that of Silverman who defines an MBI as a compound that is catalytically transformed by the enzyme to a species that prior to release from the active site renders the enzyme inactive (Silverman 1996). Mechanism-based inactivation, although rare in most enzyme systems, is much more frequent with P450 enzymes (Kent, Juschyshyn and Hollenberg 2001; Zhang and Wong 2005).

The kinetic scheme for an MBI is similar to that of a noninactivating substrate but with an additional product, the modified inactive enzyme (Scheme 5.1). After the MBI associates with the enzyme (E), catalytic turnover generates the inactivating species (MBI′) complexed with the

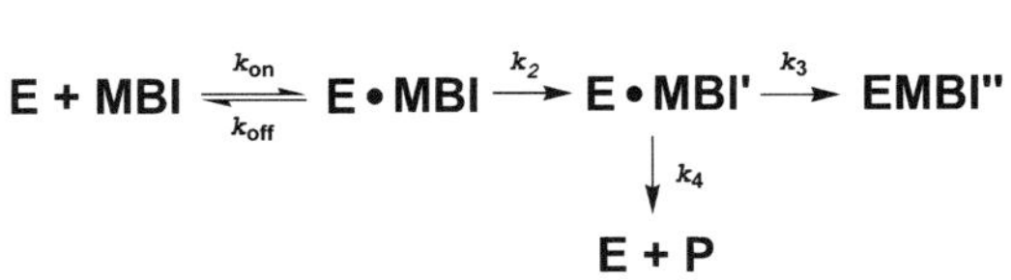

Scheme 5.1

enzyme (E•MBI′). The inactivating species may then either be released as product (P) or bind irreversibly to the enzyme, rendering it inactive (EMBI″). A more in depth description of Scheme 5.1 and how kinetic constants are derived from it has been reviewed by Silverman (1988). The key parameters which describe mechanism-based inactivation of an enzyme are: k_{inact}, the maximal inactivation rate constant; K_I, which can be considered analogous to K_m; and the partition ratio. The partition ratio is a measure of the efficiency of the MBI. It is the ratio of product release to enzyme inactivation, and is described by k_3/k_4. This ratio does not depend on the concentration of inactivator. It depends on the reactivity of MBI′, the rate of diffusion of MBI′ from the active site, and the proximity of an appropriate binding site in the enzyme active site for covalent bond formation. In the case of P450 enzymes binding may occur either with an amino acid side chain or the heme molecule.

There are several criteria that are routinely assessed to determine if a compound is an MBI of a particular P450 enzyme (Silverman 1996). These criteria and a brief rationale are listed below.

- Inactivation is dependent on catalytic turnover; that is, the compound must be metabolized to a reactive species, which then inactivates the enzyme.
- Inactivation is time dependent. Since the inactivation requires catalytic turnover the loss in enzyme activity is usually first-order with respect to time.
- Inactivation exhibits saturation kinetics.
- Inactivation is irreversible or at least quasi-irreversible.
- The enzyme is protected from inactivation through the addition of an alternate substrate. The alternative substrate will compete with the MBI and slow its metabolism and hence enzyme inactivation.
- Only one inactivator molecule is attached to each molecule of inactivated enzyme.
- The inactivation occurs prior to release of the reactive species from the active site of the enzyme. Therefore, the addition of a nucleophile such as glutathione, which will react with electrophilic reactive species released from the active site, should not affect the rate of inactivation.

The protocols that are used to test these criteria are described in detail elsewhere (Silverman 1996) and will only be partially discussed here. The classic method to study an MBI is to characterize enzyme activity in two reactions. In the primary reaction, the P450 of interest is incubated under standard conditions with varying concentrations of the putative MBI in the presence and absence of NADPH. Then at different time intervals, aliquots of the primary reaction are removed and added to a fresh reaction mixture containing NADPH and a saturating concentration of another substrate of this P450. The secondary reaction is carried out so that a minimum 20-fold dilution of the MBI occurs. If the MBI is also a potent inhibitor of the enzyme, the dilution necessary to eliminate inhibition in the secondary reaction might be too great for the accurate quantitation of enzyme activity. In this case, the removal of the MBI may be accomplished through the use of spin-column gel filtration or dialysis. Kinetic parameters for the MBI reaction may be determined from the enzyme activities measured in these experiments.

Mechanism-based inactivation is usually the result of covalent binding of a reactive intermediate to the active site of the enzyme, although tight-binding noncovalent complexes between the inactivating species and the enzyme also occur. The former are irreversible but the latter can sometimes slowly disassociate over time. Presently, it has not been clearly established when a quasi-irreversible inactivator is no longer classified as an MBI.

There are three pathways by which an MBI may inactivate a P450 enzyme: covalent modification of amino acids residues in the active site, covalent modification of the heme moiety, or destruction of the heme. When the heme is destroyed, fragments of the heme sometimes become bound to the apoprotein. Mechanism-based inactivators may also generate cross-links between the heme and the apoprotein, although this is not common. It is important to note that multiple mechanisms of inactivation may occur for one compound. For example, P450-catalyzed metabolism of the MBI may result in modification of both the heme and the apoprotein. In addition, since several factors influence enzyme inactivation, the relative contribution of different mechanisms of inactivation by an MBI may vary among different enzymes. The factors that will influence the mechanism include the site of MBI oxidation, the structure of the reactive intermediate generated, and the geometry and composition of the active site of the enzyme.

5.2.1. MBI as Tools

Over the years, MBIs have proven to be useful tools with which to study structure–function relationships of individual P450 enzymes (reviewed in Kent, Juschyshyn and Hollenberg 2001). Specifically, the use of MBIs have aided in determining the orientation of the heme in the P450 active site and in identifying regions of the P450 protein involved in substrate binding (Kent et al. 2006; Kunze et al. 1983; Ortiz de Montellano et al. 1992; Ortiz de Montellano 1995). Studies with MBIs by Ortiz de Montellano and co-workers allowed the identification of the correct orientation of the heme molecule in the active site. They concluded that although the general orientation of the heme appears to be the same in different P450s, the extent to which different regions of the heme molecule are accessible to inactivating species varies among P450 enzymes (Ortiz de Montellano 1995). Mechanism-based inactivators that result in covalent modification of the apoprotein are particularly useful for identifying amino acids in the active site that are important in substrate binding (Kent, Juschyshyn and Hollenberg 2001).

Inactivators that affect highly homologous P450 enzymes differently, such as the human P450s 2A6 and 2A13 (94% identical) and 3A4 and 3A5 (84% identical) or the rat P450s 2B1 and 2B2 (97% identical), can also play an important role in the identification of the P450s responsible for the metabolism of a particular compound *in vivo*. The use of inhibitory antibodies are usually sufficient to identify which subfamily of P450 enzymes is involved in the metabolism, but quite often these antibodies cannot distinguish between highly homologous enzymes within that subfamily.

Mechanism-based inactivators that are able to differentially inactivate highly homologous P450 enzymes such as rat P450s 2B1 and 2B2 (Kent et al. 2002b; von Weymarn, Sridar and Hollenberg 2004) and human P450s 3A4 and 3A5 (Khan et al. 2002) could be used to pinpoint which enzyme is responsible for the metabolism of a specific compound *in vivo*.

5.2.2. MBI and Drug Metabolism

Annually about two million serious adverse drug reactions occur in the US (Lazarou, Pomeranz and Corey 1998). Inhibition and/or inactivation of metabolic enzymes such as the P450 enzymes has been recognized as one of the significant causes of adverse drug–drug interactions (Wienkers and Heath 2005). Drug–drug interactions are often caused by one drug inhibiting the metabolism of another and therefore increasing the plasma concentration of the second drug. Since MBIs irreversibly inhibit an enzyme, the risk for serious drug–drug interactions may be greater for these compounds than for competitive inhibitors. Mibefradil is one example where mechanism-based inactivation may have contributed to the serious drug–-drug interactions which resulted in this drug being pulled from the market (Friedman et al. 1999). Mibefradil is a potent MBI of P450 3A4, with a K_i of 2.3 μM and a partition ratio of 1.7 (Prueksaritanont et al. 1999). It was withdrawn from the market due to potentially harmful interactions with 26 identified drugs. Reduced P450 3A4 enzyme activity was believed to play a role in many of these interactions (Friedman et al. 1999). Over the past decade the pharmaceutical industry has invested a great deal of money and effort into screening for P450 inhibition by new drug entities at early stages of the development process.

In addition to MBI-mediated drug–drug interactions, environmental factors may result in inactivation of P450 enzymes and cause adverse drug reactions. Compounds found in the diet, cigarette smoke, and air or water pollution all have the potential to cause mechanism-based inactivation and hence result in dangerous but unexpected drug reactions. Grapefruit juice is the best characterized example of a dietary exposure resulting in the mechanism-based inactivation of P450 enzymes. The influence of grapefruit juice on the pharmacokinetics of a large number of drugs is well documented (reviewed in Saito et al. 2005). Grapefruit juice increases the area under the curve (AUC) and the maximum plasma concentration (C_{max}) of orally co-administered drugs such as simvastatin, triazolam, midazolam, nitrendipine, and a number of others (Saito et al. 2005). The major cause of these effects of grapefruit juice is considered to be mechanism-based inactivation of P450 3A4 (Lown et al. 1997; Schmiedlin-Ren et al. 1997). *In vitro* studies have identified several components of grapefruit juice as inhibitors of P450 enzymes (Guo and Yamazoe 2004; Tassaneeyakul et al. 2000). Among these bergamottin and 6′,7′-dihydroxybergamottin have been well characterized as MBIs of P450 3A4 (Paine, Criss and Watkins 2004; Schmiedlin-Ren et al. 1997; Tassaneeyakul et al. 2000). 6′,7′-Dihydroxybergamottin appears to be the major contributor to grapefruit juice-mediated P450 3A4-mediated inactivation. However in other foods that contain bergamottin but not 6′,7′-dihydroxybergamottin, bergamottin is likely to contribute significantly to the inactivation of

P450 3A4 (Paine, Criss and Watkins 2005). Recently, bergamottin has been identified as a MBI of P450 2B6 (Lin, Kent and Hollenberg 2005). Therefore, grapefruit juice consumption may also cause drug–drug interactions with drugs primarily metabolized by P450 2B6. This will be discussed in the following section.

Another class of naturally occurring compounds that may result in the inactivation of drug-metabolizing P450s are isothiocyanates. These compounds, found in various cruciferous vegetables such as cabbage, watercress, broccoli, and cauliflower as thioglucoside conjugates, have been studied as cancer chemopreventive agents (reviewed in Hecht 2000). The chemopreventive properties of isothiocyanates are believed in part to be due to inhibition and inactivation of P450 enzymes that have been implicated in the bioactivation of chemical carcinogens. Notable, the same mechanisms that result in the chemopreventive properties of the isothiocyanates could also give rise to adverse drug interactions. Mechanism-based inactivation of the rat enzymes P450 2E1 and P450 2B1 by benzyl isothiocyanate has been well characterized (Goosen, Mills and Hollenberg 2001; Moreno et al. 2001). In both cases the mechanism of inactivation was covalent modification of the apoprotein. Some recent work on isothiocyanates as MBIs of P450 2A6 and P450 2A13 is discussed below.

In addition to diet, tobacco smoke is a major source of exposure to a large number of xenobiotics, and smokers clearly metabolize many drugs differently than do nonsmokers. Polycyclic aromatic hydrocarbons present in tobacco smoke are well known to induce drug-metabolizing enzymes, including P450 1A2 and 1A1 (Kroon 2006). Whether or not, mechanism-based inactivation by tobacco smoke constituent influences drug metabolism is unknown. However, we have recently demonstrated that *in vitro*, nicotine, the main addictive agent in tobacco, inactivates two human P450s, 2A6 and 2A13 (von Weymarn, Brown and Murphy 2006a). Considering tobacco smoke contains over 4000 chemicals one might suspect that further studies of the components of tobacco will result in the identification of a number of MBIs of P450 enzymes. Hence smokers may be of potentially higher risk of adverse drug reactions than are nonsmokers. In the following two sections examples of drugs, including nicotine, and dietary constituents that are MBIs of the human P450s 2A6, 2A13, and 2B6 are discussed in detail.

5.3. Inactivation of P450 2B6

The mechanism-based inactivation of P450 2B enzymes, P450 2B1 and 2B2 in rats, P450 2B4 and 2B5 in rabbit, and more recently P450 2B6 in humans, has been well studied (Kent, Juschyshyn and Hollenberg 2001; Kent et al. 2002b, 2004; Lin, Kent and Hollenberg 2005). The main focus of these studies has been on the use of MBIs as structure–function probes (Kent, Juschyshyn and Hollenberg 2001; Lin et al. 2004; von Weymarn et al. 2004). Only recently has mechanism-based inactivation of P450 2B enzymes by pharmacologically relevant drugs and dietary constituents received attention (Bumpus, Kent and Hollenberg 2006; Harleton et al. 2004; Kent et al. 2002b, 2006; Lin, Kent and Hollenberg 2005). P450 2B6 is not one of the major drug-metabolizing P450 enzymes; it typically accounts for <1% of the total P450 protein in the liver (Guengerich 2003). However, P450 2B6 is inducible and levels as high as 4% of the total P450 protein have been reported (Hanna et al. 2000; Wang et al. 2003). Recently, an increasing number of drugs that are primarily metabolized by P450 2B6 (Chang et al. 1993; Faucette et al. 2000; Ward et al. 2003) have been identified. Therefore, the potential for the inactivation of P450 2B6 to cause drug–drug interactions may be greater than previously appreciated. Mechanism-based inactivation of P450 2B6 has been characterized for a number of pharmaceutical compounds, dietary components, and synthetic compounds (Table 5.1). The discussion in this chapter will focus on five of these: 17α-ethynylestradiol (17EE), phencyclidine, efavirenz, *N*,*N*′,*N*″-triethylenethiophosphoramide (tTEPA), and bergamottin (Figure 5.1). This focus is due to both the extent of characterization of these MBIs and their possible relevance to drug–drug interactions.

P450 2B6 plays an important role in the metabolism of a number of commonly used drugs, such as cyclophosphamide (for cancer chemotherapy and autoimmune disease treatment), bupropion (an antidepressant used in smoking cessation), propofol (an anesthetic agent), and efavirenz (used to treat HIV-1) (Faucette et al. 2000; Roy et al. 1999; Ward et al. 2003). Only one of these compounds, efavirenz, inactivates P450 2B6. However, other compounds that inactivate P450 2B6 may influence the pharmacokinetic parameters of these clinically important drugs. In addition to these pharmaceutical compounds, nicotine- and the tobacco-specific carcinogen, NNK are substrates for P450 2B6 (Dicke, Skrlin and Murphy 2005; Yamazaki et al. 1999). However, while recent studies have shown that P450 2B6, if present in relatively high levels, may play a role in the metabolic activation of NNK in human liver microsomes, it is not likely to contribute significantly to nicotine metabolism (Dicke, Skrlin and Murphy 2005).

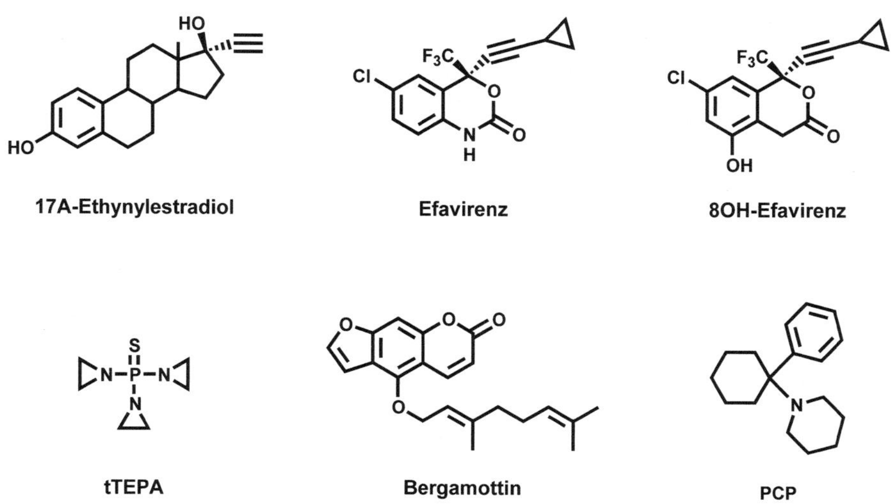

Figure 5.1 Mechanism-based inhibitors of P450 2B6.

5.3.1. 17α-Ethynylestradiol (17EE)

One of the best-characterized MBIs of P450 2B6 is 17EE, the major estrogenic component of oral contraceptives. The ethynyl group at the 17 position was introduced to increase the oral availability of the estradiol; however, it also gave rise to mechanism-based inactivation (Kent et al. 2002b; Lin, Kent and Hollenberg 2002; Lin and Hollenberg 2007). In 2002, Kent et al. reported that 17EE was a potent MBI of rat P450 2B1 and human P450 2B6, but not rat P450 2B2 and rabbit P450 2B4 (Kent et al. 2002b). Inactivation of P450 2B6 was irreversible, and time- and concentration-dependent (Figure 5.2). The apparent K_I for the inactivation of P450 2B6 was quite low, 0.8 μM; $t_{1/2}$ was 28 min. The partition ratio for the inactivation of P450 2B6 by 17EE was 13; that is, 13 molecules of 17EE were metabolized, per molecule of P450 2B6 inactivated. It was also demonstrated that P450 2B6 was protected from inactivation by alternate substrates, but the addition of exogenous nucleophiles had no effect on inactivation. Using [^{3}H]-17EE it was possible to demonstrate the formation of covalently modified P450 2B6 (EMBI″, Scheme 5.1).

The previously identified mechanism of P450 3A4 inactivation by 17EE (K_i, 18 μM; $t_{1/2}$, 25 min) was destruction of the heme (Lin, Kent and Hollenberg 2002). In contrast, inactivation of P450 2B6 by 17EE occurred through the formation of adducts to the apoprotein (Kent et al. 2002b; Kent et al. 2006). However, due to large errors in the mass assignments, it was not possible to detect a 17EE-adducted protein by liquid chromatography-mass spectrometry (LC/MS) analysis (Kent et al. 2006). In general, whole-protein LC/MS analysis of inactivated P450 2B6 has been difficult to perform (Jushchyshyn, Kent and Hollenberg 2003; Lin, Kent and Hollenberg 2005). Inactivated P450 2B6 appears to give rise to very weak signals potentially due to poor ionization or aggregation of the inactivated enzyme; therefore, the deconvolution of the whole-protein mass spectrum gives rise to a relatively large error. P450 2B1 is more easily analyzed by whole-protein LC/MS. The increase in the mass of the P450 2B1 apoprotein upon inactivation with 17EE was consistent with binding of 17EE plus

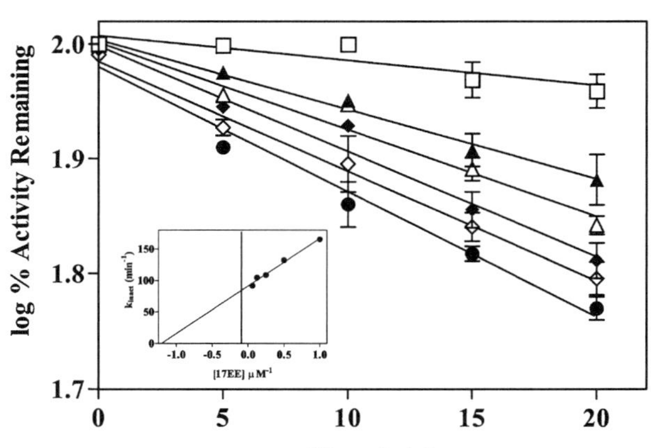

Figure 5.2 Time- and concentration-dependent inactivation of P450 2B6 7-ethoxycoumarin O-deethylation by 17-ethynylestradiol [from Kent et al. 2002b].

one oxygen atom (Kent et al. 2006). Cyanogen bromide digestion of inactivated P450 2B1 and 2B6 followed by Edman sequencing and MS analysis resulted in the identification of one adducted peptide for each protein. The authors proposed that serine 360 within this peptide was the amino acid residue modified since P450s 2B2 and 2B4 do not contain a serine at this position and they are not inactivated by 17EE. The structure of the adduct is hypothesized to be a serine ester generated from the ketene resulting from oxidation of the ethynyl group. However, the formation of this adduct has not been confirmed.

2-Hydroxyethynylestradiol formation is the primary pathway of P450 2B6-catalyzed 17EE metabolism (Kent et al. 2002b). Estriol, estrone, and two unidentified metabolites were also products of P450 2B6-mediated 17EE metabolism (Kent et al. 2002b). These same five metabolites were products of P450 2B1-catalyzed metabolism but all five were not products of P450 2B2- or P450 2B4-catalyzed metabolisms. The fact that the latter two enzymes are not inactivated during 17EE metabolism, led to the suggestion that one or both of the missing metabolites (one identified as estrone and one unidentified) might be the products of a nonbound reactive intermediate; that is, P450 2B6 and P450 2B1, but not P450s 2B2 and 2B4, catalyze the formation of the reactive metabolite responsible for enzyme inactivation. However, whether the lack of 17EE-mediated inactivation of P450s 2B2 and 2B4 is due to differences in metabolism or, as discussed in the preceding paragraph, the lack of binding to the critical residues in the active site of these two enzymes is unknown.

17EE-mediated inactivation on P450 2B6 meets all the criteria for mechanism-based inactivation and it has been shown that inactivation is due to binding of a reactive intermediate to an amino acid in the active site. What remains to be confirmed is whether or not serine 360 is the site of modification, and the structure of the amino acid adduct. The complete characterization of the protein adduct should aid in the identification of the reactive intermediate. This in turn should confirm if the differences in the sensitivity of P450 2B enzymes to 17EE-mediated inactivation are due to differences in the pathways of metabolism or the location and identity of amino acid residues in the active site.

5.3.2. Efavirenz

The reverse transcriptase inhibitor efavirenz is used in combination therapy for the treatment of HIV-1. In humans efavirenz undergoes oxidative hydroxylation to form primarily 8-hydroxyefavirenz, which may be further metabolized to 8,14-dihydroxyefavirenz (Mutlib et al. 1999). P450 2B6 is the principal catalyst of the 8-hydroxylation of efavirenz and the formation of 8,14-dihydroxyefavirenz (Ward et al. 2003). The possibility for drug interactions with efavirenz is high, since efavirenz is always used in combination therapy. In addition, patients receiving efavirenz frequently take herbal and nutritional supplements and/or drugs for the treatment of infections and other HIV-related disorders.

Efavirenz inactivated P450 2B6 in a time-, concentration-, and NADPH-dependent manner with a K_I of 30 μM and a $t_{1/2}$ of 16 min (Bumpus et al. 2005). The inactivation followed pseudo first-order kinetics. The inactivation of P450 2B6 resulted in a significant loss in both the amount of spectrally measurable enzyme and the amount of native heme. Interestingly, the inactivation was completely reversible upon 24-hour dialysis, indicating that efavirenz is probably not a true MBI of P450 2B6. The most likely cause of reversible inactivation is the formation of a metabolite-intermediate (MI) complex; therefore, the authors looked for the characteristic absorbance maximum at 455 nm that is typical for a MI complex (Chatterjee and Franklin 2003). They did not observe an absorbance maximum at 455 nm, instead they observed what appears to be a type II binding spectra with an absorption maximum of 435 nm and a minimum of 418 nm (Bumpus et al. 2005). The mechanism of the reversible inactivation of P450 2B6 by efavirenz has not been yet characterized.

Interestingly, the primary metabolite of efavirenz, 8-hydroxyefavirenz, inactivated P450 2B6 in a time-, concentration-, and NADPH-dependent manner with kinetic parameters similar to those of efavirenz (Bumpus et al. 2005). However, unlike efavirenz, 8-hydroxyefavirenz gave rise to irreversible inactivation. Further studies on the inactivation of P450 2B6 by both efavirenz and 8-hydroxyefavirenz are currently ongoing (Namandjé Bumpus, personal communication).

5.3.3. N,N′,N″-Triethylenethiophosphoramide (tTEPA)

tTEPA (Figure 5.2) was developed in the 1950s as a nonspecific antineoplastic agent used in the treatment of breast, bladder, and ovarian cancer (Maanen, Smeets and Beijnen 2000). It is also used in high-dose chemotherapy regimens when bone marrow toxicity is not an issue – for example, in a bone marrow transplantation setting. tTEPA is metabolized to its primary metabolite *N*,*N*′,*N*″-triethylenephosphoramide (TEPA) by P450 2B6 and P450 3A4 *in vitro* (Jacobson et al. 2002). TEPA is the active metabolite of tTEPA and is formed by oxidative desulfuration of tTEPA. tTEPA is often co-administered with cyclophosphamide, a chemotherapeutic pro-drug that requires P450-mediated 4-hydroxylation to exert its alkylating activity. It was observed that if tTEPA is administered prior to cyclophosphamide, the levels of 4-hydroxycyclophosphamide are greatly reduced in the plasma (Huitema et al. 2000). Reduced metabolism of cyclophosphamide was also observed in human liver microsomes when tTEPA was co-incubated with cyclophosphamide.

Two laboratories have reported that tTEPA was an MBI of P450 2B6 (Harleton et al. 2004; Richter et al. 2005). Richter et al (2005) demonstrated time-, concentration-, and NADPH-dependent loss in P450 2B6 activity in human liver microsomes and in membranes containing overexpressed P450 2B6. They reported that P450 2B6 was the only P450 enzyme out of a panel of nine that was significantly inhibited by 10 μM tTEPA. Harleton et al. (2004) used purified P450 2B6 expressed in *Escherichia coli* in their studies and also observed time-, concentration-, and NADPH-dependent inactivation. They reported a higher K_I (50 μM) than Richter et al. (3.8 μM). However, the inactivation was not linear over time for the higher tTEPA concentrations used in the study by Richter et al.(2005). Nonlinearity can significantly change the apparent kinetic parameters and could possibly account for the 10-fold difference in K_I

between the two studies. A more important difference between these two studies may be the use of different substrates to determine the extent of inactivation. The substrate used by Harleton and co-workers was 7-ethoxycoumarin, and that used by Richter and co-workers was bupropion. In the characterization of MBIs of the rat P450 2B1 it was reported that different substrates in the secondary reaction resulted in different levels of enzyme inactivation (Kent et al. 2004). A similar phenomenon with P450 2B6 could give rise to the different kinetic parameters that have been reported for tTEPA-mediated inactivation of P450 2B6.

Richter (2005) and Harleton (2004) also reported that different mechanisms were responsible for the inactivation of P450 2B6 by tTEPA. Richter et al did not detect any loss in heme integrity after inactivation and therefore concluded that inactivation was due to binding of a reactive intermediate to the apoprotein. In contrast, Harleton et al concluded that inactivation occurred by heme destruction. They detected a significant loss of intact heme using three different methods: monitoring reduced CO spectrum, quantification by high-performance liquid chromatography (HPLC) with detection at 405 nm, and pyridine hemochrome analysis,. The loss of native heme observed with the latter two methods correlated with the loss of enzyme activity. Considering the differences in analysis and kinetic results between these two studies, it is possible that inactivation of P450 2B6 by tTEPA might occur through both heme and apoprotein modification. One could reasonably propose that due to differences in substrate orientation and size, an apoprotein adduct may not result in a detectable loss in 7-ethoxycoumarin activity (measured by Harleton) but might significantly inhibit bupropion activity (measured by Richter). Therefore, Harleton et al would detect enzyme inactivation only at higher concentration of tTEPA that resulted in significant heme destruction.

These studies should draw attention to the need to be aware of the potential effect of tTEPA-mediated inactivation of P4502B6 on the efficacy of co-administered drugs (such as cyclophosphamide) that are metabolized by P450 2B6. However, based on the differing outcomes of the two studies discussed above, it is critical to determine the affect of tTEPA-mediated inactivation of P450 2B6 on cyclophosphamide 4-hydroxylation.

5.3.4. Grapefruit Juice and Bergamottin

The first clinical study of the effects of grapefruit juice on the pharmacokinetics of drugs was published in 1991 (Bailey et al. 1991). Since then many studies on grapefruit juice–drug interactions have been published including several reviews on the topic (Bailey and Dresser 2004; Dahan and Altman 2004; Greenblatt et al. 2001; Guo and Yamazoe 2004; Saito et al. 2005). Bergamottin, 6′,7′-dihydroxybergamottin, and bergapten are major furanocoumarin components in grapefruit juice and were suggested to play a role in the observed grapefruit juice–drug interactions. All three compounds have been identified as MBIs of P450 3A4 *in vitro* (He et al. 1998; Schmiedlin-Ren et al. 1997; Tassaneeyakul et al. 2000). The major mechanism of grapefruit juice interactions with most drugs is considered to be inactivation of intestinal P450 3A4 by 6′,7′-dihydroxybergamottin (Paine, Criss and Watkins 2005).

Recently, Lin et al. reported that bergamottin was an MBI of P450 2B6 (Lin, Kent and Hollenberg 2005). The inactivation was irreversible, and time-, concentration-, and NADPH-dependent. The K_I was 5 μM, but in the presence of cytochrome b_5 decreased to 0.2 μM. The partition coefficient for the inactivation of P450 2B6 by bergamottin was 2. The low K_I and partition ratio clearly demonstrate that bergamottin is a potent inactivator of P450 2B6; the most potent identified to date. Bergamottin appears to be inactivating P450 2B6 by both heme destruction and apoprotein adduct formation. The ratio of ^{14}C-bergamottin metabolite bound to apoprotein was determined to be 0.5–1. The fact that this value is less than 1:1 is likely due to the contribution of heme destruction to enzyme inactivation. As in other studies of the mechanism-based inactivation of P450 2B6, it was not possible to determine the exact mass of the apoprotein adduct by LC/MS analysis due to large errors in the mass assignment. From the LC/MS data that was obtained, the adduct appeared to contain bergamottin with two or three oxygen atoms attached to it. The potency of inactivation of P450 2B6 by bergamottin is as great, or greater than that of P450 3A4 by either bergamottin or 6′,7′-dihydroxybergamottin (He et al. 1998; Schmiedlin-Ren et al. 1997; Tassaneeyakul et al. 2000). Therefore, grapefruit juice may significantly influence drugs that are primarily metabolized by P450 2B6 as well as those metabolized by P450 3A4.

5.3.5. Phencyclidine

Phencyclidine, PCP or angel dust, became a popular drug of abuse in the 1960s. PCP was developed in the mid-1950s by Parke-Davis as an anesthetic, but due to severe psychotic side effects never made it to the market. Mechanism-based inactivation of P450 enzymes by PCP was first reported in studies with liver microsomes from phenobarbital-treated rabbits (Hoag et al. 1984). More recently, mechanism-based inactivation of human P450 2B6 was reported (Jushchyshyn, Kent and Hollenberg 2003). PCP met all the criteria for a MBI of P450 2B6 and the mechanism of inactivation appeared to be through formation of adducts to the apoprotein. The stoichiometry of binding of a PCP reactive metabolite to the P450 apoprotein was approximately 5.5 nmol PCP per nmol P450. However, when glutathione was present in the reaction mixture the stoichiometry of binding was reduced to 1:1. Neither glutathione nor CN^- was able to protect the enzyme from inactivation. The reactive intermediates responsible for the loss in activity are not trapped by glutathione, giving rise to the 1:1 stoichiometry observed in the presence of glutathione.

The formation of covalent modification of biological macromolecules during the metabolism of PCP was first observed with rabbit liver microsomes (Ward et al. 1982). The PCP iminium ion was proposed as the reactive metabolite responsible. Hoag et al. (1984) investigated the mechanism-based inactivation of rabbit liver microsomal enzymes by PCP and concluded that the iminium ion required further metabolism to inactivate these enzymes. They later showed that the PCP iminium ion was metabolized by rabbit liver microsomes in a P450-dependent manner and that this metabolism resulted in inactivation of one or more P450 enzymes (Hoag et al. 1987). Similar results have been reported with purified rat

P450 2B1 (Crowley and Hollenberg 1995). While the PCP iminium ion was the major PCP metabolite formed by the rodent P450s, P450 2B6 metabolized PCP primarily through oxidation of the cyclohexane ring (Jushchyshyn et al. 2006). The PCP iminium ion was a minor product of P450 2B6-catalyzed PCP metabolism. Interestingly, P450 3A4 and 2D6 were not inactivated by PCP although they metabolize PCP primarily to the iminium ion (Jushchyshyn et al. 2006). These data suggest that the iminium ion might not be the precursor to the reactive intermediate that inactivates P450 2B6, and it has been suggested that the true inactivating metabolite is a product of carbon hydroxylation on the PCP cyclohexane ring (Jushchyshyn et al. 2006). So despite much efforts the mechanisms of phencyclidine-mediated P450 inactivation have not yet been elucidated.

Among the other seven compounds that have been identified as MBIs of P450 2B6 (Table 5.1), three are drugs, clopidogrel, ticlopidine and tamoxifen (Richter et al. 2004; Sridar et al. 2002). These three are relatively potent, but not specific inactivators of P450 2B6; K_i values are less than 1μM. In all cases, the integrity of the heme molecule was unaffected by enzyme inactivation. Therefore, it has been proposed that the mechanism of inactivation is apoprotein modification, but no direct evidence of a protein adduct has been obtained. The mechanism of P450 2B6 inactivation for all the compounds that have been studied appears to be at least in part due to covalent modification of the apoprotein, although heme destruction clearly plays a role for some. However, neither a protein nor a heme adduct of P450 2B6 has yet been characterized.

5.4. Inactivation of Cytochrome P450 2A Enzymes

Relatively few MBIs of P450 2A6 and P450 2A13 have been identified (Table 4.1). This is partially due to the fact that these enzymes play a minor role in drug metabolism (Guengerich 2003). Only a few drugs on the market, such as valporic acid, lisigamone, 3,5-dimethyl-2-(3-pyridyl)-thiazolidin-4-one (SM-12502), and pilcarbine (Endo et al. 2007; Pelkonen et al. 2000) are primarily metabolized by P450 2A6. However, P450 2A6 is the major catalyst of nicotine metabolism (Hukkanen, Jacob III and Benowitz 2005) and both P450 2A6 and P450 2A13 are efficient catalysts of the bioactivation of a number of carcinogens (Camus et al. 1993; He et al. 2006; Jalas, Hecht and Murphy 2005; Wong et al. 2005a; Wong et al. 2005b). Therefore, MBIs of P450 2A6 and P450 2A13 have the potential to be potent cancer chemopreventive agents.

There are three members of the P450 2A subfamily in humans: P450 2A6, P450 2A13, and P450 2A7, an orphan P450 enzyme (Guengerich 2003; Su et al. 2000). P450 2A13 and P450 2A6 are 94.5% identical, differing by only 32 amino acids. P450 2A6 is primarily expressed in the liver, and P450 2A13 is expressed throughout the respiratory tract but not in the liver. These two closely related enzymes catalyze the metabolism of a number of common substrates; for example, both are efficient coumarin 7-hydroxylases. However, with other substrates, the metabolic efficiency of P450 2A6 and P450 2A13 often differs (Brown, von Weymarn and Murphy 2005; Jalas, Hecht and Murphy 2005; Murphy, Raulinaitis and Brown

2005; Su et al. 2000; Wong, Murphy and Hecht 2005). One of the more striking differences was observed for the metabolic activation of the tobacco carcinogen NNK (Su et al. 2000). P450 2A13 is a more than 500-fold more efficient catalyst of NNK metabolism than is P450 2A6. In addition, the site of substrate oxidation sometimes differs between these two enzymes. For example, P450 2A6 catalyzes the metabolism of coumarin exclusively by 7-hydroxylation, whereas P450 2A13 efficiently catalyzes both 7-hydroxylation and 3′, 4′-epoxidation of coumarin (von Weymarn and Murphy 2003).

P450 2A6 catalyzes the conversion of nicotine, the primary addictive agent present in tobacco, to cotinine, a nonaddictive metabolite (Hukkanen, Jacob III and Benowitz 2005). Inactivation of P450 2A6 should lead to slower elimination of nicotine in smokers, and since smokers are believed to titrate their smoking to maintain a minimum plasma nicotine concentration, the treatment with a P450 2A6- specific MBI might lead to a decrease in smoking (Sellers, Tyndale and Fernandes 2003b). The use of 8-methoxysporalen (8-MOP) for this purpose has been investigated and will be discussed below (Sellers, Kaplan and Tyndale 2000). A decrease in smoking, or the use of other tobacco products, would necessarily decrease exposure to tobacco carcinogens and could therefore lower cancer risk. In addition, P450 2A13 is likely the primary catalyst of NNK metabolism in the lungs of smokers (Jalas, Hecht and Murphy 2005; Wong et al. 2005). NNK is a lung carcinogen. Therefore, inactivation of P450 2A13 by a potent and specific MBI might lead to a lower risk of lung cancer, and the development of inactivators of P450s 2A6 and 2A13 may be a valid chemoprevention approach with great potential to lower the lung cancer risk in smokers.

Only a handful of MBIs of either P450 2A6 or P450 2A13 have been studied in any detail: they are listed in Table 5.1. Two additional compounds not listed, isoniazid and valporic acid, have been reported to be MBIs of P450 2A6 based on NADPH- and time-dependent inactivation, but no further characterization has been carried out (Wen et al. 2001; Wen et al. 2002). The most potent MBI of P450 2A6 is (R)-(+)-menthofuran (Figure 5.3), a component of peppermint oil (Bertea et al. 2001) and a toxic

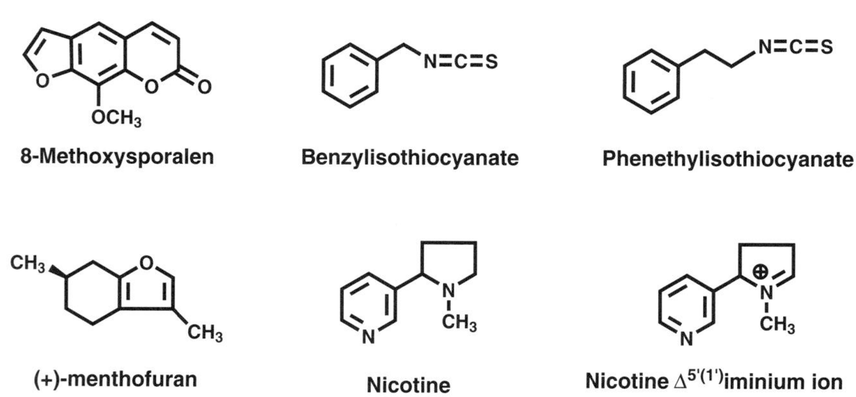

Figure 5.3 Mechanism-based inactivators of P450 2A6 and P450 2A13.

metabolite of the abortifacient (R)-(+)-pulegone. The K_I of inactivation was ~1.0 μM; k_{inact} was 0.2 min^{-1}, the partition ratio was ~3.5, and covalent modification of the apoprotein was detected (Khojasteh-Bakht et al. 1998). Menthofuran was highly selective for P450 2A6; P450s 1A2, 2D6, 2E1, and 3A4 were not inactivated at concentrations significantly higher than those that lead to inactivation of P450 2A6.

5.4.1. 8-Methoxypsoralen

The furanocoumarin 8-MOP is, like menthofuran, a potent MBI of P450 2A6, with a K_I of 0.9μM and $k_{inact.}$ of 1 min^{-1} (Koenigs et al. 1997). The partition ratio was 21, about sixfold greater than that for menthofuran. Inactivation of the enzyme occurred by formation of a covalent adduct to the apoprotein, which was detected using [^{14}C]-8-MOP (Koenigs and Trager 1998). The reactive metabolite responsible for adduct formation was proposed to be a furanoepoxide; however, the structure of the adduct has yet to be identified. More recently, we reported that 8-MOP is both an inhibitor and an MBI of P450 2A13 (von Weymarn et al. 2005). Interference from potent inhibition of P450 2A13 by 8-MOP did not allow us to determine the kinetic parameters of inactivation. However, the irreversible time-dependent inactivation of P4502A13 by 8-MOP was demonstrated by using spin-column gel filtration to remove residual 8-MOP. P450 2A13, like 2A6, was inactivated through the formation of adducts to the apoprotein. Covalently modified P450 2A13 protein was detected by electrospray LC/MS analysis of P450 2A13 following 70% inactivation by 8-MOP. The analysis detected both native P450 2A13 (theoretical mass 56,665) and a co-eluting protein (theoretical mass of 56,888) (Figure 5.4). The 232 mass difference between the proteins corresponds to the addition of one molecule of 8-MOP with an additional oxygen atom. This mass is consistent with the formation of a covalent adduct between P450 2A13 and the furanocoumarin reactive metabolite proposed by Koenigs and Trager (1998).

In experiments with human liver microsomes and enzyme-specific substrates Koenigs et al. (1997) demonstrated that in addition to P450 2A6, P450s 2C19 and P450 2E1 were inactivated by 8-MOP. In comparison to P450 2A6, inactivation of these enzymes was very modest. Therefore, at low concentrations 8-MOP appears to be a specific and potent MBI of both P450 2A6 and 2A13. Sellers et al reported that 8-MOP inhibited P450 2A6-dependent clearance of nicotine *in vivo* in human subjects (Sellers, Kaplan and Tyndale 2000). They also reported that 8-MOP increased the amount of NNK derived from cigarette smoke that was detoxified through NNAL-glucuronidation (Sellers et al. 2003a). The observed increase in NNK detoxification was attributed to a decrease in P450 2A6-mediated NNK bioactivation. However, the interpretation of these data may be more complicated. 8-MOP is a potent inhibitor of P450 1A2 (Zhang et al. 2001), and P450 1A2 may contribute significantly to hepatic NNK metabolism (Jalas, Hecht and Murphy 2005). Therefore, the observed increase in NNAL-glucuronidation could be due to 8-MOP-mediated inhibition of P450 1A2-catalyzed NNK metabolism, not 8-MOP-mediated inactivation of P450 2A6.

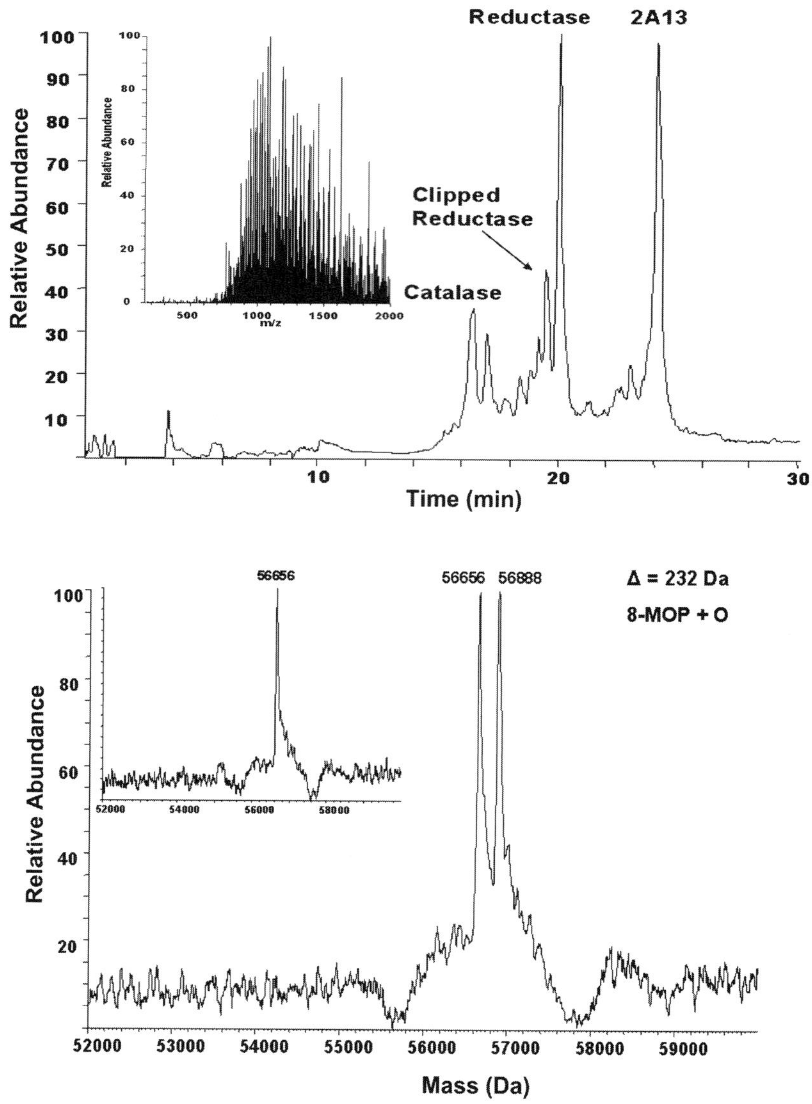

Figure 5.4 Electrospray LC/MS analysis P450 2A13 apoprotein following inactivation by 8-methoxypsoralen. *Top panel*: Total ion chromatograph of inactivated sample. *Bottom panel:* Deconvoluted spectrum of inactivated P450 2A13 (insert is an exposed control sample) (from von Weymarn et al. 2005).

5.4.2. Benzylisothiocyanate and Phenethylisothiocyanate

Isothiocyanates have been studied in some detail as chemopreventive agents of NNK-induced lung carcinogenesis, and one mechanism of action is inhibition of P450s (Hecht 2000). Isothiocyanates can inhibit P450 activity by three different mechanisms: (1) competitive inhibition, (2) inactivation without P450 catalysis, or (3) as a mechanism-based inactivator (Goosen, Mills and Hollenberg 2001; Hecht 2000; Nakajima et al. 2001). These multiple pathways of inhibition complicate the analysis of isothiocyanates as potential MBIs. However, we have demonstrated that both benzylisothiocyanate (BITC) and phenethylisothiocyanate (PEITC) inactivate P450 2A6 and 2A13 in a time- and NADPH-dependent manner (von Weymarn, Chun and Hollenberg 2006b). This is in contrast to a previous study that reported that PEITC inhibited, but did not inactivated, P450 2A6 (Nakajima et al. 2001). The kinetic parameters for the inactivation of P450 2A6 by BITC were determined. The apparent K_I of 28 μM and a k_{inact} of 0.055 min^{-1} are similar to what has been reported for P450s 2B1 and 2E1 (Goosen, Mills and Hollenberg 2001; Moreno et al. 2001). However, due to the potent inhibition of P450 2A13 by BITC, and inhibition of both P450 2A6 and P450 2A13 by PEITC, the kinetic parameters for the inactivation of P450 2A16 and 2A13 by these isothiocyanates could not be determined.

The inactivation of P450s 2A6 and 2A13 by BITC and PEITC was irreversible and both compounds inactivated the enzymes exclusively through the formation of adducts to the P450 apoprotein (von Weymarn, Chun and Hollenberg 2006b). LC/MS analysis of the inactivated P450s identified a covalently modified enzyme with an adduct that corresponded to the isothiocyanate plus one oxygen atom. Nonspecific binding of the isothiocyanate alone to the enzymes was also observed both in the absence and presence of NADPH. Due to the potent inhibition of P450s 2A6 and 2A13 by BITC and PEITC, not all the criteria of mechanism-based inactivation have been tested. However, the observed time- and NADPH-dependent irreversible activity loss, and the NADPH-dependent formation of covalent adducts to the P450 apoprotein, together with the published data characterizing BITC and PEITC as MBIs of other P450 enzymes lead us to conclude that BITC and PEITC are MBIs of both P450 2A6 and P450 2A13.

5.4.3. Nicotine and Nicotine $\Delta^{5'(1')}$iminium ion

As noted above, P450 2A6 is the primary catalyst of nicotine metabolism. The major pathway of nicotine metabolism in smokers is conversion to cotinine and subsequent metabolism to trans 3′-hydroxycotinine. The first step in the formation of cotinine is P450 2A6-catalyzed 5′-oxidation to generate the nicotine $\Delta^{5'(1')}$iminium ion (Hukkanen, Jacob III and Benowitz 2005). P450 2A6 also catalyzes the 2′ and methyl oxidation of nicotine (Figure 5.5), but these are minor pathways. Conversion of the nicotine $\Delta^{5'(1')}$iminium ion to cotinine may be catalyzed by aldehyde oxidase or P450 2A6 (Hukkanen, Jacob III and Benowitz 2005; von Weymarn, Brown and Murphy 2006b). *In vivo*, cotinine is primarily metabolized to *trans* 3′-hydroxycotinine. However, *in vitro* both P450 2A6 and P450 2A13 also catalyze the formation of 5′-hydroxycotinine and *N*-hydroxymethylnorcotinine (Figure 5.5) (Brown, von Weymarn and Murphy 2005). Surprisingly, both P450 2A6 and P450 2A13 rather quickly catalyzed the oxidation of nicotine all the way to *trans*-3′-hydroxycotinine, 5′-hydroxycotinine, and *N*-hydroxymethylnorcotinine (Murphy, Raulinaitis and Brown 2005; von Weymarn, Brown and Murphy 2006a). We have suggested that sequential oxidation of nicotine may occur without the intermediate products leaving the active site of the enzyme.

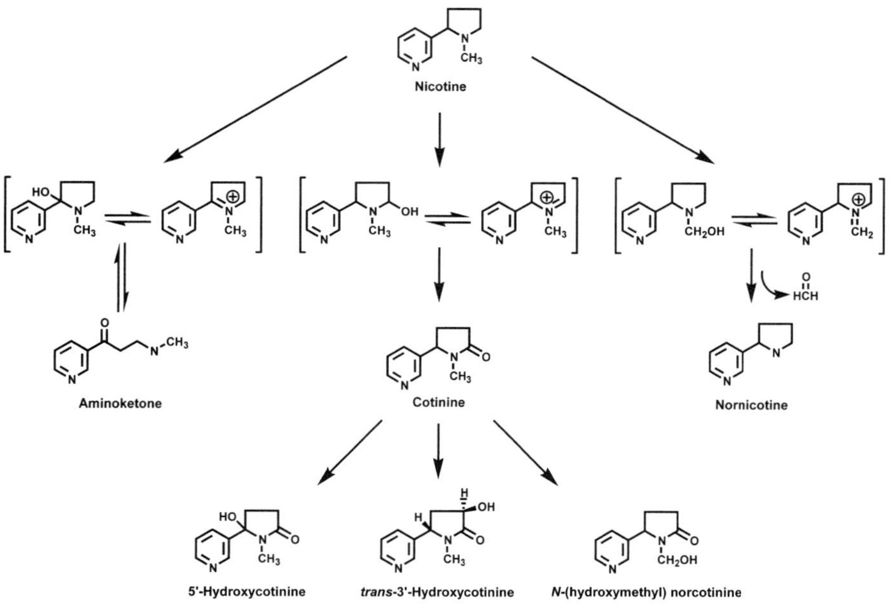

Figure 5.5 P450 2A6 and P450 2A13-catalyzed nicotine metabolism pathways.

We recently reported that nicotine irreversibly inactivates both P450 2A6 and 2A13 (von Weymarn, Brown and Murphy 2006a). The inactivation of P450 2A13 by nicotine was significantly faster than that of P450 2A6; the $t_{1/2}$ values are 7 min and 33 min, respectively. The K_I for the inactivation of P450 2A13 by nicotine is 17 μM. The K_I for the inactivation of P450 2A6 was estimated to be 21 μM. This is an estimate since inactivation was only linear over a very narrow range. The partition ratio for the inactivation of P450 2A13 by nicotine was 33. No partition ratio was determined for P450 2A6, since during the relatively long time required for complete inactivation of P450 2A6 there was significant activity loss in the absence of nicotine. Both enzymes were protected from nicotine-mediated inactivation by alternate substrates. P450 2A13 inactivation was irreversible and the exogenous nucleophile glutathione had no effect on the inactivation. Irreversibility and the effect of exogenous nucleophiles were not tested with P450 2A6. The mechanism of inactivation was investigated using [^{3}H]-nicotine; however, no adducts to either the heme or the apoprotein were observed. It was proposed that the adducts may be unstable to the denaturing acidic conditions of the HPLC analyses.

Interestingly, significant inactivation of both P450 2A6 and P450 2A13 occurred after nicotine metabolism was complete (von Weymarn, Brown and Murphy 2006a). Under conditions where 90% of the nicotine was metabolized in 2 minutes, there was only a 20% loss in activity. However, the extent of P450 2A13 inactivation continued to increase for the next 15 minutes. During those 15 min the primary metabolite, the nicotine $\Delta^{5'(1')}$iminium ion, was further metabolized to cotinine, and cotinine was metabolized to *trans* 3′-hydroxycotinine, 5′-hydroxycotinine, and *N*-hydroxymethylnorcotinine. These data lead us to suggest that the reactive species responsible for nicotine-mediated enzyme inactivation was formed during the oxidation of the $\Delta^{5'(1')}$iminium ion to cotinine. This would suggest that the nicotine $\Delta^{5'(1')}$iminium ion is an MBI of P450 2A6 and P450 2A13. We have observed time-, concentration-, and NADPH-dependent inactivation of both P450 2A6 and 2A13 by the nicotine $\Delta^{5'(1')}$iminium ion (unpublished data). The nicotine $\Delta^{5'(1')}$iminium ion did not inactivate either P450 2A6 or P450 2A13 in the absence of NADPH. Experiments are ongoing to determine the mechanism of inactivation and to begin to characterize the effects of this inactivation *in vivo* in smokers.

In summary, a number of compounds have been identified as MBIs of P450 2A6 and P450 2A13, and certainly more will be characterized in the future. It is likely that a component of grapefruit juice is an MBI of P450 2A6 (Tassaneeyakul et al. 2000) and that this compound may contribute to the observed affect of grapefruit juice on nicotine clearance (Hukkanen, Jacob III and Benowitz 2006). Mechanism-based inactivators of P450 2A6 and P450 2A13 may be useful compounds for both treating tobacco addiction and as cancer chemopreventive agents. Based on our knowledge MBIs of P450 2A enzymes, nicotine analogs and furan coumarin derivatives appear to be the type of compounds that should be explored for this purpose. It has been demonstrated in a mouse model that NNK-induced lung tumorigenesis was inhibited by 8-MOP (Takeuchi et al. 2003). Presumably the protection from NNK-induced tumors was due to either inhibition or inactivation of P450 2A5, the mouse orthologue of P450 2A6 and 2A13. P450 2A5 is an excellent catalyst of NNK bioactivation (Jalas, Hecht and Murphy 2005). Also, as discussed above, smokers administered 8-MOP decreased the number of cigarettes they smoked (Sellers, Kaplan and Tyndale 2000).

References

Alvarez-Diez, T. M., and Zheng, J. 2004. Mechanism-based inactivation of cytochrome P450 3A4 by 4-ipomeanol. Chem. Res. Toxicol. 17:150–157.

Bailey, D. G., and Dresser, G. K. 2004. Interactions between grapefruit juice and cardiovascular drugs. Am. J. Cardiovasc. Drugs 4:281–297.

Bailey, D. G., Spence, J. D., Munoz, C., and Arnold, J. M. 1991. Interaction of citrus juices with felodipine and nifedipine. Lancet 337:268–269.

Bertea, C. M., Schalk, M., Karp, F., Maffei, M., and Croteau, R. 2001. Demonstration that menthofuran synthase of mint (Mentha) is a cytochrome P450 monooxygenase: cloning, functional expression, and characterization of the responsible gene. Arch. Biochem. Biophys. 390:279–286.

Bertelsen, K. M., Venkatakrishnan, K., von Moltke, L. L., Obach, R. S., and Greenblatt, D. J. 2003. Apparent mechanism-based inhibition of human CYP2D6 in vitro by paroxetine: comparison with fluoxetine and quinidine. Drug Metab. Dispos. 31:289–293.

Brown, K. M., von Weymarn, L. B., and Murphy, S. E. 2005. Identification of *N*-(hydroxymethyl)-norcotinine as a major product of cytochrome P450 2A6, but not cytochrome P450 2A13-catalyzed cotinine metabolism. Chem. Res. Toxicol. 18:1792–1798.

Bumpus, N. N., Kent, U. M., and Hollenberg, P. F. 2006. Metabolism of efavirenz and 8-hydroxyefavirenz by P450 2B6 leads to inactivation by two distinct mechanisms. J. Pharmacol. Exp. Ther. 318:345–351.

Bumpus, N. N., Sridar, C., Kent, U. M., and Hollenberg, P. F. 2005. The naturally occurring cytochrome P450 (P450) 2B6 K262R mutant of P450 2B6 exhibits alterations in substrate metabolism and inactivation. Drug Metab. Dispos. 33:795–802.

Cai, H. and Guengerich, F. P. 2001. Reaction of trichloroethylene and trichloroethylene oxide with cytochrome P450 enzymes: inactivation and sites of modification. Chem. Res. Toxicol. 14:451–458.

Cai, Y., Baer-Dubowska, W., Ashwood-Smith, M. J., Ceska, O., Tachibana, S., and DiGiovanni, J. 1996. Mechanism-based inactivation of hepatic ethoxyresorufin O-dealkylation activity by naturally occurring coumarins. Chem. Res. Toxicol. 9:729–736.

Camus, A. M., Geneste, O., Hankakoski, P., Béréziat, J. C., Henderson, C. J., Wolf, C. R., Bartsch, H., and Lang, M. A. 1993. High variability of nitrosamine metabolism among individuals: role of cytochromes P450 2A6 and 2E1 in the dealkylation of *N*-nitrosodimethylamine and *N*-nitrosodiethylamine in mice and humans. Mol. Carcinog. 7:268–275.

Chan, W. K. and Delucchi, A. B. 2000. Resveratrol, a red wine constituent, is a mechanism-based inactivator of cytochrome P450 3A4. Life Sci. 67:3103–3112.

Chang, T. K., Chen, J., and Lee, W. B. 2001. Differential inhibition and inactivation of human CYP1 enzymes by trans-resveratrol: evidence for mechanism-based inactivation of CYP1A2. J. Pharmacol. Exp. Ther. 299:874–882.

Chang, T. K., Weber, G. F., Crespi, C. L., and Waxman, D. J. 1993. Differential activation of cyclophosphamide and ifosphamide by cytochromes P-450 2B and 3A in human liver microsomes. Cancer Res. 53:5629–5637.

Chatterjee, P., and Franklin, M. R. 2003. Human cytochrome p450 inhibition and metabolic-intermediate complex formation by goldenseal extract and its methylenedioxyphenyl components. Drug Metab. Dispos. 31:1391–1397.

Chen, Q., Ngui, J. S., Doss, G. A., Wang, R. W., Cai, X., DiNinno, F. P., Blizzard, T. A., Hammond, M. L., Stearns, R. A., Evans, D. C., Baillie, T. A., and Tang, W. 2002. Cytochrome P450 3A4-mediated bioactivation of raloxifene: irreversible enzyme inhibition and thiol adduct formation. Chem. Res. Toxicol. 15:907–914.

Chun, J., Kent, U. M., Moss, R. M., Sayre, L. M., and Hollenberg, P. F. 2000. Mechanism-based inactivation of cytochromes P450 2B1 and P450 2B6 by 2-phenyl-2-(1-piperidinyl)propane. Drug Metab. Dispos. 28:905–911.

Chun, Y. J., Ryu, S. Y., Jeong, T. C., and Kim, M. Y. 2001. Mechanism-based inhibition of human cytochrome P450 1A1 by rhapontigenin. Drug Metab. Dispos. 29:389–393.

Crowley, J. R., and Hollenberg, P. F. 1995. Mechanism-based inactivation of rat liver cytochrome P4502B1 by phencyclidine and its oxidative product, the iminium ion. Drug Metab. Dispos. 23:786–793.

Dahan, A., and Altman, H. 2004. Food–drug interaction: grapefruit juice augments drug bioavailability – mechanism, extent and relevance. Eur. J. Clin. Nutr. 58:1–9.

Dicke, K., Skrlin, S., and Murphy, S. E. 2005. Nicotine and 4-(methylnitrosamino)-1-(3-pyridyl)-butanone (NNK) metabolism by P450 2B6. Drug Metab. Dispos. 33:1760–1764.

Endo, T., Ban, M., Hirata, K., Yamamoto, A., Hara, Y., and Momose, Y. 2007. Involvement of CYP2A6 in the formation of a novel metabolite, 3-hydroxypilocarpine, from pilocarpine in human liver microsomes. Drug Metab. Dispos. 35:476–483.

Ernest, C. S., Hall, S. D., and Jones, D. R. 2005. Mechanism-based inactivation of CYP3A by HIV protease inhibitors. J. Pharmacol. Exp. Ther. 312:583–591.

Fan, P. W., Gu, C., Marsh, S. A., and Stevens, J. C. 2003. Mechanism-based inactivation of cytochrome P450 2B6 by a novel terminal acetylene inhibitor. Drug Metab. Dispos. 31:28–36.

Faucette, S. R., Hawke, R. L., LeCluyse, E. L., Shord, S. S., Yan, B. F., Laethem, R. M., and Lindley, C. M. 2000. Validation of bupropion hydroxylation as a selective marker of human cytochrome P4502B6 catalytic activity. Drug Metab. Dispos. 28:1222–1230.

Friedman, M. A., Woodcock, J., Lumpkin, M. M., Shuren, J. E., Hass, A. E., and Thompson, L. J. 1999. The safety of newly approved medicines: do recent market removals mean there is a problem? JAMA 281:1728–1734.

Goosen, T. C., Mills, D. E., and Hollenberg, P. F. 2001. Effects of benzyl isothiocyanate on rat and human cytochromes P450: identification of metabolites formed by P450 2B1. J Pharmacol. Exp. Ther. 296:198–206.

Greenblatt, D. J., Patki, K. C., von Moltke, L. L., and Shader, R. I. 2001. Drug interactions with grapefruit juice: an update. J. Clin. Psychopharmacol. 21:357–359.

Guengerich, F. P. 1990. Mechanism-based inactivation of human liver microsomal cytochrome P-450 IIIA4 by gestodene. Chem. Res. Toxicol. 3:363–371.

Guengerich, F. P. 2003. Cytochromes P450, drugs, and diseases. Mol. Interv. 3:194–204.

Guo, L. Q., and Yamazoe, Y. 2004. Inhibition of cytochrome P450 by furanocoumarins in grapefruit juice and herbal medicines. Acta Pharmacol. Sin. 25:129–136.

Ha-Duong, N. T., Dijols, S., Macherey, A. C., Goldstein, J. A., Dansette, P. M., and Mansuy, D. 2001. Ticlopidine as a selective mechanism-based inhibitor of human cytochrome P450 2C19. Biochemistry 40:12112–12122.

Hanioka, N., Ozawa, S., Jinno, H., Tanaka-Kagawa, T., Nishimura, T., Ando, M., and Sawada, J. J. 2002. Interaction of irinotecan (CPT-11) and its active metabolite 7-ethyl-10-hydroxycamptothecin (SN-38) with human cytochrome P450 enzymes. Drug Metab. Dispos. 30:391–396.

Hanna, I. H., Reed, J. R., Guengerich, F., and Hollenberg, P. F. 2000. Expression of human cytochrome P450 2B6 in *Escherichia coli:* Characterization of catalytic activity and expression levels in human liver. Arch. Biochem. Biophys. 376:206–216.

Harleton, E., Webster, M., Bumpus, N. N., Kent, U. M., Rae, J. M., and Hollenberg, P. F. 2004. Metabolism of *N,N′,N*-triethylenethiophosphoramide by CYP2B1 and CYP2B6 results in the inactivation of both isoforms by two distinct mechanisms. J. Pharmacol. Exp. Ther. 310:1011–1019.

He, K., Iyer, K. R., Hayes, R. N., Sinz, M. W., Woolf, T. F., and Hollenberg, P. F. 1998. Inactivation of cytochrome p450 3A4 by bergamottin, a component of grapefruit juice. Chem. Res. Toxicol. 11:252–259.

He, K., Woolf, T. F., and Hollenberg, P. F. 1999. Mechanism-based inactivation of cytochrome P-450-3A4 by mifepristone (RU486). J. Pharmacol. Exp. Ther. 288:791–797.

He, X. Y., Tang, L., Wang, S. L., Cai, Q. S., Wang, J. S., and Hong, J. Y. 2006. Efficient activation of aflatoxin B1 by cytochrome P450 2A13, an enzyme predominantly expressed in human respiratory tract. Int. J. Cancer 118:2665–2671.

Hecht, S. S. 2000. Inhibition of carcinogenesis by isothiocyanates. Drug Metab. Rev. 32:395–411.

Hoag, M. K., Trevor, A. J., Asscher, Y., Weissman, J., and Castagnoli, N., Jr. 1984. Metabolism-dependent inactivation of liver microsomal enzymes by phencyclidine. Drug Metab. Dispos. 12:371–375.

Hoag, M. K., Trevor, A. J., Kalir, A., and Castagnoli, N., Jr. 1987. Phencyclidine iminium ion. NADPH-dependent metabolism, covalent binding to macromolecules, and inactivation of cytochrome(s) P-450. Drug Metab. Dispos. 15:485–490.

Huitema, A. D., Kerbusch, T., Tibben, M. M., Rodenhuis, S., and Beijnen, J. H. 2000. Reduction of cyclophosphamide bioactivation by thioTEPA: critical sequence-dependency in high-dose chemotherapy regimens. Cancer Chemother. Pharmacol. 46:119–127.

Hukkanen, J., Jacob, P., III, and Benowitz, N. L. 2005. Metabolism and disposition kinetics of nicotine. Pharmacol. Rev. 57:79–115.

Hukkanen, J., Jacob, P., III, and Benowitz, N. L. 2006. Effect of grapefruit juice on cytochrome P450 2A6 and nicotine renal clearance. Clin. Pharmacol. Ther. 80:522–530.

Iwata, H., Tezuka, Y., Kadota, S., Hiratsuka, A., and Watabe, T. 2005. Mechanism-based inactivation of human liver microsomal CYP3A4 by rutaecarpine and limonin from Evodia fruit extract. Drug Metab. Pharmacokinet. 20:34–45.

Jacobson, P. A., Green, K., Birnbaum, A., and Remmel, R. P. 2002. Cytochrome P450 isozymes 3A4 and 2B6 are involved in the in vitro human metabolism of thiotepa to TEPA. Cancer Chemother. Pharmacol. 49:461–467.

Jalas, J. R., Hecht, S. S., and Murphy, S. E. 2005. Cytochrome P450 enzymes as catalysts of metabolism of 4-(methylnitrosamino)-1-(3-pyridyl)-1-butanone (NNK), a tobacco-specific carcinogen. Chem. Res. Toxicol. 18:95–110.

Jean, P., Lopez-Garcia, P., Dansette, P., Mansuy, D., and Goldstein, J. L. 1996. Oxidation of tienilic acid by human yeast-expressed cytochromes P-450 2C8, 2C9, 2C18 and 2C19. Evidence that this drug is a mechanism-based inhibitor specific for cytochrome P-450 2C9. Eur. J. Biochem. 241:797–804.

Jushchyshyn, M. I., Kent, U. M., and Hollenberg, P. F. 2003. The mechanism-based inactivation of human cytochrome P450 2B6 by phencyclidine. Drug Metab. Dispos. 31:46–52.

Jushchyshyn, M. I., Wahlstrom, J. L., Hollenberg, P. F., and Wienkers, L. C. 2006. Mechanism of inactivation of human cytochrome P450 2B6 by phencyclidine. Drug Metab. Dispos. 34:1523–1529.

Kanamitsu, S., Ito, K., Green, C. E., Tyson, C. A., Shimada, N., and Sugiyama, Y. 2000. Prediction of in vivo interaction between triazolam and erythromycin based on in vitro studies using human liver microsomes and recombinant human CYP3A4. Pharm. Res. 17:419–426.

Kassahun, K., Skordos, K., McIntosh, I., Slaughter, D., Doss, G. A., Baillie, T. A., and Yost, G. S. 2005. Zafirlukast metabolism by cytochrome P450 3A4 produces an electrophilic alpha,beta-unsaturated iminium species that results in the selective mechanism-based inactivation of the enzyme. Chem. Res. Toxicol. 18:1427–1437.

Kent, U. M., Aviram, M., Rosenblat, M., and Hollenberg, P. F. 2002a. The licorice root derived isoflavan glabridin inhibits the activities of human cytochrome P450S 3A4, 2B6, and 2C9. Drug Metab. Dispos. 30:709–715.

Kent, U. M., Juschyshyn, M. I., and Hollenberg, P. F. 2001. Mechanism-based inactivators as probes of cytochrome P450 structure and function. Curr. Drug Metab. 2:215–243.

Kent, U. M., Lin, H. L., Mills, D. E., Regal, K. A., and Hollenberg, P. F. 2006. Identification of 17-alpha-ethynylestradiol-modified active site peptides and glutathione conjugates formed during metabolism and inactivation of P450s 2B1 and 2B6. Chem. Res. Toxicol. 19:279–287.

Kent, U. M., Mills, D. E., Rajnarayanan, R. V., Alworth, W. L., and Hollenberg, P. F. 2002b. Effect of 17-alpha-ethynylestradiol on activities of cytochrome P450 2B (P450 2B) enzymes: characterization of inactivation of P450s 2B1 and 2B6 and identification of metabolites. J. Pharmacol. Exp. Ther. 300:549–558.

Kent, U. M., Pascual, L., Roof, R. A., Ballou, D. P., and Hollenberg, P. F. 2004. Mechanistic studies with *N*-benzyl-1-aminobenzotriazole-inactivated CYP2B1:

differential effects on the metabolism of 7-ethoxy-4-(trifluoromethyl)coumarin, testosterone, and benzphetamine. Arch. Biochem. Biophys. 423:277–287.

Kent, U. M., Yanev, S., and Hollenberg, P. F. 1999. Mechanism-based inactivation of cytochromes P450 2B1 and P450 2B6 by *n*-propylxanthate. Chem. Res. Toxicol. 12:317–322.

Khan, K. K., He, Y. Q., Domanski, T. L., and Halpert, J. R. 2002. Midazolam oxidation by cytochrome P450 3A4 and active-site mutants: an evaluation of multiple binding sites and of the metabolic pathway that leads to enzyme inactivation. Mol. Pharmacol. 61:495–506.

Khojasteh-Bakht, S. C., Koenigs, L. L., Peter, R. M., Trager, W. F., and Nelson, S. D. 1998. (R)-(+)-Menthofuran is a potent, mechanism-based inactivator of human liver cytochrome P450 2A6. Drug Metab. Dispos. 26:701–704.

Koenigs, L. L., Peter, R. M., Thompson, S. J., Rettie, A. E., and Trager, W. F. 1997. Mechanism-based inactivation of human liver cytochrome P450 2A6 by 8-methoxypsoralen. Drug Metab. Dispos. 25:1407–1415.

Koenigs, L. L., and Trager, W. F. 1998. Mechanism-based inactivation of P450 2A6 by furanocoumarins. Biochemistry 37:10047–10061.

Krantz, A. 1992. A classification of enzyme inhibitors. Bioorg. Med. Chem. Lett. 2:1327–1334.

Kroon, L. A. 2006. Drug interactions and smoking: raising awareness for acute and critical care providers. Crit. Care Nurs. Clin. N. Am. 18:53–62, xii.

Kunze, K. L., Mangold, B. L., Wheeler, C., Beilan, H. S., and Ortiz de Montellano, P. R. 1983. The cytochrome P-450 active site. Regiospecificity of prosthetic heme alkylation by olefins and acetylenes. J. Biol. Chem. 258:4202–4207.

Kunze, K. L., and Trager, W. F. 1993. Isoform-selective mechanism-based inhibition of human cytochrome P450 1A2 by furafylline. Chem. Res. Toxicol. 6:649–656.

Langouet, S., Furge, L. L., Kerriguy, N., Nakamura, K., Guillouzo, A., and Guengerich, F. P. 2000. Inhibition of human cytochrome P450 enzymes by 1,2-dithiole-3-thione, oltipraz and its derivatives, and sulforaphane. Chem. Res. Toxicol. 13:245–252.

Lazarou, J., Pomeranz, B. H., and Corey, P. N. 1998. Incidence of adverse drug reactions in hospitalized patients: a meta-analysis of prospective studies. JAMA 279:1200–1205.

Lin, H. L., and Hollenberg, P. F. 2007. The inactivation of cytochrome P450 3A5 by 17{alpha}-ethynylestradiol is cytochrome b5 dependent: Metabolic activation of the ethynyl moiety leads to the formation of glutathione conjugates, a heme adduct and covalent binding to the apoprotein. J. Pharmacol. Exp. Ther. 321:276–287.

Lin, H. L., Kent, U. M., and Hollenberg, P. F. 2002. Mechanism-based inactivation of cytochrome P450 3A4 by 17 alpha-ethynylestradiol: evidence for heme destruction and covalent binding to protein. J. Pharmacol. Exp. Ther. 301:160–167.

Lin, H. L., Kent, U. M., and Hollenberg, P. F. 2005. The grapefruit juice effect is not limited to cytochrome P450 (P450) 3A4: evidence for bergamottin-dependent inactivation, heme destruction, and covalent binding to protein in P450s 2B6 and 3A5. J. Pharmacol. Exp. Ther. 313:154–164.

Lin, H. L., Kent, U. M., Zhang, H., Waskell, L., and Hollenberg, P. F. 2004. The functional role of threonine-205 in the mechanism-based inactivation of P450 2B1 by two ethynyl substrates: the importance of the F helix in catalysis. J. Pharmacol. Exp. Ther. 311:855–863.

Lown, K. S., Bailey, D. G., Fontana, R. J., Janardan, S. K., Adair, C. H., Fortlage, L. A., Brown, M. B., Guo, W., and Watkins, P. B. 1997. Grapefruit juice increases felodipine oral availability in humans by decreasing intestinal CYP3A protein expression. J. Clin. Invest. 99:2545–2553.

Lu, P., Schrag, M. L., Slaughter, D. E., Raab, C. E., Shou, M., and Rodrigues, A. D. 2003. Mechanism-based inhibition of human liver microsomal cytochrome P450 1A2 by zileuton, a 5-lipoxygenase inhibitor. Drug Metab. Dispos. 31:1352–1360.

Ma, B., Prueksaritanont, T., and Lin, J. H. 2000. Drug interactions with calcium channel blockers: possible involvement of metabolite-intermediate complexation with CYP3A. Drug Metab. Dispos. 28:125–130.

Maanen, M. J., Smeets, C. J., and Beijnen, J. H. 2000. Chemistry, pharmacology and pharmacokinetics of*N*,*N*′,*N*-triethylenethiophosphoramide (ThioTEPA). Cancer Treat. Rev. 26:257–268.

Masubuchi, Y., and Horie, T. 1999. Mechanism-based inactivation of cytochrome P450s 1A2 and 3A4 by dihydralazine in human liver microsomes. Chem. Res. Toxicol. 12:1028–1032.

Masubuchi, Y., Nakano, T., Ose, A., and Horie, T. 2001. Differential selectivity in carbamazepine-induced inactivation of cytochrome P450 enzymes in rat and human liver. Arch. Toxicol. 75:538–543.

Masubuchi, Y., Ose, A., and Horie, T. 2002. Diclofenac-induced inactivation of CYP3A4 and its stimulation by quinidine. Drug Metab. Dispos. 30:1143–1148.

Mayhew, B. S., Jones, D. R., and Hall, S. D. 2000. An in vitro model for predicting in vivo inhibition of cytochrome P450 3A4 by metabolic intermediate complex formation. Drug Metab. Dispos. 28:1031–1037.

Moreno, R. L., Goosen, T., Kent, U. M., Chung, F. L., and Hollenberg, P. F. 2001. Differential effects of naturally occurring isothiocyanates on the activities of cytochrome P450 2E1 and the mutant P450 2E1 T303A. Arch. Biochem. Biophys. 391:99–110.

Murphy, S. E., Raulinaitis, V., and Brown, K. M. 2005. Nicotine 5′-oxidation and methyl oxidation by P450 2A enzymes. Drug Metab. Dispos. 13:1166–1173.

Mutlib, A. E., Chen, H., Nemeth, G. A., Markwalder, J. A., Seitz, S. P., Gan, L. S., and Christ, D. D. 1999. Identification and characterization of efavirenz metabolites by liquid chromatography/mass spectrometry and high field NMR: species differences in the metabolism of efavirenz. Drug Metab. Dispos. 27:1319–1333.

Nakajima, M., Yoshida, R., Shimada, N., Yamazaki, H., and Yokoi, T. 2001. Inhibition and inactivation of human cytochrome P450 isoforms by phenethyl isothiocyanate. Drug Metab. Dispos. 29:1110–1113.

O′Donnell, J. P., Dalvie, D. K., Kalgutkar, A. S., and Obach, R. S. 2003. Mechanism-based inactivation of human recombinant P450 2C9 by the nonsteroidal anti-inflammatory drug suprofen. Drug Metab. Dispos. 31:1369–1377.

Ohyama, K., Nakajima, M., Suzuki, M., Shimada, N., Yamazaki, H., and Yokoi, T. 2000. Inhibitory effects of amiodarone and its *N*-deethylated metabolite on human cytochrome P450 activities: prediction of in vivo drug interactions. Br. J. Clin. Pharmacol. 49:244–253.

Ortiz de Montellano, P. R. 1995. Structure, mechanism and inhibition of cytochrome P450. Drug Metab. Dispos. 23:1181–1187.

Ortiz de Montellano, P. R., Chan, W. K., Tuck, S. F., Kaikaus, R. M., Bass, N. M., and Peterson, J. A. 1992. Mechanism-based probes of the topology and function of fatty acid hydroxylases. FASEB J. 6:695–699.

Paine, M. F., Criss, A. B., and Watkins, P. B. 2004. Two major grapefruit juice components differ in intestinal CYP3A4 inhibition kinetic and binding properties. Drug Metab. Dispos. 32:1146–1153.

Paine, M. F., Criss, A. B., and Watkins, P. B. 2005. Two major grapefruit juice components differ in time to onset of intestinal CYP3A4 inhibition. J. Pharmacol. Exp. Ther. 312:1151–1160.

Palamanda, J. R., Casciano, C. N., Norton, L. A., Clement, R. P., Favreau, L. V., Lin, C., and Nomeir, A. A. 2001. Mechanism-based inactivation of CYP2D6 by 5-fluoro-2-[4-[(2-phenyl-1 H-imidazol-5-yl)methyl]-1-piperazinyl]pyrimidine. Drug Metab. Dispos. 29:863–867.

Pelkonen, O., Rautio, A., Raunio, H., and Pasanen, M. 2000. CYP2A6: a human coumarin 7-hydroxylase. Toxicology 144:139–147.

Polasek, T. M., Elliot, D. J., Lewis, B. C., and Miners, J. O. 2004. Mechanism-based inactivation of human cytochrome P4502C8 by drugs in vitro. J. Pharmacol. Exp. Ther. 311:996–1007.

Polasek, T. M., Elliot, D. J., Somogyi, A. A., Gillam, E. M., Lewis, B. C., and Miners, J. O. 2006. An evaluation of potential mechanism-based inactivation of human drug metabolizing cytochromes P450 by monoamine oxidase inhibitors, including isoniazid. Br. J Clin. Pharmacol. 61:570–584.

Pratt, R. F. 1992. On the definition and classification of mechanism-based enzyme inhibitors. Bioorg. Med. Chem. Lett. 11:1323–1326.

Prueksaritanont, T., Ma, B., Tang, C., Meng, Y., Assang, C., Lu, P., Reider, P. J., Lin, J. H., and Baillie, T. A. 1999. Metabolic interactions between mibefradil and HMG-CoA reductase inhibitors: an in vitro investigation with human liver preparations. Br. J. Clin. Pharmacol. 47:291–298.

Richter, T., Murdter, T. E., Heinkele, G., Pleiss, J., Tatzel, S., Schwab, M., Eichelbaum, M., and Zanger, U. M. 2004. Potent mechanism-based inhibition of human CYP2B6 by clopidogrel and ticlopidine. J. Pharmacol. Exp. Ther. 308:189–197.

Richter, T., Schwab, M., Eichelbaum, M., and Zanger, U. M. 2005. Inhibition of human CYP2B6 by *N,N′,N″*-triethylenethiophosphoramide is irreversible and mechanism-based. Biochem. Pharmacol. 69:517–524.

Roy, P., Yu, L. J., Crespi, C. L., and Waxman, D. J. 1999. Development of a substrate-activity based approach to identify the major human liver P-450 catalysts of cyclophosphamide and ifosfamide activation based on cDNA-expressed activities and liver microsomal P-450 profiles. Drug Metab. Dispos. 27:655–666.

Saito, M., Hirata-Koizumi, M., Matsumoto, M., Urano, T., and Hasegawa, R. 2005. Undesirable effects of citrus juice on the pharmacokinetics of drugs: focus on recent studies. Drug Safety 28:677–694.

Schmiedlin-Ren, P., Edwards, D. J., Fitzsimmons, M. E., He, K., Lown, K. S., Woster, P. M., Rahman, A., Thummel, K. E., Fisher, J. M., Hollenberg, P. F., and Watkins, P. B. 1997. Mechanisms of enhanced oral availability of CYP3A4 substrates by grapefruit constituents. Decreased enterocyte CYP3A4 concentration and mechanism-based inactivation by furanocoumarins. Drug Metab. Dispos. 25:1228–1233.

Sellers, E. M., Kaplan, H. L., and Tyndale, R. F. 2000. Inhibition of cytochrome P450 2A6 increases nicotine's oral bioavailablity and decreases smoking. Clin. Pharmacol. Ther. 68:35–43.

Sellers, E. M., Ramamoorthy, Y., Zeman, M. V., Djordjevic, M. V., and Tyndale, R. F. 2003a. The effect of methoxsalen on nicotine and 4-(methylnitrosamino)-1-(3-pyridyl)-1-butanone (NNK) metabolism in vivo. Nicotine. Tob. Res. 5:891–899.

Sellers, E. M., Tyndale, R. F., and Fernandes, L. C. 2003b. Decreasing smoking behaviour and risk through CYP2A6 inhibition. Drug Discov. Today 8:487–493.

Silverman, B. D. 1988. Kinetics of mechanisms-based inactivation. In Mechanism-based Enzyme Inactivation:Chemistry and Enzymology, pp. 3–30. Boca Raton: CRC Press.

Silverman, R. B. 1996. Mechanism-based enzyme inactivators. In Contemporary Enzyme Kinetics and Mechanisms, ed. D. L. Purich, pp. 291–334. San Diego: Academic Press.

Sridar, C., Goosen, T. C., Kent, U. M., Williams, J. A., and Hollenberg, P. F. 2004. Silybin inactivates cytochromes P450 3A4 and 2C9 and inhibits major hepatic glucuronosyltransferases. Drug Metab. Dispos. 32:587–594.

Sridar, C., Kent, U. M., Notley, L. M., Gillam, E. M., and Hollenberg, P. F. 2002. Effect of tamoxifen on the enzymatic activity of human cytochrome CYP2B6. J. Pharmacol. Exp. Ther. 301:945–952.

Su, T., Bao, Z., Zhang, Q. Y., Smith, T. J., Hong, J. Y., and Ding, X. 2000. Human cytochrome P 450 CYP2A13: Predominant expression in the respiratory tract and in high efficiency metabolic activation of a tobacco-specific carcinogen, 4-(methylnitrosamino)-1-(3-pyridyl)-1-butanone. Cancer Res. 60:5074–5079.

Takeuchi, H., Saoo, K., Yokohira, M., Ikeda, M., Maeta, H., Miyazaki, M., Yamazaki, H., Kamataki, T., and Imaida, K. 2003. Pretreatment with 8-methoxypsoralen, a potent human CYP2A6 inhibitor, strongly inhibits lung tumorigenesis induced by 4-(methylnitrosamino)-1-(3-pyridyl)-1-butanone in female A/J mice. Cancer Res. 63:7581–7583.

Tassaneeyakul, W., Guo, L. Q., Fukuda, K., Ohta, T., and Yamazoe, Y. 2000. Inhibition selectivity of grapefruit juice components on human cytochromes P450. Arch. Biochem. Biophys. 378:356–363.

von Weymarn, L., and Murphy, S. E. 2003. CYP 2A13-catalyzed coumarin metabolism, comparison to CYP2A5 and CYP2A6. Xenobiotica 33:73–81.

von Weymarn, L. B., Brown, K. M., and Murphy, S. E. 2006a. Inactivation of CYP2A6 and CYP2A13 during nicotine metabolism. J. Pharmacol. Exp. Ther. 316:295–303.

von Weymarn, L. B., Chun, J. A., and Hollenberg, P. F. 2006b. Effects of benzyl and phenethyl isothiocyanate on P450s 2A6 and 2A13: potential for chemoprevention in smokers. Carcinogenesis 27:782–790.

von Weymarn, L. B., Sridar, C., and Hollenberg, P. F. 2004. Identification of amino acid residues involved in the inactivation of cytochrome P450 2B1 by two acetylenic compounds: the role of three residues in nonsubstrate recognition sites. J. Pharmacol. Exp. Ther. 311:71–79.

von Weymarn, L. B., Zhang, Q. Y., Ding, X., and Hollenberg, P. F. 2005. Effects of 8-methoxypsoralen on cytochrome P450 2A13. Carcinogenesis 26:621–629.

Voorman, R. L., Maio, S. M., Payne, N. A., Zhao, Z., Koeplinger, K. A., and Wang, X. 1998. Microsomal metabolism of delavirdine: evidence for mechanism-based inactivation of human cytochrome P450 3A. J. Pharmacol. Exp. Ther. 287:381–388.

Wang, H., Faucette, S. R., Gilbert, D., Jolley, S. L., Sueyoshi, T., Negishi, M., and LeCluyse, E. L. 2003. Glucocorticoid receptor enhancement of pregnane X receptor-mediated CYP2B6 regulation in primary human hepatocytes. Drug Metab. Dispos. 31:620–630.

Wang, Y. H., Jones, D. R., and Hall, S. D. 2004. Prediction of cytochrome P450 3A inhibition by verapamil enantiomers and their metabolites. Drug Metab. Dispos. 32:259–266.

Ward, B. A., Gorski, J. C., Jones, D. R., Hall, S. D., Flockhart, D. A., and Desta, Z. 2003. The cytochrome P450 2B6 (CYP2B6) is the main catalyst of efavirenz primary and secondary metabolism: implication for HIV/AIDS therapy and utility of efavirenz as a substrate marker of CYP2B6 catalytic activity. J. Pharmacol. Exp. Ther. 306:287–300.

Ward, D. P., Trevor, A. J., Kalir, A., Adams, J. D., Baillie, T. A., and Castagnoli, N., Jr. 1982. Metabolism of phencyclidine. The role of iminium ion formation in covalent binding to rabbit microsomal protein. Drug Metab. Dispos. 10:690–695.

Wen, X., Wang, J. S., Kivisto, K. T., Neuvonen, P. J., and Backman, J. T. 2001. In vitro evaluation of valproic acid as an inhibitor of human cytochrome P450 isoforms: preferential inhibition of cytochrome P450 2C9 (CYP2C9). Br. J. Clin. Pharmacol. 52:547–553.

Wen, X., Wang, J. S., Neuvonen, P. J., and Backman, J. T. 2002. Isoniazid is a mechanism-based inhibitor of cytochrome P450 1A2, 2A6, 2C19 and 3A4 isoforms in human liver microsomes. Eur. J. Clin. Pharmacol. 57:799–804.

Wienkers, L. C., and Heath, T. G. 2005. Predicting in vivo drug interactions from in vitro drug discovery data. Nat. Rev. Drug Discov. 4:825–833.

Wong, H. L., Murphy, S. E., and Hecht, S. S. 2005. Cytochrome P450 2A-catalyzed metabolic activation of structurally similar carcinogenic nitrosamines: *N′*-nitrosonornicotine enantiomers, *N*-nitrosopiperidine, and *N*-nitrosopyrrolidine. Chem. Res. Toxicol. 18:61–69.

Wong, H. L., Zhang, X., Zhang, Q. Y., Gu, J., Ding, X., Hecht, S. S., and Murphy, S. E. 2005. Metabolic activation of the tobacco carcinogen 4-(methylnitrosamino)-(3-pyridyl)-1-butanone by cytochrome p450 2A13 in human fetal nasal microsomes. Chem. Res. Toxicol. 18:913–918.

Yamazaki, H., Inoue, K., Hashimoto, M., and Shimada, T. 1999. Roles of CYP2A6 and CYP2B6 in nicotine C-oxidation by human liver microsomes. Arch. Toxicol. 73:65–70.

Zhang, W., Kilicarslan, T., Tyndale, R. F., and Sellers, E. M. 2001. Evaluation of methoxsalen, tranylcypromine, and tryptamine as specific and selective CYP2A6 inhibitors in vitro. Drug Metab. Dispos. 29:897–902.

Zhang, Z. Y., and Wong, Y. N. 2005. Enzyme kinetics for clinically relevant CYP inhibition. Curr. Drug Metab. 6:241–257.

Zhao, X. J., Jones, D. R., Wang, Y. H., Grimm, S. W., and Hall, S. D. 2002. Reversible and irreversible inhibition of CYP3A enzymes by tamoxifen and metabolites. Xenobiotica 32:863–878.

6

CYP2E1 – Biochemical and Toxicological Aspects and Role in Alcohol-Induced Liver Injury

Arthur I. Cederbaum
Department of Pharmacology and Biological Chemistry, Mount Sinai School of Medicine, New York, 10029, USA
e-mail: Arthur.cederbaum@mssm.edu

Keywords: CYP2E1 · Alcohol Liver Disease · Oxidative Stress · Lipid Peroxidation · HepG2 Cells

6.1. Cytochrome P450 and Oxidative Stress

The cytochrome P450 enzymes are a superfamily of hemeproteins that serve as terminal oxidases in the mixed-function oxidase system for metabolizing various endogenous substrates, such as steroids and fatty acids, and xenobiotics including drugs, toxins, and carcinogens (Guengerich 1987). Many different enzymes belong to this P450 family; P450s are present in virtually all living organisms. A systematic nomenclature system was developed for the P450 family which is based on the sequence identity of the different P450 sequences (Nebert et al. 1991; Nelson et al. 1996). The enzymes are named CYP for cytochrome P450, followed by an Arabic number denoting the family (more than 40% identity on the amino acid sequence level), a letter designating the subfamily (more than 55% identity), and finally an Arabic numeral representing the individual gene in the subfamily. The P450s catalyze many different chemical reactions including monooxygenation (insertion of an atom of oxygen into the substrate), peroxidation, reduction, dealkylation, epoxidation, and dehalogenation (Porter and Coon 1991; Rendic and Dicarlo 1997; Guengerich 2001). Many different compounds of diverse structure can be metabolized by P450 enzymes. A major function of P450-catalyzed reactions is to convert a compound into a more polar metabolite that can be easily excreted directly by the organism or conjugated by phase II enzymes into more polar excretable metabolites. With some compounds, for example, carbon tetrachloride or acetaminophen, metabolism by P450 can give rise to toxic metabolites which damage cells. For P450s to function catalytically, flavoprotein reductases such as NADPH-cytochrome P450 reductase,

A.A. Elfarra (ed.), *Advances in Bioactivation Research*, DOI: 10.1007/978-0-387-77300-1_6,

adrenodoxin, adrenodoxin reductase, are necessary to transfer electrons from NADPH or NADH to reduce the heme from the ferric redox state to the ferrous state. The latter is necessary to bind molecular oxygen to form the oxygenated P450 complex that catalyzes the diverse chemical reactions mentioned above (Lewis and Pratt 1998). Cytochrome b5 may also play an important role in electron transfer to certain P450s.

It is important to recognize that oxygen activation by P450, necessary for the enzymes catalytic function, can also result in the production of reactive-oxygen species (ROS). Small amounts of the superoxide anion radical (O_2^-) can be produced from decay of the oxygenated P450 complex, while hydrogen peroxide (H_2O_2) can form from either dismutation of O_2^- or from decay of the peroxy P450 complex (Loida and Sligar 1993; Kuthan and Ullrich 1982; White 1991). Reactive oxygen species have been implicated in many of the major diseases that plague mankind, including the toxicity of O_2 itself; hyperbaric O_2; ischemia-reperfusion injury; cardiovascular diseases; atherosclerosis; carcinogenesis; diabetes; neurodegenerative diseases, including Parkinsons disease and Alzheimer's disease; toxicity of heavy metals, for example, iron; asbestos injury; radiation injury; vitamin deficiency; drug (e.g., redox cycling agents) toxicity; aging; inflammation; smoke toxicity; emphysema; and toxicity of acute and chronic ethanol treatment (Knight 1998; Kehrer 1993; Bondy 1992; Nordman, Riviere and Rouach 1992; Cederbaum 2001). Reactive-oxygen species can be produced from many systems in cells including the mitochondrial respiratory chain (Chance, Sies and Boveris 1979); the cytochrome P450s (White 1991; Blanck et al. 1991); oxidative enzymes such as xanthine oxidase, aldehyde oxidase, cyclooxygenase, monoamine oxidase, the NADPH oxidase complex (Toykuni 1999; De Groot 1994); autooxidation of heme proteins such as ferrohemoglobin or myoglobin or biochemicals such as catecholamines, quinones, or tetrahydrobiopterins. In addition to these cellular sources of ROS, environmental sources of ROS include radiation, UV light, smoke, and certain drugs which are metabolized to radical intermediates or which can redox cycle. Reactive oxygen species are toxic to cells because they can react with most cellular macromolecules inactiving enzymes or denaturing proteins, causing DNA damage such as strand breaks, base removal, or base modifications which can result in mutation, peroxidation of lipids which can result in destruction of biological membranes and produce reactive aldehydic products such as malondialdehyde or 4-hydroxynonenal (Nakazawa, Genka and Fujishima 1996; McCord 1998). A variety of enzymatic and nonenzymatic mechanisms have evolved to protect cells against ROS, including the superoxide dismutases, which remove O_2^-; catalase and the glutathione (GSH) peroxidase system which remove H_2O_2; glutathione transferases which can remove reactive intermediates and lipid aldehydes, metallothioneins, heme oxygenase, thioredoxin which remove various ROS; ceruloplasmin and ferritin which help remove metals such as iron which promote oxidative reactions; nonenzymatic, low-molecular-weight antioxidants such as GSH itself, vitamin E, ascorbate (vitamin C), vitamin A, ubiquinone, uric acid, bilirubin (Halliwell 1999; Yu 1994). Oxidative stress or toxicity by ROS reflects a balance between the rates of production of ROS compared to the rates of removal of ROS plus repair of damaged cellular macromolecules. While excess ROS can cause toxicity, macrophages and neutrophils contain an NADPH oxidase which produces ROS to destroy foreign organisms (Rosen et al. 1995), and the enzyme myeloperoxidase catalyzes a reaction between H_2O_2 and chloride to produce the powerful oxidant hypochlorite (bleach) to help destroy foreign invaders. In addition, ROS at low concentrations, especially H_2O_2, may be important in signal transduction mechanisms in cells, and thus be involved in cellular physiology and metabolism (Lander 1997).

6.2. Alcohol, Oxidative Stress and Cell Injury

The ability of acute and chronic ethanol treatment to increase production of ROS and enhance peroxidation of lipids, protein, and DNA has been demonstrated in a variety of systems, cells, and species, including humans. Much has been learned about alcohol metabolism, the various enzymes and pathways involved, and how alcohol, directly via its metabolism, or indirectly via its solvent-like action affecting cellular membranes impacts on cell function. Yet, despite this tremendous growth in understanding alcohol metabolism and actions, the mechanism(s) by which alcohol causes cell injury are still not clear. A variety of leading mechanisms have been briefly summarized (Cederbaum 2001; Bondy 1992; Nordman, Riviere and Rouach 1992), and it is likely that many of them ultimately converge as they reflect a spectrum of the organism's response to the myriad of direct and indirect actions of alcohol. A major mechanism that is a focus of considerable research is the role of lipid peroxidation and oxidative stress in alcohol toxicity. Many pathways have been suggested to play a key role in how ethanol induces "oxidative stress". Some of these include redox state changes (decrease in the $NAD^+/NADH$ redox ratio) produced as a result of ethanol oxidation by alcohol and aldehyde dehydrogenases; production of the reactive product acetaldehyde as a consequence of ethanol oxidation by all major oxidative pathways; damage to mitochondria which results in decreased ATP production; direct or membrane effects caused by hydrophobic ethanol interaction with either phospholipids or protein components or enzymes; ethanol-induced hypoxia, especially in the pericentral zone of the liver acinus as oxygen is consumed in order for the liver to detoxify ethanol via oxidation; ethanol effects on the immune system, and altered cytokine production; ethanol-induced increase in bacterial-derived endotoxin with subsequent activation of Kupffer cells; ethanol induction of CYP2E1; ethanol mobilization of iron which results in enhanced levels of low-molecular-weight non-heme iron; effects on antioxidant enzymes and chemicals, particularly mitochondrial and cytosolic glutathione; one-electron oxidation of ethanol to the 1-hydroxy ethyl radical; conversion of xanthine dehydrogenase to the xanthine oxidase form. Again, many of these pathways are not exclusive of one another and it is likely that several, indeed many, systems contribute to the ability of ethanol to induce a state of oxidative stress.

What is the evidence that ethanol-induced oxidative stress plays a role in cell injury? While many studies have shown increases in lipid peroxidation or protein carbonyl formation by alcohol, it is not always clear if these are causes of or consequences of the alcohol-induced tissue injury. Nevertheless, there are many studies which show that administration of antioxidants or iron chelators or GSH-replenishing agents can prevent or ameliorate the toxic actions of alcohol. The most convincing data that oxidative stress contributes to alcohol-induced liver injury comes from the studies using the intragastric infusion model of alcohol administration. In these studies, alcohol-induced liver injury was associated with enhanced lipid peroxidation, protein carbonyl formation, formation of the 1-hydroxyethyl radical, formation of lipid radicals, and decreases in hepatic antioxidant defense especially GSH (Knecht et al. 1995; Tsukamoto and Lu 2001; Iimuro et al. 2000; Nanji et al. 1994; Morimoto et al. 1994). Replacement of polyunsaturated fat (required for lipid peroxidation to occur) with saturated fat or medium chain triglycerides in the diets fed to rats intragastrically, lowered or prevented the lipid peroxidation, and the alcohol-induced liver injury. Thus, alcohol plus polyunsaturated fat was required for the injury to occur. Addition of iron, known to generate OH and promote oxidative stress, to these diets exacerbated the liver injury (Tsukamoto et al. 1995). Importantly, addition of antioxidants such as vitamin E, ebselen, superoxide dismutase, GSH precursors, prevented the alcohol-induced liver injury. Because alcohol-induced liver injury has been linked to oxidative stress, we investigated the effect of a compromised antioxidant defense system, copper–zinc superoxide dismutase (Sod1) deficiency on alcohol-induced liver injury (Kessova et al. 2003). C57BL/SV129 wild-type and Sod1 knockout mice were fed dextrose or ethanol (10% total calories) liquid diets for 3 weeks. Histological evaluation of the liver showed the development of liver injury ranging from mild to extensive centrilobular necrosis and inflammation. Alanine aminotransferase levels were elevated only in the Sod1 knockouts fed ethanol and not in the other three groups (Figure 6.1). Hepatic ATP levels were lowered only in the Sod1 knockout mice fed ethanol (Figure 6.1), and oxidative and nitrosative stress was found in their livers. Thus a rather moderate ethanol consumption promoted oxidative stress and liver injury in Sod1 knockout mice indicating that compromised antioxidant defense promotes alcohol liver injury.

In addition to these in vivo studies, in vitro studies with hepatocytes also showed that ethanol can produce oxidative stress and hepatocyte toxicity. Studies with isolated hepatocytes from control rats or chronic ethanol-fed rats indicated that ethanol metabolism via alcohol dehydrogenase results in an increase in ROS production, hepatocyte injury, and apoptosis, reactions blocked by antioxidants (Adachi and Ishii 2002; Bailey and Cunningham 2002). Studies in our laboratory with HepG2 cell lines expressing CYP2E1 showed that addition of ethanol or polyunsaturated fatty acids (PUFAs) or iron, or depletion of GSH, resulted in cell toxicity, increased oxidative stress, and mitochondrial damage, reactions prevented by antioxidants (Wu and Cederbaum 1999). Since CYP2E1 plays a role in ethanol-induced oxidant stress and is a minor pathway of ethanol oxidation,

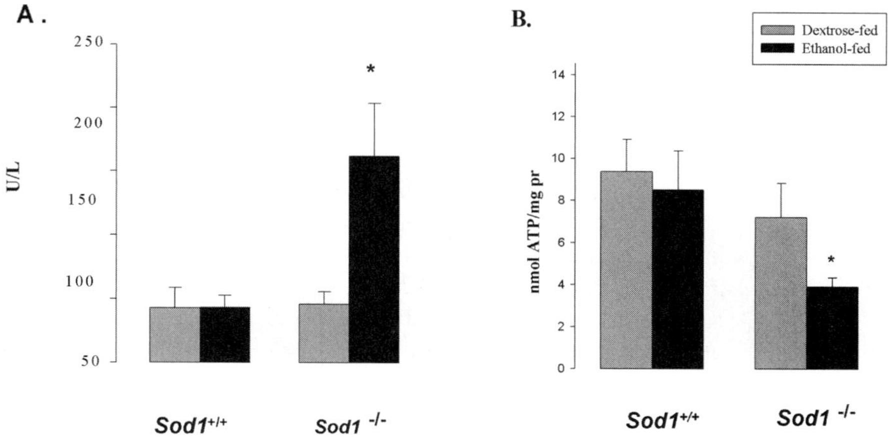

Figure 6.1 Levels of serum ALT (**A**) and hepatic ATP (**B**) in *Sod1*$^{+/+}$ and *Sod1*$^{-/-}$ mice fed ethanol or dextrose diets. * indicates $P < 0.05$ compared with correspondent control, using one-way ANOVA followed by Student–Newman–Keuls post-hoc test.

the biochemical and toxicological properties of CYP2E1 will form the basis for the remainder of this review.

6.3. CYP2E1 and the Microsomal Ethanol-Oxidizing System

Alcohol dehydrogenase is the major enzyme pathway for oxidizing ethanol to acetaldehyde. The morphological observations that chronic ethanol treatment causes proliferation of the liver smooth endoplasmic reticulum (ER) suggested that ethanol, similar to certain xenobiotics which are metabolized by cytochrome P450, may also be metabolized by P450 (Lieber 1999). A microsomal ethanol-oxidizing system (MEOS) was characterized by Lieber and associates and shown to be dependent on P450 (Lieber 1997). The K_m for ethanol oxidation by the MEOS (about 10 mM) was about an order of magnitude greater than the K_m for ethanol by alcohol dehydrogenase. Acetaldehyde is the product resulting from ethanol oxidation by MEOS, and it is clear that MEOS represents a minor pathway of ethanol oxidation, probably accounting for less than 10% of the liver capacity to oxidize ethanol (Lieber and DeCarli 1972). Importantly, activity of MEOS is enhanced after chronic ethanol treatment, partly due to an increased total content of P450, and partly due to induction of CYP2E1, a member of the P450 family with high catalytic activity with ethanol (Lieber 1997). Induction of MEOS may play an important role in the metabolic tolerance found after chronic ethanol treatment, that is, the increased capacity to oxidize ethanol. While there was early controversy over the nature of MEOS, the purification of an ethanol-inducible form of P450 from rabbit liver microsomes firmly established the role of P450 in MEOS (Koop et al. 1982). Ethanol-inducible P450s have been isolated from many species and while several P450s may be induced by ethanol, the major inducible P450 is now referred to as CYP2E1.

6.3.1. CYP2E1 Localization

CYP2E1 is mainly found in the liver but significant amounts are also found in most organs, including the brain (Hansson et al. 1990). Within the liver acinus, the levels of CYP2E1 are highest in the centrilobular zone of the liver (Ingelman-Sundberg et al. 1988). This is of interest because toxins such as ethanol, acetaminophen, nitrosamines, and carbon tetrachloride preferentially destroy the centrilobular liver region. CYP2E1 is expressed mainly in the hepatocytes of the liver; however, significant amounts are also found in the Kupffer cells (Koop, Chernosky and Brass 1991), and hepatocyte and Kupffer cell CYP2E1 are inducible, for example, by ethanol. CYP2E1, like other xenobiotic-metabolizing P450s, is mainly located in the membrane of the ER, where it is anchored and retained through its hydrophobic NH_2-terminus, leaving the large COOH-terminal domain including the catalytic site exposed to the cytosol. CYP2E1 has also been detected in other cellular compartments such as the plasma membrane (Loeper et al. 1990, 1993; Wu and Cederbaum 1992). CYP2E1 located at the plasma membrane has been suggested to play a role in the immune-mediated hepatotoxicity observed in patients suffering from alcoholic liver disease (ALD) (Eliasson and Kenna 1996; Bourdi et al. 1996; Lytton et al. 1999). CYP2E1 was shown to be transported out of the ER to the Golgi apparatus, with subsequent transfer to the plasma membrane (Neve et al. 1996; Neve and Ingelman-Sundberg 2000). Removal or modification of the hydrophobic NH_2-terminal transmembrane domain of CYP2E1 resulted in specific targeting to the mitochondria. After mitochondrial import and processing, a soluble and catalytically active protein, called Δ2E1 ($M_r \approx 40$ kD), was formed. Low levels of Δ2E1 were also observed in mitochondria isolated from rat liver, thus showing that Δ2E1 is present in vivo. Removal or modification of the NH_2-terminus of CYP2E1 results in the exposure of a mitochondrial targeting signal that directs the protein to the mitochondria. The mitochondrial targeting signal was identified and demonstrated to be located between amino acid residues 74 and 95, an area rich in positively charged amino acid residues and also containing a hydrophobic region (Neve and Ingelman-Sundberg 1999).

6.3.2. CYP2E1 Substrates

Perhaps the most important endogenous substrate of CYP2E1 is acetone which is converted to acetol and methylglyoxal three-carbon intermediates which can ultimately produce glucose (Koop and Casazza 1985). Blood levels of acetone under fasting conditions were elevated up to 50-fold in transgenic mice lacking CYP2E1 as compared to wild-type mice indicating the critical role of CYP2E1 in acetone metabolism (Bondoc et al. 1999). Other endogenous compounds that can be metabolized by CYP2E1 include fatty acids such as linoleic and arachidonic acids (AA) (Laethem et al. 1993) and lipid peroxidation-derived hydrocarbon gases such as pentane and hexane (Terelius and Ingelman-Sundberg 1986). With respect to exogenous substrates, CYP2E1 metabolizes a variety of small, hydrophobic substrates including solvents such as chloroform and carbon tetrachloride, aromatic hydrocarbons such as benzene and toluene, alcohols such as ethanol and pentanol, aldehydes such as acetaldehyde, halogenated anesthetics such as enflurane and halothane, nitrosamines such as *N,N*-dimethylnitrosamine and drugs such as chlorzoxazone and acetaminophen. Table 6.1, adapted from Koop (1992), Lieber (1997), Raucy, Kraner and Lasker (1993), Tanaka et al. (2000), Ronis et al. (1996), Bolt et al. (2003), summarizes some of the substrates which are effectively metabolized by CYP2E1. From a toxicological point of view, interest in CYP2E1 revolves around the ability of this P450 to metabolize and activate many toxicologically important compounds such as ethanol, carbon tetrachloride, acetaminophen, benzene, halothane, and many other halogenated substrates. Procarcinogens including nitrosamines and azo compounds are effective substrates for CYP2E1; for example, CYP2E1 is a low K_m dimethylnitrosamine demethylase in contrast to other forms of P450 which exhibit a high K_m for dimethylnitrosamine (Yang et al. 1990). Toxicity by the above compounds is enhanced after induction of CYP2E1, for example, by ethanol treatment, and toxicity is reduced by inhibitors of CYP2E1 or in CYP2E1 knockout mice (Lee et al. 1996). Of the substrates mentioned in Table 6.1, chlorzoxazone is of special value as its hydroxylated product can readily be assayed in the blood and the ratio of 6-hydroxychlorzoxazone/chlorzoxazone is widely used to assess the approximate levels of CYP2E1 in humans, including alcoholics (Girre et al. 1994).

Molecular oxygen itself is likely to be a most important substrate for CYP2E1. CYP2E1, relative to several other P450 enzymes, displays high NADPH oxidase activity as it appears to be poorly coupled with NADPH-cytochrome P450 reductase (Gorsky, Koop and Coon 1984; Ekstrom and Ingelman-Sundberg 1989). CYP2E1 was the most efficient P450 enzyme in the initiation of NADPH-dependent lipid peroxidation in reconstituted membranes among five different P450 forms investigated. Furthermore, anti-CYP2E1 immunoglobulin G (IgG) inhibited microsomal oxidase activity and microsomal lipid peroxidation dependent on P450, but not lipid peroxidation initiated by the action of NADPH-cytochrome P450 reductase (Ekstrom and Ingelman-Sundberg 1989). In our laboratory, we found that microsomes isolated from rats fed ethanol chronically were about twofold to threefold more reactive in generating superoxide radical and H_2O_2, and in the presence of ferric complexes, in generating hydroxyl radical and undergoing lipid peroxidation (Dicker and Cederbaum 1987; Klein et al. 1983; Puntarulo and Cederbaum 1988; Rashba-Step, Turro and Cederbaum 1993). CYP2E1 levels were elevated about threefold to fivefold in the liver microsomes after feeding rats the Lieber–DeCarli diet for 4 weeks. Mixed-function oxidase systems produce an oxidant that reacts with proteins to inactivate them and to generate protein carbonyls, a consequence of oxidation of certain amino acids such as histidine residues. This inactivation sensitizes the protein for eventual degradation by cellular proteinases and is important in protein turnover. Microsomes isolated from the ethanol-fed rats were twice as reactive as those isolated from pair-fed or chow-fed rats in catalyzing inactivation of added enzymes, such as lactic dehydrogenase, alcohol dehydrogenase, or pyruvic kinase, in the presence of ferric-ATP or ferric-citrate (Dicker and Cederbaum 1988). Similarly, microsomes isolated from the ethanol-fed

Table 6.1 Substrates metabolized/activated by CYP2E1.

Alcohols, aldehydes, ketones	Aromatic compounds	Ethers	Fatty Acids	Halogenated and nonhalogenated alkanes and alkenes	Nitrosamines, azocompounds	Reducible substrates
Acetaldehyde	Acetaminophen	Diethyl ether	Arachidonic acid (ω-1 and ω-2 hydroxylation)	Acetoacetate	Azoxymethane	*t*-Butylhydroxy-peroxide
Butanol	Aniline	Methyl *t*-butyl ether		Acetol	*N*,*N*-Diethylnitrosamine	Carbon tetrachloride
2-Butanone	Benzene		Lauric acid (ω-1 hydroxylation)	Acetone	*N*,*N*-Dimethylnitrosamine	Chromium [Cr(VI)]
Ethanol	Bromobenzene			Acetonitrile (+ catalase)	Methylazoxymethanol	Oxygen
Glycerol	Caffeine			Acrylonitrile	*N*-Nitroso-2,3-dimethyl morpholine	
Isopropanol	Capsaicin			1,3-Butadiene	*N*-Nitrosopyrrolidine	
Methanol	Chlorzoxazone			Chloroform		
Pentanol	3-Hydroxypyridine			Chloromethane		

Propanol	Isoniazid		Dibromoethane
	Phenol		Dichloromethane
	p-Nitrophenol		1,1-Dichloroethane
	Pyrazole		1,1-Dichloroethylene
	Pyridine		1,2-Dichloropropane
	Styrene		*N*,*N*-Dimethylacetamide
	Tamoxifen		*N*,*N*-Dimethylformamide
	Toluene		Enflurane
			Ethane
			Ethyl carbamate
			Ethylene dichloride
			Halothane
			Hexane
			Methylenechloride
			N-Methylformamide
			Pentane
			Thioacetamide
			Trichloroethylene
			Vinyl bromide
			Vinyl chloride

rats were more reactive in catalyzing DNA strand cleavage when plasmid DNA was added to the microsomal incubation system (Kukielka and Cederbaum 1994).

In all the above systems, the enhanced effectiveness of microsomes isolated from the ethanol-fed rats was prevented by addition of chemical inhibitors of CYP2E1 and by polyclonal antibody raised against CYP2E1 purified from pyrazole-treated rats, confirming that the increased activity in these microsomes was due to CYP2E1. Validation for the production of the appropriate oxidant (e.g., hydroxyl radical) was obtained by use of appropriate antioxidant molecules (e.g., catalase, superoxide dismutase, competitive hydroxyl radical-scavenging agents, vitamin E, glutathione).

CYP2E1 is a minor pathway of ethanol oxidation as it catalyzes the two-electron oxidation of ethanol to acetaldehyde. Interestingly, acetaldehyde is also a substrate for CYP2E1 and is oxidized to acetate; thus, CYP2E1 can, at least theoretically, catalyze the oxidation of ethanol to acetate (Terelius et al. 1991). However, this oxidation is likely to be negligible in the presence of ethanol, the substrate which generates acetaldehyde (Wu, Salmela and Lieber 1998). CYP2E1 can also promote the one-electron oxidation of ethanol to the 1-hydroxyethyl radical (Albano et al. 1987, 1991). The mechanism for this oxidation is not clear but appears to involve the oxidase activity of CYP2E1 rather than a direct metabolism by CYP2E1, since production of the hydroxyethyl radical is inhibited by ROS scavengers such as superoxide dismutase and catalase (Knecht, Thurman and Mason 1993; Rao et al. 1996). Detection of the 1-hydroxyethyl radical in the bile after administration of ethanol to rodents has been the most valuable assay for determining ethanol-induced radical formation and oxidant stress in vivo (Knecht et al. 1995; Reinke et al. 1987). Formation of the 1-hydroxylethyl radical may play a role in the development of liver damage produced by ethanol, perhaps via formation of protein adducts with subsequent autoantibody formation (Albano et al. 1996; Clot et al. 1996).

6.3.3. CYP2E1 Polymorphisms

The CYP2E1 gene is polymorphically distributed and 10 polymorphic loci on the human CYP2E1 gene have been reported (Harada et al. 2001). No significant difference was observed in drinking behavior and susceptibility to alcohol in terms of frequencies of genotypes and alleles among Japanese subjects (Itoga et al. 1999). To date, there does not appear to be any relationship between allelic forms of the CYP2E1 gene and the incidence of ethanol-mediated liver cirrhosis. No differences in gene expression were observed when reporter constructs of various CYP2E1 variant alleles were transfected into transformed cell lines (Badger et al. 2003). Many epidemiologic studies have been carried out to try to relate various CYP2E1 polymorphic alleles to numerous types of cancers (stomach, lung, colorectal, pancreatic, hepatic, renal, oval), but obvious and significant relationships have been difficult to observe. For a recent review on CYP2E1 polymorphisms, the reader is referred to Bolt, Koos and Their (2003).

6.3.4. Induction of CYP2E1

Many of the substrates for CYP2E1 can induce their own metabolism. This was initially observed with ethanol, which is a substrate for CYP2E1 and elevates CYP2E1 levels (Lieber 1997, 1999). In fact, these two properties explain the ability of ethanol to inhibit the metabolism of certain substrates when the alcohol is present; that is, ethanol and the substrate compete for oxidation by CYP2E1, and for ethanol to increase the metabolism of substrates when it is no longer present to compete, but the ethanol treatment elevated the levels of the CYP2E1 catalyst. Ethanol can be oxidized by other P450s besides CYP2E1, notably CYPs 3A and IA, and ethanol treatment can elevate the levels of these CYPs (Asai et al. 1996; Salmela et al. 1998). A variety of heterocyclic compounds such as imidazole, pyridine, pyrazole, 4-methylpyrazole (4-MP), thiazole, and isoniazid have been shown to elevate CYP2E1 levels as do solvents such as dimethylsulfoxide, various alcohols, benzene, and acetone (Song et al. 1986, 1996, Song 1995). These low-molecular-weight compounds have been used in vivo or in vitro to elevate or help prevent loss of CYP2E1 under tissue culture conditions, and their mode of mechanism will be discussed below.

CYP2E1 can also be induced under a variety of metabolic or nutritional conditions. For example, CYP2E1 levels were elevated in chronically obese, overfed rats and in rats fed a high-fat diet (Raucy et al. 1991; Yun et al. 1992). Somewhat paradoxical, in rats levels of CYP2E1 were increased by fasting and by prolonged starvation (Hong et al. 1987; Johansson et al. 1990). Diabetes has been reported to increase the expression of CYP2E1 mRNA and protein levels several fold (Woodcroft et al. 2002). This may be related to actions of insulin which downregulated CYP2E1 expression at the post-transcriptional level in a rat hepatoma cell line (DeWaziers et al. 1995; Peng and Coon 1998) and in rat hepatocyte culture (Woodcroft and Novak 1997). CYP2E1 levels were elevated in liver and kidney microsomes of rats treated with streptozocin (Shimojo et al. 1993). CYP2E1 induction in diabetes may be associated with the elevated production of ketone bodies (Bellward et al. 1987). The carbohydrate content of the diet influences CYP2E1 levels as a low-carbohydrate diet increased the extent of induction of MEOS by ethanol (Teschke, Moreno and Petrides 1981) and high-fat/low-carbohydrate diets resulted in the highest levels of CYP2E1 induced by ethanol (Yoo et al. 1991). In this respect, it is interesting that alcohol-induced liver injury is magnified in diets with very low levels of carbohydrate and high levels of fat (Badger et al. 1998; Lindros and Jarvelainen 1998).

Besides insulin, other hormones can affect CYP2E1 levels. Hypophysectomy and triiodothyronine increase CYP2E1 protein and mRNA levels in contrast to insulin which lowers them (Peng and Coon 1998; Hong et al. 1990). In primary rat hepatocyte cultures, glucagon lowered CYP2E1 levels by accelerating turnover of the CYP2E1 protein by a cyclic AMP-dependent process (Eliasson, Mkrtachian and Ingelman-Sunberg 1992). Testosterone increased renal but not hepatic, CYP2E1 levels (Hoivik et al. 1995).

Nonalcoholic steatohepatitis (NASH) is a condition characterized by hepatomegaly, elevated serum aminotransferase levels, and a histologic picture similar to alcoholic hepatitis (Reid 2001). Oxidative stress and lipid peroxidation is one of the critical factors involved in the genesis and probably the progression of NASH (Weltman et al. 1998). In a mouse model of NASH, hepatic CYP2E1 was upregulated, and this was associated with a dramatic increase in total lipid peroxide levels that were substantially inhibited by anti-CYP2E1 antibody (Leclereq et al. 2000). However, it is now recognized that NASH also develops in CYP2E1 knockout mice as other CYPs, notably CYP4A10 and CYP4A14 were upregulated (Leclereq et al. 2000). An integrated concept whereby either CYP2E1 or CYP4A or both play key roles in ROS production and contribute centrally to the pathogenesis of NASH was recently proposed (Robertson, Leclereq and Farrell 2001).

6.3.5. Regulation of CYP2E1

Considerable data have been reported elucidating the molecular mechanism of CYP2E1 regulation by exogenous compounds as well as during pathophysiological conditions. CYP2E1 is regulated by multiple, distinct regulatory mechanisms (Koop and Tierney 1990; Ronis et al. 1991; Song 1995, Song et al. 1996). The CYP2E1 gene is under transcriptional control during development. In rats, immediately after birth, it is activated and is maximally transcribed within the first week. Upon fasting or induced diabetes, the mRNA for 2E1 is increased several fold (Song et al. 1987). It was suggested, from nuclear run-on transcription assays, that this increase is due to post-transcriptional mRNA stabilization. Although these mechanisms have been established, the regulation of CYP2E1 by the small diverse group of chemicals is less clear. At one fixed time point (24 h) after administration of ethanol, acetone, or pyrazole to rats, Song et al. found that mRNA levels did not increase (Song et al. 1986). The mechanism of induction was, therefore, suggested to be at the level of protein degradation. Unlike other major classes of cytochrome P450 (especially, class I–IV family members) which can be transcriptionally activated by their respective inducers, CYP2E1 is not transcriptionally activated by an acute bolus dose or chronic administration of ethanol, acetone, or other exogenous inducing agents. Although elevation of CYP2E1 mRNA levels has been reported (Tsutsumi et al. 1989), most investigators reported little induction or slight reduction of CYP2E1 mRNA level after ethanol administration (Song et al. 1986, 1996; Johansson et al. 1988). From in vivo data of CYP2E1 turnover in rats chronically treated with acetone (Song et al. 1989) and in vitro hepatocyte culture systems (Eliasson, Johansson and Ingelman-Sundberg 1988; Wu et al. 1990), exogenous CYP2E1 inducers such as acetone, ethanol, imidazole, and 4-MP were shown to increase CYP2E1 by protein stabilization. Using in vivo radiolabeling of CYP2E1 followed by immunopurification, the turnover rate of CYP2E1 was determined. Under normal conditions, CYP2E1 was degraded by two phases with a short half-life of 7 h and a longer half-life of 37 h However, after chronic acetone administration, the rapid phase of degradation was abolished, while the slower phase with the same half-life of 37 h was still observed. These data indicated that acetone, a substrate of CYP2E1, stabilizes the enzyme by inhibiting the rapid phase of its degradation (Song et al. 1989).

However, different results have been reported to suggest alternative mechanisms of CYP2E1 regulation. Tsutsumi et al. (1993) reported that ethanol induces CYP2E1 by increasing the rate of CYP2E1 protein synthesis without changing its half-life (a single half-life of 27 h). It was also suggested that CYP2E1 may be degraded in the ER (Eliasson, Johansson and Ingelman-Sundberg 1990). Furthermore, ethanol, at high concentrations (>300 mg dl^{-1}) achieved by the intragastric infusion model, induced the CYP2E1 gene transcriptionally (Ronis et al. 1993). It is of interest to note that ethanol (up to 1.5 M concentration) did not change the level of CYP2E1 mRNA despite a fivefold elevation of CYP2E1 protein and its activity in a FGC-4 hepatoma culture system (McGehee et al. 1994). The various differences discussed above may result from different model systems utilized. Using an in vivo rat model of alcohol withdrawal, Roberts et al. (1994, 1995) recently reported that ethanol increases CYP2E1 by protein stabilization. This phenomenon was observed not only in the liver but also other extrahepatic tissues such as kidney, brain, and intestine. In addition, CYP2E1 protein stabilization appeared dependent upon blood alcohol or acetone concentration. Furthermore, a turnover study, using in vivo radiolabeling of CYP2E1 with (^{14}C) $NAHCO_3$ and immunopurification, demonstrated that ethanol treatment abolished the rapid phase of CYP2E1 degradation while biphasic degradation of CYP2E1 was observed in the control animals (Roberts, Shoaf and Song 1995).

Our laboratory has investigated the increase in CYP2E1 levels by ligands such as pyrazole or 4-MP. Under a variety of reaction conditions (dose, time after in vivo administration) or co-administration with streptozotocin which stabilizes CYP2E1 mRNA, or administration to neonates in which active CYP2E1 transcription is occurring, pyrazole and 4-MP elevated liver and kidney CYP2E1 immunoreactive protein and catalytic activity in the absence of an increase in CYP2E1 mRNA levels (Winters and Cederbaum 1992; Wu and Cederbaum 1993a,b). In isolated rat hepatocyte cultures, CYP2E1 mRNA and protein levels and CYP2E1 catalytic activity rapidly declined with time in culture. Addition of pyrazole or 4-MP slowed the decline in CYP2E1 protein and activity, without any effect on CYP2E1 mRNA levels (Wu et al. 1990). Similarly, McGhee et al. (1994) reported the half-life of CYP2E1 in a hepatoma cell line to be 1.8 h in the absence of ethanol and 45 h in the presence of ethanol. In our HepG2 cell model, the half-life of CYP2E1 was about 3 h, and this was increased by glycerol, DMSO, ethanol, and 4-MP (Yang and Cederbaum 1997a). It is clear that a major level of regulation of CYP2E1 formation appears to be post-transcriptional as various substrates and ligands increase the content of CYP2E1 by protection against rapid degradation by intracellular proteolytic pathways.

What triggers CYP2E1 turnover and the nature of the proteases responsible for its degradation is not clear. Two different pathways have been reported in the literature. Ingelman-Sundberg and co-workers reported that cAMP-dependent phosphorylation of CYP2E1 is followed by heme loss and subsequent apoprotein degradation by serine proteases present in the ER which exhibit proteolytic activities, in vitro, toward detergent-solubilized rat liver CYP2E1 (Eliasson, Johansson and Ingelman-Sundberg 1990; Eliasson, Mkrtachian and Ingelman-Sundberg 1992; Zhukov, Werlinder and Ingelman-Sundberg 1993). Substrates and ligands are postulated to prevent CYP2E1 from rapid degradation by blocking the recognition sites of phosphorylation. Tierney, Haas and Koop (1992) using an in vivo mouse model showed that 2E1 inactivated by CCl_4 and 3-aminotriazole was rapidly removed from the ER. In this model they detected production of high-molecular-weight microsomal proteins after CCl_4 treatment believed to be ubiquitin conjugates. Roberts (1997) using an in vitro microsomal system plus a 105 000 $\times$ g supernatant fraction found that the loss of CYP2E1 was accompanied by the appearance of high-molecular-weight material, some which reacted with anti-ubiquitin IgG, suggesting that ubiquitin conjugates may target CYP2E1 for rapid proteolysis. CYP2E1 may be labilized by oxidant stress as inhibition of electron transfer by inhibition of the NADPH-cytochrome P450 reductase increased the stability of CYP2E1 (Zhukov and Ingelman-Sundberg, 1999).

In our laboratory, CYP2E1 degradation was studied in HepG2 cells which stably and constitutively express CYP2E1. When the cells were incubated for 2 days in the presence of CYP2E1 ligands such as ethanol, DMSO, glycerol, pyrazole or 4-MP, CYP2E1 steady-state levels were increased several-fold as shown by immunoblot analysis and by enhanced oxidation of *p*-nitrophenol (Yang and Cederbaum 1997a). Levels of cytochrome b_5 or activities of NADPH-cytochrome P450 reductase or NADH-cytochrome b_5 reductase were not affected by the ligand (glycerol) treatment suggesting some selectivity for effects on CYP2E1 compared to other microsomal enzymes which comprise the mixed-function oxidase system (Yang and Cederbaum 1997a,b). Levels of CYP2E1 mRNA were not increased by the ligands. Expression of CYP2E1 mRNA is under control of the long terminal repeats of the retroviral promoter in the HepG2 cells. These results showed that ethanol and other CYP2E1 ligands increase the content and activity of CYP2E1 in this HepG2 cell model without any effect on CYP2E1 mRNA. To evaluate CYP2E1 turnover in the HepG2 cells, pulse-chase experiments or addition of cyclohexmide to inhibit new protein synthesis followed by examination of the degradation rates of the remaining CYP2E1 protein were carried out. The half-life of CYP2E1 was 3 (pulse-chase) or 5 (cycloheximide) h in the absence of ligand, whereas in the presence of the ligand, 60–80% of the original para nitrophenol (PNP) oxidation activity and CYP2E1 levels remained 24 h after addition of cyclohexmide or after addition of excess cold methionine. In contrast to results with ethanol, dimethyl sulfoxide (DMSO), 4-MP, or glycerol, not all CYP2E1 substrates stabilize the enzyme against degradation; addition of 2-mM CCl_4 caused a marked increase in the loss of CYP2E1 catalytic activity and content (Yang and Cederbaum 1997a). CCl_4 has long been known to inactivate CYP2E1 and enhance its degradation (Tierney, Haas and Koop 1992; Sohn et al. 1991). These experiments appear to suggest that ethanol and the other ligands elevate CYP2E1 levels by stabilizing the enzyme against rapid proteolysis.

6.3.6. CYP2E1 and the Proteasome Complex

What are the proteolytic systems responsible for CYP2E1 turnover and prevented from their action on CYP2E1 by ethanol? Microsomes isolated from these cells showed a very slow rate of CYP2E1 degradation suggesting that a protease in the ER is not a likely candidate for the rapid degradation of CYP2E1. Several inhibitors of lysosomal protease had little or no effect on CYP2E1 degradation. In order to evaluate a role for the proteasome complex in the degradation of CYP2E1, the effect of the substrate analogue Czb-Ile-Glu (otBu)-Ala-Leucinal (PSI) on CYP2E1 degradation and content was determined. PSI inhibits the chymotrypsin-like activity of the proteasome. Calpeptin inhibitor, a peptidyl aldehydic nonproteasomal cytosolic protease inhibitor, was also evaluated to try to minimize the possibility of nonspecific effects by PSI. PSI proved to be effective in preventing CYP2E1 degradation, whereas calpeptin inhibitor provided little or no protection (Yang and Cederbaum 1997a). PSI, added in vitro at concentrations up to 300 μM, had no effect on oxidation of PNP by microsomes, suggesting that PSI was not acting as a ligand or substrate for CYP2E1. Theoretically, one consequence of diminishing the proteolytic degradation rate of CYP2E1 by PSI should be the steady-state accumulation of CYP2E1 within the cells. Treatment of the HepG2 cells with PSI caused a concentration-dependent increase in levels of CYP2E1 apoprotein as shown by the Western blot analysis in Figure 6.2. Taken as a whole, these results indicate that the human CYP2E1 has a short half-life span and substrates can significantly modify its turnover rate in the intact cells. The proteasome proteolytic pathway appears to be involved in the degradation process of CYP2E1 in this model. Importantly, Bardag-Gorce et al. (2002) recently showed that the rapid loss of CYP2E1, which occurs in vivo after the ethanol inducer is withdrawn, could be blocked by the proteasome inhibitor PS-341, thus establishing the critical role of the proteasome in regulating CYP2E1 turnover in vivo.

In view of the importance of the proteasome complex in the turnover of CYP2E1, the effect of chronic ethanol treatment on activity or content of the proteasome would be important to determine, since inhibition of this degradation complex would cause an increase in CYP2E1 levels. Studies by French and collaborators indeed showed that chronic ethanol administration in the intragastric infusion model produced a decrease in activity of the proteasome (Donohue et al. 1998; Fatաccioli et al. 1999). This inhibition may also cause oxidized, damaged proteins to accumulate in the liver and thereby contribute to ethanol-induced hepatomegaly. To specifically determine the role of CYP2E1 in the chronic ethanol-induced

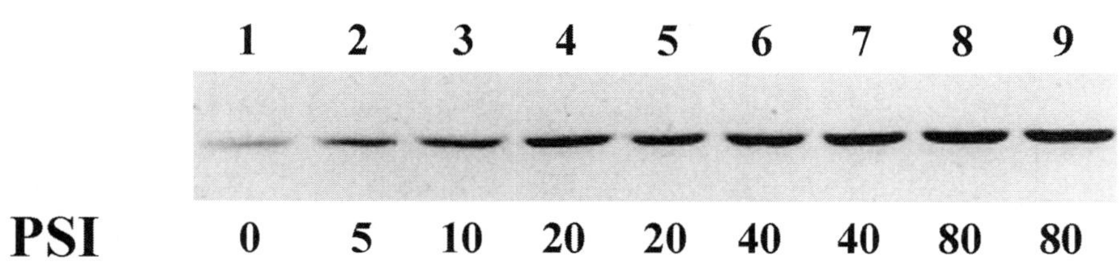

Figure 6.2 Proteasome inhibitor elevates steady-state levels of CYP2E1.

lowering of proteasome activity, CYP2E1 knockout mice were treated with ethanol; whereas ethanol lowered proteasomal activity in the wild-type mice, activity was not affected in the CYP2E1-knockout mice (Bardag-Gorce et al. 2000). It was suggested that CYP2E1-dependent ROS production and lipid peroxidation may be responsible for the decrease in proteasome activity. We recently showed that in HepG2 cells that constitutively express CYP2E1, inhibition of the proteasome with lactacystin and other typical inhibitors potentiated the toxicity caused by addition of a PUFA, AA, or by depletion of GSH (Perez and Cederbaum 2003). Potentiation of toxicity by the proteasome inhibitors was associated with an increased oxidative damage as reflected by elevated lipid peroxidation, protein carbonyls, and protein nitrotyrosine adducts and could be prevented by antioxidants. Lactacystin also potentiated AA toxicity in hepatocytes isolated from pyrazole-treated rats with elevated levels of CYP2E1. Thus, the proteasome plays an important role in CYP2E1 turnover and removal of oxidized, damaged proteins and subsequently in CYP2E1-mediated toxicity.

6.4. The CYP2E1 Knockout Mouse

The development of the CYP2E1 knockout mouse has been of great value in establishing the role of CYP2E1 in the toxicity of various hepatotoxins such as acetaminophen, benzene, acrylonitrile, or styrene (Lee et al. 1996; Wang, Chanas and Ghanayem 2002; Carlson 2004). These mice have been used to validate that hydroxylation of *p*-nitrophenol may be used as a specific probe for CYP2E1 (Wolf et al. 2004). Levels of acetone were strikingly elevated under fasting conditions in CYP2E1 null mice, indicating the critical role of CYP2E1 in acetone metabolism (Bondoc et al. 1999). It has been reported that alcohol-induced liver damage occurred in CYP2E1 null mice to the same extent as in wild-type controls, indicating that CYP2E1 does not play a role in alcohol liver injury (Kono et al. 1999). However, others have shown that ethanol-induced oxidative stress and inactivation of the proteasome complex was completely prevented in these mice (Bardag-Gorce et al. 2000). This is further discussed below. Recently, a CYP2E1-humanized transgenic mouse model that expresses functional and inducible human CYP2E1 was described (Cheung et al. 2005). Comparisons between CYP2E1-humanized mice, CYP2E1 null mice and wild-type mice will allow a determination of whether actions of human CYP2E1 are similar to those of mouse CYP2E1 in vivo. Indeed, the CYP2E1-humanized mouse model was successfully used to characterize acetaminophen toxicity by human CYP2E1 (Cheung et al. 2005).

6.5. CYP2E1 and Alcohol-Induced Liver Injury

Since CYP2E1 can generate ROS during its catalytic cycle, and its levels are elevated by chronic treatment with ethanol, CYP2E1 has been suggested as a major contributor to ethanol-induced oxidant stress, and to ethanol-induced liver injury. Initial suggestions for a role for CYP2E1 in alcoholic liver injury arose from studies with the intragastric model of ethanol feeding in which prominent induction of CYP2E1 occurs and in which significant alcohol liver injury occurs (Tsukamoto et al. 1995; Morimoto et al. 1994; Nanji et al. 1994). In these models, large increases in microsomal lipid peroxidation have been observed and the ethanol-induced liver pathology has been shown to correlate with CYP2E1 levels and elevated lipid peroxidation (Castillo et al. 1992; Ronis et al. 1993; Nanji et al. 1994; Morimoto et al. 1994). Experimentally, a decrease in CYP2E1 induction was found to be associated with a reduction in alcohol-induced liver injury (French et al. 1997; Kim, Kwak and Kim 1997). CYP2E1 inhibitors such as diallyl sulfide (DAS) (Morimoto et al. 1993), phenethyl isothiocyanate (PIC), (Morimoto et al. 1995; Albano et al. 1996) and chlormethiazole (Gouillon et al. 2000), blocked the lipid peroxidation and ameliorated the pathologic changes in ethanol-fed rats. Polyenylphosphatidylcholine (PPC), another compound exerting anti-CYP2E1 properties (Aleynik et al. 1999), was effective in opposing alcohol-induced oxidative stress (Lieber et al. 1997). A strong association between dietary carbohydrate, enhanced CYP2E1 induction, and hepatic necrosis was observed. No liver injury was found if carbohydrate levels were elevated (Korourian et al. 1999). It was concluded that diet is an important factor in toxicity mediated by ethanol because of modulation of the levels of CYP2E1 (Korourian et al. 1999). Ethanol consumption in liquid diets does not cause liver injury. However, micro- and macrovesicular steatosis, occasional inflammatory foci, and a threefold increase in transaminase levels was observed in a nutritionally adequate ethanol-containing liquid diet with a carbohydrate content of 5.5%; no changes were found if the level of carbohydrate was elevated to 11% (Lindros and Jarvelainen 1998; Li et al. 2001). Thus, dietary and nutritional factors play a key role in the toxic actions of ethanol to the liver, in part, due to modulation of the levels of CYP2E1. Recently, a CYP2E1 transgenic mouse model was developed that overexpressed CYP2E1. When treated with ethanol, the CYP2E1-overexpressing mice displayed higher transaminase levels and histological features of liver injury compared with the control mice (Morgan, French and Morgan 2002). We developed an adenoviral vector which expresses human CYP2E1 and showed that infection of HepG2 cells with this adenovirus potentiated acetaminophen toxicity as compared to HepG2 cells infected with a LacZ-expressing adenovirus (Bai and Cederbaum 2004). Administration of the CYP2E1 adenovirus in vivo to mice produced significant liver injury compared to the LacZ-infected mice as reflected by histopathology, markers of oxidative stress and, as shown in Figure 6.3, elevated transaminase levels (Bai and Cederbaum 2006).

On the other hand, studies by Thurman and colleagues have presented powerful support for a role for endotoxin, activation of Kupffer cells and cytokines such as TNFα in the alcohol-induced liver injury found with the intragastric infusion model (Yin et al. 1999; Wheeler and Thurman 2001). They suggested that CYP2E1 may not play a role in alcohol liver injury based upon studies with gadolinium chloride or CYP2E1 knockout mice (Kono et al. 1999; Koop et al. 1997). However, in contrast to their observations, others have reported that gadolinium chloride does indeed decrease levels of several P450 enzymes, including CYP2E1, and lowered

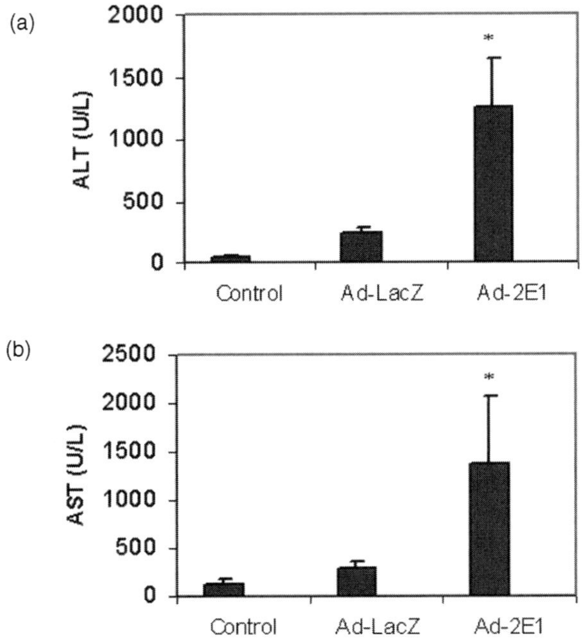

Figure 6.3 Adenovirus-mediated overexpression of CYP2E1 causes liver toxicity in mice.

the induction of CYP2E1 by ethanol (Badger et al. 1997; Jarvelainen et al. 2000). With respect to the CYP2E1 knockouts, only "early" alcohol-induced injury was studied (Tsukamoto 2000). Moreover, Leclereq et al. (2000) using the same knockout mice observed that other CYPS, notably CYP4A10 and CYP4A14, were upregulated in the CYP2E1 knockout but not the wild-type mice; these CYPS were, like CYP2E1, active generators of reactive oxygen and catalysts of lipid peroxidation, and in the absence of CYP2E1 served as alternative initiators of oxidative stress. Activity of NADPH-cytochrome P450 reductase was elevated 2.5-fold by alcohol treatment in the CYP2E1 knockouts; this enzyme can generate ROS, thus, as discussed by Tsukamoto (2000), induction by ethanol of other CYPs or of the reductase in the CYP2E1 knockout mice might have served as alternative sources of oxidative stress in these mice, especially in the absence of CYP2E1. Another possible consideration is that the relative level of CYP2E1 to total P450 in mice (12 pmol per mg protein for controls, 60 pmol per mg after ethanol treatment) is much lower than the CYP2E1-to-total P450 ratio in rats (about 40 pmol mg^{-1} and 800 pmol mg^{-1}, respectively (Bardag-Gorce et al. 2000; Badger et al. 2003). However, it was recently suggested that the metabolism of several CYP substrates, including those for CYP2E1, was similar between mice and rats (Arteel 2003). French and collaborators found that the ethanol-induced oxidative inactivation of the proteasome and increase in oxidized proteins (but not fatty liver) was completely prevented in these CYP2E1 knockout mice (Bardag-Gorce et al. 2000). Clearly, further studies are necessary to resolve the above discrepancies. As mentioned earlier, it is likely that several mechanisms contribute to alcohol-induced liver injury, and that ethanol-induced oxidant stress is likely to arise form several sources, including CYP2E1, mitochondria, and activated Kupffer cells.

6.6. Biochemical and Toxicological Properties of CYP2E1 in HepG2 Cells

As discussed above, major interest in CYP2E1 reflects the ability of this enzyme to oxidize ethanol; to generate reactive products from ethanol oxidation, for example, acetaldehyde and the 1-hydroxyethyl radical; to activate various agents (CCl_4, acetaminophen, benzene, halothane, halogenated alkanes, alcohol) to reactive products; to generate ROS; and to be "induced" by ethanol (as well as several low-molecular-weight agents), and under a variety of nutritional and pathophysiological conditions. An approach that our laboratory has utilized to try to understand basic effects and actions of CYP2E1 is to establish cell lines that constitutively express human CYP2E1. HepG2 cell lines, which overexpress CYP2E1, were established either by retroviral infection methods (MV2E1-9 cells, or E9 cells) or by plasmid transfection methods (E47 cells) (Dai et al. 1993; Chen and Cederbaum 1998). Hepatotoxins such as CCl_4 or acetaminophen were more toxic in E9 cells than control HepG2 cells validating the utility of the model to study CYP2E1-dependent toxicity (Dai and Cederbaum 1995a,b). We have characterized the toxicity of ethanol, PUFAs such as AA and iron in the E9 and E47 cell lines (Wu and Cederbaum 1996, 1999; Chen, Galleano and Cederbaum 1997; Sakurai and Cederbaum 1998). Concentrations of ethanol or AA or iron which were toxic to the CYP2E1-expressing cells had no effect on control HepG2 cells not expressing CYP2E1 or to HepG2 cells expressing a different P450, CYP3A4 (3A4 cells). Toxicity to CYP2E1-expressing cells was found when GSH was depleted by treatment with 1-buthionine sulfoximine (BSO) (Wu and Cederbaum 2001a). Inhibitors of CYP2E1 prevented the toxicity by the above treatments. Antioxidants such as vitamin E, trolox, and ascorbate also prevented toxicity found when the CYP2E1-expressing E9 HepG2 cells were treated with either ethanol or AA (Figure 6.4). The above treatments of CYP2E1-expressing cells with ethanol, AA, iron, or BSO resulted in an increase in oxidative stress to the cells as reflected by increased lipid peroxidation and enhanced dichlorofluorescein fluorescence. In other studies, we observed that (Caro and Cederbaum 2001) low concentrations of iron and AA that are not cytotoxic by themselves can act as priming or sensitizing factors for CYP2E1-dependent loss of viability in HepG2 cells or rat hepatocytes. This synergistic toxicity was associated with elevated lipid peroxidation and could be prevented by antioxidants which prevent lipid peroxidation. Damage to mitochondria by CYP2E1-derived oxidants seems to be an early event in the overall pathway of cellular injury. Relatively low concentrations of iron or AA were effective in promoting toxicity in the CYP2E1-expressing cells, supporting the suggestion that interactions between CYP2E1 and iron and PUFAs may lower the threshold concentrations for these reactive nutrients for inducing a state of oxidative stress, which may play a role in the development of alcohol-induced liver injury.

Addition	Percent Viability	
	Ethanol	Arachidonic Acid
None	64	40
5 mM N-Acetylcysteine	93	55
5 mM Thiourea	104	N/A
25 μM Tocopherol Phosphate	86	89
25 μM DPPD	91	89
50 μM Trolox	110	75
1 mM Ascorbic Acid	N/A	90

Figure 6.4 Effects of antioxidants on ethanol and arachidonic acid toxicity in MV2E1-9 cells.

To extend the results with the HepG2 cells to primary hepatocytes, cultures of hepatocytes from rats treated with pyrazole to elevate levels of CYP2E1 and from saline controls were evaluated. Many of the basic findings described above for E9 and E47 cells were recapitulated in the hepatocytes from the pyrazole-treated rats (called pyrazole hepatocytes); that is, AA or iron or AA plus iron were more toxic to pyrazole hepatocytes than saline control hepatocytes (Wu and Cederbaum 2000, 2001b; Caro and Cederbaum 2001). Ethanol was weakly toxic, but even this was greater in the pyrazole hepatocytes. Toxicity was associated with increased lipid peroxidation and could be prevented by antioxidants and the CYP2E1 inhibitor diallylsulfide.

Adaptation to oxidant stimuli is critical for short- and long-term survival of cells exposed to oxidative stress. While much of the focus on CYP2E1 has been from a toxicology point of view, the possibility that the hepatocyte attempts to respond to increased levels of CYP2E1 by upregulation of protective factors has not been studied. We found, to our surprise, that the E47 cells had higher GSH levels than CYP3A4-expressing HepG2 cells or control HepG2 cells (Mari and Cederbaum 2000). Increases in GSH were due to activation of the genes encoding the heavy and light subunits of gamma glutamyl cysteine synthetase (GCLC and GCLM). These increases in the E47 cells were prevented by inhibitors of CYP2E1 and were also found in hepatocytes from pyrazole-treated rats with elevated levels of CYP2E1 as compared to saline-treated controls (Mari and Cederbaum 2000; Nieto, Mari and Cederbaum 2003). The increase in GSH and GCLC and GCLM mRNA were prevented by antioxidants, suggesting that ROS generated by CYP2E1 were responsible for the upregulation of these antioxidant genes. GCLC and GCLM mRNA expression and protein levels were further increased when E47 cells were challenged with substrates for CYP2E1 or prooxidants, which further elevated oxidative stress, such as ethanol, AA, and Fe+AA. The increase in mRNA in treated E47 cells was blocked by antioxidants and by a CYP2E1 inhibitor. The transcriptional upregulation mediated by CYP2E1-derived ROS seems to operate through a redox-sensitive element (ARE4) localized 3.1 kb upstream of the transcription start site in the GCLC gene (Nieto, Mari and Cederbaum 2003). The mechanisms controlling the induction of genes by oxidative stress involve the activation of transcription factors, such as NF-kβ, AP-1, and Nrf2, which could mediate such inductions (Morel and Barouki 1999), but this remains to be evaluated.

There was also a twofold increase in the content and activity of catalase, cytosolic glutathione transferase, and microsomal glutathione transferase in the E47 cells due to activation of their respective genes (Mari and Cederbaum 2001). Figure 6.5 shows that heme oxygenase 1 protein levels and activity was twofold higher in the CYP2E1-expressing E47 cells as compared to control C34 HepG2 cells or to HepG2 cells expressing a different cytochrome P450, CYP3A4. The elevated heme oxygenase 1 activity and protein level in the E47 cells is associated with high CYP2E1 levels and activity in these cells compared to the C34 or CYP3A4 cells (Gong et al. 2003). These activations in the E47 cells were prevented by antioxidants, suggesting that ROS generated by CYP2E1 were responsible for the upregulation of these antioxidant genes. Indeed, the E47 cells, because of this activation of antioxidant genes, were less sensitive to toxicity by added H_2O_2 or menadione or 4-hydroxynonenal than were control cells. We believe that the upregulation of these antioxidant genes may reflect an adaptive mechanism to remove CYP2E1-derived oxidants.

Hepatic stellate cells (HSCs) are central to the fibrotic response of the liver to injury, and ROS activate stellate cells. Since CYP2E1 produces ROS, ethanol-induced CYP2E1 expression may promote collagen type I biosynthesis by stellate cells. However, CYP2E1 is mostly present in hepatocytes, whereas stellate cells contain low levels of CYP2E1. Accordingly, a co-culture model involving HepG2 cells and stellate cells was developed (Nieto, Friedman and Cederbaum 2002a,b) in which the

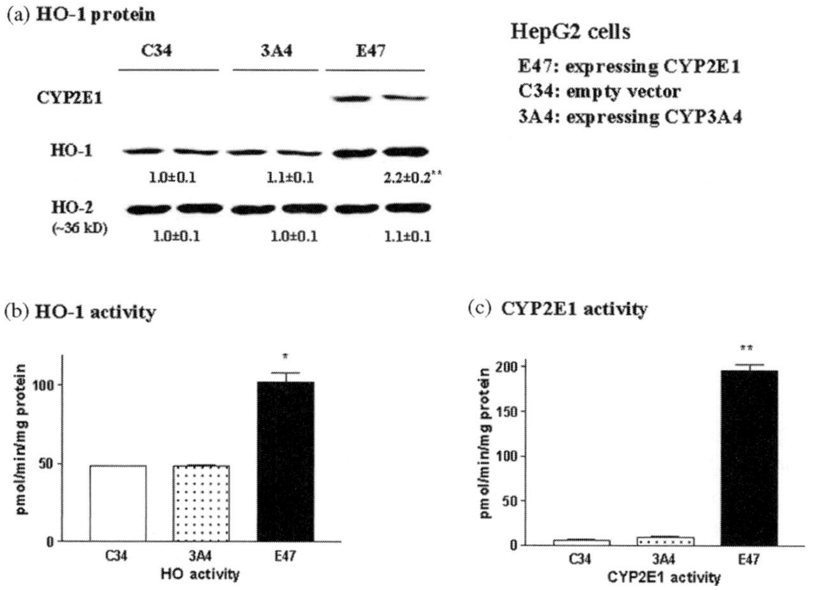

Figure 6.5 HO-1 protein and HO activity are increased in E47 cells. (**a**) HO-1 protein. (**b**) HO-1 activity. (**c**) CYP2E1 activity.

HepG2 cells and the stellate cells were separated from each other by an insert; therefore, the experimental protocol was designed to evaluate whether mediators (ROS, cytokines, growth factors) produced by HepG2 cells diffuse to the HSC and affect collagen type I protein levels. There was a time-dependent increase in collagen type I when stellate cells were co-incubated with C34 control cells, which was further elevated when stellate cells were co-incubated with CYP2E1-overexpressing E47 cells. E47 plus stellate cell co-cultures secreted much more type I collagen protein. These experiments suggest that CYP2E1-overexpressing E47 cells generate diffusible mediators that promote type I collagen synthesis and release by stellate cells. Catalase and vitamin E markedly decreased type I collagen synthesis by both co-cultures and completely blocked the increased collagen production by the E47 co-culture. These results suggest that E47 cells release ROS, such as H_2O_2 and lipid peroxidation products, that stimulate type I collagen synthesis by stellate cells.

Work from several laboratories has indicated that mitochondrial damage may represent a common early event in cell injury caused by toxic agents (Susin, Zamzami and Kroemer 1998). Mitochondrial damage is initially manifested by a decrease in mitochondrial membrane potential ($\Delta\psi_m$) followed by ATP depletion (Orrenius, Ankarcrona and Nicotera 1996; Trost and Lemasters 1996). Two major processes are likely candidates as mechanism for a loss of $\Delta\psi_m$: nonspecific damage to the inner mitochondrial membrane or a more specific process, the permeability transition, due to the opening of mitochondrial permeability pore. Mitochondrial membrane potential was assessed by flow cytometry after double staining with rhodamine 123 and propidium iodide (PI). Exposure of E47 cells to BSO (Mari, Bai and Cederbaum 2002), AA (Perez and Cederbaum 2001), and Fe+AA (Caro and Cederbaum 2001) increased the percentage of cells that showed low rhodamine 123 fluorescence but were not stained with PI. This population refers to cells that are still viable but with damaged mitochondria, showing that these CYP2E1-dependent models of toxicity affect mitochondria before the onset of cell death (i.e., early event). This early mitochondrial damage was prevented by antioxidants, linking oxidative stress to mitochondrial damage. That mitochondria are an important target for CYP2E1-mediated oxidative stress is suggested by the fact that overexpression of mitochondrial catalase is capable of protecting cells that overexpress CYP2E1 against the toxicity induced by BSO, AA, and Fe+AA (Mari, Bai and Cederbaum 2002; Bai and Cederbaum 2001; Wu and Cederbaum 2002). If the decrease of mitochondrial membrane potential depends on the opening of the permeability transition pore, then a specific inhibitor should decrease the loss of mitochondrial membrane potential induced by the toxic agents. Cyclosporin A inhibited the loss of $\Delta\psi_m$ and the toxicity in CYP2E1-expressing cells exposed to AA, AA+Fe, and BSO (Caro and Cederbaum 2002; Wu and Cederbaum 2001, 2002), suggesting a role for the permeability transition on mitochondrial depolarization and subsequent toxicity. Additional evidence for increased mitochondrial damage in CYP2E1-overexpressing cells include the following: depletion of GSH decreased oxygen uptake in permeabilized E47 cells with all respiratory substrates, and vitamin E prevented this decrease (Chen and Cederbaum 1998). In CYP2E1-overexpressing cells treated with

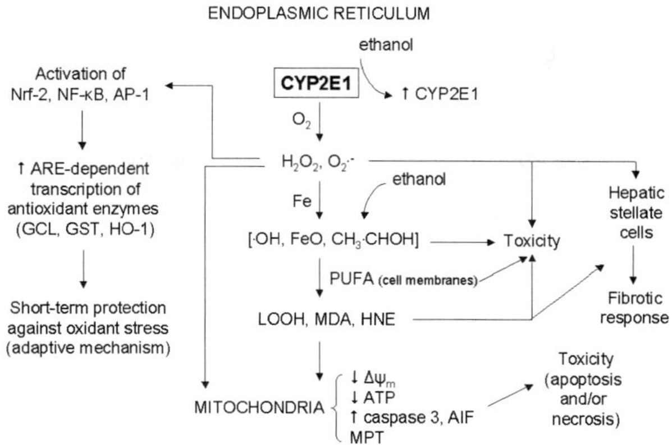

Figure 6.6 Scheme for CYP2E1 toxicity in HepG2 cells.

BSO + Fe-NTA, levels of ATP were lowered, and this was associated with a decreased rate of oxygen consumption by permeabilized cells with substrates donating electrons to complexes I, II, and IV of the respiratory chain. This mitochondrial damage was prevented by vitamin E (Sakurai and Cederbaum 1998). Damage to mitochondria is an important event in the CYP2E1-dependent toxicity.

A working model of CYP2E1-dependent oxidative stress and toxicity is shown in Figure 6.6. Ethanol increases levels of CYP2E1, largely by a post-transcriptional mechanism involving enzyme stabilization against degradation. CYP2E1, a loosely coupled enzyme, generates ROS such as O_2^- and H_2O_2 during its catalytic cycle. In the presence of iron, which is increased after ethanol treatment, more powerful oxidants including OH, ferryl species, and 1-hydroxyethyl radical are produced. Initially, the liver cells respond to the CYP2E1-related oxidative stress by transcriptionally inducing various antioxidant enzymes. Ultimately, these protective mechanisms are overwhelmed and the cells become sensitive to the CYP2E1-generated oxidants. These various oxidants can promote toxicity by protein oxidation and enzyme inactivation, oxidative damage to the DNA, and disturbing cell membranes via lipid peroxidation and production of reactive lipid aldehydes, such as malondialdehyde and 4-hydroxynonenal. Mitochondria appear to be among the critical cellular organelles damaged by CYP2E1-derived oxidants. A decrease of $\Delta\psi_m$ likely due to the mitochondrial membrane permeability transition causes release of proapoptotic factors resulting in apoptosis. Decrease in ATP levels will cause necrosis. We believe that the linkage between CYP2E1-dependent oxidative stress, mitochondrial injury, and GSH homeostasis contribute to the toxic actions of ethanol on the liver.

6.7. Future Perspectives

With respect to alcohol-induced liver injury, such injury is likely to be a multifactorial process involving several mechanisms. Future studies are required to further clarity how alcohol produces oxidative stress in various tissues. Some of the major proposed systems require more detailed mechanism; for example, how ethanol-derived NADH itself or when reoxidized in the mitochondrial respiratory chain produces ROS. What is the role of ethanol metabolism or ethanol metabolites such as acetaldehyde (or NADH) in the production of ROS, and how is oxidative stress produced by ethanol in tissues with limited ethanol metabolism?

The role of CYP2E1 in the toxic effects of ethanol requires further study as this remains a controversial issue. This is significant not only from a mechanistic point of view but perhaps from a therapeutic treatment approach. If indeed CYP2E1-induced oxidative stress plays a central role in alcohol-induced hepatic damage, possible strategies for preventing this stress may be effective in attempts to minimize the hepatotoxicity of ethanol in humans. The CYP2E1 inhibitors which were partially effective in preventing ethanol-induced liver injury are not entirely selective and may be toxic. There is a need for the development of selective, nontoxic inhibitors of CYP2E1 that could be used in vivo. Inhibitors such as phenylisothiocyanate, diethyldithiocarbamate, and DAS are often toxic at concentrations needed to inhibit CYP2E1, especially in vivo. They are also not selective as they can function as antioxidants or have other actions: for example, DAS can induce heme oxygenase-1 (Gong, Hu and Cederbaum 2004). *S*-adenosyl-L-methionine is hepatoprotective against several toxins and can inhibit CYP2E1; however, the K_I for inhibiting CYP2E1 was high, therefore *S*-adenosyl-L-methionine is not likely to be an effective inhibitor of CYP2E1 in vivo (Caro and Cederbaum 2005). YH439 is a novel synthetic compound inhibiting CYP2E1 (but also other P450s) that is currently being evaluated as a hepatoprotective agent (Choi et al. 1996; Jeong et al. 1996). Actually, natural agents inhibiting CYP2E1, including DAS (from garlic) mentioned above, phenylethylisothiocyanate and sulforaphane (presents in cruciferous vegetables), (Barcelo et al. 1996) and bergamottin (found in the essential oils of grapefruit and orange) (He et al. 1998) have been proposed as possible candidates for minimizing the ethanol-induced hepatotoxicity (McCarty 2001).

The regulation of CYP2E1 protein levels is complex, being observed at the transcriptional and post-transcriptional levels; more mechanistic details as to how ethanol modulates CYP2E1 levels would be important to define, for example, effects on activity of the proteasome, ubiquitination, and how ethanol stabilizes CYP2E1. What are the factors which trigger the rapid turnover of CYP2E1? This is a key question to help understand why CYP2E1 turns over so rapidly. Chronic ethanol treatment decreases activity of the proteasome (Bardag-Gorce et al. 2000; Donohue et al. 1998); is this part of the mechanism by which ethanol increases the content of CYP2E1? Is ubiquitination of CYP2E1 required for its degradation by the proteasome (Huan et al. 2004)? This is not clear and has important implications with respect to the mechanism of CYP2E1 turnover, the role of the 20S versus the 26S proteasome complex, the role of accessory chaperones (e.g., heat shock proteins), how ethanol and other low molecular ligands act to stabilize CYP2E1 (e.g., preventing labilization, ubiquitination, and access to the proteasome core).

Most information on the biochemical and pharmacological actions of CYP2E1 is derived from studies with rodents and rabbits, and cultured hepatocytes: extrapolation to human studies will obviously be necessary. A major advance in this direction will be the humanized CYP2E1 transgenic mouse model (Cheung et al. 2005). The role of polymorphic forms of CYP2E1 on its expression, activity, and actions requires further understanding, as current literature suggests some possible relationships with certain types of cancers, but not with alcohol toxicity. Are there other endogenous substrates for CYP2E1? At present, acetone and some fatty acids (ω-hydroxylation catalyzed by CYP2E1) appear to be physiological substrates for CYP2E1, but further study should be carried out, because altered metabolism of such putative endogenous substrates, if any, could contribute to the cellular actions associated with activated CYP2E1. CYP2E1 is present, although at relatively low levels, in other tissues (e.g., kidney, lung, brain, and gastrointestinal tract). Much less is known about the actions of CYP2E1 under various pathophysiological conditions or after chronic ethanol exposure in these tissues. There is much current interest in synergistic interactions between alcohol and hepatitis B or hepatitis C virus, especially with respect to generating oxidative stress. The role of CYP2E1 in such synergistic interactions would be important to explore in view of the many chemicals and conditions that are known to elevate CYP2E1.

Acknowledgement. Studies in the author's laboratory were supported by Grants from the National Institute on Alcohol Abuse and Alcoholism.

References

Adachi, M., and Ishii, H. 2002. Role of mitochondria in alcoholic liver injury. Free Rad. Biol. Med. 32:487–491.

Albano, E., Tomasi A., Goria-Gatti, L., Poli G., Vannini A., and Dianzani M. U. 1987. Free radical metabolism of alcohols in rat liver microsomes. Free Rad. Res. Commun. 3:243–253.

Albano, E., Tomasi, A., Persson, J. O., Terelius, Y., Goria-Gatti, L., Ingelman-Sundberg, M., and Dianzani, M. U. 1991. Role of ethanol-inducible cytochrome P-450 (P-450IIE1) in catalysis of the free radical activation of aliphatic alcohols. Biochem. Pharmacol. 41:1895–1902.

Albano, E., Clot, P., Morimoto, M., Tomasi, A., Ingelman-Sundberg, M., and French, S. 1996. Role of cytochrome P4502E1-dependent formation of hydroxyethyl free radicals in the development of liver damage in rats intragastrically fed with ethanol. Hepatology 23:155–163.

Aleynik, M. K., Leo, M. A., Aleynik, S. I., and Lieber, C. S. 1999. Polyenylphosphatidyl-choline opposes the increase of cytochrome P4502E1 by ethanol and corrects its iron-induced decrease. Alcoholism: Clin. Exp. Res. 23:96–100.

Arteel, G. E. 2003. Oxidants and antioxidants in alcohol-induced liver disease. Gastroenerology 124:778–790.

Asai, H., Imaoka, S., Kuroki, T., Monna, T., and Funae, Y. 1996. Microsomal ethanol oxidizing system activity by human hepatic cytochrome P-450s. J. Pharmacol. Exp. Ther. 277:1004–1009.

Badger, D. A., Kuester, R. K., Sauer, J. M., and Sipes, L. G. 1997. Gadolinium chloride reduces cytochrome p450: relevance to chemical induced hepatotoxicity. Toxicology 121:143–153.

Badger, T. M.., Korourian, S., Hakkak, R., Ronnis, M. J. J., Ingelman-Sundberg, M., Shelnutt, S. R., and Waldron, J. 1998. Carbohydrate deficiency as a possible factor in ethanol-induced hepatic necrosis. Alcohol. Clin. Exp. Res. 22:742.

Badger, T. M., Ronis, M. J. J., Seitz, H. K., Albano, E., Ingelman-Sundberg, M., and Lieber, C. S. 2003. Alcohol metabolism: role in toxicity and carcinogenicity. Alcohol. Clin. Exp. Res. 27:336–347.

Bai, J. X., and Cederbaum, A. I. 2001. Adenovirus-mediated overexpression of catalase in the cytosolic or mitochondrial compartment protects against cytochrome P450 2E1-dependent toxicity in HepG2 cells. J. Biol. Chem. 276:4315–4321.

Bai, J. X., and Cederbaum, A. I. 2004. Adenovirus-mediated overexpression of CYP2E1 increases sensitivity of HepG2 cells to acetaminophen induced cytotoxicity. Mol. Cell. Biochem. 262:165–176.

Bai, J. X., and Cederbaum, A. I. 2006. Adenovirus-mediated expression of CYP2E1 produces liver toxicity in mice. Toxicol. Sci. 91:365–371.

Bailey, S. M., and Cunningham, C. C. 2002. Contribution of mitochondria to oxidative stress associated with alcoholic liver disease. Free Rad. Biol. Med. 32:11–16.

Barcelo, S., Gardiner, J. M., Gescher, A., and Chipman, J. K. 1996. CYP2E1-mediated mechanism of antigenotoxicity of the broccoli constituent sulforaphane. Carcinogenesis 17:277–282.

Bardag-Gorce, F., Yuan, Q. X., Li, J., French, B. A., Fang, C., Ingelman-Sundberg, M., and French, S. W. 2000. The effect of ethanol-induced cytochrome P450 2E1 on the inhibition of proteasome activity by alcohol. Biochem. Biophys. Res. Commun. 279:23–29.

Bardag-Gorce, F., Li, J., French, B. A., and French, S. W. 2002. Ethanol withdrawal induced CYP2E1 degradation in vivo, blocked by the proteasomal inhibitor PS-341. Free Rad. Biol. Med. 32:17–21.

Bellward, G. D., Chang, T., Rodrigues, J. H., McNeil J. H., Maines, S., Ryan, D. E., Levin, W., and Thomas, P. E., 1987. Hepatic cytochrome P-450j induction in the spontaneously diabetic BB rat. Mol. Pharmacol. 33:140–143.

Blanck, J., Ristau, O., Zhukov, A. A., Archakov, A. L., Rein, H., and Ruckpaul, K. 1991. Cytochrome P450 spin state and leakiness of the monooxygenase pathway. Xenobiotica 21:121–135.

Bolt, M., Koos, P. H., and Their, R., 2003. The cytochrome P450 isoenzyme CYP2E1 in the biological processing of industrial chemicals. Int. Arch. Occup. Environ. Health 76:174–185.

Bondoc, F. Y., Bao, Z., Hu, W. Y., Gonzalez, F. J., Wang, Y., Yang, C. S., and Hong, J. Y. 1999. Acetone catabolism by cytochrome P450 2E1: studies with CYP2E1-null mice. Biochem. Pharmacol. 58:461–463.

Bondy, S. C. 1992. Ethanol toxicity and oxidative stress. Toxicol. Lett. 63:231–242.

Bourdi, M., Chen, W., Peter, R. M., Martin, J. L., Buters, J. T., Nelson, S. D., and Pohl, L. R. 1996. Human cytochrome P450 2E1 is a major autoantigen associated with halothane hepatitis. Chem. Res. Toxicol. 9:1159–1166.

Carlson, G. P. 2004. Comparison of the susceptibility of wild type and CYP2E1 knockout mice to the hepatotoxic and neurotoxic effects of styrene and styrene oxide. Toxicol. Lett. 150:335–339.

Caro, A. A., and Cederbaum, A. I. 2001. Synergistic toxicity of iron and arachidonic acid in HepG2 cells overexpressing CYP2E1. Mol. Pharmacol. 60:742–752.

Caro, A. A., and Cederbaum, A. I. 2002. Role of calcium and calcium-activated proteases in CYP2E1-dependent toxicity in HepG2 cells. J. Biol. Chem. 277:104–113.

Caro, A. A., and Cederbaum, A. I. 2005. Inhibition of CYP2E1 catalytic activity in vitro by *S*-adenosyl-L-methionine. Biochem. Pharmacol. 69:1081–1093.

Castillo, T., Koop, D. R., Kamimura, S., Triadafilopoulos, G., and Tsukamoto, H. 1992. Role of cytochrome P4502E1 in ethanol, carbon tetrachloride and iron-dependent microsomal lipid peroxidation. Hepatology 16:992–996.

Cederbaum, A. I. 2001. Introduction serial review: alcohol, oxidative stress and cell injury. Free Rad. Biol. Med. 31:1524–1526.

Chance, B., Sies, H., and Boveris, A. 1979. Hydroperoxide metabolism in mammalian organisms. Physiol. Rev. 59:527–604.

Chen, Q., and Cederbaum, A. I. 1998. Cytotoxicity and apoptosis produced by cytochrome P4502E1 in HepG2 cells. Mol. Pharmacol. 53:638–648.

Chen, Q., Galleano, M., and Cederbaum, A. I. 1997. Cytotoxicity and apoptosis produced by arachidonic acid in HepG2 cells over-expressing human cytochrome P4502E1. J. Biol. Chem. 272:14532–14541.

Cheung, C., Yu A. M., Ward, J. M., Krausz, K. W., Akiyama, T. E., Feigenbaum, L., and Gonzalez, F. J. 2005. The CYP2E1 humanized transgenic mouse; role of CYP2E1 in acetaminophen toxicity. Drug Metab. Disp. 33: 449–457.

Choi, E. Y., Kim, S. G., Lee, J. W., Yoo, J. K., Shin, J. K., and Kim, N. D. 1996. Suppression of rat hepatic cytochrome P4502E1 expression by YH439, an experiment hepatoprotectant: protective role against hepatic injury. Biochem. Pharmacol. 52:1219–1225.

Clot, P., Albano, E., Eliasson E., Tabone, M., Arico, S., Israel, Y., Moncada, C., and Ingelman-Sundberg, M. 1996. Cytochrome P4502E1 hydroxyethyl radical adducts as the major antigen in autoantibody formation among alcoholics. Gastroenterology 111:206–216.

Dai, Y., and Cederbaum, A. I. 1995a. Cytotoxicity of acetaminophen in human cytochrome P4502E1-transfected HepG2 cells. J. Pharmacol. Exp. Ther. 273:1497–1505.

Dai, Y., and Cederbaum, A. I. 1995b. Inactivation and degradation of human cytochrome P4502E1 by CC14 in a transfected HepG2 cell line. J. Pharmacol. Exp. Ther. 275:1614–1622.

Dai, Y., Rashba-Step, J., and Cederbaum, A. I. 1993. Stable expression of human cytochrome P4502E1 in HepG2 cells: characterization of catalytic activities and production of reactive oxygen intermediates. Biochemistry 32:6928–6937.

De Groot, H. 1994. Reactive oxygen species in tissue injury. Hepatogastroenterology 41:328–332.

DeWaziers, I., Garlatti, M., Bouguet, J., Beaune, P. H., and Barouki, R. 1995. Insulin down-regulates cytochrome P-450 2B and 2E expression at the posttranscriptional level in the rat hepatoma cell line. Mol. Pharmacol. 47:474–479.

Dicker, E., and Cederbaum, A. I. 1987. Hydroxyl radical generation by microsomes after chronic ethanol consumption. Alcohol. Clin. Exp. Res. 11:309–314.

Dicker, E., and Cederbaum, A. I. 1988. Increased oxygen radical dependent inactivation of metabolic enzymes by liver microsomes after chronic ethanol consumption. FASEB J. 2:2901–2906.

Donohue, T. M., Zetterman, R. K., Zhang-Gouilon, Z. Q., and French, S. W. 1998. Peptidase activities of the multicatalytic protease in rat liver after voluntary and intragastric ethanol administration. Hepatology 28:486–491.

Ekstrom G., and Ingelman-Sundberg, M. 1989. Rat liver microsomal NADPH-supported oxidase activity and lipid peroxidation dependent on ethanol-inducible cytochrome P-450 (P-450IIE1). Biochem. Pharmacol. 38: 1313–1319.

Eliasson, E., and Kenna, J. G. 1996. Cytochrome P450 2E1 is a cell surface autoantigen in halothane hepatitis. Mol. Pharmacol. 50:573–582.

Eliasson, E., Johansson, I., and Ingelman-Sundberg, M. 1988. Ligand-dependent maintenance of ethanol-inducible cytochrome P450 in primary hepatocyte cell culture. Biochem. Biophys. Res. Commun. 150:436–443.

Eliasson, E., Johansson, I., and Ingelman-Sundberg, M. 1990. Substrate-hormone, and cAMP-regulated cytochrome P450 degradation. Proc. Natl. Acad. Sci. U.S.A. 87:3225–3229.

Eliasson, E., Mkrtachian, S., and Ingelman-Sundberg, M. 1992. Hormone-and substrate-regulated intracellular degradation of cytochrome P450(2E1) involving MgATP-activated rapid proteolysis in the endoplasmic reticulum membranes. *J. Biol. Chem.* 267:15765–15769.

Fataccioli, V., Andraud, E., Gentil, M., French, S. W., and Rouach, H. 1999. Effects of chronic ethanol administration on rat liver proteasome activities: relationship with oxidative stress. Hepatology 29:14–20.

French, S. W., Morimoto, M., Reitz, R. C., Koop, D., Klopfenstein, B., Estes, K., Clot, P., Ingelman-Sundberg, M., and Albano, E. 1997. Lipid peroxidation, CYP2E1 and arachidonic acid metabolism in alcoholic liver disease in rats. J. Nutr. 127:907S–911S.

Girre, C., Lucas, D., Hispard, F. R., Menez, C., Dally, S., and Menez, J. P. 1994. Assessment of cytochrome P4502E1 in induction in alcoholic patients by chlorzoxazone pharmacokinetics. Biochem. Pharmacol. 47:1503–1508.

Gong, P., Cederbaum, A. I., and Nieto, N. 2003. Increased expression of cytochrome P4502E1 induces heme oxygenase 1 through ERK MAPK pathway. J. Biol. Chem. 278:29693–29700.

Gong P., Hu, B., and Cederbaum, A. I. 2004. Diallyl sulfide induces heme oxygenase 1 through MAPK pathway. Arch. Biochem. Biophys. 432:252–260.

Gorsky, L. D., Koop, D. R., and Coon, M. J. 1984. On the stoichiometry of the oxidase and monooxygenase reactions catalyzed by liver microsomal cytochrome P450. J. Biol. Chem. 259:6812–6817.

Gouillon, Z., Lucas, D., Li, J., Hagbjork, A. L., French, B. A., Fu, P., Fang, C., Ingelman-Sundberg, M., Donohue, T. M. Jr., and French, S. W. 2000. Inhibition of ethanol-induced liver disease in the intragastric feeding rat model by chlormethiazole. Proc. Soc. Exp. Biol. Med. 224:302–308.

Guengerich, F. P. 1987. Mammalian cytochrome P450. Boca Raton, FL: CRC Press.

Guengerich, F. P. 2001. Common and uncommon cytochrome P450 reactions related to metabolism and chemical toxicity. Chem. Res. Toxicol. 14:611–650.

Halliwell, B. 1999. Antioxidant defense mechanisms: from the beginning to the end. Free Rad. Res. 31:261–272.

Hansson, T., Tindberg, N., Ingelman-Sundberg, M., and Kohler, C. 1990. Regional distribution of ethanol-inducible cytochrome P-450 IIE1 in the rat brain. Neuroscience 34:451–463.

Harada, S., Agarwal D. P., Nomura, F., and Higuchi, S. 2001. Metabolic and ethnic determinants of alcohol-related drinking habits and vulnerability to alcohol-related disorder. Alcohol. Clin. Exp. Res. 25:71S–75S.

He, K., Iyer, K. R., Hayes, R. N., Sinz, M. W., Woolf, T. F., and Hollenberg, P. F. 1998. Inactivation of cytochrome P4503A4 by bergamottin, a component of grapefruit juice. Chem. Res. Toxicol. 11:252–259.

Hoivik, D. J., Manautou, J. E., Tveit, A., Hart., S. G., Khairallah, E. A., and Cohen S. D. 1995. Gender-related differences in susceptibility to acetaminophen induced protein arylation and nephrotocicity in the CD-1 mouse. Toxicol Appl. Pharmacol. 130:257–271.

Hong, J. Y., Pan, J., Gonzalez, F. J., Gelboin, H. V., and Yang, C. S. 1987. The induction of a specific form of cytochrome P-450 (P-450 j) by fasting. Biochem. Biophys. Res. Commun. 142:1077–1083.

Hong, J. Y., Ning, S. M., Ma, B. L., Lee, M. J., Pan, J. M., and Yang C. S. 1990. Roles of pituitary hormones in the regulation of hepatic cytochrome P-450IIE1 in rats and mice. Arch. Biochem. Biophys. 28:132–138.

Huan, J. Y., Streicher, J. M., Bleyle, L. A., and Koop. D. R. 2004. Proteasome-dependent degradation of cytochromes P4502E1 and 2B1 expressed in tetracycline-regulated Hela cells. Toxicol. Appl. Pharamcol. 199:332–343.

Iimuro, Y., Bradford, B. U., Yamashina, S., Rusyn, I., Nakagami, M., Enomoto, N., Kono, H., Frey, W., Forman, D., Brenner, D., and Thurman, R. G. 2000. The glutathione precursor L-2-oxothiazolidine-4-carboxylic acid protects against liver injury due to chronic enteral ethanol exposure in the rat. Hepatology 31:391–398.

Ingelman-Sundberg, M., Johansson, I., Penttilä, K. E., Glaumann, H., and Lindros, K. O. 1988. Centrilobular expression of ethanol-inducible cytochrome P-450 (IIE1) in rat liver. Biochem. Biophys. Res. Commun. 157:55–60.

Itoga, S., Nomura, F., Harada, S., Tsusumi, M., Takase, S., and Nakai, T. 1999. Mutation in the exon and exon–intron junction regions of human cytochrome P4502E1 gene and alcoholism. Alcoholism Clin. Exp. Res. 23:13S–16S.

Jarvelainen, H. A., Fang, C., Ingelman-Sundberg, M., Lukkan, T. A., Sippel, H., and Lindros, K. O. 2000. Kupffer cell inactivation alleviates ethanol-induced steatosis and CYP2E1 induction but not inflammatory responses in rat liver. J. Hepatol. 32:900–910.

Jeong, K. S., Lee, I. J., Roberts, B. J., Soh, Y., Yoo, J. K., Lee, J. W., and Song, B. J. 1996. Transcriptional inhibition of cytochrome P4502E1 by a synthetic compound, YH 439. Arch. Biochem. Biophys. 326:137–144.

Johansson, I., Ekstrom, G., Scholte, B., Puzycki, D., Jorvall, H., and Ingelman-Sundberg, M. 1988. Ethanol, fasting and acetone-inducible cytochromes P450 in rat liver. Biochemistry 27:1925–1934.

Johansson, I., Lindros, K. O., Eriksson, H., and Ingelman-Sundberg, M. 1990. Transcriptional control of CYP2E1 in the perivenous liver region and during starvation. Biochem. Biophys. Res. Commun. 173:331–338.

Kehrer J. P. 1993. Free radicals as mediators of tissue injury and disease. Crit. Rev. Toxicol. 23:21–48.

Kessova, I., Ho,Y., Thung, S., and Cederbaum, A. I. 2003. Alcohol-induced liver injury in mice lacking copper,zinc superoxide dismutase. Hepatology 38:1136–1145.

Kim, N. D., Kwak, M. K., and Kim, S. G. 1997. Inhibition of cytochrome P4502E1 expression by 2-(allylthio) pyrazine a protential chemo-protective agent: hepatoprotective effects. Biochem. Pharmacol. 53:261–269.

Klein, S. M., Cohen, G., Lieber, C. S., and Cederbaum, A. I. 1983. Increased microsomal oxidation of hydroxyl radical scavenging agents and ethanol after chronic consumption of ethanol. Arch. Biochem. Biophys. 223:425–433.

Knecht, K. T., Thurman, R. G., and Mason, R. P. 1993. Role of superoxide and trace transition metals in the production of α-hydroxyethyl radical from ethanol by microsomes from alcohol dehydrogenase-deficient deermice. Arch. Biochem. Biophys. 303:339–348.

Knecht, K. T., Adachi, Y., Bradford, B., Iimuro, Y., Kadiiska, M., Qun-Hue, X., and Thurman, R. G. 1995. Free radical adducts in the bile of rats treated chronically with intragastric alcohol. Mol. Pharmacol. 47:1028–1034.

Knight J. A. 1998. Free radicals: their history and current status in aging and disease. Ann. Clin. Lab. Sci. 28:331–346.

Kono, H., Bradford, B. U., Yin, M., Sulik, K. K., Koop, D. R., Peters, J. M., Gonzalez, F. J., McDonald, T., Dikalova, A., Kadiiska, M. B., Mason, R. P., and Thurman, R. G. 1999. CYP2E1 is not involved in early alcohol-induced liver injury. Am. J. Physiol. 277:G1259–G1267.

Koop, D. R. 1992. Oxidative and reductive metabolism by cytochrome P4502E1. FASEB J. 6:724–730.
Koop, D. R., and Casazza, J. P. 1985. Identification of ethanol-inducible P-450 isozyme 3a as the acetone and acetol monooxygenase of rabbit microsomes. J. Biol. Chem. 260:13607–13612.
Koop, D. R., and Tierney, D. J. 1990. Multiple mechanisms in the regulation of ethanol-inducible cytochrome P450IIE1. Bioessay 12:429–435.
Koop, D. R., Morgan, E. T., Tarr, G. E., and Coon, M. J. 1982. Purification and characterization of a unique isozyme of cytochrome P450 from liver microsomes of ethanol-treated rabbits. J. Biol. Chem. 257:8472–8480.
Koop, D. R., Chernosky, A., and Brass, E. P. 1991. Identification and induction of cytochrome P4502E1 in rat Kupffer cells. J. Pharmacol. Exp. Ther. 258:1072–1076.
Koop, D. R., Klopfenstein, B., Iimuro, Y., and Thurman, R. G. 1997. Gadolinium chloride blocks alcohol-dependent liver tocicity in rats treated chronically with intragastric alcohol despite the induction of CYP2E1. Mol. Pharmacol. 51:944–950.
Korourian, S., Hakkak, R., Ronis, M. J., Shelnut, S. R., Waldron, J., Ingelman-Sundberg, M., and Badger, T. M. 1999. The effects of enteral nutrition and chronic alcohol on hepatic necrosis. Toxicol. Sci. 47:110–117.
Kukielka, E., and Cederbaum, A. I. 1994. DNA strand cleavage as a sensitive assay for the production of hydroxyl radical by microsomes: role of CYP2E1 in the increased activity after ethanol treatment. Biochem. J. 302:773–779.
Kuthan, H., and Ullrich, V. 1982. Oxidase and oxygenase function of the microsomal cytochrome P450 monooxygenase system. Eur. J. Biochem. 126:583–588.
Laethem, R. M., Balazy, M., Falck, J. R., Laethem, C. L., and Koop, D. R. 1993. Formation of 19(*S*)-, 19(*R*)-, and 18(*R*)- hydroxyeicosatetraenoic acids by alcohol-inducible cytochrome P450 2E1. J. Biol. Chem. 268:12912–12918.
Lander, H. M. 1997. An essential role for free radicals and derived species in signal transduction. FASEB J. 11:118–124.
Leclereq, I. A., Farrell G. C., Field, J., Bell, D. R., Gonzalez, F. J., and Robertson, G. R. 2000. CYP2E1 and CYP4A as microsomal catalysts of lipid peroxides in murine nonalcoholic steatohepatitis. J. Clin. Invest.105:1067–1075.
Lee, S. S. T., Buters, J. T. M., Pineau, T., Fernandez-Salguero, P., and Gonzalez, F. J. 1996. Role of CYP2E1 in the hepatotoxicity of acetaminophen. J. Biol. Chem. 271:12063–12067.
Lewis, D. F. V., and Pratt, J. M. 1998. The P450 catalytic cycle and oxygenation mechanism. Drug Metab. Rev. 30:739–786.
Li, J., French, B. A., Riley, N., Bardag-Gorce, F., Fu, P., and French, S. W. 2001. Oral low carbohydrate liquid diet induces experimental steatohepatitis in the rat. Exp. Mol. Pathol. 71:132–136.
Lieber, C. S. 1997. Cytochrome P4502E1; its physiological and pathological role. Physiol. Rev. 77:517–544.
Lieber, C. S. 1999. Microsomal ethanol oxidizing system: the first 30 years – a review. Alcohol. Clin. Exp. Res. 23:991–1007.
Lieber, C. S., and DeCarli, L. M. 1972. The role of the hepatic microsomal ethanol oxidizing system for ethanol metabolism in vivo. J. Pharmacol. Exp. Ther. 181:279–287.
Lieber, C. S., Leo, M. A., Aleynik, S. I., Aleynik, M. K., and DeCarli, L. M. 1997. Polyenylphosphatidylcholine decreases alcohol-induced oxidative stress in the baboon. Alcohol. Clin. Exp. Res. 21:375–379.
Lindros K., and Jarvelainen, H. 1998. A new oral low-carbohydrate alcohol liquid diet producing liver lesions: a preliminary account. Alcohol 33:347–353.

Loeper, J., Descatoire, V., Maurice, M., Beaune, P., Feldmann, G., Larrey, D., and Pessayre, D. 1990. Presence of functional cytochrome P-450 on isolated rat hepatocytes plasma membrane. Hepatology 11:850–858.

Loeper, J., Decatoire, V., Maurice, M., Beaune, P., Belghiti, J., Houssin, D., Ballet, F., Feldmann G., Guengerich, F. P., and Pessayre, D. 1993. Cytochromes P-450 in human hepatocytes plasma membrane: recognition by several autoantibodies. Gastroeterology 104:203–216.

Loida, P. J., and Sligar, S. G. 1993. Molecular recognition in cytochrome P450: mechanism for the control of uncoupling reactions. Biochemistry 32:11530–11538.

Lytton, S. D., Helander, A., Zhang-Gouillon, Z. Q., Stokkeland K., Bordone R., Arico, S., Albano, E., French, S. W., and Ingelman-Sundberg, M. 1999. Autoantibodies against cytochromes P-4502E1 and P-4503A in alcoholics. Mol. Pharmacol. 55:223–233.

Mari, M., and Cederbaum, A. I. 2000. CYP2E1 overexpression in HepG2 cells induces glutathione synthesis by transcriptional activation of glutamyl cysteine synthetase. J. Biol. Chem. 275:15563–15571.

Mari, M., and Cederbaum, A. I. 2001. Induction of catalase, alpha and microsomal glutathione S-transferases in CYP2E1-overexpressing HepG2 cells and protection against short-term oxidative stress. Hepatology 33:652–661.

Mari, M., Bai, J., and Cederbaum, A. I. 2002. Adenovirus-mediated overexpression of catalase in the cytosolic or mitochondrial compartments protects against toxicity caused by glutathione depletion in HepG2 cells expressing CYP2E1. J. Pharmacol. Exp. Ther. 301:111–118.

McCarty, M. F. 2001. Inhibition of CYP2E1 with natural agents may be a feasible strategy for minimizing the hepatotoxicity of ethanol. Med. Hypothesis 56:8–11.

McCord, J. 1998. Iron, free radicals and oxidative injury. Semin. Hematol. 35:5–12.

McGehee, R. E., Jr. Ronis, M. J. J., Cowherd, R. M., Ingelman-Sundberg, M., and Badger, T. M. 1994. Characterization of cytochrome P450-2E1 induction in a rat hepatoma FGC-4 cell model by ethanol. Biochem. Pharmacol. 48:1823–1833.

Morel, Y., and Barouki, R. 1999. Repression of gene expression by oxidative stress. Biochem. J. 342:481–496.

Morgan, K., French, S. W., and Morgan, T. R. 2002. Production of a cytochrome P450 2E1 transgenic mouse and initial evaluation of alcoholic liver damage. Hepatology 36:122–134.

Morimoto, M., Hagbjork, A. L., Nanji, A. A., Ingelman-Sundberg, M., Lindros, K. O., Fu, P. C., Albano, E., and French, S. W. 1993. Role of cytochrome P450 2E1 in alcoholic liver disease pathogenesis. Alcohol 10:459–464.

Morimoto, M., Zern, M. A., Hagbjork, A. L., Ingelman-Sundberg, M., and French, S. W. 1994. Fish oil, alcohol and liver pathology: role of cytochrome P450 2E1. Proc. Soc. Exp. Biol. Med. 207:197–205.

Morimoto, M., Hagbjork, A. L., Wan, Y. J., Fu, P. C., Clot, P., Albano, E., Ingelman-Sundberg, M., and French, S. W. 1995. Modulation of experimental alcohol-induced liver disease by cytochrome P450 2E1 inhibitors. Hepatology 21:1610–1617.

Nakazawa, J., Genka, C., and Fujishima, M. 1996. Pathological aspects of active oxygens/free radicals. Jpn. J. Physiol. 46:15–32.

Nanji, A. A., Zhao, S., Sadrzadeh S. M. H., Dannenberg, A. J., Tahan, S. R., and Waxman, D. J. 1994. Markedly enhanced cytochrome P4502E1 induction and lipid peroxidation is associated with severe liver injury in fish oil–ethanol-fed rats. Alcohol. Clin. Exp. Res 18:1280–1285.

Nebert, D. W., Nelson, D. R., Coon, M. J., Estabrook, R. W., Feyereisen, R., Fujii-Kuriyama, Y., Gonzalez, F. J., Guengerich, F. A. P., Gunsalus, I. C., and Johnson, E. F. 1991. The P450 superfamily: update on new sequences, gene mapping, and recommended nomenclature. DNA Cell Biol. 10:1–14.

Nelson, D. R., Koymans, L., Kamataki, T., Stegeman, J. J., Feyereisen, R., Waxman, D. J., Waterman, M. R., Gotoh, O., Coon, M. J., Estabrook, R. W., Gunsalus, I. C., and Nebert, D. W. 1996. P450 superfamily: update on new sequences, gene mapping, accession numbers and nomenclature. Pharmacogenetics 6:1–42.

Neve, E. P. A., and Ingelman-Sundberg, M. 1999. A soluble NH_2-terminally truncated catalytically active form of rat cytochrome P450 2E1 targeted to liver mitochondria. FEBS Lett. 460:309–314.

Neve, E. P. A., and Ingelman-Sundberg, M. 2000. Molecular basis for the transport of cytochrome P450 2E1 to the plasma membrane. J. Biol. Chem. 275: 17130–17135.

Neve, E. P. A., Eliasson, E., Pronzato, M. A., Albano, E., Marinari, U., and Ingelman-Sundberg, M. 1996. Enzyme-specific transport of rat liver cytochrome P450 to the golgi apparatus. Arch. Biochem. Biophys. 333:459–465.

Nieto, N., Friedman, S. L., and Cederbaum, A. I. 2002a. Cytochrome P450 2E1-derived reactive oxygen species mediate paracrine stimulation of collagen I protein synthesis by hepatic stellate cells. J. Biol. Chem. 277:9853–9864.

Nieto, N., Friedman, S. L., and Cederbaum, A. I. 2002b. Stimulation and proliferation of primary rat hepatic stellate cells by cytochrome P4502E1-derived reactive oxygen species. Hepatology 35:62–73.

Nieto, N., Mari, M., and Cederbaum, A. I. 2003. Cytochrome P4502E1 responsiveness in the promoter of glutamate-cysteine ligase catalytic subunit. Hepatology 37:96–106.

Nordman, R., Riviere, C., and Rouach, H. 1992. Implication of free radical mechanisms in ethanol-induced cellular injury. Free Rad. Biol. Med. 12:219–240.

Orrenius S., Ankarcrona M., and Nicotera, P. 1996. Mechanisms of calcium-related cell death. Adv. Neurol. 71:137–151.

Peng, H. M., and Coon, M. J. 1998. Regulation of rabbit cytochrome P-450 2E1 expression in HepG2 cells by insulin and thyroid hormone. Mol. Pharmacol. 54:740–747.

Perez, M. J., and Cederbaum, A. I. 2001. Spin trapping agents (TEMPOL and POBN) protect HepG2 cells over-expressing CYP2E1 against arachidonic acid toxicity. Free Rad. Biol. Med. 30:734–746.

Perez, M. J., and Cederbaum, A. L. 2003. Proteasome inhibition potentiates CYP 2E1-mediated toxicity in HepG2 cells. Hepatology 37:1395–1404.

Porter, T. D., and Coon, M. J. 1991. Cytochrome P450: multiplicity of isoforms, substrates and catalytic and regulatory mechanisms. J. Biol. Chem. 266:13469–13472.

Puntarulo, S., and Cederbaum A. I. 1988. Increased NADPH-dependent chemiluminescence by microsomes after chronic ethanol consumption. Arch. Biochem. Biophys. 266:435–445.

Rao, D. N. R., Yang, M. X., Lasker, J. M., and Cederbaum, A. I. 1996. 1-Hydroxyethyl radical formation during NADPH- and NADH-dependent oxidation of ethanol by human liver microsomes. Mol. Pharmacol. 49:814–821.

Rashba-Step, J., Turro, N. J., and Cederbaum, A. I. 1993. Increased NADPH- and NADH-dependent production of superoxide and hydroxyl radical by microsomes after chronic ethanol treatment. Arch. Biochem. Biophys. 300:401–408.

Raucy, J. L., Lasker, J. M., Kramer, J. C., Salazer, D. E., Lieber, C. S., and Corcoran, G. B. 1991. Induction of P-450IIE1 in the obese rat. Mol. Pharmacol. 39:275–280.

Raucy, J. L., Kraner, J. C., and Lasker, J. M. 1993. Bioactivation of halogenated hydrocarbons by cytochrome P4502E1. Crit. Rev. Toxicol. 23:1–20.

Reid, A. E. 2001. Nonalcoholic steatohepatitis. Gastroenterology 121:710–723.

Reinke, L., Lai, E. K., DuBose, C. M., McCay, P. B., and Janzen, E. G. 1987. Reactive free radical generation in vivo in heart and liver of ethanol fed rats: correlations with radical formation in vitro. Proc. Natl. Acad. Sci. U.S.A. 84:8223–8227.

Rendic, S., and DiCarlo, F. 1997. Human cytochrome P450 enzymes: a status report summarizing their reactions, substrates, inducers, and inhibitors. Drug Metab. Rev. 29:413–580.

Roberts, B. J. 1997. Evidence of proteasome-mediated cytochrome P450 degradation. J. Biol. Chem. 272:9771–9778.

Roberts, B. J., Shoaf, S. E., Jeong, K. S., and Song, B. J. 1994. Induction of CYP2E1 in liver, kidney, brain, and intestine during chronic ethanol administration and withdrawal: evidence that CYP2E1 possesses a rapid phase half-life of 6 hours or less. Biochem., Biophys. Res. Commun. 205:1064–1071.

Roberts, B. J., Shoaf, S. E., and Song, B. J. 1995. Rapid changes in cytochrome P4502E1 (CYP2E1) activity and other P40 isozymes following ethanol withdrawal in rat. Biochem. Pharmacol. 49:1665–1673.

Roberts, B. J., Song, B. J., Soh, Y., Park, S. S., and Shoaf, S. E. 1995. Ethanol induces CYP2E1 by protein stabilization: role of ubiquitin conjugation in the rapid degradation for CYP2E1. J. Biol. Chem. 270:29632–29635.

Robertson, G. R., Leclereq, I. A., and Farrell, G. C. 2001. Nonalcoholic steatohepatitis II: cytochrome P-450 enzymes and oxidative stress. Am. J. Physiol. Gastrointest. Liver Physiol. 281:G1135–G1139.

Ronis, M. J. J., Johansson, I., Hultenby, K., Lagercrants, J., Glaumann, H., and Ingelman-Sundberg, M. 1991. Acetone-regulated synthesis and degradation of cytochrome P4502E1 and cytochrome 2B1 in rat liver. Eur. J. Biochem. 198:383–389.

Ronis, M. J. J., Huange, J., Crouch, J., Mercadao, C., Irby, D., Valentine, C. R., Lumpkin, C. K., Ingelman-Sundberg, M., and Badger, T. M. 1993. Cytochrome P450 CYP2E1 induction during chronic alcohol exposure occurs by a two-step mechanism associated with blood alcohol concentrations in rats. J. Pharmacol. Exp. Ther. 264:944–950.

Ronis, M. J. J., Lindros K. O., and Ingelman-Sundberg, M. 1996. The CYP2E subfamily. In Cytochromes P450. Metabolic and Toxicological Aspects, ed. C. Ioannides, pp. 211–239. New York: CRC Press.

Rosen, G. M., Pou, S., Ramos, C. L., Cohen, M. S., and Britigan, B. E. 1995. Free radicals and phagocytic cells. FASEB J. 9:200–209.

Sakurai, K., and Cederbaum, A. I. 1998. Oxidative stress and cytotoxicity induced by ferric-nitrilotriacetate in HepG2 cells expressing CYP2E1. Mol. Pharmacol. 54:1024–1035.

Salmela, K. S., Kessova, I. G., Tsyrlov, I. B., and Lieber, C. S. 1998. Respective roles of human cytochrome P-4502E1, 1A2, and 3A4 in the hepatic microsomal ethanol oxidizing system. Alcohol. Clin. Exp. Res. 22:2125–2132.

Shimojo, N., Ishizaki, T., Imaoka, S., Funae, Y., Fujii, S., and Okuda, K. 1993. Changes in amounts of cytochrome P-450 isozymes and levels of catalytic activities in hepatic and renal microsomes of rats with streptozocin-induced diabetes. Biochem. Pharmacol. 46:621–627.

Sohn, D. H., Yun, Y. P., Park, K. S., Veech, R. L., and Song, B. J. 1991. Posttranscriptional reduction of cytochrome P450IIE1 by CCl_4 its substrate. Biochem. Biophys. Res. Commun. 179:449–454.

Song, B. J. 1995. Gene structure and multiple regulations of the ethanol-inducible cytochrome P4502E1 (CYP2E1) subfamily. In Alcohol and Hormones, vol. 6., ed. R. R. Watson, pp. 177–192. Totowa: Humana Press.

Song, B. J., Gelboin, H. V., Park, S. S., Yang, C. S., and Gonzalez, F. J. 1986. Complementary DNA and protein sequences of ethanol-inducible rat and human cytochrome P450s: transcriptional and posttranscriptional regulation of the rat enzyme. J. Biol. Chem. 261:16689–16697.

Song, B. J., Matsunaga, T., Hardwich, J. P., Park, S. S., Veech, R. L., Yang, C. S., Gelboin, H. V., and Gonzalez, F. J. 1987. Stabilization of cytochrome P450 J mRNA in the diabetic rat. Mol. Endocrinol. 1:542–547.

Song, B. J., Veech, R. L., Park, S. S., Gelboin, H. V., and Gonazalez, F. J. 1989. Induction of rat hepatic *N*-nitrosodimethylamine demethylase by acetone is due to protein stabilization. J. Biol. Chem. 264:3568–3572.

Song , B. J., Cederbaum, A. I., Koop, D. R., Ingelman-Sundberg, M., and Nanji, A. 1996. Ethanol-inducible cytochrome P450 (CYP2E1): biochemistry, molecular biology and clinical relevance. Alcohol. Clin. Exp. Res. 20(Suppl.):138A–146A.

Susin, S. A., Zamzami, N., and Kroemer, G. 1998. Mitochondria as regulators of apoptosis: doubt no more. Biochim. Biophys. Acta 1366:151–165.

Tanaka, E., Terada, M., and Misawa, S. 2000. Cytochrome P450 2E1: its clinical and toxicological role. J. Clin. Pharm. Ther. 25:165–175.

Terelius, Y., and Ingelman-Sundberg, M. 1986. Metabolism of *n*-pentane by ethanol-inducible cytochrome P-450 in liver microsomes and reconstituted membrane. Eur. J. Biochem. 161:303–308.

Terelius, Y., Norsten-Hoog, C., Cronholm, T., and Ingelman-Sundberg, M. 1991. Acetaldehyde as a substrate for ethanol-inducible cytochrome P-450 (CYP2E1). Biochem. Biophys. Res. Commun. 179:689–694.

Teschke, R., Moreno, F., and Petrides, A. S. 1981. Hepatic microsomal ethanol oxidizing system (MEOS): respective roles of ethanol and carbohydrates for the enhanced activity after chronic alcohol consumption. Biochem. Pharmacol. 30:1745–1751.

Tierney, D. J., Haas, A. L., and Koop, D. R. 1992. Degradation of cytochrome P4502E1: selective loss after labilization of the enzyme. Arch. Biochem. Biophys. 293:9–16.

Toykuni, S. 1999. Reactive oxygen species-induced molecular damage and its application in pathology. Pathology Inter. 49:91–102.

Trost, L. C., and Lemasters, J. J. 1996. The mitochondrial permeability transition: a new pathophysiological mechanism for Reye's syndrome and toxic liver injury. J. Pharmacol. Exp. Ther. 278:1000–1005.

Tsukamoto, H. 2000. CYP2E1 and ALD. Hepatology 32:154–155.

Tsukamoto, H., and Lu, S. C. 2001. Current concepts in the pathogenesis of alcoholic liver injury. FASEB J. 15:1335–1349.

Tsukamoto, H., Horne, W., Kamimura, S., Niemela, O., Parkkila, S., Yla-Herttuala, S., and Brittenham, G. M. 1995. Experimental liver cirrhosis induced by alcohol and iron. J. Clin. Invest. 96:620–630.

Tsutsumi, M., Lasker, J., Shimizu, M., Rosman, A. S., and Lieber, C. S. 1989. The interlobular distribution of ethanol-inducible P4502E1 in rat and human liver. Hepatology 10:437–446.

Tsutsumi, M, Lasker, J. M., Takahasi, T., and Lieber, C. S. 1993. In vivo induction of hepatic P4502E1 by ethanol: role of increased enzymes synthesis. Arch. Biochem. Biophys. 394:209–218.

Wang, M., Chanas, B., and Ghanayem, B. I. 2002. Cytochrome P4502El is essential for acrylonitrile metabolism to cyanide: comparative studies using CYP2E1-null and wild-type mice. Drug Metab. Disp. 30:911–917.

Weltman, M., Farrell, G., Hall P., Ingelman-Sundberg, M., and Liddle, C. 1998. Hepatic cytochrome P450 2E1 is increased in patients with nonalcoholic steatohepatitis. Hepatology 27:128–133.

Wheeler, M. D., and Thurman, R. G. 2001. The role of Kupffer cell oxidant production in early ethanol-induced liver disease. Free Rad. Biol. Med. 31:1544–1549.

White, R. E. 1991. The involvement of free radicals in the mechanisms of monooxygenases. Pharmacol. Ther. 49:21–42.

Winters, D. K., and Cederbaum, A. I. 1992. Time course characterization of the induction of cytochrome P450 2E1 by pyrazole and 4-methylpyrazole. Biochim. Biophys. Acta. 1117:15–24.

Wolf, K. K., Wood, S. G., Bement, J. L, Sinclair, P. R., Wrighton, S. A., Jeffery, E., Gonzalez, F. J., and Sinclair, J. F. 2004. Role of mouse CYP2E1 in the *o*-hydroxylation of *p*-nitrophenol. Drug Metab. Disp. 32:681–684.

Woodcroft, K. J., and Novak, R. F. 1997. Insulin effects on CYP 2E1, 2B, 3A, and 4A expression in primary cultured rat hepatocytes. Chem. Biol. Interact. 107:75–91.

Woodcroft, K. J., Hafner, M. S., and Novak, R. F. 2002. Insulin signaling in the transcriptional and posttranscriptional regulation of CYP 2E1 expression. Hepatology 35:263–273.

Wu, D., and Cederbaum, A. I. 1992. Presence of functionally active cytochrome P-450IIE1 in the plasma membrane of rat hepatocytes. Hepatology 15:515–524.

Wu, D., and Cederbaum, A. I. 1993a. Combined effects of streptozotocin-induced diabetes plus-4 methylpyrazole treatment on rat liver cytochrome P450 2E1. Arch. Biochem. Biophys. 302:175–182.

Wu, D., and Cederbaum, A. I. 1993b. Induction of liver cytochrome P450 2E1 by pyrazole and 4-methylpyrazole in neonatal rats. J. Pharmacol. Exp. Ther. 264:1468–1473.

Wu, D., and Cederbaum, A. I. 1996. Ethanol toxicity to a transfected HepG2 cell line expressing human cytochrome P450 2E1. J. Biol. Chem. 271:23914–23919.

Wu, D., and Cederbaum, A. I. 1999. Ethanol-induced apoptosis to stable HepG2 cell lines expressing human cytochrome P450 2E1. Alcohol. Clin. Exp. Res. 23:67–76.

Wu, D., and Cederbaum, A. I. 2000. Ethanol and arachidonic acid produce toxicity in hepatocytes from pyrazole-treated rats with high levels of CYP2E1. Mol. Cell. Biochem. 204:157–167.

Wu, D., and Cederbaum, A. I. 2001a. Removal of glutathione produces apoptosis and necrosis in HepG2 cells overexpressing CYP2E1. Alcohol. Clin. Exp. Res. 25:619–628.

Wu, D., and Cederbaum, A. I. 2001b. Sodium salicylate increases CYP2E1 levels and enhances arachidonic acid toxicity in HepG2 cells and cultured rat hepatocytes. Mol. Pharmacol. 59:795–805.

Wu, D., and Cederbaum, A. I. 2002. Cyclosporin protects against arachidonic acid toxicity in rat hepatocytes: role of CYP2E1 and mitochondria. Hepatology 35:1420–1430.

Wu, D., Clejan, L. A., Potter, B., and Cederbaum, A. I. 1990. Rapid decrease of cytochrome P-450IIE1 in primary hepatocyte culture and its maintenance by added 4-methypyrazole. Hepatology 12:1379–1389.

Wu, Y., Salmela, K., and Lieber, C. S. 1998. Microsomal acetaldehyde oxidation is negligible in the presence of ethanol. Alcohol. Clin. Exp. Res. 22:1165–1169.

Yang, M. X., and Cederbaum, A. I. 1997a. Characterization of cytochrome P450 2E1 turnover in transfected HepG2 cells expressing human CYP2E1. Arch. Biochem. Biophys. 341:25–33.

Yang, M. X., and Cederbaum, A. I. 1997b. Glycerol increases content and activity of human cytochrome P450 2E1 in a transduced HepG2 cell line by protein stabilization. Alcohol. Clin. Exp. Res. 21:340–347.

Yang, C. S., Yoo, J. S. H., Ishizaki, H., and Hong, J. 1990. Cytochrome P450IIE1. Roles in nitrosamine metabolism and mechanisms of regulation. Drug Metab. Rev. 22:147–159.

Yin, M., Wheeler, M. D., Kono, H., Bradford, B. U., Galluci, R. M., Luster, M. I., and Thurman, R. G. 1999. Essential role of TNFα in alcohol-induced liver injury in mice. Gastroenterology 117:942–952.

Yoo, J., Ning, S. M., Pantuck, C. B., Pantuck, E. J., and Yang, C. S. 1991. Regulation of hepatic microsomal cytochrome P-450 2E1 level by dietary lipids and carbohydrates in rats. J. Nutr. 121:959–965.

Yu, B. P. 1994. Cellular defenses against damage from reactive oxygen species. Physiol. Rev. 74:139–162.

Yun, Y., Casazza, J. P., Sohn, D. H., Veech, R. L., and Song, B. J. 1992. Pretranslational activation of cytochrome P450IIE during ketosis induced by a high fat diet. Mol. Pharmacol. 41:474–479.

Zhukov, A., and Ingelman-Sundberg, M. 1999. Relationship between cytochrome P450 catalytic cycling and stability. Biochem. J. 340:453–458.

Zhukov, A., Werlinder, V., and Ingelman-Sundberg, M. 1993. Purification and characterization of two membrane bound serine proteases from rat liver microsomes active in degradation of cytochrome P450. Biochem. Biophys. Res. Commun. 197:221–228.

7

One- and Two-Electron-Mediated Reduction of Quinones: Enzymology and Toxicological Implications

David Siegel, Phillip Reigan and David Ross

Department of Pharmaceutical Sciences, School of Pharmacy, University Colorado Denver, Denver, CO 80262, USA

e-mail: david.ross@uchsc.edu

Keywords: Quinines · Cytochrome P450 Reductase · Cytochrome b_5 Reductase · Xanthine Oxidoreductase · Quinone Oxidoreductase 1 and 2 · Mitochrondrial Reductases · Carbonyl Reductases · Mitomycin C · Porfiromycin

7.1. Enzymology of Quinone Reduction

Quinones can undergo one- or two-electron reductions to generate semiquinone and hydroquinone derivatives, respectively (Gutierrez 2000; Butler 1998; Ross et al. 1996; O'Brien 1991; Powis 1987). The importance of these reactions from a toxicological perspective depends on the chemical properties of the semiquinone and hydroquinone, the oxygen tension, and the ability of the organ system or cell to remove or metabolize the semiquinone or hydroquinone generated. This review will focus on the enzymology and toxicological implications associated with both one- and two-electron-mediated reduction of quinones.

In the following sections, enzymes associated with either one- or two-electron reductions of quinones (Figure 7.1) will be briefly summarized.

7.1.1. Cytochrome P450 Reductase

NADPH-cytochrome P450 reductase (CPR; NADPH-ferrihemoprotein reductase, EC 1.6.2.4) is the electron-donor flavoprotein for the multi-component monooxygenase system, in which reducing equivalents from NADPH ultimately are transferred to molecular oxygen, found in the endoplasmic reticulum (microsomes) of most eukaryotic cells (Shen, Sem and Kasper 1999). Fundamentally, the monooxygenase system consists of CPR and one of many cytochrome P450 isozymes (Williams and Kamin 1962; Phillips and Langdon 1962), involved in the metabolism of many

A.A. Elfarra (ed.), *Advances in Bioactivation Research*, DOI: 10.1007/978-0-387-77300-1_7,

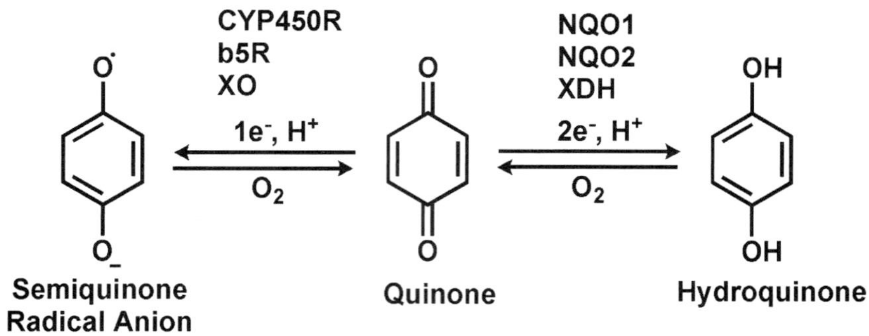

Figure 7.1 The generation of semiquinone and hydroquinone intermediates from one- or two-electron reduction of quinones.

drugs, dietary substances, the synthesis of steroid hormones, and other extracellular lipid signaling molecules. Consistent with its many functions in the cell, CPR is a widely expressed protein, present at some level in all tissues examined. It is most abundant in the liver, where the cytochrome P450 system is highly expressed. Mechanistically, CPR accepts a pair of electrons from NADPH as a hydride ion, with flavinadenine dinucleotide (FAD) and flavin mononucleotide (FMN) being the point of entry and exit, respectively, and transfers these electrons to cytochrome P450. Cytochromes P450, in turn, utilizes these reducing equivalents for the hydroxylation of a variety of substrates. The redox potentials of each flavin half-reaction in the native enzyme have been determined by potentiometric titrations (Iyanagi, Makino and Mason 1974; Vermilion and Coon 1978). The enzyme cycles between $1e^-$ and $3e^-$ reduced levels (or $2e^-$ and $4e^-$), with the one-electron reduced semiquinone of the FMN being the highest oxidation state during catalytic turnover (Masters et al. 1965; Backes and Reker-Backes 1988).

The ability of CPR to reduce quinones to the semiquinone radical is related to their one-electron reduction potential. The analysis of a large number of quinones demonstrated a correlation between their rate of reduction by CPR and their one-electron reduction potential (Butler and Hoey 1993). This correlation, however, is true for quinones with one-electron reduction potentials between –400 mV and –165 mV, while quinones with reduction potentials more positive than –165 mV underwent predominantly two-electron reduction by NADPH directly without the participation of the enzyme (Butler and Hoey 1993). In another study, the rate of reduction of a series of quinones increased as the one-electron redox couple was increased up to a limiting value of >–100 mV (Nemeikaite-Ceniene et al. 2003).

7.1.2. Cytochrome b_5 Reductase

NADH-cytochrome b_5 reductase (b5R, NADH-methemoglobin reductase, EC 1.6.2.2) and cytochrome b_5 are integral membrane proteins with cytosolic active domains and have been implicated as components of a number of systems, where essentially, b5R catalyzes the two-electron transfer from NADH to cytochrome b_5 through the enzyme-bound FAD cofactor (Strittmatter 1965; Iyanagi 1977). In human erythrocytes, these proteins are components of the major methemoglobin reducing system (Hultquist and Passon 1971; Schwartz and Jaffe 1978). The confusion over the nomenclature of b5R as a diaphorase related to NQO1 has recently been clarified (Vasiliou, Ross and Nebert 2006).

While there has not been an extensive study published on the relationship between the one-electron reduction potential and the rate of reduction by b5R there is evidence using a limited number of quinones suggesting that the higher the one-electron reduction potential the slower the rate of reduction by b5R (Powis and Appel 1980). These studies also demonstrated that there was no correlation between the octanol/H_2O partition coefficient of a series of quinones and their rate of reduction by b5R (Powis and Appel 1980).

7.1.3. Xanthine Oxidoreductase (Xanthine Dehydrogenase, Xanthine Oxidase)

Xanthine oxidoreductase (XOR), a member of the molybdenum hydroxylase flavoprotein family, exists in two interconvertable forms, xanthine dehydrogenase (XDH, EC 1.1.1.204) and xanthine oxidase (XO, EC 1.1.3.22) (Amaya et al. 1990; Della Corte et al. 1969). The functional distinction between XDH and XO is the preference of each for the reducing substrate. Xanthine oxidase uses molecular oxygen efficiently, as an electron acceptor, reducing molecular oxygen by a single electron, but has negligible reactivity with NAD^+. Xanthine dehydrogenase however prefers NAD^+ to molecular oxygen, reducing NAD^+ by a direct two-electron reduction, but is able to use the latter in the course of turnover (Hille and Nishino 1995). Xanthine dehydrogenase isolated from mammalian sources can be either reversibly converted to XO by sulfhydryl modification or irreversibly converted to XO by limited proteolysis (Harris, Sanders and Massey 1999; Amaya et al. 1990; Battelli, Lorenzoni and Stripe 1973; Nishino 1994). Physiologically, XOR is the key rate-limiting enzyme in the catabolism of purines, both XDH and XO catalyze the oxidation of hypoxanthine to xanthine and xanthine to uric acid, which introduces reducing equivalents into the enzyme. The reoxidation of the molybdenum center occurs via electron transfer to the two iron–sulfur redox-active centers of the enzyme and ultimately to the FAD-site where electrons are removed from the enzyme by reaction with NAD^+ in the case of XDH or with molecular oxygen for XO (Hille 1996; Hille and Massey 1981).

In mammalian tissues XOR exists mainly in the XDH form; however, when O_2 levels decrease, due to an insult, such as ischemia, XDH may be converted to XO which is considered to be important in the pathogenesis of ischemia/reperfusion injury (McCord 1985). During reperfusion, when O_2 levels return to normal, reduction of oxygen by XO yields the superoxide anion, O_2^-, and hydrogen peroxide, H_2O_2, (Terada et al. 1991; Brown et al. 1988) and other reactive-oxygen species (ROS). These reactive-oxygen metabolites have been implicated in diseases characterized by ischemia/reperfusion injury (Linas, Whittenburg and Repine 1990; Sussman and Bulkley 1990; Petrone et al. 1980).

Xanthine oxidase is a one-electron and XDH is a two-electron transfer enzyme and therefore either the semiquinone and hydroquinone forms of the quinone drug can be formed (Figure 7.1). Anthracyclines such as doxorubicin, daunomycin, and marcellomycin are reduced by XOR to the corresponding semiquinone under aerobic conditions (Pan and Bachur 1980). Mitomycin C is reduced by XOR under aerobic conditions to the semiquinone radical with consequent formation of ROS (Pan et al. 1984). Conversely, anaerobic conditions lead to the formation of 2,7-diaminomitosene, a DNA alkylating metabolite (Gustafson and Pritsos 1992). The activation of a number of quinone drugs, such as mitomycin C, by one-electron reduction by XO or two-electron reduction by XDH, at the FAD site, has also been reported (Maliepaard et al. 1995; Pritsos and Gustafson 1994; Komiyama, Kikuchi and Sugiura 1986; Pan et al. 1984).

The relationship between the quinone one-electron reduction potential and the rate of reduction by XO under a nitrogen atmosphere and in air has been studied using a series of 2,5- *bis*(1-aziridinyl)-1,4-benzoquinone analogs. Under nitrogen, the rate of reduction of these quinones by XO correlated with the one-electron reduction potential as well as steric factors (Lusthof et al. 1990). However, when similar studies were performed in air, substantially higher quinone concentrations (>25 μM) were required presumably to outcompete O_2 for electrons donated by XO (Lusthof et al. 1990).

7.1.4. NAD(P)H:quinone Oxidoreductase 1

NAD(P)H:quinone oxidoreductase 1 (NQO1, DT-diaphorase, EC 1.6.99.2) is a homodimeric flavoprotein that catalyzes two-electron reduction of a wide range of substrates (Lind et al. 1990). In addition, NQO1 has also been shown to catalyze the four-electron reduction of methyl red (Wu et al. 1997; Chen, Hwang and Deng 1993). The enzyme is characterized by its ability to utilize either NADH or NADPH as reducing cofactors and inhibition by the anticoagulant dicumarol (Hollander and Ernster 1975). Recently, a number of indolequinone-containing mechanism-based inhibitors such as ES936 and MAC220 have been developed and these compounds have demonstrated potent and specific inactivation of NQO1 without affecting the activities of other reductases including NQO2 (Dehn et al. 2003; Siegel et al. unpublished data). The enzymatic mechanism of quinone reduction proceeds through a "ping-pong" type mechanism, whereby NAD(P)H binds to the enzyme, reduces the protein-bound flavin, and leaves the protein prior to substrate binding and subsequent reduction (Li et al. 1995). NQO1 displays a wide, species-specific substrate spectrum, including quinones and their glutathione metabolites, quinoneimines, and several azo- and nitroaromatic compounds. The four-electron reduction of nitroaromatic compounds to the hydroxylamine derivatives has been proposed to occur through the cooperative behavior of the two subunits (Cenas et al. 2001).

Expression of NQO1 protein has been detected primarily in epithelial cells in tissues such as lung, breast, and colon as well as in vascular endothelium and adipocytes (Siegel and Ross 2000). Humans, unlike rodents, dogs, and monkeys, do not express high levels of NQO1 in the normal liver

(Strassburg et al. 2002; Siegel and Ross 2000), but humans do express high levels of NQO1 in hepatic tumors (Cresteil and Jaiswal 1991). A similar finding has been seen in the pancreas which has very low NQO1 expression in normal pancreatic tissue but NQO1 expression increases significantly as the tissue becomes neoplastic (Lyn-Cook et al. 2006; Dehn et al. unpublished data). In addition to pancreatic cancer, there are high levels of NQO1 in most epithelial-derived solid tumors (Siegel and Ross 2000; Schlager and Powis 1990) and this has made NQO1 an attractive target for the bioactivation of many quinone-based antitumor drugs (see below). NQO1 is highly inducible and NQO1 protein levels in tissues can be influenced by a number of environmental and dietary factors (Munday, Smith and Munday 1999a; Sreerama, Hedge and Sladek 1995; De Long, Prochaska and Talalay 1986). A major factor governing the levels of NQO1 protein expression in tissues is the NQO1*2 polymorphism. The NQO1*2 polymorphism has been characterized as a C-to-T base pair substitution at position 609 of the human cDNA that results in a proline-to-serine amino acid substitution at position 187 in the mutant NQO1 protein (Traver et al. 1997) Genotype–phenotype studies have shown that individuals homozygous for the NQO1*2 polymorphism are deficient in NQO1 due to enhanced ubiquitination and proteasomal degradation of the mutant protein (Siegel et al. 2001). In humans the absence of NQO1 has been linked to increased rates of cancer, most notably leukemias (Ross and Siegel 2004). This is supported by studies using NQO1 knockout mice that demonstrated increased bone marrow myeloid hyperplasia in NQO1-deficient mice compared to wild-type mice (Iskander and Jaiswal 2005). NQO1 knockout mice were also more susceptible to menadione-induced toxicities confirming a role for NQO1 in quinone detoxification (Radjendirane et al. 1998).

The rate at which a substrate is reduced by NQO1 cannot be predicted by the one-electron reduction potential. Studies using a series of substituted aziridinylbenzoquinones found no correlation between the one-electron reduction potential and the ability to undergo reduction by NQO1 (Nemeikaite-Ceniene et al. 2003; Gibson et al. 1992), while another study found no correlation between the half-wave reduction potentials of quinone epoxides and hydroxy-, methyl-, methoxy-, and glutathionyl-substituted naphthoquinones and their rate of reduction by NQO1 (Buffinton et al. 1989; Brunmark et al. 1988). In addition, there was no correlation between the two-electron reduction potential and rate of reduction of a series of aziridinylbenzoquinone by NQO1 (Hargreaves et al. 1999).

7.1.5. NRH:quinone Oxidoreductase 2

NRH:quinone oxidoreductase 2 (NQO2, EC 1.10.99.2) is a cytosolic homodimeric flavoprotein that demonstrates 49% amino acid homology with NQO1 (Jaiswal et al. 1990). An update of the NQO gene family has recently been published (Vasiliou, Ross and Nebert 2006). The major difference between the two enzymes is a 43-amino-acid deletion in the C terminus of NQO2 (Jaiswal et al. 1990). NQO2 carries out the direct two- and four-electron reduction of substrates similar to NQO1; however,

NQO2 is more efficient at catalyzing the four-electron reduction of methyl red compared to NQO1 (Wu et al. 1997). A major difference between NQO1 and NQO2 is their ability to utilize reduced pyridine nucleotide cofactors. NQO2 cannot utilize NADPH as a reducing cofactor and NADH is a very poor substrate for NQO2 (Wu et al. 1997). NQO2, however, can efficiently utilize reduced ribosyl- and *N*-alkyldihydronicotinamides as reducing cofactors, including dihydronictinamide riboside (NRH, Knox et al. 2000). NRH can be synthesized from NADH by enzymatic cleavage using phosphodiesterases and phosphatases (Friedlos et al. 1992). Inhibitors of NQO1 such as dicumarol, cibacron blue, ES936, and MAC220 do not inhibit NQO2 (Wu et al. 1997; Siegel and Ross unpublished data); however, NQO2 activity can be inhibited by polyphenolic compounds such as quercetin and resveratrol (Buryanovskyy et al. 2004; Wang et al. 2004; Wu et al. 1997). NQO2 has also been shown to interact with antimalarial quinolines such as primaquine, quinacrine, and chloroquine. Interestingly, it has been shown that primaquine binds to the oxidized form of NQO2 while quinacrine and chloroquine bind to the reduced form of NQO2 (Kwiek, Haystead and Rudolph 2004). Another notable feature of NQO2 is that it can bind melatonin, and NQO2 has been characterized as the melatonin MT_3 binding site (Nosjean et al. 2000). NQO2 is expressed in many human tissues most notably in human liver (Strassburg et al. 2002; Jaiswal 1994), testis (Long and Jaiswal 2000) and red blood cells (Graves et al. 2002). NQO2 activity or protein expression has been detected in many human tumor cells including K562 human leukemia cells and human melanoma cell lines (Hsieh et al. 2005; Buryanovskyy et al. 2004). As observed previously in studies with NQO1 knockout mice, studies using NQO2 knockout mice also demonstrated increased bone marrow myeloid hyperplasia in NQO2-deficient mice compared to wild-type mice (Iskander and Jaiswal 2005; Long et al. 2002). Unlike NQO1 knockout mice, NQO2-deficient animals demonstrated significantly less menadione-induced hepatic toxicity suggesting a positive role for NQO2 in menadione-induced toxicities (Long et al. 2002).

7.1.6. Mitochondrial Reductases

Mitochondria contain a number of enzymes capable of quinone metabolism. NADH:ubiquinone oxidoreductase (complex I) is believed to play an important role in quinone toxicity. This enzyme is a large multisubunit complex consisting of 42 different polypeptide chains including a FMN-containing subunit and six iron–sulfur centers. Complex I catalyzes the transfer of a hydride ion from NADH to FMN through a series of iron–sulfur centers and finally to ubiquinone to generate ubiquinol (Lenaz et al. 2006). NADH: ubiquinone oxidoreductase is responsible for the majority of superoxide generated in mitochondria (Grivennikova and Vinogradov 2006) and NADH :ubiquinone oxidoreductase may play a central role in neurodegenerative diseases such as Parkinson's (Keeney et al. 2006). Another source of quinone reduction in mitochondria is complex II (succinate dehydrogenase). This complex contains five polypeptide chains with one bound FAD and two iron–sulfur centers. Complex II functions by passing electrons from succinate to FAD and then through the iron–sulfur centers to ubiquinone to generate ubiquinol

(Cecchini 2003). Succinate dehydrogenase also catalyzes the oxidation of succinate to fumarate in the Kreb's cycle (Cecchini 2003).

7.1.7. Carbonyl Reductases

Carbonyl reductases (EC 1.1.1.1.81, CBR1, CBR2, CBR3) are monomeric cytosolic enzymes, able to catalyze the NADPH-dependent reduction of a variety of xenobiotic ketones and quinones (Wermuth et al. 1988; Wermuth et al. 1982; Ris and von Wartburg 1981; Wermuth 1981). The human enzyme is a monomer of 277 amino acid residues and was named carbonyl reductase (gene name CBR1) owing to its properties to reduce efficiently various endogenous and xenobiotic carbonyl compounds. Human CBR1 is expressed in a wide variety of tissues, with high levels found in liver, placenta, and the central nervous system (CNS), consistent with a possible protective role against toxic carbonyls (Wirth and Wermuth 1992). The xenobiotic substrates known to be metabolized by CBR1 include *ortho*-quinones derived from polycyclic aromatic hydrocarbons or *para*-quinones, such as menadione (Wermuth et al. 1986), as well as a broad spectrum of xenobiotic carbonyls, such as anthracyclines, metyrapone, or the carcinogen 4-methylnitrosamino-1-(3-pyridyl)-1-butanone (Wermuth 1981; Atalla, Breyer-Pfaff and Maser 2000). The enzyme fulfills an important role in the phase I metabolism of xenobiotics; human CBR1A is the major hepatic reductase of quinones, suggesting a major role in detoxification of these compounds (Wermuth et al. 1986). This is in contrast to the metabolic preference in rat liver, where NQO1 is the major quinone reductase. However, in the absence of superoxide dismutase (SOD), quinone reduction by CBR1 leads to redox cycling, with generation of superoxide anion and semiquinone radicals mediated through one-electron transfer from the reduced hydroquinones to molecular oxygen (Jarabak and Harvey 1993). Thus, CBR1 is an important determinant in the metabolism of quinones; however, a possible protective role against quinone toxicity exerted by CBR1 depends on expression and activity of SOD and further metabolism, reactivity, and excretion of the hydroquinone formed.

7.1.8. Other Enzymes

A wide variety of flavin-containing proteins have been shown to participate in quinone metabolism. Examples include glutathione reductase and thioredoxin reductase, both of which are cytosolic, selenium-containing flavoproteins, catalyzing the reduction of disulfide bonds utilizing NADPH as the reducing cofactor (Mustacich and Powis 2000). Nitric oxide synthase is another flavoprotein that can participate in quinone metabolism. Nitric oxide synthase is a heme-containing flavoprotein whose carboxy terminus demonstrates significant sequence homology with CPR (Iyanagi 2005). Recently, all the three isoforms of nitric oxide synthetase (NOS), whose reductase domains have a high sequence homology with P450 reductase, have also been demonstrated as being capable of one-electron reduction of quinones (Kumagai et al. 1998). Lipoamide dehydrogenase is a member of the pyridine nucleotide disulfide oxidoreductase family. Proteins in this family are homodimers with each subunit containing a

FAD cofactor and a redox active disulfide (Arscott et al. 1997). Lipoamide dehydrogenase is a component of the 2-oxo acid dehydrogenase complexes and is responsible for catalyzing the NAD^+-dependent oxidation of dihydrolipoamide in these complexes. Lipoamide dehydrogenase has been shown to operate in reverse and reduce quinones via a ping-pong mechanism utilizing NADH as the electron donor (Vienozinskis et al. 1990).

7.2. Toxicological Implications of Quinone Reduction

7.2.1. One-Electron Reduction of Quinones and Redox Cycling

The reaction of semiquinones with oxygen to produce superoxide depends on the one-electron reduction potential of the semiquinone radical relative to the oxygen/superoxide couple but may also depend on reaction conditions and removal of products by secondary reactions (Wardman 2001; Gutierrez 2000; Halliwell and Gutteridge 1985; Lusthof et al. 1992). The redox potential of the oxygen/superoxide couple has been estimated at –155 mV (Wardman 2001) and –137 mV (Petlicki and van de Ven 1998). A useful tabulation of redox potentials of biologically relevant molecules and their application can be found in Halliwell and Gutteridge (1999). The semiquinone radical can also disproportionate to form a half mole equivalent of both quinone and hydroquinone, so this reaction represents an alternate fate for the semiquinone radical (Butler 1998). However, many semiquinones do react rapidly with molecular oxygen to produce superoxide. This reaction can initiate and sustain the production of ROS and reactive-nitrogen species (RNS), leading to lipid peroxidation, protein adducts, and DNA modifications, followed by a cascade of altered cellular responses and defense mechanisms (Figure 7.2). Consequently, metabolism of quinones by one-electron reductases has been regarded as a toxification step. The other major point of toxicological relevance with respect to this reaction is its cyclical nature. The interaction of semiquinone with oxygen regenerates the quinone substrate, so under aerobic conditions and in the presence of reductases with sufficient concentrations of reduced pydridine nucleotide cofactors, a cycling reaction can ensue generating large quantities of superoxide radical, hydrogen peroxide, and other aggressive oxygen and nitrogen species formed by downstream reactions (Figure 7.2). This process is referred to as redox or futile cycling (Figure 7.2).

7.2.2. Two-Electron Reduction of Quinones

Two-electron-mediated reduction of quinones is often viewed as a detoxification reaction since it removes an electrophilic quinone from a biological system and bypasses one-electron reduction leading to the production of ROS and oxidative stress. The hydroquinone is generally more water soluble and more easily excreted However, as will be described in subsequent sections, whether the generation of a hydroquinone is truly a detoxification step depends on the stability and pharmacological reactions of the hydroquinone generated.

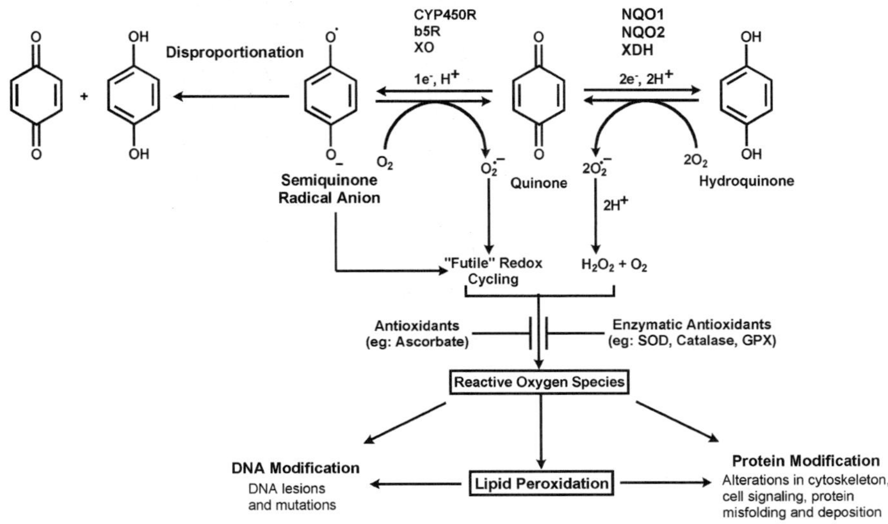

Figure 7.2 Pathways of quinone metabolism and toxicity.

7.2.2.1. Detoxification of Benzene-Derived Quinones

The benzene metabolite hydroquinone can undergo peroxidase-catalyzed oxidation to generate 1,4-benzoquinone, a metabolite that has been shown to directly alkylate DNA and protein (Levay, Ross and Bodell 1993; Thomas et al. 1990; Schlosser and Kalf 1989). Reduction of 1,4-benzoquinone by NQO1, however, regenerates hydroquinone and this reaction prevents the cellular damage induced by 1,4-benzoquinone. The role of the two-electron reductase NQO1 in protection against hydroquinone-induced cytotoxicity in cellular systems is well established. For example, the treatment of KG1A human promyeloblastic cells with hydroquinone resulted in induction of NQO1 and subsequent protection against hydroquinone-induced apoptosis (Moran, Siegel and Ross 1999). Furthermore, the role of NQO1 in protection against benzene toxicity has been studied using NQO1 knockout mice exposed to benzene. In these studies NQO1-deficient mice developed more hematotoxicity when compared to wild-type mice following benzene exposure (Bauer et al. 2003). A role for NQO1 in protection against benzene toxicity in human populations has emerged as well from epidemiological studies that have demonstrated an increased risk for benzene-induced hematotoxicites in individuals lacking NQO1 due to homozygous expression of the NQO1*2 polymorphism (Rothman et al. 1997).

7.2.2.2. Cellular Protection by Generation of Antioxidant Quinones via Two-Electron Reduction

Lipophilic antioxidant quinones such as α-tocopherol quinone and ubiquinone (Figure 7.3) are a special type of quinone that when reduced by two electrons to the corresponding hydroquinone generates stable lipophilic antioxidants that aid in the protection of lipid membranes against peroxidative damage. α-Tocopherolquinone can be generated following oxidation of α-tocopherol (Liebler, Kaysen and Kennedy 1989) and reduction to α-tocopherolhydroquinone has been shown to be carried out by

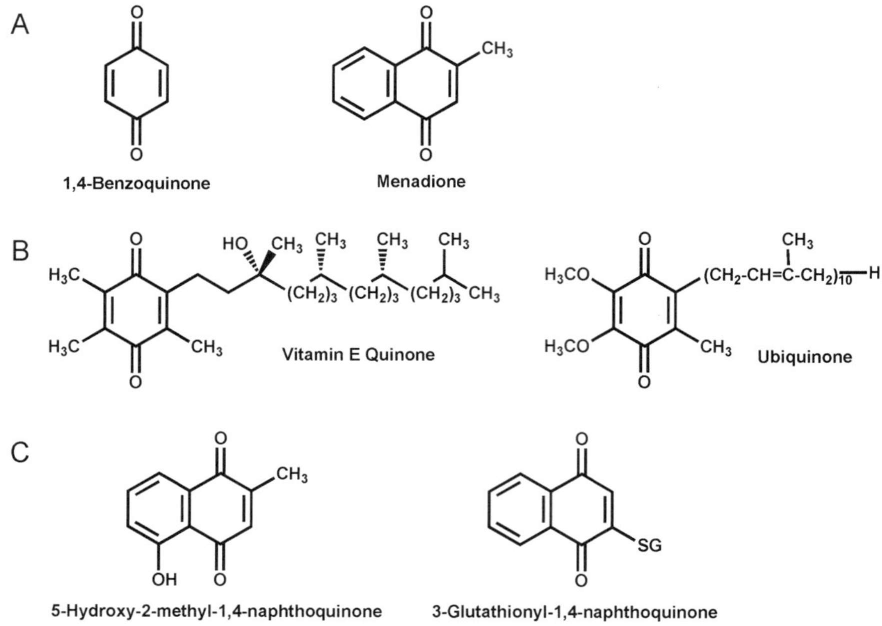

Figure 7.3 The structure of selected quinones that undergo: (**a**) detoxification by two-electron reduction, (**b**) reduction to a more potent hydroquinone antioxidant, and (**c**) activation by two-electron reduction.

NQO1 (Siegel et al. 1997) as well as by complex I of the mitochondrial respiratory chain (Gregor et al. 2006). Microsomal enzymes such as CPR and b5R have also been shown to generate α-tocopherolhydroquinone (Gregor et al. 2006). Besides the role of an electron carrier in the mitochondrial electron transport chain, ubiquinone can also be reduced to a stable hydroquinone and embedded into lipid membranes to protect against lipid peroxidation (Frei, Kim and Ames 1990).

7.2.2.3. Naphthoquinones: Toxification or Detoxification Depending on the Properties of the Hydroquinone

The generation of a hydroquinone metabolite does not always result in quinone detoxification. The two-electron reduction of naphthoquinones by enzymes such as NQO1 can produce hydroquinones that are resistant to autooxidation, but depending on the particular naphthoquinone examined may also produce hydroquinones that rapidly undergo autooxidation generating large quantities of ROS. For napthoquinones like menadione (2-methyl-1,4-naphthoquinone), reduction to a relatively stable hydroquinone metabolite has been shown to be a detoxification pathway by directly competing with one-electron reductases such as CPR. The one-electron reduction of menadione by these flavoproteins generates a semiquinone radical that rapidly reacts with oxygen generating substantial quantities of ROS (Mishin, Pokrovsky and Lyakhovich 1976). In experiments using isolated rat hepatocytes significantly more menadione-induced oxidative damage was observed in cells pretreated with the NQO1 inhibitor dicumarol compared to cells that did not receive the inhibitor (Thor et al.1982). Interestingly, studies in Chinese hamster ovary cell lines engineered to overexpress a range of NQO1 activities showed that there was a threshold level of NQO1 activity above which offered no greater level of protection against menadione toxicity (De Haan et al. 2002). A role for the two-electron reduction of menadione as a detoxification pathway was further confirmed in studies using NQO1 knockout mice where the absence of NQO1 led to a dramatic decreased in survival following multiple doses of menadione (Radjendirane et al. 1998). Since naphthoquinones have both alkylating and redox activities they have been evaluated as potential antitumor drugs. The anticancer activities of a series of 1,4-naphthoquinones was tested against a series of four human cancer cells lines and in terms of quantitative structure–activity relationships (QSARs) cytotoxicity largely depended upon the hydrophobicity of the naphthoquinone (Verma 2006)

A study using a variety of substituted 1,4-naphthoquinones demonstrated that the rate of autooxidation of hydroquinones formed following reduction by purified NQO1 was influenced to a large degree by the presence of hydroxy and glutathionyl substituents (Buffinton et al. 1989). For example, the rate of menadione autooxidation could be increased significantly by the addition of hydroxy and glutathionyl substituents (Buffinton et al. 1989). Therefore, as a rule the two-electron reduction of naphthoquinones does not always results in detoxification since minor chemical modifications to the naphthoquinone molecule can result in dramatic changes in redox behavior. Other factors that will influence the redox behavior of naphthoquinones include quinone concentration, pH, and the level of superoxide (Munday 2000; Ollinger et al. 1990). Studies by Munday et al. have shown that following reduction by NQO1 the rate of autooxidation for alkyl, alkoxy, hydroxyl, and amino derivatives was decreased in the presence of SOD, while in similar experiments, SOD had no effect on the rate of autooxidation of halogenated compounds (Munday 2000). Since NQO1 has been shown to have superoxide-reducing activity increasing NQO1 levels could also inhibit autooxidation in a manner similar to SOD (Siegel et al. 2004), and in cell-free experiments increasing the concentration of NQO1 was shown to inhibit menadiol autooxidation (Munday 2004). A pivotal role for the two-electron reduction of naphthoquinones by NQO1 in vivo can be seen from studies in rats pretreated with inducers that increase the levels of NQO1 in tissues. As expected, the induction of NQO1 in tissues by BHA decreased the toxicity of menadione but conversely, increasing the tissue levels of NQO1 increased the hemolytic anemia induced by 2-hydroxy-1,4-naphthoquinone (Munday, Smith and Munday 1999b; Munday, Smith and Munday 1998). Thus, prediction of whether NQO1 contributes to activation or deactivation of naphthoquinones requires a detailed knowledge of hydroquinone properties, the cellular context in which it is generated, and other enzyme activities, such as SOD.

7.3. Bioreductive Activation of Antitumor Quinones

The generation of cytotoxic hydroquinones within cancer cells is know as bioreductive activation and has become the basis for the development of a wide variety of both natural and synthetic quinones as chemotherapeutic agents. This type of therapy exploits the high levels of quinone reductases,

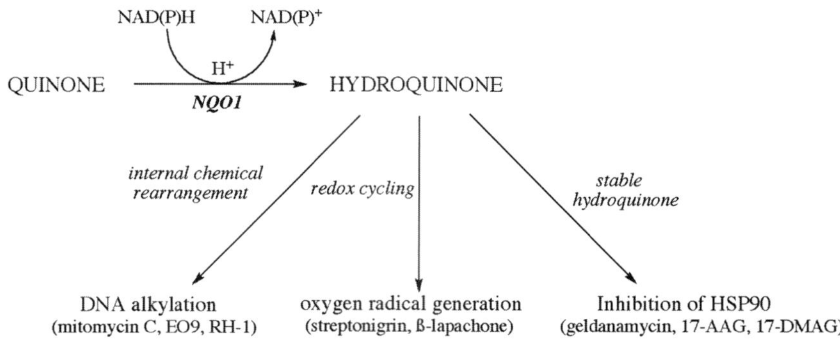

Figure 7.4 The role of two-electron reduction in the bioreductive activation of antitumor quinones.

particularly NQO1, in most solid tumors as a means of targeting drug activation to cancer cells (Ross et al. 1996; Ross et al. 1994; Ross et al. 1993). Following two-electron reduction in cancer cells by enzymes, such as NQO1, antitumor quinones can inflict cellular damage in at least three separate ways (Figure 7.4). Reduction to a hydroquinone can promote intramolecular chemical rearrangements leading to the generation of monofunctional and bifunctional DNA alkylating agents. Secondly, the generation of large quantities of ROS by the intracellular redox cycling of antitumor quinones is another mechanism whereby quinones can exert anticancer activity (Figure 7.4). Finally, the generation of a hydroquinone can have a more pronounced effect against a particular intracellular target and exert an improved therapeutic effect.

7.3.1. Mitomycins

Mitomycin C is inactive until reduced by enzymes such as NQO1 (Siegel et al. 1992), NQO2 (Jamieson et al. 2006; Celli et al. 2006), or XDH (Gustafson and Pritsos 1992). Under hypoxic conditions, XO, CPR, and b5R can also bioactivate mitomycin C (Hodnick and Sartorelli 1993; Pan et al. 1984, see above). A relationship between the reduction potential of a series of mitomycins and cytotoxicity has been observed (Pan and Gonzalez 1990). The bioactivation of mitomycin C by NQO1 has been shown to be pH-dependent where substantially more metabolism and DNA crosslinking were observed as the reaction pH was decreased (Siegel et al. 1992). At higher pH values, mitomycin C was shown to inactivate NQO1 by directly alkylating amino acid residues on the protein (Siegel et al. 1993). Despite mechanism-based inhibition of NQO1 by mitomycin C at high pH values, studies have shown that NQO1 does play an essential role in the bioactivation of mitomycin C in vivo (Fleming et al. 2002; Gan et al. 2001). The *N*-methyl aziridine analogue of MMC, porfiromycin, is a potent antitumor agent that also undergoes pH-dependent metabolism as the result of mechanism-based inhibition of NQO1 in a manner similar to mitomycin C (Siegel et al. 1993). This is in contrast to mitomycin A and B which did not demonstrate mechanism-based inhibition of NQO1 and underwent bioreductive activation by NQO1 under both acidic and basic conditions (Ross et al. 1993).

7.3.2. Diazirdinyl 1,4-benzoquinones

The diaziridinyl 1,4-benzoquinones are another class of bioreductive DNA alkylating quinones that, following metabolism by two-electron reductases, generate the hydroquinone species facilitating aziridinyl ring opening leading to monofunctional and bifunctional DNA alkylation (King, Wong and Loo 1984). AZQ (2,5-diaziridinyl-3,6-*bis*-(carboethoxyamino)-1,4-benzoquinone) was the first of these compounds to enter clinical trials and was designed primarily to cross the blood–brain barrier for the treatment of pediatric brain tumors (Curt et al. 1983). AZQ was shown to be bioactivated rather poorly by NQO1 (Gibson et al. 1992; Siegel et al. 1990) and this led to the design and synthesis of a series of diaziridinyl 1,4-benzoquinones that were more efficiently bioactivated by NQO1 and from these compounds RH-1 (2,5-diaziridinyl-3-hydroxymethyl-6-methyl-1, 4-benzoquinone) has emerged as the lead compound and is currently in clinical trials (Danson et al. 2007; Winski et al. 1998). RH-1 has been shown to undergo very efficient reduction by NQO1 and to induce more DNA crosslinking and cytotoxicity in NQO1-rich cancer cells compared to NQO1-deficient cells (Dehn, Inayat-Hussain and Ross 2005; Dehn, Winski and Ross 2004). It has also been shown using human isogenic cancer cell lines that differ only in the level of NQO1 protein and activity that sensitivity to RH-1 correlated with the level of NQO1 activity. However, there was a threshold level of NQO1 activity and increasing NQO1 activity above this value did not lead to an increase in cytotoxicity (Winski et al. 2001). Studies have also shown that RH-1 can also be reduced by CPR to semiquinone and hydroquinone species leading to both DNA strand breaks and DNA-crosslinking (Nemeikaite-Ceniene et al. 2003). However, studies in human cancer cell lines engineered to overexpress CRP did not demonstrate any significant increase in cytotoxicity following treatment with RH-1 suggesting a limited role for this enzyme in RH-1 bioactivation (Begleiter et al. 2007).

7.3.3. Indolequinones

EO9 is an indolequinone antitumor drug that was developed to undergo bioreductive activation similar to mitomycin C but despite robust antitumor activity against human cancer cell lines with high levels of NQO1 activity EO9 failed to demonstrate a significant antitumor response in clinical trials (Pavlidis et al. 1996; Dirix et al. 1996). The three active centers, the vinylic group at C-2, the hydroxymethyl group at C-3, and the aziridinyl group at C-5 are possibly activated upon reduction of the quinone group of EO9. DNA interstrand crosslinking was observed by indoloquinone following reductive activation with XO (Maliepaard et al. 1995).

A structure/activity study of a series of indolequinones concluded that slight modifications of the indolequinone structure resulted in substantial variations in activation and cytotoxicity after reduction by NQO1 (Swann et al. 2001; Beall et al. 1998). These studies also demonstrated that NQO1 can bioactivate these compounds more efficiently under aerobic conditions while under hypoxia, the one-electron reduction of these indolequinones is an important pathway in bioactivation (Jafar et al. 2003; Naylor et al. 1998).

Indolequinones have also been used to target NQO1 and induce cytotoxicity in human pancreatic cancer cells. A series of indolequinones based on the structure of ES936 (5-methoxy-1,2-dimethyl-3-[(4-phenoxy)methyl]-indole-4,7-dione) demonstrated potent mechanism-based inhibition of NQO1 without affecting the activities of other reductases such as NQO2, CPR, or b5R (Dehn et al. 2003; Siegel et al. unpublished data). Since high levels of cellular NQO1 can scavenge superoxide (Siegel et al. 2004), indolequinones were developed to selectively inhibit NQO1 and increase levels of superoxide leading to increased cell death of pancreatic tumor cells (Reigan et al. 2007; Cullen et al. 2003). However, in studies using a series of indolequinones, despite greater than 95% inactivation of NQO1 in pancreatic cancer cells, there was no correlation between NQO1 inhibition and ability to induce cytotoxicity suggesting that indolequinones may have molecular targets in addition to NQO1 (Reigan et al. 2007).

7.3.4. Streptonigrin

The generation of ROS, and in particular the hydroxyl radical, in close association with DNA can produce large quantities of DNA strand breaks resulting in the loss of genomic integrity and cell death. Streptonigrin is an example of a redox-cycling quinone antitumor antibiotic isolated from cultures of *Streptomyces flocculus* (Marsh, Garretson and Wesel 1961). Streptonigrin has multiple metal binding sites and can interact with a variety of metals to produce streptonigrin-metal-DNA complexes (White 1977). The reduction of the quinone moiety in streptonigrin by either one or two electrons generates the semiquinone radical or hydroquinone, respectively. In the presence of oxygen both forms will rapidly autooxidize to produce ROS and the parent quinone (Beall et al. 1994; Bachur et al. 1979). During autooxidation the presence of metal ions bound to streptonigrin catalyze the generation of hydroxyl radicals via Fenton-type reactions in close proximity to DNA resulting in large quantities of DNA single- and double-strand breaks (Sugiura, Kuwahara and Suzuki 1984). Streptonigrin was shown to be reduced very efficiently by NQO1 to the corresponding hydroquinone in cell-free systems (Beall et al. 1994), and in studies with human isogenic cancer cell lines streptonigrin was more cytotoxic to NQO1-expressing cells compared to NQO1-null cells (Beall et al. 1996).

7.3.5. ß-Lapachone

β-lapachone (3,4-dihydro-2,2-dimethyl-2*H*-naphtho[1,2-*b*]-pyran-5,6-dione) is another example of a redox-cycling quinone antitumor drug. β-lapachone was isolated from the bark of the lapacho tree (*Tabebuia avellanedae*) and has been reported to possess a wide range of pharmacological properties, including antiviral, antiparasitic, and antitumor activities (Planchon et al. 1995; Schuerch and Wehrli 1978; Boveris et al. 1978). β-lapachone can inhibit topoisomerase I and prevent DNA repair induced by methylating agents and radiation (Boothman and Pardee 1989; Boorstein and Pardee 1984). However, the treatment of cells with β-lapachone also results in the generation of large quantities of hydrogen peroxide due to the redox cycling of the quinone. An interesting finding was that in a variety of human cancer cell lines the sensitivity to β-lapachone correlated with intracellular hydrogen peroxide generation; cell lines that generated high levels of hydrogen peroxide were sensitive to β-lapachone while cell lines with low levels of hydrogen peroxide were resistant (Chau et al. 1998). These data suggest that the ability to undergo bioreductive activation to either semiquinone or hydroquinone species and subsequent redox cycling are required for β-lapachone to exert maximal cytotoxicity. In studies using cell sonicates, the addition of β-lapachone resulted in the oxidation of greater than stoichiometric equivalents of reduced pyridine nucleotide cofactors and the rate of cofactor oxidation was dependent upon the activity of NQO1 (Pink et al. 2000). Subsequent studies in cell lines and human xenograft tumors grown in mice have shown that NQO1 is the principle determinant of β-lapachone cytotoxicity (Ough et al. 2005; Pink et al. 2000).

7.3.6. Benzoquinone Hsp90 Inhibitors

A third mechanism whereby the two-electron reduction of quinones to hydroquinones can induce cytotoxicity is through the generation of a stable hydroquinone with unique pharmacological properties (Figure 7.4). An example of this type of bioreductive activation can be seen with the benzoquinone ansamycin class of HSP90 inhibitors which includes geldanamycin, 17-AAG, 17-DMAG, and 17AG. These compounds are characterized by a quinone moiety attached to a large planer macrocyclic ansa bridge structure (Figure 7.5). The benzoquinone ansamycins represent a class of compounds that disrupt multiple pathways involved in tumor cell proliferation (Goetz et al. 2003). It has been shown that these compounds bind to an N-terminal ATP-binding site in heat shock protein 90 (HSP90) preventing ATP binding and hydrolysis (Grenert et al. 1997). The inability of HSP90 to utilize ATP prevents the protein from assisting in the folding and maturation of critical oncogenic and regulatory proteins (Powers and Workman 2006; Goetz et al. 2003). Geldanamycin, the prototype for this class of compounds, is a natural product isolated from cultures of *Streptomyces hygrosopicus* (BeBoer and Dietz 1976). In clinical trials geldanamycin induced unacceptable levels of hepatotoxicity; therefore, a second generation of benzoquinone ansamycin compounds were developed that include 17-AAG and 17-AG. These compounds were selected because they induced less toxicity in animal studies but still retained the ability to inhibit HSP90 (Behrsing et al. 2005; Schulte and Neckers 1998). In studies using a variety of human cancer cell lines treated with 17-AAG there was a positive correlation between 17-AAG sensitivity and NQO1 activity suggesting a role for quinone reduction by NQO1 in the mechanism of action of the benzoquinone ansamycins (Kelland et al. 1999). Subsequent studies using purified recombinant NQO1 demonstrated that the benzoquinone ansamycins could be reduced by NQO1 to their corresponding hydroquinone species (Guo et al. 2005, 2006) and in studies using purified yeast and human HSP90 the hydroquinone species induced substantially greater inhibition of HSP90 when compared to the quinone form (Guo et al. 2005, 2006). Molecular modeling studies also confirmed that when reduced to their corresponding hydroquinones the benzoquinone

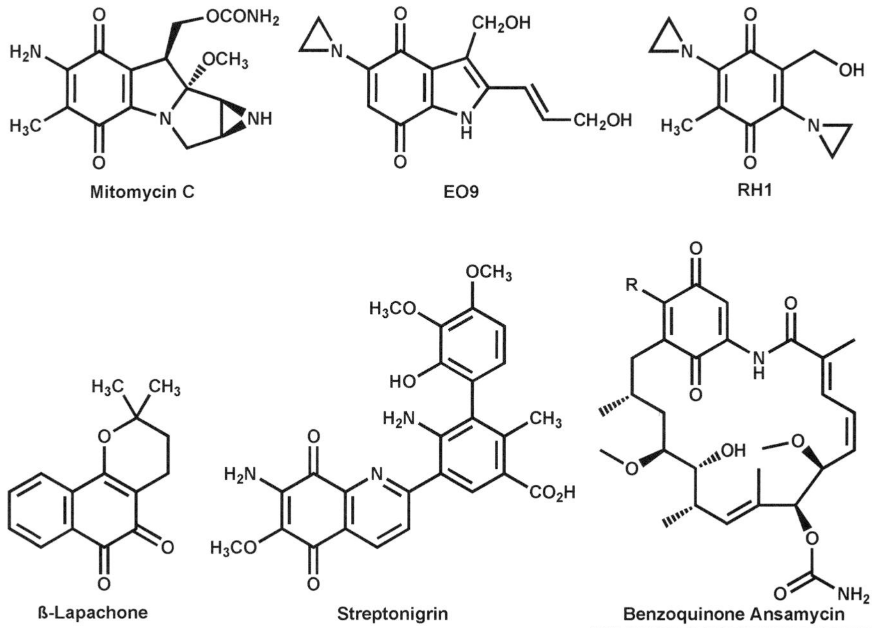

Compound	R (17-Substitutent)
GM	OCH_3
17AAG	$NHCH_2CHCH_2$
17AG	NH_2
17DMAG	$NHCH_2CH_2N(CH_3)_2$

Figure 7.5 The structures of antitumor quinones that undergo bioreductive activation.

ansamycins exhibited a stronger binding interaction with the ATP-binding site in HSP90 (Guo et al. 2005, 2006). In studies using isogenic human cancer cell lines that differ only in the expression of NQO1, the reduction of 17-AAG to the corresponding hydroquinone was seen exclusively in cells expressing NQO1 and formation of the hydroquinone could be inhibited by pretreating the cells with an NQO1 inhibitor (Guo et al. 2005). In addition, these experiments also showed that cells expressing NQO1 were more sensitive to 17-AAG and sensitivity correlated with the marked degradation of HSP90 client proteins (Guo et al. 2005). Recently, the more active and water-soluble hydroquinone of 17-AAG has been formulated into a stable product and is currently in clinical trials (Sydor et al. 2006). While the reduction of benzoquinone ansamycins by NQO1 to their corresponding hydroquinones generates more potent HSP90 inhibitors, one-electron reduction will form an unstable semiquinone radical that in the presence of oxygen may redox cycle back to the quinone-generating ROS. Studies have shown that geldanamycin can undergo CPR-mediated reduction to the semiquinone radical that reacts spontaneously with oxygen to regenerate the quinone and in the process generates superoxide (Dikalov, Landmesser and Harrison 2002; Benchekroun, Myers and Sinha 1994). The ability of geldanamycin to undergo one-electron reduction by enzymes such as CPR in the liver may play a role in the hepatotoxicity observed in patients treated with geldanamycin in clinical trials.

7.3.7. The Case of Hypoxia-Activated Quinone Prodrugs: Therapeutic Exploitation of One-Electron Reduction of Quinines

Despite the association of one-electron cycling of semiquinones with oxidative stress and toxicity, one-electron reduction of quinones with subsequent generation of ROS may be a more desirable outcome from a toxicological perspective than accumulation of potentially toxic semiquinone radicals (Sartorelli 1988). As explained by Wardman, for drug efficacy as a hypoxic cytotoxin, the damaging effect of the reactive product under hypoxia must be greater than the toxicity resulting from oxygen-cycling reactions under aerobic conditions (Wardman 2001). This reaction has been exploited for therapeutic purposes and has been employed in the design of antitumor quinones to kill hypoxic cell fractions in tumors. Quinone analogues were among the first compounds explored as hypoxia-selective tumour-activated prodrugs. After one-electron reduction of a quinone species to the semiquinone radical anion (Belcourt et al. 1996), dependent on the redox potential of the semiquinone, it can be back-oxidized by molecular oxygen in normal well-perfused cells. Under hypoxic conditions, however, the semiquinone radical is not back-oxidized, accumulates, and can lead to cellular damage potentially resulting in hypoxia-selective cytotoxicity (Everett et al. 1998; Sartorelli 1988). For example, the *N*-methyl aziridine analogue of MMC, porfiromycin, is a potent antitumor agent, which shows greater hypoxic selectivity (Belcourt et al. 1996). The reduction of porfiromycin to the semiquinone radical anion can be reversed by molecular oxygen, but under hypoxia this undergoes complex fragmentation to a reactive species that binds to DNA (Figure 7.6) via guanine–guanine crosslinks in the major groove (Pan and Iracki 1988).

Mitomycin C and porfiromycin are naturally occurring prototypes of bioreductive anticancer prodrugs. Since their discovery, various reductively activated prodrugs have been developed based on the mechanism of action revealed by these hypoxically activated cytotoxins. In addition, many hypoxia-targeting hybrid drugs have been designed that incorporate quinones and nitroaromatics (triggers) connected to cytotoxic units (effectors) through linker units. Upon activation, such hybrid drugs are designed to release strong alkylating agents, for example, cyclophosphoramide (Denny 2005).

7.4. Summary

In summary, a wide range of one- and two-electron reductases are capable of metabolizing quinones. Both semiquinones and hydroquinones formed by one- and two-electron reductions, respectively, may be unstable to oxygen and undergo redox-cycling reactions in the presence of adequate oxygen and enzymatic cofactor. Metabolism of quinones to hydroquinone derivatives may result in either toxification or detoxification depending on the properties of the hydroquinone generated, and good examples of both reactions have been documented. Both the one- and two-electron-mediated reduction of quinones have been utilized to target cancers. One-electron reduction has been employed in the targeting of hypoxic fractions in tumors

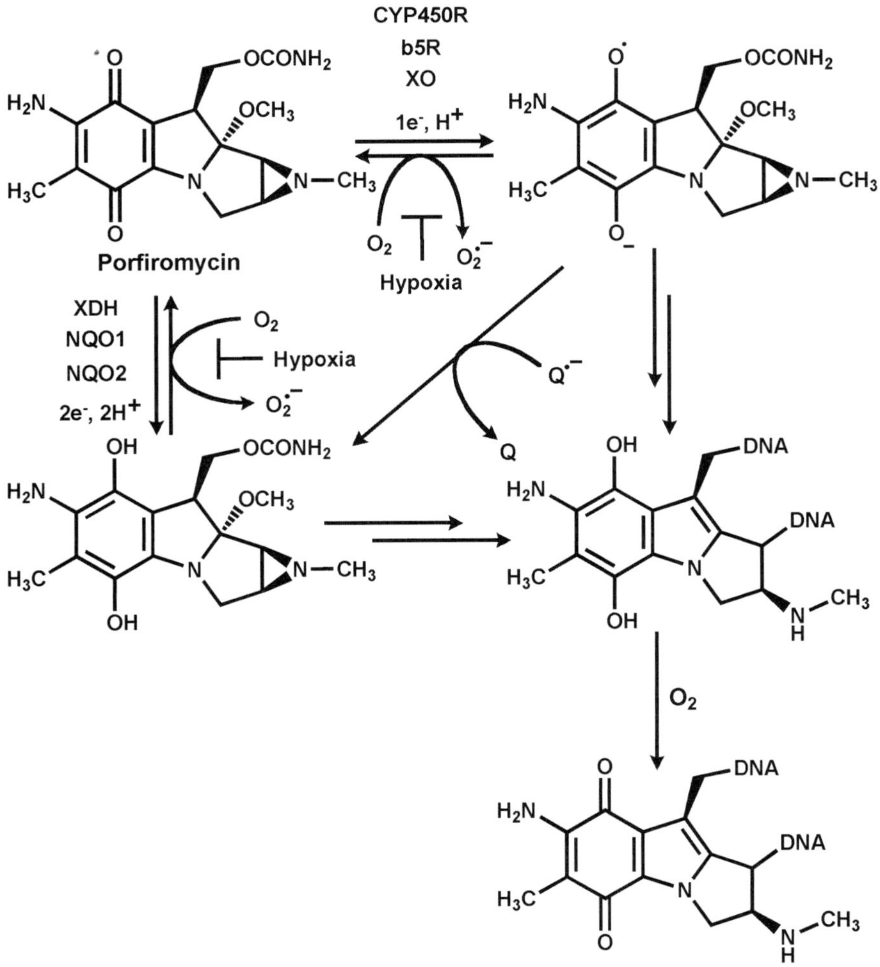

Figure 7.6 Porfiromycin bioactivation and DNA modifications.

while the presence of elevated levels of two-electron reductases such as NQO1 in tumors has led to the design of anticancer quinones that can be activated specifically in neoplasic cells.

Acknowledgements. The authors are supported by H.H.S. grants CA51210, CA114441, E09554, and NS44613.

References

Amaya, Y., Yamazaki, K., Sato, M., Noda, K., Nishino, T., and Nishino, T. 1990. Proteolytic conversion of xanthine dehydrogenase from the NAD-dependent type to the O2-dependent type. Amino acid sequence of rat liver xanthine dehydrogenase and identification of the cleavage sites of the enzyme protein during irreversible conversion by trypsin. J. Biol. Chem. 265:14170–14175.

Arscott, L. D., Gromer, S., Schirmer, R. H., Becker, K and Williams, C. H. Jr. 1997. The mechanism of thioredoxin reductase from human placenta is similar to the mechanisms of lipoamide dehydrogenase and glutathione reductase and is

distinct from the mechanism of thioredoxin reductase from Escherichia coli. Proc. Natl. Acad. Sci. U. S. A. 94:3621–3626.
Atalla, A., Breyer-Pfaff, U., and Maser, E. 2000. Purification and characterization of oxidoreductases catalyzing carbonyl reduction of the tobacco-specific nitrosamine 4-methylnitrosamino-1-(3-pyridyl)-1-butanone (NNK) in human liver cytosol. Xenobiotica 30:755–769.
Bachur, N. R., Gordon, S. L., Gee, M. V., and Kon, H. 1979. NADPH cytochrome P-450 reductase activation of quinone anticancer agents to free radicals. Proc. Natl. Acad. Sci. U.S.A. 76:954–957.
Backes, W. L., and Reker-Backes, C. E. 1988. The effect of NADPH concentration on the reduction of cytochrome P-450 LM2. J. Biol. Chem. 263:247–253.
Battelli, M. G., Lorenzoni, E., and Stripe, F. 1973. Milk xanthine oxidase type D (dehydrogenase) and type O (oxidase). Purification, interconversion and some properties. Biochem. J. 131:191–198.
Bauer, A. K., Faiola, B., Abernethy, D. J., Marchan, R., Pluta, L. J., Wong, V. A., Roberts, K., Jaiswal, A. K., Gonzalez, F. J., Butterworth, B. E, Borghoff, S., Parkinson, H., Everitt, J., and Recio, L. 2003. Genetic susceptibility to benzene-induced toxicity: role of NADPH: quinone oxidoreductase-1. Cancer Res. 63:929–935.
Beall, H. D., Liu, Y., Siegel, D., Bolton, E. M., Gibson, N. W., and Ross, D. 1996. Role of NAD(P)H:quinone oxidoreductase (DT-diaphorase) in cytotoxicity and induction of DNA damage by streptonigrin. Biochem. Pharmacol. 51:645–652.
Beall, H. D., Winski, S., Swann, E., Hudnott, A. R., Cotterill, A. S., O'Sullivan, N., Green, S. J., Bien, R., Siegel, D., Ross, D., and Moody, C. J. 1998. Indolequinone antitumor agents: correlation between quinone structure, rate of metabolism by recombinant human NAD(P)H:quinone oxidoreductase, and in vitro cytotoxicity. J. Med. Chem. 41:4755–4766.
Beall, H. D., Mulcahy, R. T., Siegel, D., Traver, R. D., Gibson, N. W., and Ross, D. 1994. Metabolism of bioreductive antitumor compounds by purified rat and human DT-diaphorases. Cancer Res. 54:3196–3201.
BeBoer, C., and Dietz, A. 1976. The description and antibiotic production of *Streptomyces hygroscopicus* var. Geldanus. J. Antibiot. (Tokyo) 29:1182–1188.
Begleiter A., Leith, M. K., Patel, D., and Hasinoff, B. B. 2007. Role of NADPH cytochrome P450 reductase in activation of RH1. Cancer Chemother. Pharmacol. 60:713–723.
Behrsing, H. P., Amin, K., Ip, C., Jimenez, L., and Tyson, C. A. 2005. In vitro detection of differential and cell-specific hepatobiliary toxicity induced by geldanamycin and 17-allylaminogeldanamycin in rats. Toxicol. In Vitro 19:1079–1088.
Belcourt, M. F., Hodnick, W. F., Rockwell, S., and Sartorelli, A. C. 1996. Differential toxicity of mitomycin C and porfiromycin to aerobic and hypoxic Chinese hamster ovary cells overexpressing human NADPH:cytochrome c (P-450) reductase. Proc. Natl. Acad. Sci. U.S.A. 93:456–460.
Benchekroun, N. M., Myers, C. E., and Sinha, B. K. 1994. Free radical formation by ansamycin benzoquinone in human breast tumor cells: implications for cytotoxicity and resistance. Free Rad. Biol. Med. 17:191–200.
Boorstein, R. J., and Pardee, A. B. 1984. Beta-lapachone greatly enhances MMS lethality to human fibroblasts. Biochem. Biophys. Res. Commun. 118:828–834.
Boothman, D. A., and Pardee, A. B. 1989. Inhibition of radiation-induced neoplastic transformation by beta-lapachone. Proc. Natl. Acad. Sci. U.S.A. 86:4963–4967.
Boveris, A., Docampo, R., Turrens, J. F., and Stoppani, A. O. 1978. Effect of beta-lapachone on superoxide anion and hydrogen peroxide production in *Trypanosoma cruzi*. Biochem. J. 175:431–439.
Brown, J. M., Terada, L. S., Grosso, M. A., Whitmann, G. J., Velasco, S. E., Patt, A., Harken, A. H., and Repine, J. E. 1988. Xanthine oxidase produces

hydrogen peroxide which contributes to reperfusion injury of ischemic, isolated, perfused rat hearts. J. Clin. Invest. 81:1297–1301.
Brunmark, A., Cadenas, E., Segura-Aguilar, J., Lind, C., and Ernster, L. 1988. DT-diaphorase-catalyzed two-electron reduction of various *p*-benzoquinone- and 1,4-naphthoquinone epoxides. Free Rad. Biol. Med. 5:133–143.
Buffinton, G. D., Ollinger, K., Brunmark, A., and Cadenas, E. 1989. DT-diaphorase-catalysed reduction of 1,4-naphthoquinone derivatives and glutathionyl-quinone conjugates. Effect of substituents on autoxidation rates. Biochem. J. 257:561–571.
Buryanovskyy, L., Fu, Y., Boyd, M., Ma, Y., Hsieh, T. C., Wu, J. M., and Zhang, Z. 2004. Crystal structure of quinone reductase 2 in complex with resveratrol. Biochemistry 43:11417–11426.
Butler, J. 1998. Redox cycling antitumor drugs. In DNA and Free Radicals. Techniques, Mechanisms and Applications, eds. B. Halliwell, and O. I. Aruoma, pp. 131–154. London: OICA International.
Butler, J., and Hoey, B. M. 1993. The one-electron reduction potential of several substrates can be related to their reduction rates by cytochrome P-450 reductase. Biochim. Biophys. Acta 1161:73–78.
Cecchini, G. 2003. Function and structure of complex II of the respiratory chain. Annu. Rev. Biochem. 72:77–109.
Celli, C. M., Tran, N., Knox, R., and Jaiswal, A. K. 2006. NRH:quinone oxidoreductase 2 (NQO2) catalyzes metabolic activation of quinines and anti-tumor drugs. Biochem. Pharmacol. 72:366–376.
Cenas, N., Nemeikaite-Ceniene, A., Sergediene, E., Nivinskas, H., Anusevicius, Z., and Sarlauskas, J. 2001. Quantitative structure–activity relationships in enzymatic single-electron reduction of nitroaromatic explosives: implications for their cytotoxicity. Biochim Biophys Acta 1528:31–38.
Chau, Y. P., Shiah, S. G., Don, M. J., and Kuo, M. L. 1998. Involvement of hydrogen peroxide in topoisomerase inhibitor beta-lapachone-induced apoptosis and differentiation in human leukemia cells. Free Rad. Biol. Med. 24:660–670.
Chen, S., Hwang, J., and Deng, P. S. 1993. Inhibition of NAD(P)H:quinone acceptor oxidoreductase by flavones: a structure–activity study. Arch. Biochem. Biophys. 302:72–77.
Cresteil, T., and Jaiswal, A. K. 1991. High levels of expression of the NAD(P)H:-quinone oxidoreductase (NQO1) gene in tumor cells compared to normal cells of the same origin. Biochem. Pharmacol. 42:1021–1027.
Cullen, J. J., Hinkhouse, M. M., Grady, M., Gaut, A. W., Liu, J., Zhang, Y. P., Weydert, C. J., Domann, F. E., and Oberley, L. W. 2003. Dicumarol inhibition of NADPH:quinone oxidoreductase induces growth inhibition of pancreatic cancer via a superoxide-mediated mechanism. Cancer Res. 63:5513–5520.
Curt, G. A., Kelley, J. A., Kufta, C. V., Smith, B. H., Kornblith, P. L., Young, R. C., and Collins, J. M. 1983. Phase II and pharmacokinetic study of aziridinylbenzoquinone [2,5-diaziridinyl-3,6-bis(carboethoxyamino)-1,4-benzoquinone, diaziquone, NSC182986] in high-grade gliomas. Cancer Res. 43:6102–6105.
Danson, S., Ranson, M., Denneny, O., Cummings, J., and Ward, T. H. 2007. Validation of the comet-X assay as a pharmacodynamic assay for measuring DNA cross-linking produced by the novel anticancer agent RH1 during a phase I clinical trial. Cancer Chemother. Pharmacol. 60:851–861.
De Haan, L. H., Boerboom, A. M., Rietjens, I. M., van Capelle, D., De Ruijter, A. J., Jaiswal, A. K., and Aarts, J. M. 2002. A physiological threshold for protection against menadione toxicity by human NAD(P)H:quinone oxidoreductase (NQO1) in Chinese hamster ovary (CHO) cells. Biochem. Pharmacol. 64:1597–1603.
De Long, M. J., Prochaska, H. J., and Talalay, P. 1986. Induction of NAD(P)H:-quinone reductase in murine hepatoma cells by phenolic antioxidants, azo dyes,

and other chemoprotectors: a model system for the study of anticarcinogens. Proc. Natl. Acad. Sci. U.S.A. 83:787–791.

Dehn, D. L., Inayat-Hussain, S. H., and Ross, D. 2005. RH1 induces cellular damage in an NAD(P)H:quinone oxidoreductase 1-dependent manner: relationship between DNA cross-linking, cell cycle perturbations, and apoptosis. J. Pharmacol. Exp. Ther. 313:771–779.

Dehn, D. L., Siegel, D., Swann, E., Moody, C. J., and Ross, D. 2003. Biochemical, cytotoxic, and genotoxic effects of ES936, a mechanism-based inhibitor of NAD(P)H:quinone oxidoreductase 1, in cellular systems. Mol. Pharmacol. 64:714–720.

Dehn, D. L., Winski, S. L., and Ross, D. 2004. Development of a new isogenic cell-xenograft system for evaluation of NAD(P)H:quinone oxidoreductase-directed antitumor quinones: evaluation of the activity of RH1. Clin. Cancer Res. 10:3147–3155.

Della Corte, E., Gozzetti, G., Novello, F., and Stirpe, F. 1969. Properties of the xanthine oxidase from human liver. Biochim. Biophys. Acta 191:164–166.

Denny, W. A. 2005. Hypoxia-activated anticancer drugs. Expert Opin. Ther. Pat. 15:635–646.

Dikalov, S., Landmesser, U., and Harrison, D. G. 2002. Geldanamycin leads to superoxide formation by enzymatic and non-enzymatic redox cycling. Implications for studies of Hsp90 and endothelial cell nitric-oxide synthase. J. Biol. Chem. 277:25480–25485.

Dirix, L. Y., Tonnesen, F., Cassidy, J., Epelbaum, R., ten Bokkel Huinink, W. W., Pavlidis, N., Sorio, R., Gamucci, T., Wolff, I., Te Velde, A., Lan, J., and Verweij, J. 1996. EO9 phase II study in advanced breast, gastric, pancreatic and colorectal carcinoma by the EORTC Early Clinical Studies Group. Eur. J. Cancer 32:2019–2022.

Everett, S. A., Naylor, M. A., Nolan, J., Patel, K. B., and Wardman, P. 1998. Indolequinone bioreductive drugs: kinetic factors which influence selectivity for hypoxia. Anticancer Drug Des. 13:635–653.

Fleming, R. A., Drees, J., Loggie, B. W., Russell, G. B., Geisinger, K. R., Morris, R. T., Sachs, D., and McQuellon, R. P. 2002. Clinical significance of a NAD(P)H: quinone oxidoreductase 1 polymorphism in patients with disseminated peritoneal cancer receiving intraperitoneal hyperthermic chemotherapy with mitomycin C. Pharmacogenetics 12:31–37.

Frei, B., Kim, M. C., and Ames, B. N. 1990. Ubiquinol-10 is an effective lipid-soluble antioxidant at physiological concentrations. Proc. Natl. Acad. Sci. U.S. A. 87:4879–4883.

Friedlos, F., Jarman, M., Davies, L. C., Boland, M. P., and Knox, R. J. 1992. Identification of novel reduced pyridinium derivatives as synthetic co-factors for the enzyme DT diaphorase (NAD(P)H dehydrogenase (quinone), EC 1.6.99.2). Biochem. Pharmacol. 44:25–31.

Gan, Y., Mo, Y., Kalns, J. E., Lu, J., Danenberg, K., Danenberg, P., Wientjes, M. G., and Au, J. L. 2001. Expression of DT-diaphorase and cytochrome P450 reductase correlates with mitomycin C activity in human bladder tumors. Clin. Cancer Res. 7:1313–1319.

Gibson, N. W., Hartley, J. A., Butler, J., Siegel, D., and Ross, D. 1992. Relationship between DT-diaphorase-mediated metabolism of a series of aziridinylbenzoquinones and DNA damage and cytotoxicity. Mol. Pharmacol. 42:531–536.

Goetz, M. P., Toft, D. O., Ames, M. M., and Erlichman, C. 2003. The Hsp90 chaperone complex as a novel target for cancer therapy. Ann. Oncol. 14:1169–1176.

Graves, P. R., Kwiek, J. J., Fadden, P., Ray, R., Hardeman, K., Coley, A. M., Foley, M., and Haystead, T. A. 2002. Discovery of novel targets of quinoline drugs in the human purine binding proteome. Mol. Pharmacol. 62:1364–1372.

Gregor, W., Staniek, K., Nohl, H., and Gille, L. 2006. Distribution of tocopheryl quinone in mitochondrial membranes and interference with ubiquinone-mediated electron transfer. Biochem. Pharmacol. 71:1589–1601.

Grenert, J. P., Sullivan, W. P., Fadden, P., Haystead, T. A., Clark, J., Mimnaugh, E., Krutzsch, H., Ochel, H. J., Schulte, T. W., Sausville, E., Neckers, L. M., and Toft, D. O. 1997. The amino-terminal domain of heat shock protein 90 (hsp90) that binds geldanamycin is an ATP/ADP switch domain that regulates hsp90 conformation. J. Biol. Chem. 272:23843–23850.

Grivennikova, V. G., and Vinogradov, A. D. 2006. Generation of superoxide by the mitochondrial Complex I. Biochim. Biophys. Acta 1757:553–561.

Guo, W., Reigan, P., Siegel, D., Zirrolli, J., Gustafson, D., and Ross, D. 2005. Formation of 17-allylamino-demethoxygeldanamycin (17-AAG) hydroquinone by NAD(P)H:quinone oxidoreductase 1: role of 17-AAG hydroquinone in heat shock protein 90 inhibition. Cancer Res. 65:10006–10015.

Guo, W., Reigan, P., Siegel, D., Zirrolli, J., Gustafson, D., and Ross, D. 2006. The bioreduction of a series of benzoquinone ansamycins by NAD(P)H:quinone oxidoreductase 1 to more potent heat shock protein 90 inhibitors, the hydroquinone ansamycins. Mol. Pharmacol. 70:1194–1203.

Gustafson, D. L., and Pritsos, C. A. 1992. Bioactivation of mitomycin C by xanthine dehydrogenase from EMT6 mouse mammary carcinoma tumors. J. Natl. Cancer Inst. 84:1180–1185.

Gutierrez, P. L. 2000. The metabolism of quinone-containing alkylating agents: free radical production and measurement. Front. Biosci. 5:629–638.

Halliwell, B., and Gutteridge, J. M. 1985. The importance of free radicals and catalytic metal ions in human diseases. Mol. Aspects Med. 8:89–193.

Halliwell, B., and Gutteridge, J. M. 1999. Radical chemistry: thermodynamics and kinetics. In Free Radicals in Biology and Medicine, pp. 39–48. Oxford: Oxford University Press.

Hargreaves, R. H., O'Hare, C. C., Hartley, J. A., Ross, D., Butler, J. 1999. Cross-linking and sequence-specific alkylation of DNA by aziridinylquinones. 3. Effects of alkyl substituents. J. Med. Chem. 42:2245–2250.

Harris, C. M., Sanders, S. A., and Massey, V. 1999. Role of the flavin midpoint potential and NAD binding in determining NAD versus oxygen reactivity of xanthine oxidoreductase. J. Biol. Chem. 274:4561–4569.

Hille, R. 1996. The mononuclear molybdenum enzymes. Chem. Rev. 96: 2757–2816.

Hille, R., and Massey, V. 1981. Studies on the oxidative half-reaction of xanthine oxidase. J. Biol. Chem. 256: 9090–9095.

Hille, R., and Nishino, T. 1995. Flavoprotein structure and mechanism. Xanthine oxidase and xanthine dehydrogenase. FASEB J. 9:995–1003.

Hodnick, W. F., and Sartorelli, A. C. 1993. Reductive activation of mitomycin C by NADH:cytochrome b_5 reductase. Cancer Res. 53:4907–4912.

Hollander, P. M., and Ernster, L. 1975. Studies on the reaction mechanism of DT diaphorase. Action of dead-end inhibitors and effects of phospholipids. Arch. Biochem. Biophys. 169:560–567.

Hsieh, T. C., Wang, Z., Hamby, C. V., and Wu, J. M. 2005. Inhibition of melanoma cell proliferation by resveratrol is correlated with upregulation of quinone reductase 2 and p53. Biochem. Biophys. Res. Commun. 334:223–230.

Hultquist, D. E., and Passon, P. G. 1971. Catalysis of methaemoglobin reduction by erythrocyte cytochrome b_5 and cytochrome b_5 reductase. Nat. New Biol. 229:252–254.

Iskander, K., and Jaiswal, A. K. 2005. Quinone oxidoreductases in protection against myelogenous hyperplasia and benzene toxicity. Chem. Biol. Interact. 30:153–154.

Iyanagi, T. 1977. Redox properties of microsomal reduced nicotinamide adenine dinucleotide-cytochrome b_5 reductase and cytochrome b_5. Biochemistry 16:2725–2730.

Iyanagi, T. 2005. Structure and function of NADPH-cytochrome P450 reductase and nitric oxide synthase reductase domain. Biochem. Biophys. Res. Commun. 338:520–528.

Iyanagi, T., Makino, N., and Mason, H. S. 1974. Redox properties of the reduced nicotinamide adenine dinucleotide phosphate-cytochrome P-450 and reduced nicotinamide adenine dinucleotide-cytochrome b_5 reductases. Biochemistry 13:1701–1710.

Jaffar, M., Phillips, R. M., Williams, K. J., Mrema, I., Cole, C., Wind, N. S., Ward, T. H., Stratford, I. J., and Patterson, A. V. 2003. 3-substituted-5-aziridinyl-1-methylindole-4,7-diones as NQO1-directed antitumouragents: mechanism of activation and cytotoxicity in vitro. Biochem. Pharmacol. 66:1199–1206.

Jaiswal, A. K. 1994. Human NAD(P)H:quinone oxidoreductase2. Gene structure, activity, and tissue-specific expression. J. Biol. Chem. 269:14502–14508.

Jaiswal, A. K., Burnett, P., Adesnik, M., and McBride, O. W. 1990. Nucleotide and deduced amino acid sequence of a human cDNA (NQO2) corresponding to a second member of the NAD(P)H:quinone oxidoreductase gene family. Extensive polymorphism at the NQO2 gene locus on chromosome 6. Biochemistry 29:1899–1906.

Jamieson, D., Tung, A. T., Knox, R. J., and Boddy, A. V. 2006 Reduction of mitomycin C is catalysed by human recombinant NRH:quinone oxidoreductase 2 using reduced nicotinamide adenine dinucleotide as an electron donating co-factor. Br. J. Cancer 95:1229–33.

Jarabak, J., and Harvey, R. G. 1993. Studies on three reductases which have polycyclic aromatic hydrocarbon quinones as substrates. Arch. Biochem. Biophys. 303:394–401.

Keeney, P. M., Xie, J., Capaldi, R. A., Bennett, J. P. 2006. Parkinson's disease brain mitochondrial complex I has oxidatively damaged subunits and is functionally impaired and misassembled. J. Neurosci. 26:5256–5264.

Kelland, L. R., Sharp, S. Y., Rogers, P. M., Myers, T. G., and Workman, P. 1999. DT-Diaphorase expression and tumor cell sensitivity to 17-allylamino, 17-demethoxygeldanamycin, an inhibitor of heat shock protein 90. J. Natl. Cancer Inst. 91:1940–1949.

King, C. L., Wong, S. K., and Loo, T. L. 1984. Alkylation of DNA by the new anticancer agent 3,6-diaziridinyl-2,5-bis(carboethoxyamino)-1,4-benzoquinone (AZQ). Eur. J. Cancer Clin. Oncol. 20:261–264.

Knox, R. J., Jenkins, T. C., Hobbs, S. M., Chen, S., Melton, R. G., and Burke, P. J. 2000. Bioactivation of 5-(aziridin-1-yl)-2,4-dinitrobenzamide (CB 1954) by human NAD(P)H quinone oxidoreductase 2: a novel co-substrate-mediated antitumor prodrug therapy. Cancer Res. 60:4179–4186.

Komiyama, T., Kikuchi, T., and Sugiura, Y. 1986. Interactions of anticancer quinone drugs, aclacinomycin A, adriamycin, carbazilquinone, and mitomycin C, with NADPH-cytochrome P-450 reductase, xanthine oxidase and oxygen. J. Pharmacobiodyn. 9:651–664.

Kumagai, Y., Midorikawa, K., Nakai, Y., Yoshikawa, T., Kushida, K., Homma-Takeda, S., and Shimojo, N. 1998. Inhibition of nitric oxide formation and superoxide generation during reduction of LY83583 by neuronal nitric oxide synthase. Eur. J. Pharmacol. 360:213–218.

Kwiek, J. J., Haystead, T. A., and Rudolph, J. 2004. Kinetic mechanism of quinone oxidoreductase 2 and its inhibition by the antimalarial quinolines. Biochemistry 43:4538–4547.

Levay, G., Ross, D., and Bodell, W. J. 1993. Peroxidase activation of hydroquinone results in the formation of DNA adducts in HL-60 cells, mouse bone marrow macrophages and human bone marrow. Carcinogenesis 14:2329–2334.

Lenaz, G., Fato, R., Genova, M. L., Bergamini, C., Bianchi, C., and Biondi, A. 2006. Mitochondrial Complex I: structural and functional aspects. Biochim. Biophys. Acta 2006 1757:1406–20.

Li, R., Bianchet, M. A., Talalay, P., and Amzel, L. M. 1995. The three-dimensional structure of NAD(P)H:quinone reductase, a flavoprotein involved in cancer chemoprotection and chemotherapy: mechanism of the two-electron reduction. Proc. Natl. Acad. Sci. U.S.A. 92:8846–8850.

Liebler, D. C., Kaysen. K. L., and Kennedy, T. A. 1989. Redox cycles of vitamin E: hydrolysis and ascorbic acid dependent reduction of 8a-(alkyldioxy)tocopherones. Biochemistry 28:9772–9777.

Linas, S. L., Whittenburg, D., and Repine, J. E. 1990. Role of xanthine oxidase in ischemia/reperfusion injury. Am. J. Physiol. 258:F711–F716.

Lind, C., Cadenas, E., Hochstein, P., and Ernster, L. 1990. DT-diaphorase: purification, properties, and function. Methods Enzymol. 186:287–301.

Long, D. J., and Jaiswal, A. K. 2000. Mouse NRH:quinone oxidoreductase (NQO2): cloning of cDNA and gene- and tissue-specific expression. Gene. 252:107–117.

Long, D. J., Iskander, K., Gaikwad, A., Arin, M., Roop, D. R., Knox, R., Barrios, R., and Jaiswal, A. K. 2002. Disruption of dihydronicotinamide riboside:quinone oxidoreductase 2 (NQO2) leads to myeloid hyperplasia of bone marrow and decreased sensitivity to menadione toxicity. J. Biol. Chem. 277: 46131–46139.

Lusthof, K. J., Richter, W., de Mol, N. J., Janssen, L. H., Verboom, W., and Reinhoudt, D. N. 1990. Reductive activation of potential antitumor *bis*(aziridinyl)benzoquinones by xanthine oxidase: competition between oxygen reduction and quinone reduction. Arch. Biochem. Biophys. 277:137–142.

Lusthof, K.J., de Mol, N. J., Richter, W., Janssen, L. H., Butler, J., Hoey, B. M., Verboom W. and Reinhoudt, D. N. 1992. Redox cycling of potential antitumor aziridinyl quinones. Free Radic. Biol. Med. 13:599–608.

Lyn-Cook, B. D, Yan-Sanders, Y., Moore, S., Taylor, S., Word, B., and Hammons, G. J. 2006. Increased levels of NAD(P)H: quinone oxidoreductase 1 (NQO1) in pancreatic tissues from smokers and pancreatic adenocarcinomas: a potential biomarker of early damage in the pancreas. Cell Biol. Toxicol. 22:73–80.

Maliepaard, M., Wolfs, A., Groot, S. E., de Mol, N. J., and Janssen, L. H. 1995. Indoloquinone EO9: DNA interstrand cross-linking upon reduction by DT-diaphorase or xanthine oxidase. Br. J. Cancer 71:836–839.

Marsh, W. S., Garretson, A. L., and Wesel, E. M. 1961. Streptonigrin, an antitumor agent produced by strains of *Streptomyces flocculus*. I. Microbiological studies. Antibiot. Chemother. 11:151–157.

Masters, B. S., Bilimoria, M. H., Kamin, H., and Gibson, Q. H. 1965. The mechanism of 1- and 2-electron transfers catalyzed by reduced triphosphopyridine nucleotide-cytochrome c reductase. J. Biol. Chem. 240:4081–4088.

McCord, J. M. 1985. Oxygen-derived free radicals in postischemic tissue injury. N. Engl. J. Med. 312:159–163.

Mishin, V., Pokrovsky, A., and Lyakhovich, V. V. 1976. Interactions of some acceptors with superoxide anion radicals formed by the NADPH-specific flavoprotein in rat liver microsomal fractions. Biochem. J. 154:307–310.

Moran, J. L., Siegel, D., and Ross, D. 1999. A potential mechanism underlying the increased susceptibility of individuals with a polymorphism in NAD(P)H:quinone oxidoreductase 1 (NQO1) to benzene toxicity. Proc. Natl. Acad. Sci. U.S.A. 96:8150–8155.

Munday, R. 2000. Autoxidation of naphthohydroquinones: effects of pH, naphthoquinones and superoxide dismutase. Free Rad. Res. 32:245–253.

Munday, R. 2004. Activation and detoxification of naphthoquinones by NAD(P)H:-quinone oxidoreductase. Methods. Enzymol. 382:364–380.
Munday, R., Smith, B. L., and Munday, C. M. 1998. Effects of butylated hydroxyanisole and dicoumarol on the toxicity of menadione to rats. Chem. Biol. Interact. 108:155–170.
Munday, R., Smith, B. L., and Munday, C. M. 1999a. Effect of butylated hydroxyanisole on the toxicity of 2-hydroxy-1,4-naphthoquinone to rats. Chem. Biol. Interact. 117:241–256.
Munday, R., Smith, B. L., and Munday, C. M. 1999b. Effect of inducers of DT-diaphorase on the toxicity of 2-methyl- and 2-hydroxy-1,4-naphthoquinone to rats. Chem. Biol. Interact. 123:219–237.
Mustacich, D., and Powis, G. 2000. Thioredoxin Reductase. Biochem. J.346:1–8.
Naylor, M. A., Swann, E., Everett, S. A., Jaffar, M., Nolan, J., Robertson, N., Lockyer, S. D., Patel, K. B., Dennis, M. F., Stratford, M. R, Wardman, P., Adams, G. E., Moody, C. J., and Stratford, I. J. 1998. Indolequinone antitumor agents: reductive activation and elimination from (5-methoxy-1-methyl-4, 7-dioxoindol-3-yl)methyl derivatives and hypoxia-selective cytotoxicity in vitro. J. Med. Chem. 41:2720–31.
Nemeikaite-Ceniene, A., Sarlauskas, J., Anusevicius, Z., Nivinskas, H., and Cenas, N. 2003. Cytotoxicity of RH1 and related aziridinylbenzoquinones: involvement of activation by NAD(P)H:quinone oxidoreductase (NQO1) and oxidative stress. Arch Biochem. Biophys. 416:110–118.
Nishino, T. 1994. The conversion of xanthine dehydrogenase to xanthine oxidase and the role of the enzyme in reperfusion injury. J. Biochem. (Tokyo). 116:1–6.
Nosjean, O., Ferro, M., Coge, F., Beauverger, P., Henlin, J. M., Lefoulon. F., Fauchere. J. L., Delagrange, P., Canet, E., and Boutin, J. A. 2000. Identification of the melatonin-binding site MT3 as the quinone reductase 2. J. Biol. Chem. 275:31311–31317.
Ollinger, K., Buffinton, G. D., Ernster, L., and Cadenas, E. 1990. Effect of superoxide dismutase on the autoxidation of substituted hydro- and semi-naphthoquinones. Chem. Biol. Interact. 73:53–76.
Ough, M., Lewis, A., Bey, E. A., Gao, J., Ritchie, J. M., Bornmann, W., Boothman, D. A., Oberley, L. W., and Cullen, J. J. 2005. Efficacy of beta-lapachone in pancreatic cancer treatment: exploiting the novel, therapeutic target NQO1. Cancer Biol. 4:95–102.
O'Brien, P. J. 1991. Molecular mechanisms of quinone cytotoxicity. Chem. Biol. Interact. 80:1–41.
Pan, S. S., and Bachur, N. R. 1980. Xanthine oxidase catalyzed reductive cleavage of anthracycline antibiotics and free radical formation. Mol. Pharmacol. 17:95–99.
Pan, S. S., and Gonzalez, H. 1990. Mitomycin antibiotic reductive potential and related pharmacological activities. Mol. Pharmacol. 37:966–970.
Pan, S. S., and Iracki, T. 1988. Metabolites and DNA adduct formation from flavoenzyme-activated porfiromycin. Mol. Pharmacol. 34:223–228.
Pan, S. S., Andrews, P. A., Glover, C. J., and Bachur, N. R. 1984. Reductive activation of mitomycin C and mitomycin C metabolites catalyzed by NADPH-cytochrome P-450 reductase and xanthine oxidase. J. Biol. Chem. 259:959–966.
Pavlidis, N., Hanauske, A. R., Gamucci, T., Smyth, J., Lehnert, M., te Velde, A., Lan, J., and Verweij, J. 1996. A randomized phase II study with two schedules of the novel indoloquinone EO9 in non-small-cell lung cancer: a study of the EORTC Early Clinical Studies Group (ECSG). Ann. Oncol. 7:529–531.
Petlicki, J., and van de Ven, T. G. M. 1998. The equilibrium between the oxidation of hydrogen peroxide by oxygen and the dismutation of peroxyl or superoxide radicals in aqueous solutions in contact with oxygen. J. Chem. Soc. Faraday Transactions 94:2763–2769.

Petrone, W. F., English, D. K., Wong, K., and McCord, J. M. 1980. Free radicals and inflammation: superoxide-dependent activation of a neutrophil chemotactic factor in plasma. Proc. Natl. Acad. Sci. U.S.A. 77:1159–1163.

Phillips, A. H., and Langdon, R. G. 1962. Hepatic triphosphopyridine nucleotide-cytochrome *c* reductase: isolation, characterization, and kinetic studies. J. Biol. Chem. 237:2652–2660.

Pink, J. J., Planchon, S. M., Tagliarino, C., Varnes, M. E., Siegel, D., and Boothman, D. A. 2000. NAD(P)H:Quinone oxidoreductase activity is the principal determinant of beta-lapachone cytotoxicity. J. Biol. Chem. 275:5416–5424.

Planchon, S. M., Wuerzberger, S., Frydman, B., Witiak, D. T,, Hutson, P., Church, D. R., Wilding, G., and Boothman, D. A. 1995. Beta-lapachone-mediated apoptosis in human promyelocytic leukemia (HL-60) and human prostate cancer cells: a p53-independent response. Cancer Res. 55:3706–3711.

Powers, M. V., and Workman, P. 2006. Targeting of multiple signaling pathways by heat shock protein 90 molecular chaperone inhibitors. Endocr. Relat. Cancer 13:S125-S135.

Powis, G. 1987. Metabolism and reactions of quinoid anticancer agents. Pharmacol. Ther. 35:57–162.

Powis, G., and Appel, P. L. 1980. Relationship of the single-electron reduction potential of quinones to their reduction by flavoproteins. Biochem. Pharmacol. 29:2567–2572.

Pritsos, C. A., and Gustafson, D. L. 1994. Xanthine dehydrogenase and its role in cancer chemotherapy. Oncol. Res. 6:477–481.

Radjendirane, V., Joseph, P., Lee, Y. H., Kimura, S., Klein-Szanto, A. J., Gonzalez, F. J., and Jaiswal, A. K. 1998. Disruption of the DT diaphorase (NQO1) gene in mice leads to increased menadione toxicity. J. Biol. Chem. 273:7382–7389.

Reigan, P., Colucci, M. A., Siegel, D., Chiloux, A., Moody, C. J., Ross, D. (2007) Development of indolequinone mechanism-based inhibitors of NAD(P)H:quinone oxidoreductase 1 (NQO1): NQO1 inhibition and growth inhibitory activity in human pancreatic MIA PaCa-2 cancer cells. Biochemistry. 46:5941–5950.

Ris, M. M., and von Wartburg, J. P. 1973. Heterogeneity of NADPH-dependent aldehyde reductase from human and rat brain. Eur. J. Biochem. 37:69–77.

Ross, D., and Siegel, D. 2004. NAD(P)H:quinone oxidoreductase 1 (NQO1, DT-diaphorase), functions and pharmacogenetics. Methods Enzymol. 382:115–144.

Ross, D., Beall, H. D., Siegel, D., Traver, R. D., and Gustafson, D. L. 1996. Enzymology of bioreductive drug activation. Br. J. Cancer 27:S1–8.

Ross, D., Beall, H., Traver. R. D., Siegel, D., Phillips, R. M., and Gibson, N. W. 1994. Bioactivation of quinones by DT-diaphorase, molecular, biochemical, and chemical studies. Oncol. Res. 6:493–500.

Ross, D., Siegel, D., Beall, H., Prakash, A. S., Mulcahy, R. T., and Gibson, N. W. 1993. DT-diaphorase in activation and detoxification of quinones. Bioreductive activation of mitomycin C. Cancer Metastasis Rev. 12:83–101.

Rothman, N., Smith, M. T., Hayes, R. B., Traver, R. D., Hoener, B., Campleman, S., Li, G. L., Dosemeci, M., Linet, M., Zhang, L., Xi, L., Wacholder, S., Lu, W., Meyer, K. B., Titenko-Holland, N., Stewart, J. T., Yin, S., and Ross, D. 1997. Benzene poisoning, a risk factor for hematological malignancy, is associated with the NQO1 609C>T mutation and rapid fractional excretion of chlorzoxazone. Cancer Res. 57:2839–2842.

Sartorelli, A. C. 1988. Therapeutic attack of hypoxic cells of solid tumors: Presidential Address. Cancer Res. 48:775–778.

Schlager, J. J., and Powis, G. 1990. Cytosolic NAD(P)H:(quinone-acceptor)-oxidoreductase in human normal and tumor tissue: effects of cigarette smoking and alcohol. Int. J. Cancer 45:403–409.

Schlosser, M. J., and Kalf, G. F. 1989. Metabolic activation of hydroquinone by macrophage peroxidase. Chem. Biol. Interact. 72:191–207.
Schuerch, A. R., and Wehrli, W. 1978. Beta-lapachone, an inhibitor of oncornavirus reverse transcriptase and eukaryotic DNA polymerase-alpha. Inhibitory effect, thiol dependence and specificity. Eur. J. Biochem. 84:197–205.
Schulte, T. W., and Neckers, L. M. 1998. The benzoquinone ansamycin 17-allylamino-17-demethoxygeldanamycin binds to HSP90 and shares important biologic activities with geldanamycin. Cancer Chemother. Pharmacol. 42:273–279.
Schwartz, J. M., and Jaffe, E. R. 1978. Hereditary methemoglobinemia with deficiency of NADH-dehydrogenase. In The Metabolic Basis of Inherited Disease (ed 4), eds. J. B. Stanbury, J. B. Wyngaarden, and D. S. Fredrickson, p. 1452. New York: McGraw-Hill.
Shen, A. L., Sem, D. S., and Kasper, C. B. 1999. Mechanistic studies on the reductive half-reaction of NADPH-cytochrome P450 oxidoreductase. J. Biol. Chem. 274:5391–5398.
Siegel, D., and Ross, D. 2000. Immunodetection of NAD(P)H:quinone oxidoreductase 1 (NQO1) in human tissues. Free Rad. Biol. Med. 29:246–253.
Siegel, D., Anwar, A., Winski, S. L., Kepa, J. K., Zolman, K. L., and Ross, D. 2001. Rapid polyubiquitination and proteasomal degradation of a mutant form of NAD(P)H:quinone oxidoreductase 1. Mol. Pharmacol. 59:263–268.
Siegel, D., Beall, H., Kasai, M., Arai, H., Gibson, N. W., and Ross, D. 1993. pH-Dependent inactivation of DT-diaphorase by mitomycin C and porfiromycin. Mol. Pharmacol. 44:1128–1134.
Siegel, D., Beall, H., Senekowitsch, C., Kasai, M., Arai, H., Gibson, N. W., and Ross, D. 1992. Bioreductive activation of mitomycin C by DT-diaphorase. Biochemistry 31:7879–7885.
Siegel, D., Bolton, E. M., Burr, J. A., Liebler, D. C., and Ross, D. 1997. The reduction of alpha-tocopherolquinone by human NAD(P)H: quinone oxidoreductase: the role of alpha-tocopherolhydroquinone as a cellular antioxidant. Mol. Pharmacol. 52:300–305.
Siegel, D., Gibson, N. W., Preusch, P. C., and Ross, D. 1990. Metabolism of diaziquone by NAD(P)H:(quinone acceptor) oxidoreductase (DT-diaphorase): role in diaziquone-induced DNA damage and cytotoxicity in human colon carcinoma cells. Cancer Res. 50:7293–7300.
Siegel, D., Gustafson, D. L., Dehn, D. L., Han, J. Y., Boonchoong, P., Berliner, L. J., and Ross, D. 2004. NAD(P)H:quinone oxidoreductase 1: role as a superoxide scavenger. Mol. Pharmacol. 65:1238–1247.
Sreerama, L., Hedge, M. W., and Sladek, N. E. 1995. Identification of a class 3 aldehyde dehydrogenase in human saliva and increased levels of this enzyme, glutathione S-transferases, and DT-diaphorase in the saliva of subjects who continually ingest large quantities of coffee or broccoli. Clin. Cancer Res. 1:1153–1163.
Strassburg, A., Strassburg, C. P., Manns, M. P., and Tukey, R. H. 2002. Differential gene expression of NAD(P)H:quinone oxidoreductase and NRH:quinone oxidoreductase in human hepatocellular and biliary tissue. Mol. Pharmacol. 61:320–325.
Strittmatter, P. 1965. The reaction sequence in electron transfer in the reduced nicotinamide adenine dinucleotide-cytochrome b_5 reductase system. J. Biol. Chem. 240:4481–4487.
Sugiura, Y., Kuwahara, J., and Suzuki, T. 1984. DNA interaction and nucleotide sequence cleavage of copper-streptonigrin. Biochim. Biophys. Acta 782:254–261.
Sussman, M. S., and Bulkley, G. B. 1990. Oxygen-derived free radicals in reperfusion injury. Methods Enzymol. 186:711–723.

Swann, E., Barraja, P., Oberlander, A. M., Gardipee, W. T., Hudnott, A. R., Beall, H. D., and Moody, C. J. 2001. Indolequinone antitumor agents: correlation between quinone structure and rate of metabolism by recombinant human NAD(P)H:quinone oxidoreductase. Part 2. J. Med. Chem. 44:3311–3319.

Sydor, J. R., Normant, E., Pien, C. S., Porter, J. R., Ge, J., Grenier, L., Pak, R. H., Ali, J. A., Dembski, M. S., Hudak, J., Patterson, J., Penders, C., Pink, M., Read, M., Sang. J., Woodward, C., Zhang, Y., Grayzel, D. S., Wright, J., Barrett, J. A., Palombella, V. J., Adams, J., and Tong, J. K. 2006. Development of 17-allylamino-17 demethoxygeldanamycin hydroquinone hydrochloride (IPI-504), an anti-cancer agent directed against Hsp 90. Proc. Natl. Acad. Sci. U.S.A. 103: 17408–17413.

Terada, L. S., Willingham, I. R., Rosandich, M. E., Leff, J. A., Kindt, G. W., and Repine, J. E. 1991. Generation of superoxide anion by brain endothelial cell xanthine oxidase. J. Cell. Physiol. 148:191–196.

Thomas, D. J., Sadler, A., Subrahmanyam, V. V., Siegel, D., Reasor, M. J., Wierda, D., and Ross, D. 1990. Bone marrow stromal cell bioactivation and detoxification of the benzene metabolite hydroquinone: comparison of macrophages and fibroblastoid cells. Mol. Pharmacol. 37:255–262.

Thor, H., Smith, M. T., Hartzell, P., Bellomo, G., Jewell, S. A., and Orrenius, S. 1982. The metabolism of menadione (2-methyl-1,4-naphthoquinone) by isolated hepatocytes. A study of the implications of oxidative stress in intact cells. J. Biol. Chem. 257:12419–12425.

Traver, R. D., Siegel, D., Beall, H. D., Phillips, R. M., Gibson, N. W., Franklin, W. A., and Ross, D. 1997. Characterization of a polymorphism in NAD(P)H:quinone oxidoreductase (DT-diaphorase). Br. J. Cancer 75:69–75.

Vasiliou, V., Ross, D., and Nebert, D. W. 2006. Update of the NAD(P)H:quinone oxidoreductase (NQO) gene family. Hum. Genom. 2:329–335.

Verma RP. 2006. Anti-cancer activities of 1,4-naphthoquinones: a QSAR study. Anticancer Agents Med. Chem. 6:489–499.

Vermilion, J. L., and Coon, M. J. 1978 Purified liver microsomal NADPH-cytochrome P-450 reductase. Spectral characterization of oxidation–reduction states. J. Biol. Chem. 253:2694–2704.

Vienozinskis, J., Butkus, A., Cenas, N. and Kulys, J.1990. The mechanism of the quinone reductase reaction of pig heart lipoamide dehydrogenase. Biochem. J. 269:101–105.

Wang, Z, Hsieh, T. C., Zhang, Z., Ma, Y., and Wu, J. M. 2004. Identification and purification of resveratrol targeting proteins using immobilized resveratrol affinity chromatography. Biochem. Biophys. Res. Commun. 323:743–749.

Wardman, P. 2001. Electron transfer and oxidative stress as key factors in the design of drugs selectively active in hypoxia. Curr. Med. Chem. 8:739–761.

Wermuth, B. 1981. Purification and properties of an NADPH-dependent carbonyl reductase from human brain. Relationship to prostaglandin 9-ketoreductase and xenobiotic ketone reductase. J. Biol. Chem. 256:1206–1213.

Wermuth, B., Bohren, K. M., Heinemann, G., and von Wartburg, J. P., Gabbay, K. H. 1988. Human carbonyl reductase. Nucleotide sequence analysis of a cDNA and amino acid sequence of the encoded protein. J. Biol. Chem. 263:16185–16188.

Wermuth, B., Burgisser, H., Bohren, K., and von Wartburg, J. P. 1982. Purification and characterization of human-brain aldose reductase. Eur. J. Biochem. 127:279–284.

Wermuth, B., Platts, K. L., Seidel, A., and Oesch, F. 1986. Carbonyl reductase provides the enzymatic basis of quinone detoxication in man. Biochem. Pharmacol. 35:1277–1282.

White, J. R. 1977. Streptonigrin-transition metal complexes: binding to DNA and biological activity. Biochem. Biophys. Res. Commun. 77:387–391.

Williams, C. H. Jr, and Kamin, H. 1962. Microsomal triphosphopyridine nucleotide-cytochrome c reductase of liver. J. Biol. Chem.. 237:587–595.
Winski, S. L., Hargreaves, R. H., Butler, J., and Ross, D. 1998. A new screening system for NAD(P)H:quinone oxidoreductase (NQO1)-directed antitumor quinones: identification of a new aziridinylbenzoquinone, RH1, as a NQO1-directed antitumor agent. Clin. Cancer Res. 4:3083–3088.
Winski, S. L., Swann, E., Hargreaves, R. H., Dehn, D. L., Butler, J., Moody, C. J., and Ross, D. 2001. Relationship between NAD(P)H:quinone oxidoreductase 1 (NQO1) levels in a series of stably transfected cell lines and susceptibility to antitumor quinones. Biochem. Pharmacol. 61:1509–1516.
Wirth, H., and Wermuth, B. 1992. Immunohistochemical localization of carbonyl reductase in human tissues. J. Histochem. Cytochem. 40:1857–63.
Wu, K., Knox, R., Sun, X. Z., Joseph, P., Jaiswal, A. K., Zhang, D., Deng, P. S., and Chen, S. 1997. Catalytic properties of NAD(P)H:quinone oxidoreductase-2 (NQO2), a dihydronicotinamide riboside dependent oxidoreductase. Arch. Biochem. Biophys. 347:221–228.

8

Lipoxidation-Derived Electrophiles as Biological Reactive Intermediates

De Lin and Lawrence M. Sayre
Department of Chemistry, Case Western Reserve University, Cleveland, OH 44106, USA
e-mail: lms3@po.cwru.edu

Keywords: Hydroxynonenal (HNE) · Oxononenal (ONE) · Lipid Oxidation · Malondialdehyde · Acrolein

8.1. Introduction Generation of Lipoxidation-Derived Electrophiles

A key process in mammalian biochemistry is the peroxidation (dioxygenation) of polyunsaturated fatty acids (PUFAs), in their free or esterified forms, to their corresponding hydroperoxy derivatives. This reaction involves both enzymatic and nonenzymatic pathways. The PUFAs in lipoproteins and membranes are the most susceptible cellular constituents to oxidative stress damage. The condition of oxidative stress results in a free-radical chain peroxidation process, initiated by abstraction of the *bis*-allylic hydrogen atom. The resulting pentadienyl radical reacts at one terminus or the other with oxygen, to give a peroxy radical, which then abstracts a second *bis*-allylic hydrogen to complete the chain. The enzymatic peroxidation pathways are catalyzed by lipoxygenases (LOXs), which constitute a heterogeneous family of enzymes responsible for the biosynthesis of leukotrienes, important mediators of inflammatory and anaphylactic disorders (Werz and Steinhilber 2005; Steinhilber 1999). The different LOXs are classified by the positional specificity of oxygen addition, two possibilities in the case of linoleic acid and four in the case of arachidonic acid. At least one LOX has been implicated in atherosclerosis, and is capable of oxidizing low-density lipoprotein (LDL) to its atherogenic form. The hydroperoxide products of the enzymatic and nonenzymatic pathways are basically the same, but the difference is that the latter is randomized in terms of both regiochemistry and stereochemistry.

A.A. Elfarra (ed.), *Advances in Bioactivation Research*, DOI: 10.1007/978-0-387-77300-1_8,

Regardless of their mechanism of formation, the initial lipid hydroperoxide products are only metastable, and can decompose through the catalytic action of transition metal ions, mainly iron and copper. In this process, the reduced forms, Fe(II) or Cu(I), induce reductive cleavage of the peroxide unit, and the resulting oxidized forms, Fe(III) and Cu(II), are re-reduced at the expense of cellular reducing stores (e.g., ascorbate or cysteine). It has also been reported that ascorbate can support a nonmetal-catalyzed decomposition of lipid hydroperoxides (Lee, Oe and Blair 2001). The process of peroxide decomposition can be divided into two categories: one that involves retention of the carbon backbone (Figure 8.1), and the other that involves chain cleavage (Figure 8.2) to generate monofunctional and bifunctional reactive aldehyde moieties (Spiteller et al. 2001; Gardner 1989).

Peroxidation of the 1,4-pentadienyl stretches of unsaturation in PUFA chains results in two "mirror image" 1,3-pentadienyl hydroperoxide intermediates (Figures 8.1 and 8.2, two alternate choices for R and R′). In the case of retention of the full PUFA carbon backbone, this translates into the expectation that there will be two possible regioisomers for every possible unsymmetrically oxygenated end-product, for example, two regioisomers for each of the *trans*-epoxy-oxo-(*E*)-octadecenoic acid series (EKODE-I and EKODE-II; Figure 8.1). On the other hand, when chain cleavage occurs, this results in two sets of aldehydes for each type of reactive moiety generated, one containing the methyl terminus of the acyl chain, and the other containing the carboxyl terminus (Kamido et al. 1995; Gu et al. 2003; Gugiu and Salomon 2003; Deng and Salomon 2000). Some of these pairs demonstrated to arise from linoleic acid (Spiteller et al. 2001) are 4-hydroxy-2-nonenal (HNE) and 9-hydroxy-12-oxo-10-dodecenoic acid (HODA); 4-oxo-2-nonenal (ONE) and 9-keto-12-oxo-10-dodecenoic acid (KODA); 2,4-decadienal (DDE) and 13-oxo-9,11-tridecadienoic acid; 2-hydroxyheptanal and 9-hydroxy-10-oxodecanoic acid; and 2-octenal and 11-oxo-8-undecenoic acid. However, the carboxyl-terminus analog of 4,5-epoxy-2-decenal (EDE), 13-oxo-9,10-epoxy-11-tridecaenoic acid, has not yet been reported.

Small aldehydes with neither a methyl or carboxy terminus have also been detected in lipid peroxidation, including malondialdehyde (MDA), glyoxal (Fu et al. 1996), and acrolein (Uchida et al. 1998a,b; Uchida 1999).

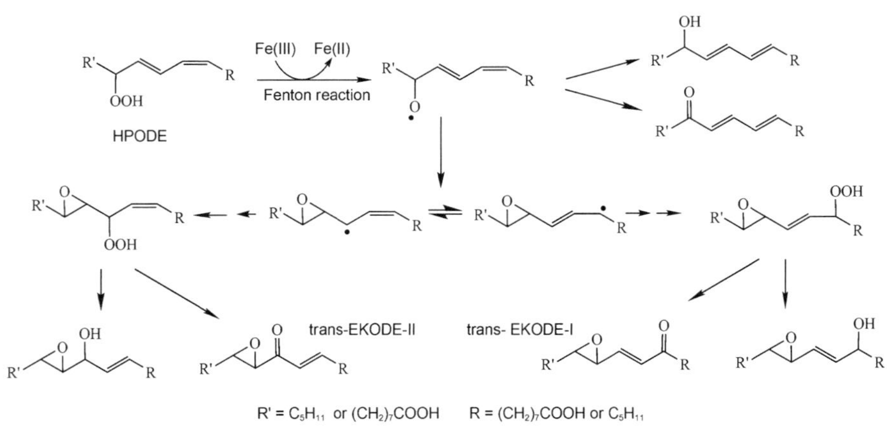

Figure 8.1 Pathways for decomposition of linoleate-derived hydroperoxides without chain cleavage.

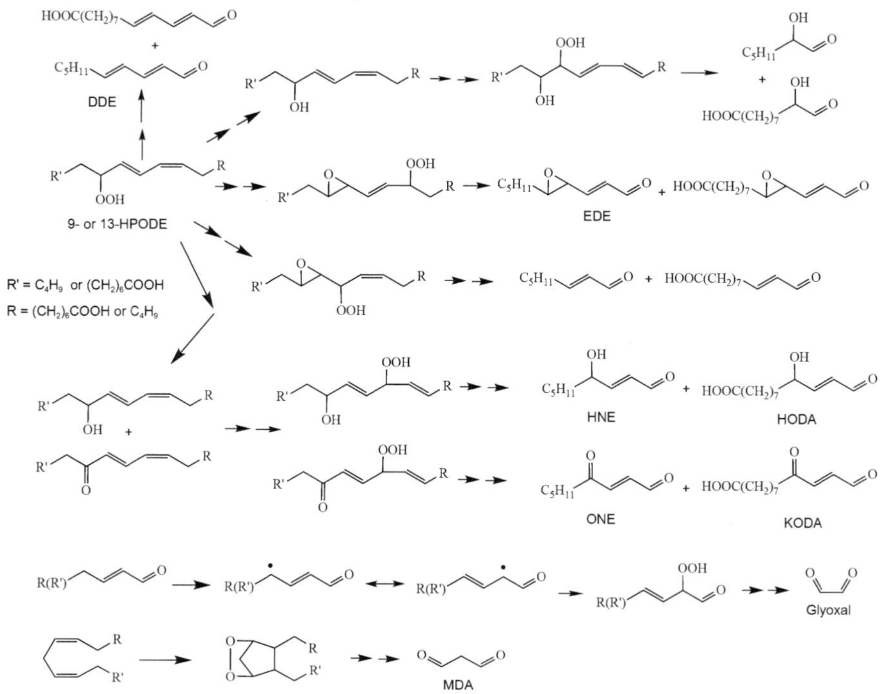

Figure 8.2 Pathways for decomposition of PUFA hydroperoxides with chain cleavage.

Possible routes to the former two are shown in Figure 8.2, though potential pathways to the formation of acrolein from intermediates of PUFA oxidation have yet to be established. It should be noted that glyoxal can form also from various glycoxidation pathways, MDA can form in prostaglandin biosynthesis, and acrolein can form from the amine oxidase-mediated metabolism of the polyamine spermine.

During the past few decades, there has been an intensive effort directed at ascertaining the nature of protein and DNA modification (Burcham 1998; Bartsch 1999; Marnett, Riggins and West 2003; Bartsch and Nair 2004) by lipoxidation (LPO)-derived electrophiles, and evidence is accumulating for their being causally involved in many pathophysiological effects associated with oxidative stress in cells and tissues in vivo (Sayre, Smith and Perry 2001). Early interest in the nature of LPO-mediated protein and DNA modification focused on MDA. More recently, the greatest effort has been directed at HNE, a readily diffusible and selective electrophile, which is a key mediator of oxidative stress (Esterbauer, Schaur and Zollner 1991). HNE has achieved the status of the best-recognized and most-studied cytotoxic product of lipid peroxidation (Uchida 2003). Recently, the 4-keto cousin of HNE, ONE, was demonstrated to be a direct product of lipid oxidation (Lee and Blair, 2000; Spiteller et al. 2001), arising independently and not from oxidation of HNE (HNE and ONE appear not to interconvert metabolically). Studies in our labs and others (see below) have characterized the side-chain-modifying chemistry of ONE, a more reactive protein modification and crosslinking agent than HNE. Other important products of lipid peroxidation capable of modifying proteins include: MDA

(1,3-propanedial); acrolein; simple 2-enals; 2,4-dienals; 2-hydroxyaldehydes; and 4,5-epoxy-2-enals.

The principal protein side-chain adducts modified by LPO-derived electrophiles are Cys, His, and Lys. The guanidino group of Arg is highly basic and the conjugate acid is therefore normally unreactive toward electrophilic agents. On the other hand, 1,2-dicarbonyl compounds are standard chemical modification agents for Arg side-chains, and these moieties are generated during glycoxidation events or in the Maillard reaction of reducing sugars with Lys side-chains. The ability of Arg to be modified by 1,2-dicarbonyl compounds probably reflects the fact that the low level of monoadducted guanidino formed in equilibrium is "trapped" by more irreversible chemistry that occurs upon intramolecular cyclization of a second guanidino nitrogen with the second carbonyl functionality. 1,2-Dicarbonyl or related bifunctional reactivity can potentially be generated from LPO-derived electrophiles, suggesting the possibility for the occurrence of Arg modification in some cases.

The search for the nature of DNA nucleobase modification was driven by the early finding that certain LPO-derived electrophiles, such as acrolein, also a known environmental toxin, are mutagenic both in vitro and in vivo. The most common types of adducts generated are those that result in bridging of the 1 and N^2 nitrogen positions of guanosine or the 1 and N^6 nitrogen positions of adenosine by C1 and C3 of α,β-unsaturated aldehydes (two regiochemistries possible), generating the so-called (substituted) propano adducts. Bridging across these same positions by two carbons to give the so-called etheno adducts is also observed under peroxidizing conditions (Chen and Chung 1994). Other noncrosslink and crosslink nucleobase adducts are formed by the various, mainly bifunctional LPO-derived aldehydes.

The chemistry of protein and DNA modification is described below in the context of different families of reactive moieties. It is most important to recognize that among the many model studies that have resulted in elucidation of adduct structures, in only limited cases has there been documentation that the protein or DNA adducts form in vivo. In the case of protein modifications, evidence for in vivo appearance of adducts has come mainly from immunochemical studies using highly specific antibodies. Verification of the presence of DNA adducts in vivo has depended not only on immunochemical methods but also polyethyleneimine cellulose thin-layer chromatography (TLC) or high-performance liquid chromatography (HPLC) methods with ^{32}P-postlabeling. The high sensitivity of mass spectrometry makes this approach the most likely method to see increased applications in the coming years for detection of in vivo adducts.

8.2. Chemistry of Protein and Polynucleotide Covalent Modification

8.2.1. Malondialdehyde

Malondialdehyde has entertained major historical significance, as it constitutes the principal aldehyde detected in the thiobarbituric acid reactive substances (TBARS) assay for lipid peroxidation (Esterbauer, Schaur and

Zollner 1991). Although other lipid-derived aldehydes give a positive TBARS signal, MDA partitions so efficiently into the water phase relative to more lipophilic LPO products that the TBARS measurement constitutes a reasonable definition of released MDA. Although the ability of MDA to modify proteins should be limited by its existence at physiological pH mainly in the form of its "inert" resonance-stabilized enolate anion conjugate base, MDA nonetheless appears capable of forming an array of protein adducts, associated with crosslinking and a characteristic fluorescence (ex/em 390–400 nm/460–470 nm). The most obvious crosslink would be the Lys–Lys *bis*-Schiff base **1a**, which would exist as its resonance-stabilized 1-amino-3-iminopropene tautomer **1b**. Evidence that this crosslink is at least reversibly formed in solution is supported by the isolation of the corresponding propano di-lysine derivative following borohydride reduction (Requena et al. 1997). At the same time, however, the extent to which **1** contributes to long-lived crosslinking of protein by MDA has been questioned (Slatter, Murray and Bailey 1998), and it would have to form first from accumulation of the mono-Schiff base adduct, shown to exist in its resonance-stabilized enamino form **2** (Uchida et al. 1997). The latter does form in considerable amounts on protein Lys residues, but because of the resonance, it might have low reactivity toward condensation with a second Lys amino group. One thing for sure is that the *bis*-Schiff base adduct cannot explain the MDA-derived fluorescence that develops in its reaction with proteins, as shown by independent synthesis of the 1-amino-3-iminopropene moiety (Itakura and Uchida 2001).

Work by others to determine the nature of the MDA-derived fluorophore in model studies under physiomimetic conditions led to the isolation of strongly fluorescent 4-methyl-1,4-dihydropyridine-3,5-dicarboxaldehyde Lys adducts **3** (Kikugawa and Beppu 1987, Nair et al. 1988). A retrosynthetic analysis of this structure indicates the need for two MDA molecules along either side of the ring, tied together by a C_2 fragment that must result from breakdown of a third MDA molecule (Slatter, Murray and Bailey 1998). Consistent with this proposal, the same structure is generated in higher yield from a mixture of MDA and acetaldehyde (Xu et al. 1997). Antibodies to the MDA–acetaldehyde protein adducts (referred to as "MAA" adducts), which include **3** and **4**, have been shown to recognize elevated circulating titers of these adducts in cases of chronic ethanol administration to rats and in humans with alcoholic liver disease, associated with the severity of liver damage (Tuma 2002).

Fluorophore **3** would not explain the protein crosslinking potential of MDA, and further studies using a model lysine-containing peptide led to the characterization of another fluorescent MDA adduct, in this case a dihydropyridinyl pyridinium Lys–Lys crosslink **5** derived from four molecules of MDA (Itakura, Uchida and Osawa 1996). Because of the need for convergence of four MDA molecules, the extent to which adduct **5** contributes to MDA-derived fluorescence and crosslinking is unclear. Another group identified a nonfluorescent imidazole-based Lys–Arg crosslink **6** derived from a single MDA molecule (Slatter, Avery and Bailey 2004).

Interest in the possible reactions of MDA with DNA has dated back more than 30 years (Mukai and Goldstein 1976), though the fact that MDA, rather than some impurity generated in its preparation, is the actual mutagen was

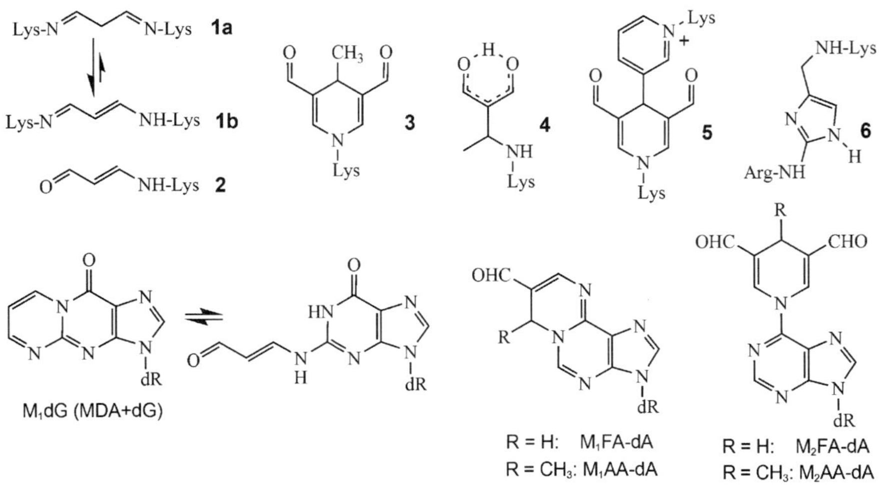

Figure 8.3 MDA adducts of protein side-chain and nucleobases.

confirmed only two decades ago (Basu and Marnett1983). The reaction between MDA and guanine nucleosides was reported to form M_1dG (Marnett et al. 1986). This adduct (Figure 8.3) was later shown to exist in equilibrium with its ring-opened tautomer (Mao et al. 1999). A mouse monoclonal antibody to M_1dG adducts was found to detect this lesion in the DNA of bacteria treated with sufficient MDA to result in expression of mutations (Sevilla et al. 1997). The M_1dG lesion was found to induce sequence-dependent frameshift mutations and base pair substitutions in bacteria and in mammalian cells, suggesting its possible role in human disease (VanderVeen et al. 2003). In additional model studies, fluorescent 2′-deoxyadenosine adducts (M_1FA-dA, M_2FA-dA; or M_1AA-dA, M_2AA-dA) were identified in the reaction of deoxyadenosine with MDA in the presence of formaldehyde or acetaldehyde (Le Curieux et al. 2000).

8.2.2. Glyoxal

It is known that glyoxal adducts on proteins arise not only from the Maillard reaction of reducing sugars with amines (Glomb and Monnier 1995), but also from lipid peroxidation (Mlakar and Spiteller 1994, 1996; Loidl-Stahlhofen and Spiteller 1994). As in the case of MDA, the most obvious crosslink would be a Lys–Lys *bis*-Schiff base (Figure 8.4). Indeed, the ethano di-lysine reduction product of the latter was identified followed by borohydride reduction (Glomb and Monnier 1995), suggesting that the *bis*-Schiff base represents at least an equilibrium state when proteins and glyoxal are present together in relatively high concentration. However, the main Lys modification that survives after some time is N^{ϵ}-(carboxymethyl)-lysine (CML) (Glomb and Monnier 1995), the mechanism of formation of which involves an intramolecular Cannizzaro rearrangement of the aldehyde hydrate of the mono Lys Schiff base. The finding that CML is also generated when proteins are exposed to PUFAs undergoing metal-catalyzed oxidation supported that fact that glyoxal or a glyoxal-donating intermediate is generated during PUFA peroxidation (Fu et al. 1996).

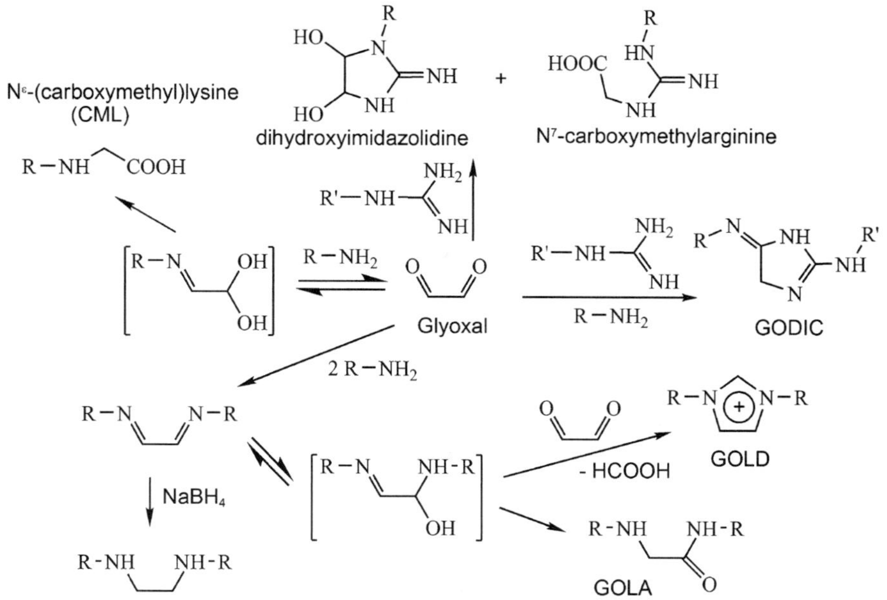

Figure 8.4 Protein modifications formed from glyoxal.

The *bis*-Schiff base is nonetheless important in that it, or its carbinolamine equilibrium form, must be an intermediate in the formation of the Lys–Lys crosslink "glyoxal lysine dimer" (GOLD) (Frye et al. 1998), the formation of which requires a second glyoxal molecule, and the Cannizzaro rearrangement product "glyoxal lysine amide" (GOLA) (Glomb and Pfahler 2001). Glyoxal also modifies arginine, producing dihydroxyimidazolidine and N^7-carboxymethylarginine (Glomb and Lang 2001). In addition, the Lys–Arg crosslink structure GODIC was identified in the incubation of glyoxal with a mixture of Lys and Arg analogs under physiological conditions (Chellan and Nagaraj 2001; Wells-Knecht, Brinkmann and Baynes 1995). The various glyoxal adducts such as CML and GOLD have been found in vivo, using either immunochemical methods (Castellani et al. 2001), or by liquid chromatography–mass spectrometry (LC–MS) techniques (Frye et al. 1998) following complete acid hydrolysis of tissue homogenates (e.g., lens proteins and skin collagen).

Glyoxal was also found to modify DNA and nucleosides, preferentially involving guanine and producing a five-membered ring fused between 1(N) and N^2 by an ethylene glycol moiety (gx-dG) (Shapiro and Hachmann 1966). Additional glyoxal-derived nucleoside adducts, such as the hydroxyacetyl adduct of deoxycytodine (gdC, Figure 8.5), and crosslinks, like dA-gx-dG, dC-gx-dG and dG-gx-dG, were detected to form in physiologic conditions on the basis of UV and MS (Kasai, Iwamoto-Tanaka and Fukada 1998). However, only recently were the latter dG-based glyoxal crosslinks isolated under preparative conditions and their structures elucidated by nuclear magnetic resonance (NMR) (Figure 8.8; Brock et al. 2004). Utilizing a monoclonal antibody to the

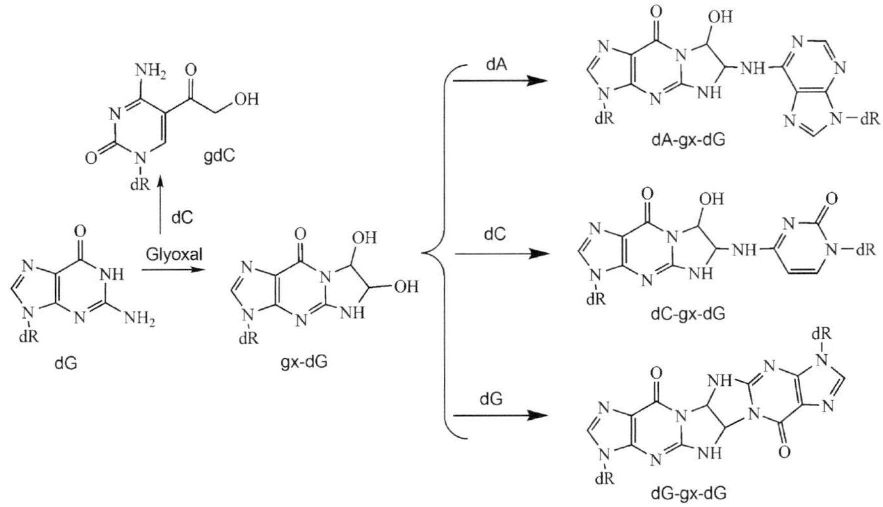

Figure 8.5 Nucleobase adducts and crosslinks formed by glyoxal.

gdC adduct, glyoxal-associated DNA lesions were measured in peripheral blood mononuclear cells of human volunteers taking vitamin C (Cooke et al. 2003), which has been suggested to result in elevated levels of lipid peroxidation products.

8.2.3. 2-Hydroxyalkanals

The most abundant 2-hydroxyalkanal found in tissue is 2-hydroxyheptanal, which has been found in the oxidation of the ω-6 PUFAs linoleic and arachidonic acids (Loidl-Stahlhofen and Spiteller 1994). 2-Hydroxybutanal has also been detected in the oxidation of the ω-3 PUFAs linolenic and docosahexaenoic acid (Mlakar and Spiteller 1994; Kawai, Takeda and Terao 2007). In model studies, free 2-hydroxyheptanal was found to be quite unstable, but reversible Schiff base formation with amines was demonstrated by reductive trapping with sodium borohydride (Figure 8.6; Kern and Spiteller 1996). A fluorescent 3-hydroxypyridinium (3-HOPy) was isolated upon prolonged incubation of amines or lysine derivatives with 2-hydroxyaldehydes, both by our laboratory (Liu and Sayre 2003) and another group (Itakura and Uchida 2003). The latter workers also obtained immunochemical evidence for the existence of the 3-HOPy epitope in atherosclerotic lesions of the human aorta (Itakura et al. 2003). 2-Hydroxyaldehydes correspond to the simplest "reducing sugar", and the mechanism of 3-HOPy formation undoubtedly involves two sequences of Schiff base formation and subsequent Amadori rearrangement, in succession (Figure 8.6). On the basis of the lack of bifunctional unsaturation in 2-hydroxyaldehydes, one would not expect any obvious reaction with DNA, and no such modifications have so far been reported.

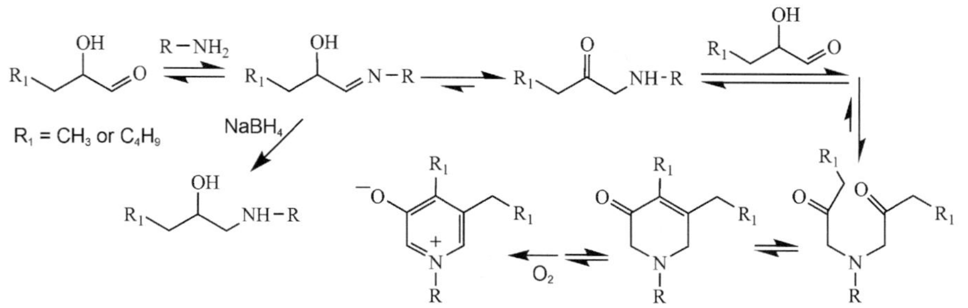

Figure 8.6 Lysine modification by 2-hydroxyaldehydes.

8.2.4. Levuglandins

Levuglandins (LGs) (Figure 8.7), levulinaldehyde (4-oxopentanal) derivatives with prostaglandin side-chains, were postulated to be generated by nonenzymatic rearrangements of prostanoid endoperoxides (Salomon 2005). A number of regioisomers of these compounds are generated, with nomenclature based on that used for prostaglandins. On the basis of the well-known Paal–Knorr condensation of γ-dicarbonyl compounds with amines to form pyrroles, one would expect the reaction of LGs with proteins to result in pyrrole derivatives on Lys side-chains. Quantitation of protein-based levuglandin E2 (LGE_2)-derived pyrroles was accomplished through colorimetric derivatization with *p*-(dimethylamino)benzaldehyde, Ehrlich's reagent (Iyer, Kobierski and Salomon 1994). However, LG-derived pyrroles are highly susceptible to oxidation because of their electron-rich property. It was thus found that LGE_2-derived pyrroles are readily oxidized by air to relatively stable end-products, lactams and hydroxylactams, through MS analysis (Brame et al. 1999). These adducts have been identified in vivo in a variety of oxidative stress states (Salomon 2005). Levuglandins were also found to be potent crosslinkers of proteins (Jirousek, Murthi and Salomon 1990; Salomon 2005), possibly arising from the generation of electrophilic moieties in the oxidation of the initially formed Lys-based pyrroles. The exact nature of the crosslinking has not been structurally established.

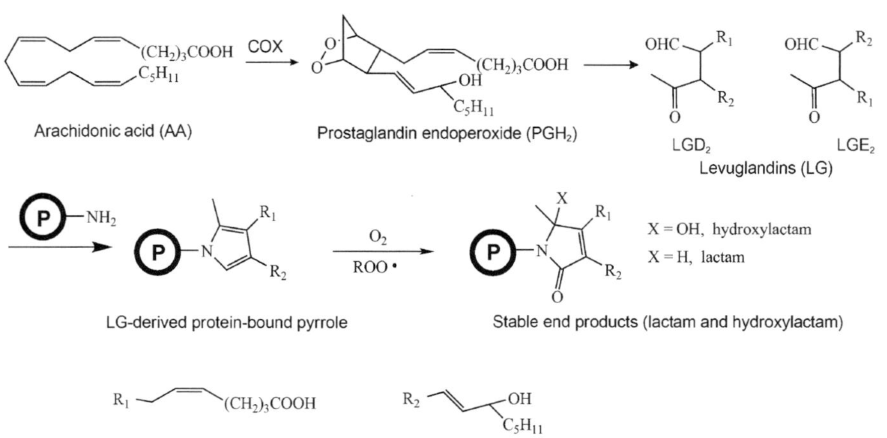

Figure 8.7 Generation of levuglandins and their modification of lysine side-chains.

On the basis of the finding that LGE_2 inhibits mitosis and microtubule assembly (Murthi, Salomon and Sternlicht 1990), the ability of these reactive molecules to modify DNA was investigated. Indeed, LGE_2 was found to produce DNA–protein crosslinks in mammalian cells (Murthi et al. 1993), though the exact nature of the crosslink chemistry remains unidentified.

8.2.5. Acrolein, 2-Alkenals, and 2,4-Dienals

The 2-alkenals represent a large group of aldehydes containing two electrophilic reaction centers, a Michael addition-reactive C=C and the C=O group. Michael additions were suggested to occur with the sulfhydryl group of cysteine, the imidazole group of histidine, and the amino group of lysine in proteins. In particular, (*E*)-2-octenal was documented to adduct to His residues of bovine serum albumin (Alaiz and Giron 1994). Acrolein is thought to be the strongest electrophile among these aldehydes and shows the highest reactivity with nucleophiles in proteins (Esterbauer , Schaur and Zollner 1991). The higher reactivity of acrolein relative to the chain-extended 2-alkenals undoubtedly reflects the steric accessibility of the unsubstituted β-carbon. The bifunctional nature suggests that 2-alkenals could potentially crosslink proteins, and this has been found to be the case, with acrolein being the most potent crosslinking agent (Zhang et al. 2003).

The chemical nature of crosslinking and noncrosslinking modification of proteins by 2-alkenals is an ongoing field of investigation. The formation of the 3-formyldihydropyridine-lysine (FDP-lysine) adduct (Figure 8.8) was first reported in the case of acrolein-modified lysine (Uchida et al. 1998a). This adduct represents the sequential conjugate addition of a single Lys residue to two molecules of the 2-alkenal, possibly reflecting equilibrium generation of an initial monoadduct that has not been characterized as a stable end-product. An alternate course for reaction of a single lysine with

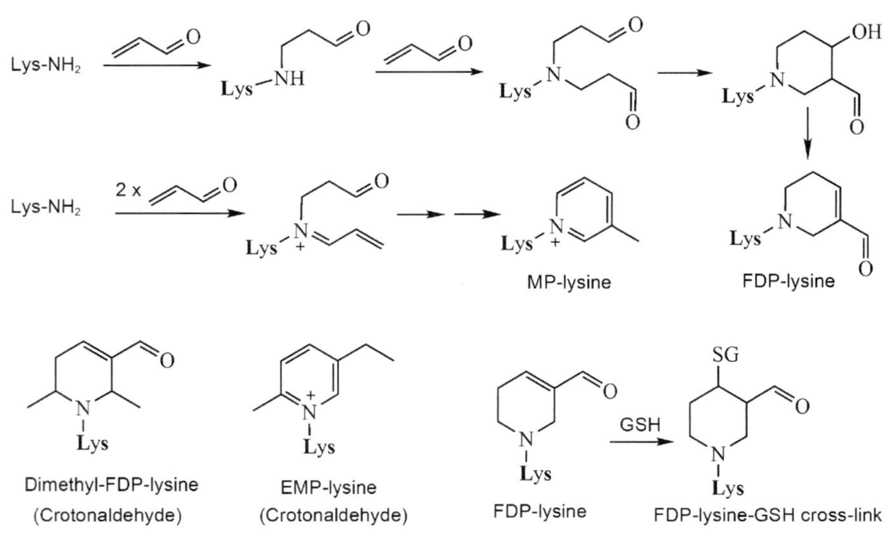

Figure 8.8 Lysine modification by acrolein/crotonaldehyde and Lys–GSH crosslinking.

two molecules of acrolein was identified to give a methylpyridinium structure (MP-lysine) (Ichihashi et al. 2001, Furuhata et al. 2003). Antibodies recognizing the acrolein–lysine protein adducts were found to recognize neurons specifically in Alzheimer's disease (Calingasan, Uchida and Gibson 1999) as well as atherosclerotic lesions from a human aorta (Uchida et al. 1998b), in which intense positivity was associated primarily with macrophage-derived foam cells and the thickening neointima of arterial walls.

The FDP- and pyridinium-type adducts were later also detected in the incubation of lysine derivatives with other 2-alkenals, such as crotonaldehyde (Figure 8.8), 2-pentenal, and 2-hexenal (Ichihashi et al. 2001). The structural connectivity of the crotonaldehyde-derived 2,5-disubstituted pyridinium adduct confirms that the latter represents the equivalent of one Michael addition and one Schiff base formation, though the mechanistic details have not been totally elucidated. Although pyridinium-type adducts were less preferentially formed than FDP-type adducts in model reactions of acrolein and crotonaldehyde with lysine derivatives, the pyridinium structures were actually the major antigenic adducts generated in acrolein- or crotonaldehyde-modified protein (Ichihashi et al. 2001, Furuhata et al. 2003).

It was later recognized that the FDP adduct was itself a reactive electrophile (α,β-unsaturated aldehyde) and thus could undergo Michael addition by a protein-based electrophile, resulting in protein–protein crosslinking. In this regard, the FDP-lysine adduct was reported to react with free sulfhydryl groups (e.g., of glutathione (Figure 8.8)) and represented a new mechanism of Lys–Cys-based protein crosslinking by acrolein (Furuhata et al. 2002).

Studies by Novotny's group on the reaction of model Lys-containing peptides with 2-hexenal were reported to yield not only 2,5-disubstituted pyridinium structures but also 3,4-disubstituted pyridinium adducts that appear to reflect condensation of the Lys ε-amino group with the C1 carbonyl group (Schiff base formation) of both molecules of 2-alkenal (Figure 8.9; Baker et al. 1998; Baker, Wiesler and Novotny 1999). Structural assignment was on the basis of NMR and mass spectrometry. Although this shift in adduct structure toward double Schiff base-like condensation probably reflects the lower tendency of the extended-chain 2-alkenal toward Michael addition relative to acrolein, as expected on steric grounds, these other studies involved higher concentrations of reactants, and more complex pyridinium structures representing condensation of one or two molecules of Lys with three molecules of aldehyde were also obtained.

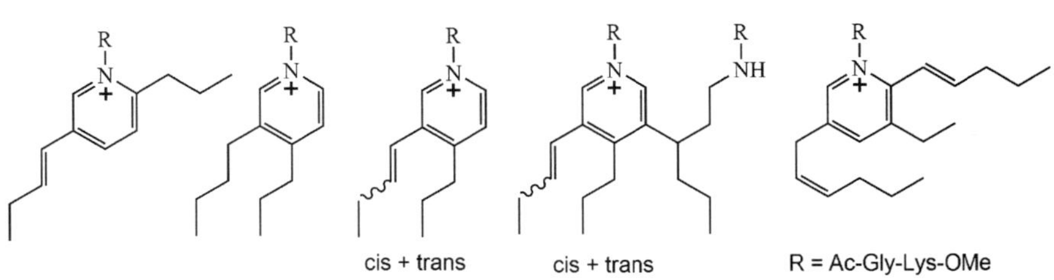

Figure 8.9 Structures of adducts formed from lysine-containing peptides and 2-hexenal.

It should be pointed out that one of the most abundant products of lipid oxidation is the simple aldehyde hexanal. Although this molecule lacks Michael adduct reactivity and its reactions with proteins would presumably be limited to Schiff base formation (reversibly) on Lys amino groups, it is known that more complex end-products are generated (Smith et al. 1999), including pyridiniums (Kato et al. 1986) and some fluorescent moieties of unknown structure (Stapelfeldt and Skibsted 1996). The most likely route to such products involves an amine-catalyzed aldol-like condensation to generate initial 2:1 aldehyde–amine adducts bearing α,β-unsaturation as an early step.

On the basis of the rich modification chemistry induced by α,β-unsaturated aldehydes, one would think that 2,4-dienals, such as DDE, a major product of oxidation of linoleic acid (Spiteller et al. 2001), would also modify proteins, and with perhaps more complicated mechanisms and structures due to the additional unsaturation. We found that DDE has about the same protein crosslinking ability as HNE (Zhang et al. 2003). However, the nature of protein modification by DDE has not been thoroughly investigated.

Acrolein is reactive with DNA bases, and cyclic 1,N^2-propanodeoxyguanosine adducts (Acr-dG1-3, Figure 8.10) have been characterized (Chung, Young and Hecht 1984). Similar adducts were also detected when deoxyguanosine was exposed to PUFAs undergoing oxidation (Pan and Chung 2002). Although HNE has one more functional group (4-hydroxy), it shares with simple 2-enals the same type of modification of deoxyguanosine. The Acr, Cro, and HNE adducts have been detected as endogenous DNA lesions in rodent and human tissues (Chung et al. 2003). Although the results showed that HNE-dG adducts are preferentially formed in a sequence-specific manner at a mutational hotspot in human cancers, these lesions were shown to be readily repairable. Acrolein also modifies deoxyadenosine, generating a similar propano adduct (Acr-dA, Figure 8.10) (Smith et al. 1990). Formation of this adduct in vivo was demonstrated immunohistochemically in the nuclei of the proximal tubular cells of rat kidney in a model for oxidative stress using a carcinogenic iron chelate (Kawai et al. 2003).

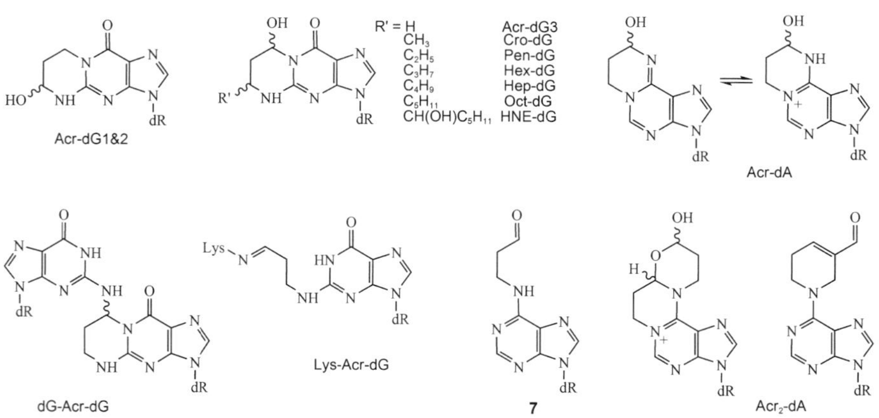

Figure 8.10 Deoxyguanosine/deoxyadenosine adducts and dG-dG and Lys-dG crosslinks generated by acrolein and various 2-alkenals.

The generation of acrolein adduct Acr-dG3 serves as an intermediate to the formation of the interchain DNA crosslink dG-Acr-dG (Figure 8.10), which could be isolated from enzymatically digested acrolein-treated DNA as well as by direct treatment of Acr-dG3 with dG (Kozekov et al. 2001). In addition, crosslinking between lysine-containing peptides and deoxyguanosine-containing oligodeoxynucleotides was reported to occur via a Schiff base linkage (Kurtz and Lloyd 2003). Very recently, three acrolein–deoxyadenosine adducts in addition to the previously identified propano adduct were identified from modification of calf thymus DNA (Figure 8.10), a ring-opened propano adduct **7** and two adducts (Acr_2-dA) that contain two molecules each of acrolein (Pawlowicz et al. 2006).

As discussed in the introduction, etheno purine DNA adducts have been identified in vivo and appear to arise from a variety of exogenous and endogenous chemical agents, including intermediates generated during lipid peroxidation (Chen and Chung 1994). Although simple 2-enals give rise to the propano adducts described in Figure 8.10, exposure of DNA to 2-enals in the presence of epoxidizing agents, including peroxy intermediates of lipid peroxidation, results in the generation of the more mutagenic etheno adducts. That these adducts arise from epoxy derivatives was shown by the fact that the independently synthesized epoxide arising from HNE (2,3-epoxy-4-hydroxynonanal), a potent mutagen unlike its parent HNE, generated the etheno adducts shown in Figure 8.11 (Chen et al. 1998). Both unsubstituted and substituted etheno adducts are seen. Other 2,3-epoxyalkanals give rise to the same chemistry.

Although some workers have found that cytotoxicity arising from the 2,4-dienal DDE involves a nonapoptotic mechanism (Cabre et al. 2003), other workers have observed DDE to exhibit genotoxic effects (Hansen, Even and Geneviere 2004; Chang, Lo and Lin 2005), suggesting its ability to modify DNA. Curiously, DDE has not been reported to give rise to propano DNA adducts analogous to those seen above from 2-alkenals. However, a number of substituted etheno adducts have been reported to form when deoxyadenosine is exposed to DDE in the presence of peroxides or H_2O_2 (Carvalho et al. 1998, 2000). In these cases (Figure 8.12), it appears that the actual DNA-modifying agents are again the 2,3-epoxides

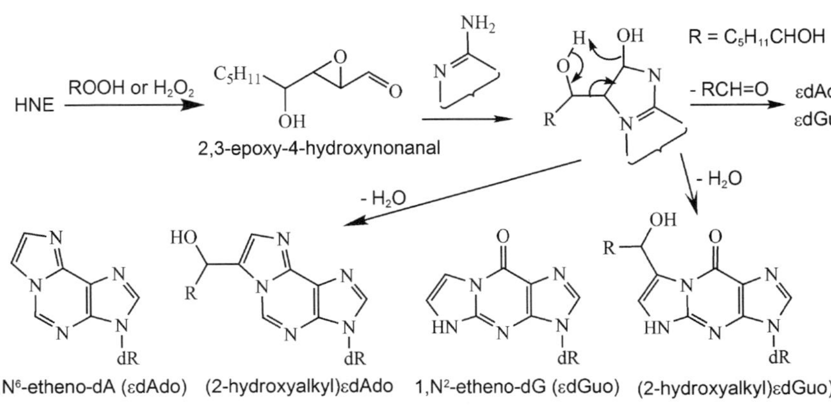

Figure 8.11 Generation of etheno DNA nucleobase adducts from 2-enals under epoxidizing conditions.

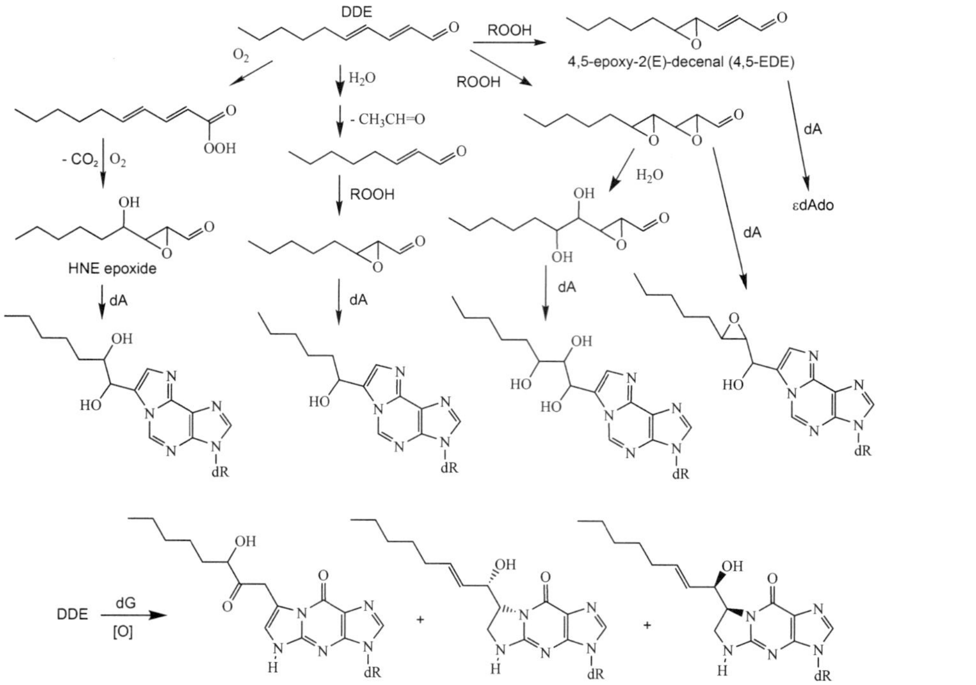

Figure 8.12 Deoxyadenosine and deoxyguanosine adducts derived from reaction with DDE under oxidizing conditions.

that form from epoxidation reactions that could occur under physiological conditions. The unsubstituted etheno adducts εdAdo and εdGuo and additional substituted deoxyguanosine etheno adducts (Figure 8.12) were found to form under similar reaction conditions (Loureiro et al. 2000, 2004). Unlike the parent etheno adducts, the substituted forms of DDE-derived etheno adducts have yet to be observed in vivo.

Despite the realization that 2,3-epoxyalkanals can serve as source of unsubstituted etheno adducts εdAdo and εdGuo (Figure 8.12), these same DNA lesions are also found to form from the independently synthesized peroxidation metabolite of DDE, 4,5-epoxy-2(*E*)-decenal (4,5-EDE) (Lee, Oe and Blair 2002). These workers were able to exclude contamination by any 2,3-epoxy compound, suggesting that there is an alternate mechanistic route to the etheno adducts from that depicted in Figure 8.12. 4,5-EDE has been observed to be generated directly from peroxidation of the ω-6 PUFAs linoleic and arachidonic acids.

8.2.6. HNE, ONE, HODA, KODA

Our laboratory has had a major focus on HNE, a highly reactive bifunctional aldehyde, that is a major product of oxidation of ω-6 polyunsaturated (linoleoyl and arachidonyl) chains. The propensity of HNE to form Michael adducts with nucleophilic amino acids (Figure 8.13) represents the dominant initial reaction pathway of HNE with proteins and underlies the ability of HNE to inactivate a large number of thiol-dependent enzymes, in

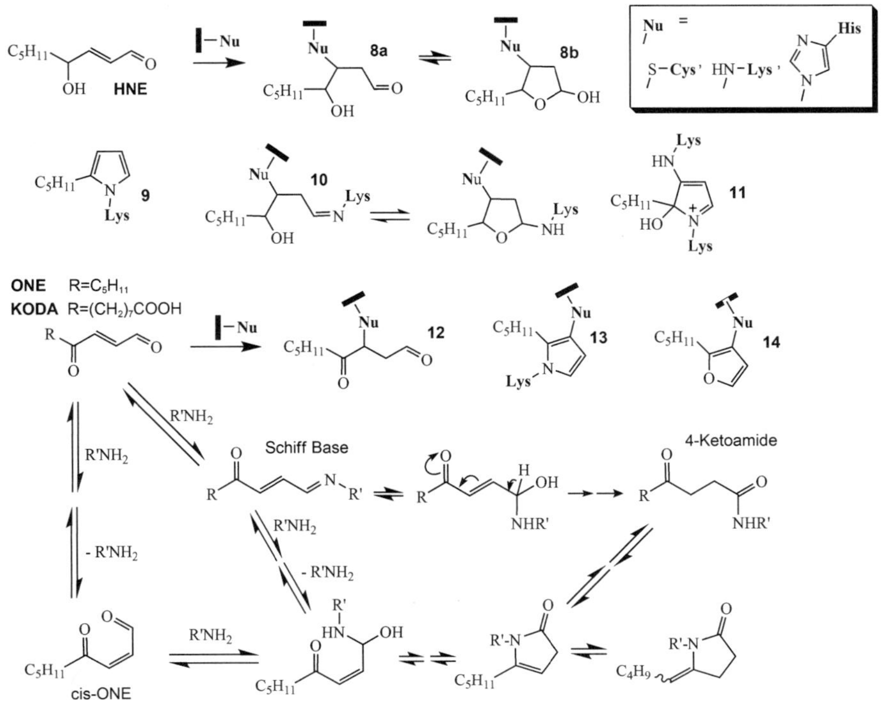

Figure 8.13 Protein side-chain modification by HNE and ONE.

particular cysteine proteases (Esterbauer , Schaur and Zollner 1991; Witz 1989; Uchida and Stadtman 1992, 1993). Unlike simple α,β-unsaturated aldehydes, the Michael adducts **8a** in this case are stabilized in the form of cyclic hemiacetals **8b** (Esterbauer, Ertl and Scholz 1976). Antibodies raised to HNE-treated protein, thought to recognize mainly HNE Michael adducts, have documented the presence of HNE modifications in vivo in diseases associated with oxidative stress (Ando et al. 1998; Yoritaka et al. 1996, Wataya et al. 2002).

Although HNE Michael adducts formed with Cys and His are stable to isolation, Michael adducts to Lys ε-amino groups are formed reversibly (Nadkarni and Sayre 1995), and can be isolated only following reductive trapping with $NaBH_4$. Our efforts to characterize an irreversibly formed HNE-lysine adduct led to the discovery of HNE-derived 2-pentylpyrroles **9** (Sayre et al. 1993, 1996), that we termed the first example of an "advanced lipoxidation end-product" (ALE). This pyrrole has been documented as a marker of oxidative stress in numerous disease states, including atherosclerosis (Salomon et al. 2000), Alzheimer's disease (Montine et al. 1997a,b; Sayre et al. 1997), Alexander's disease (Castellani et al. 1998), and Parkinsons disease (Castellani et al. 2002).

The bifunctional aspect of HNE allows it in theory to crosslink proteins by conjugate addition of Cys, His, or Lys at C3 and Schiff base condensation with Lys at the C1 carbonyl, for example, **10** (Uchida and Stadtman 1993; Friguet, Stadtman and Szweda 1994; Cohn et al. 1996). However, we found that such adduct, like the simple lysine Michael adduct, is reversibly formed (Nadkarni and Sayre 1995). Our efforts to characterize stable adducts that would rationalize the known protein crosslinking activity of HNE (Cohn et al. 1996, Montine et al. 1996), led to the discovery of a fluorescent four-electron oxidation product, 2-hydroxy-2-pentyl-1,2-dihydropyrrol-3-one iminium **11**, that has the same lysine–lysine connectivity as **10**, but arises via an independent mechanistic pathway (Xu and Sayre 1998; Xu, Liu and Sayre 1999). The same Lys–Lys crosslink was reported by another group (Itakura, Osawa and Uchida 1998), and immunochemically identified in HNE-treated protein (Tsai et al. 1998) and in-vitro-oxidized LDL (Xu, Liu and Sayre 2000). In the effort to confirm the structure of **11** by independent synthesis, we found that the 4-keto cousin of HNE, ONE, gives rise to **11** in much higher yield (Xu and Sayre 1998). Soon thereafter, ONE was demonstrated to be a direct product of lipid oxidation in its own right (Lee and Blair 2000; Spiteller et al. 2001). Subsequent work showed that **11** (ex/em 360/430 nm) plays a key role in HNE-induced protein crosslinking, and is the main contributor to the fluorescence that arises when proteins are exposed to HNE (and ONE) (Xu et al. 1999; Xu, Liu and Sayre 1999).

ONE has been found to be more reactive than HNE with protein nucleophiles (Doorn and Petersen 2002,2003; Lin et al. 2005) and in protein crosslinking (Zhang et al. 2003), and to be equal to (West et al. 2004) or somewhat more toxic (Lin et al. 2005) than HNE to cells in culture. Although levels of the more reactive ONE in tissues in oxidative stress has not been quantified in the same manner as has HNE, the presence of ONE in the circulation was evidenced by its being trapped as an ascorbate adduct detected in human plasma (Sowell, Frei and Stevens 2004). In addition to **11**, ONE forms simple 4-ketoaldehyde Michael adducts **12** of Cys, His, or Lys that can exist as such or undergo Paal–Knorr condensation with a Lys amino group, affording 3-substituted pyrrole crosslinks **13** (Zhang et al. 2003; Oe et al. 2003a). The Cys–Lys and His–Lys crosslinks are quite stable, though the Lys–Lys version readily suffers oxidation. In the absence of the possibility for condensation with Lys residues, the ONE-derived 4-ketoaldehydes appear to cyclize to furans **14** (Zhang et al. 2003; Yocum et al. 2005). The formation on proteins of HNE and ONE adducts characterized in model studies has been confirmed by immunochemical (Uchida et al. 1993, 1995; Sayre et al. 1996; Hashimoto et al. 2003) and MS studies (Bruenner, Jones and German 1995; Bolgar, Yang and Gaskell 1996; Grace et al. 1996; Alderton et al. 2003; Fenaille, Guy and Tabet 2003; Liu, Minkler and Sayre 2003, Carini, Aldini and Facino 2004; Fenaille, Tabet and Guy 2004; Isom et al. 2004; Aldini et al. 2005; Orioli et al. 2005; Yocum et al. 2005).

More recently, our focus on the initial reactions between ONE and HNE with amines led to the finding that ONE is biased toward equilibrium formation of C1 carbonyl Schiff bases (Figure 8.13), whereas HNE is biased toward equilibrium formation of the Michael adduct, as verified by trapping with $NaBH_4$ (Lin et al. 2005). On the basis of this understanding and the finding by MS that ONE nonetheless forms adducts on Lys side-chains with the molecular weight change expected of the Michael adduct, we found that the ONE-Lys Schiff base can be transformed to a stable ketoamide end-product (Figure 8.13) that is isomeric with the Michael adduct (Sayre et al. 2006; Zhu and Sayre 2007a,b). Thus, the

Lys adducts that appear to be Michael adducts by MS are actually 4-ketoamides. These ketoamides also appear to be in slow equilibrium with two isomeric pyrrolinones that form from Lys and *cis*-ONE (Figure 8.13), generated by an addition–elimination isomerization sequence (Sayre et al. 2006; Zhu and Sayre 2007a,b).

As discussed in the introductory section, generation of HNE and ONE from linoleic acid has a "mirror image" counterpart in the generation of the analogous carboxy-terminating aldehydes HODA and KODA (also referred to as DODE, Lee et al. 2005), respectively (Figure 8.2). Thus, one may expect the same variety of protein side-chain adducts to form from these reactive aldehydes. Indeed, the KODA-derived Lys 4-ketoamide (Figure 8.13) has been found in addition to the ONE-derived 4-ketoamide when proteins are exposed to peroxidizing linoleic acid (Zhu and Sayre 2007b). There are certainly free fatty acids that circulate in biological tissues, and protein and DNA adducts of carboxy-terminating reactive aldehydes can form from these. However, most PUFAs in biological systems are either esterified to cholesterol (e.g., in lipoproteins) or to (primarily) the sn-2 position of phospholipids in membranes. In the latter case, peroxidation results in the generation of the so-called "core" aldehydes as reactive truncated forms of phospholipids. Reactive aldehydes in the matrix of the membrane are most likely to target membrane proteins, unless the reactive sn-2 chains are released by lipases.

As discussed earlier, α,β-unsaturated aldehydes like acrolein induce the formation of protein–DNA crosslinks via a lysine-directed Schiff base (Kurtz and Lloyd 2003). Confirmatory structural evidence for such crosslink in the case of HNE (dG-HNE-Lys; Figure 8.14) was obtained recently in our group on the basis of a model study using $NaBH_4$ reduction and structural elucidation by NMR and MS. At the same time, this model study identified additional crosslinks dT-HNE-Lys and dG-HNE-His in their reduced forms by MS (Yuan 2006).

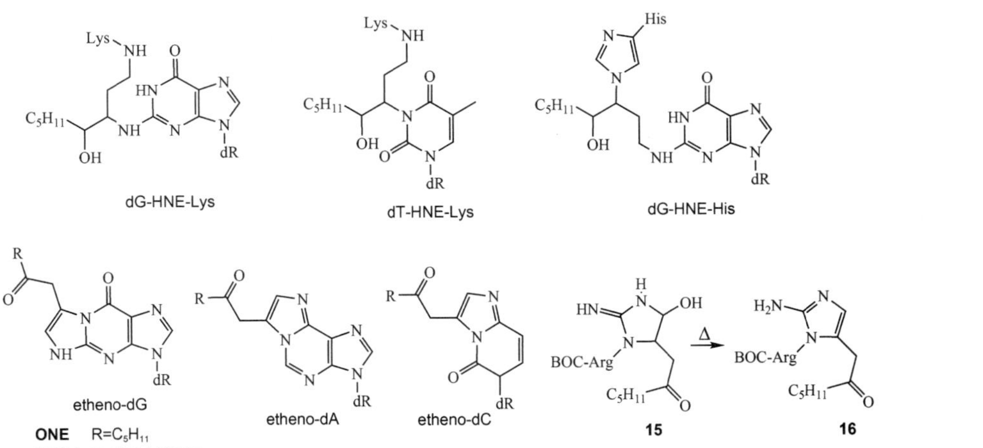

Figure 8.14 Reduced HNE-derived protein–DNA base crosslinks, ONE nucleobase adducts, and ONE Arg adducts seen in model studies.

As might be expected based on the presence of the additional reactive 4-oxo group, ONE modifies DNA bases more readily than does HNE. The structures of these adducts have been identified in a series of papers by the group of Ian Blair (Rindgen et al. 2000; Pollack et al. 2003). Unlike simple α,β-unsaturated aldehydes that form propano-adducts with nucleotides, ONE modification results in a series of substituted etheno-adducts, as shown in Figure 8.14. Similar dG, dA, and dC adducts were found for KODA (DODE) (Lee et al. 2005). Whereas all these adducts reflect the initial oxidation of linoleic acid to 13(*S*)-hydroperoxy-9,11-(*Z*,*E*)-octadecadienoic acid, analogous adducts with R = $(CH_2)_3COOH$ are formed from oxidation of arachidonic acid through the intermediacy of 5(*S*)-hydroperoxy-6,8,11,14-(*E*,*Z*,*Z*,*Z*)-eicosatetraenoic acid (Jian et al. 2005a).

On the basis of the ability of ONE to modify the guanidino moiety of dG and the amidino moiety of dA, it was suggested that ONE might similarly modify the Arg side-chain. Indeed, the reversible generation of an imidazolinone imine **15** was demonstrated on the basis of its $NaBH_4$ reductive trapping and its irreversible dehydration under heat (80°C) to an aminoimidazole adduct **16** (Oe et al. 2003b). However, the nonphysiological conditions needed for stable adduct formation in this case raises a question about its potential in vivo significance.

The congeners of HNE and ONE that derive from ω-3 rather than from ω-6 PUFAs are 4-hydroxy-2-hexenal (HHE) and 4-oxo-2-hexenal (OHE), respectively. The adducts from these aldehydes may serve as more important markers in tissues that are rich in the ω-3 PUFAs such as the nervous system. Although less work has been devoted to detecting the protein and nucleobase adducts of these congeners, the chemistry should be the same. Most work conducted has focused on immunochemical detection of HHE–protein adducts in diseased tissues using antibodies that have been raised to HHE-treated protein and are assumed to recognize HHE Michael adducts (as in the case of HNE) (Shibata et al. 2004; Tanito et al. 2005). In one case using a monoclonal antibody selected against the HHE–His Michael adduct, this biomarker was shown to be generated in copper-oxidized LDL, and to be present in atherosclerotic lesions, in which intense positivity was associated primarily with macrophage-derived foam cells (Yamada et al. 2004). As far as OHE is concerned, most work on this compound has focused on evidence for its mutagenic potential (Kawai, Matsuno and Kasai 2006), most probably associated with adduction to dG (Maekawa et al. 2006).

8.2.7. EKODE

The most abundant epoxyoxooctadecenoic acids that arise from mild oxidation of linoleic acid are *trans*-9,10-epoxy-13-oxo-11(*E*)-octadecenoic acid and *trans*-12,13-epoxy-9-oxo-11(*E*)-octadecenoic acid (Gardner and Kleiman 1981, Gardner and Crawford 1981), which we have recently named *trans*-EKODE-Ia and *trans*-EKODE-Ib (Figure 8.1) (Lin 2007). On the other hand, when the EKODEs are synthesized from reduction of the 13- and 9-hydroperoxides, oxidation of the resulting alcohols to the dienone, and epoxidation with MCPBA, the major products obtained apparently have the *cis*-epoxy stereochemistry (Hidalgo, Zamora and

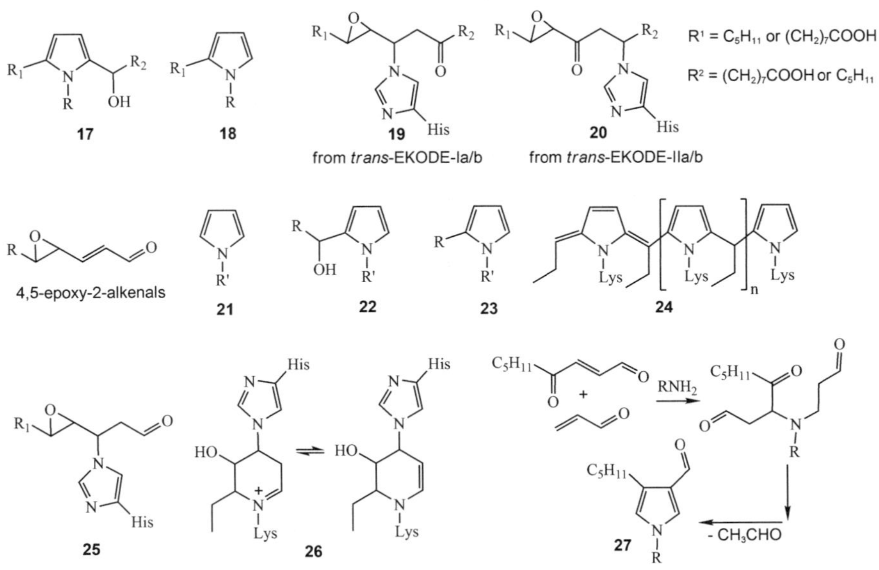

Figure 8.15 Protein adducts arising from EKODE isomers, 4,5-epoxy-2-alkenals, and acrolein+ONE.

Vioque 1992), we refer to as *cis*-EKODE-Ia and *cis*-EKODE-Ib. The methyl esters of these latter two EKODEs were found to react with amino acid derivatives to produce pyrroles **17** containing the full EKODE carbon skeleton as well as pyrroles **18** (Figure 8.15) which have split off either the methyl or carboxyl tail of EKODE as the corresponding aldehyde, through a retrocondensation process (Zamora et al. 2005).

More recently, isomeric EKODE histidine Michael adducts **19** and **20** (Figure 8.15) were found to represent a dominant family of protein modifications generated during mild nonenzymatic oxidation of linoleic acid (Lin 2007). Reaction of the independently synthesized EKODE isomers with His models revealed that all are capable of forming stable Michael adducts, though the EKODE-II series of analogs was found to be more reactive.

8.2.8. 4,5-Epoxy-2-alkenals

The reaction of 4,5-epoxy-2-alkenals with amines and amino acid derivatives has been widely studied. For reactions relevant protein lysine side-chains, N-substituted pyrroles **21**, N-substituted 2-(1-hydroxyalkyl)-pyrroles **22** (Zamora and Hidalgo 1994), and 2-alkylpyrroles **23** (Zamora and Hidalgo 2005) were isolated and characterized from the reaction under different conditions of 4,5-epoxy-2(*E*)-heptenal (EHE), the epoxyenal in this family that arises from peroxidation of ω-3 PUFAs. Moreover, the N-substituted 2-(1-hydroxyalkyl)pyrroles **22** are unstable and can polymerize to form lipofuscin-like polypyrroles **24** which results in protein crosslinking (Hidalgo and Zamora 1993). Furthermore, the reduced form of EHE histidine Michael adducts **25** were identified after borohydride reduction (Zamora, Alaiz and Hidalgo1999). Recently, EHE-derived His–Lys crosslinking was reported, and the reduced form of the Lys–His crosslink structure **26** was isolated and identified (Lin 2007).

The 10-carbon epoxyenal *trans*-4,5-epoxy-2(*E*)-decenal (EDE), which arises from peroxidation of ω-6 PUFAs linoleic and arachidonic acids, gives rise to the analogous lysine adducts as seen for EHE (Zamora and Hidalgo 2005). We already discussed above the fact that DNA adducts arising from DDE under peroxidizing conditions can arise from various epoxide metabolites, of DDE, including EDE.

8.2.9. Multicomponent LPO-Derived Protein Adducts

The generation of lysine adducts from MDA, glyoxal, acrolein, crotonaldehyde, and 2-hydroxyalkanals described above that involve condensation of two (or more) molecules of aldehyde with a single lysine group (Figures 8.3, 8.4, 8.6, 8.8, and 8.9) has been documented to occur in vivo (antibody recognition of several of them has been observed). However, since it is much more likely that any given Lys would encounter two different aldehydes, one is led to the hypothesis that the major 2:1 aldehyde–Lys adducts formed in vivo would be those incorporating two different aldehyde molecules. When the two different aldehydes are congeners of one another (e.g., acrolein/crotonaldehyde or 2-hydroxyheptanal/2-hydroxybutanal) the adduct structure would be the same (Figures 8.6 and 8.8), though the length of the alkyl "arms" would differ. In this case, significant crossreactivity of antibodies might be expected. However, when two different aldehyde types are considered, there is now the chance for formation of unique adduct types that are not seen with either aldehyde alone.

As "proof of principle" we carried out an incubation of an amine Lys surrogate with a 1:1 mixture of the two reactive aldehydes acrolein and ONE. By analyzing this reaction compared to incubations containing only one of the other aldehydes, a major unique adduct was isolated and structurally characterized to be a novel 3-formyl-4-pentylpyrrole **27** (Figure 8.15). This adduct reflects two sequential conjugate additions, cyclization and apparent elimination of $CH_3CH=O$ (Quan 2006, Sayre et al. 2006).

8.3. Functional Biological Consequences of Nonenzymatic LPO

The majority of data on the biological activities of lipid peroxidation products reflects the hundreds of studies that have been performed on HNE. HNE exhibits a wide array of biological activities, from disruption of calcium homeostasis (Camandola, Poli and Mattson 2000) to inhibition of the proteasome (Friguet and Szweda 1997, Okada et al. 1999, Hyun et al. 2002, Grune and Davies 2003, Ferrington and Kapphahn 2004). Several studies have defined the cytotoxic effects of HNE and ONE to represent primarily induction of apoptosis (Kruman et al. 1997, Herbst et al. 1999, Ji et al. 2001, West et al. 2004; Jian et al. 2005b), including such role in in vitro models of neurodegeneration (Lovell and Markesbery 2006). In addition, there is increasing evidence that HNE may act as a signaling molecule (Keller and Mattson 1998; Lu et al. 2002; Forman, Dickinson and Iles 2003; Awasthi et al. 2003; Kumagai et al. 2004; Laurora et al. 2005), including regulation of kinases (Leonarduzzi, Robbesyn and Poli 2004;

Dozza et al. 2004), activation of adenylate cyclase, increasing protein tyrosine phosphorylation, and promotion of cell proliferation. It has become clear the HNE simultaneously affects multiple stress signaling pathways, which represent potential mechanisms through which HNE alters cellular viability and response to damage (West and Marnett 2005). In contrast, DDE appears to induce cytotoxic effects through a necrotic mechanism, at least in smooth muscle cells (Cabre et al. 2003). Most biological effects of LPO-derived 2-enals are blunted by increasing the concentration of cellular reduced GSH, but there is evidence that the GSH adduct of HNE may have biological activity in its own right (Awasthi et al. 2004).

Although the mechanisms responsible for the biological properties of HNE remain unclear, it seems certain that these represent largely covalent interactions with cellular targets. It is known that modification by HNE interferes with the function of numerous enzymes (Ferrali et al. 1980; Uchida and Stadtman 1993; Siems, Hapner and van Kuijk 1996; Ji, Kozak and Marnett 2001; Ishii et al. 2003), including lysosomal proteases responsible for metabolism of oxidatively modified LDL (O'Neil et al. 1997, Okada et al. 1999), and the endoplasmic reticulum chaperone, protein disulfide isomerase (PDI) (Carbone et al. 2005), which is responsible for promoting correct disulfide formation in newly synthesized proteins. Indirect evidence that covalent modification of proteins by HNE contributes to its cytotoxic effects is that the levels of HNE–protein conjugates parallel parameters of toxicity in cell culture (Malecki et al. 2000) and in experimental animal models of brain injury (Zhang et al. 1999). Further evidence is that the rank order of potency of HNE and various reactive aldehyde analogs to inhibit cell growth and cause apoptosis correlates with electrophilic reactivity of the analogs (Haynes et al. 2000). It has been shown that the neurotoxicity of acrolein and various analogs in synaptosomes correlates with loss of free protein sulfhydryl groups (Lopachin et al. 2007). A novel aspect of the molecular actions of at least some aldehydes, for example, acetaldehyde and acrolein, is their reaction with the cysteine ligands of zinc sites in proteins and concomitant zinc release (Hao and Maret 2006).

HNE, ONE, and other 2-enals are substrates for the aldehyde-metabolizing enzymes aldose reductase and alcohol and aldehyde dehydrogenases. In some cases, metabolism is straightforward and represents a detoxication pathway, such as for the action of aldose reductase on HNE, ONE, and MDA (Doorn, Srivastava and Petersen 2003; Srivastava et al. 1999). However, in other cases (e.g., human mitochondrial aldehyde dehydrogenase) the aldehydes may additionally cause inhibition through enzyme modification (Mitchell and Petersen 1991; Doorn, Hurley and Petersen 2006; Mitchell and Petersen 1988). Mitochondrial aldehyde dehydrogenase is also inhibited by MDA (Hjelle, Grubbs and Petersen 1982).

At least some toxic effects of HNE appear to reflect an indirect effect of HNE in stimulating mitochondrial production of reactive-oxygen species (ROS), and, through depletion of reduced GSH stores, by increasing the susceptibility to other primary toxic insults (Keller, Hanni and Markesbery 1999). However, stimulation of mitochondrial ROS production most likely reflects covalent modification of electron transport proteins, since HNE analogs with weaker protein-modifying capacity exert little effect on mitochondria. If the net sum of protein modification and possible crosslinking by LPO-derived aldehydes occurs to an extent that causes them to be resistant to proteolytic turnover (possibly explaining how they inhibit the proteasome), this can result in accumulation of high-molecular-weight aggregates that typify a large number of neurodegenerative diseases (Dalle-Donne et al. 2006).

Overall, there have been some excellent recent reviews on the interplay between metabolism of LPO-derived aldehydes, their mechanisms of mutagenicity and cytotoxicity, and their potential for affecting signal transduction and gene expression (O'Brien, Siraki and Shangari 2005; Del Rio, Stewart and Pellegrini 2005).

8.4. Conclusions

The foregoing discussion has summarized the variety of covalent-binding chemistries possible for the range of known LPO-derived electrophiles. Although efforts in the future will continue to focus on qualitative and quantitative analysis of the in vivo occurrence of defined adducts in various disease states, it must also be recognized that identification of adducts in vivo does not necessarily imply the adducts are playing a functional role in that disease state. Moreover, whereas oxidative stress has long been linked to the cell death (e.g., in neurodegeneration), whether it is a primary cause or merely a downstream consequence of the degenerative process is still an open question (Andersen 2004). Despite increased reliance on in vitro and in vivo models of disease to decipher the mechanistic relationship between oxidative stress and cytotoxic events linked to DNA modification, the genotoxic and mutation-inducing potential of specific PUFA oxidation cascades remains poorly defined (Lim et al. 2003). The complexity in this field is further heightened when there appears to be disagreement for an individual aldehyde, for example, acrolein, as to whether the principal mechanism of toxicity represents apoptosis (Tanel and Averill-Bates 2005) or necrosis (Liu-Snyder et al. 2006). Thus, a good deal of work remains to be needed to unravel the full pathophysiologic consequences of reactive intermediates generated during lipid oxidation.

Acknowledgements. Work carried out in the authors' laboratory was supported by National Institutes of Health grants AG14249, HL53315, and AG15885, and by the Alzheimer's Association.

References

Alaiz, M., and Giron, J. 1994. Modification of histidine residues in bovine serum albumin by reaction with (*E*)-2-octenal. J. Agric. Food Chem. 42:2094–2098.

Alderton, A. L., Faustman, C., Liebler, D. C., and Hill, D. W. 2003. Induction of redox instability of bovine myoglobin by adduction with 4-hydroxy-2-nonenal. Biochemistry 42:4398–4405.

Aldini, G., Dalle-Donne, I., Vistoli, G., Maffei Facino, R., and Carini, M. 2005. Covalent modification of actin by 4-hydroxy-trans-2-nonenal (HNE): LC-ESI-MS/MS evidence for Cys374 Michael adduction. J. Mass Spectrom. 40:946–954.

Andersen, J. K. 2004. Oxidative stress in neurodegeneration: cause or consequence? Nat. Med. 10 Suppl:S18–25.

Ando, Y., Brannstrom, T., Uchida, K., Nyhlin, N., Nasman, B., Suhr, O., Yamashita, T., Olsson, T., El Salhy, M. Uchino, M., and Ando, M. 1998. Histochemical detection of 4-hydroxynonenal protein in Alzheimer amyloid. J. Neurol. Sci. 156:172–176.

Awasthi, Y. C., Sharma, R., Cheng, J. Z., Yang, Y., Sharma, A., Singhal, S. S., and Awasthi, S. 2003. Role of 4-hydroxynonenal in stress-mediated apoptosis signaling. Mol. Aspects Med. 24:219–230.

Awasthi, Y. C., Yang, Y., Tiwari, N. K., Patrick, B., Sharma, A., Li, J., and Awasthi, S. 2004. Regulation of 4-hydroxynonenal-mediated signaling by glutathione S-transferases. Free Rad. Biol. Med. 37:607–619.

Baker, A. G., Wiesler, D., and Novotny, M. V. 1999. Tandem mass spectrometry of model peptides modified with trans-2-hexenal, a product of lipid peroxidation. J. Am. Soc. Mass Spectrom. 10:613–624.

Baker, A., Zidek, L., Wiesler, D., Chmelik, J., Pagel, M., and Novotny, M. V. 1998. Reaction of *N*-acetylglycyllysine methyl ester with 2-alkenals: an alternative model for covalent modification of proteins. Chem. Res. Toxicol. 11:730–740.

Bartsch, H. 1999. Keynote address: exocyclic adducts as new risk markers for DNA damage in man. IARC Sci. Publ. 150:1–16.

Bartsch, H., and Nair, J. 2004. Oxidative stress and lipid peroxidation-derived DNA-lesions in inflammation driven carcinogenesis. Cancer Detect. Prev. 28:385–391.

Basu, A. K., and Marnett, L. J. 1983. Unequivocal demonstration that malondialdehyde is a mutagen. Carcinogenesis 4:331–333.

Bolgar, M. S., Yang, C. Y., and Gaskell, S. J. 1996. First direct evidence for lipid/protein conjugation in oxidized human low density lipoprotein. J. Biol. Chem. 271:27999–28001.

Brame, C. J., Salomon, R. G., Morrow, J. D., and Roberts, L. J. 2nd 1999. Identification of extremely reactive gamma-ketoaldehydes (isolevuglandins) as products of the isoprostane pathway and characterization of their lysyl protein adducts. J. Biol. Chem. 274:13139–13146.

Brock, A. K., Kozekov, I. D., Rizzo, C. J., and Harris, T. M. 2004. Coupling products of nucleosides with the glyoxal adduct of deoxyguanosine. Chem. Res. Toxicol. 17:1047–1056.

Bruenner, B. A., Jones, A. D., and German, J. B. 1995. Direct characterization of protein adducts of the lipid peroxidation product 4-hydroxy-2-nonenal using electrospray mass spectrometry. Chem. Res. Toxicol. 8:552–559.

Burcham, P. C. 1998. Genotoxic lipid peroxidation products: their DNA damaging properties and role in formation of endogenous DNA adducts. Mutagenesis 13:287–305.

Cabre, A., Girona, J., Vallve, J. C., Heras, M., and Masana, L. 2003. Cytotoxic effects of the lipid peroxidation product 2,4-decadienal in vascular smooth muscle cells. Atherosclerosis 169:245–250.

Calingasan, N. Y., Uchida, K., and Gibson, G. E. 1999. Protein-bound acrolein: a novel marker of oxidative stress in Alzheimer's disease. J. Neurochem. 72:751–756.

Camandola, S., Poli, G., and Mattson, M. P. 2000. The lipid peroxidation product 4-hydroxy-2,3-nonenal increases AP-1-binding activity through caspase activation in neurons. J. Neurochem. 74:159–168.

Carbone, D. L., Doorn, J. A., Kiebler, Z., and Petersen, D. R. 2005. Cysteine modification by lipid peroxidation products inhibits protein disulfide isomerase. Chem. Res. Toxicol. 18:1324–1331.

Carini, M., Aldini, G., and Facino, R. M. 2004. Mass spectrometry for detection of 4-hydroxy-trans-2-nonenal (HNE) adducts with peptides and proteins. Mass Spectrom. Rev. 23:281–305.

Carvalho, V. M., Asahara, F., Di Mascio, P., de Arruda Campos, I. P., Cadet, J., and Medeiros, M. H. 2000. Novel 1,*N*(6)-etheno-2′-deoxyadenosine adducts from lipid peroxidation products. Chem. Res. Toxicol. 13:397–405.

Carvalho, V. M., Di Mascio, P., de Arruda Campos, I. P., Douki, T., Cadet, J., and Medeiros, M. H. 1998. Formation of 1,*N*6-etheno-2′-deoxyadenosine adducts by trans,trans-2, 4-decadienal. Chem. Res. Toxicol. 11:1042–1047.

Castellani, R. J., Harris, P. L., Sayre, L. M., Fujii, J., Taniguchi, N., Vitek, M. P., Founds, H., Atwood, C. S., Perry, G., and Smith, M. A. 2001. Active glycation in neurofibrillary pathology of Alzheimer disease: *N*(epsilon)-(carboxymethyl) lysine and hexitol-lysine. Free Rad. Biol. Med. 31:175–180.

Castellani, R. J., Perry, G., Harris, P. L., Cohen, M. L., Sayre, L. M., Salomon, R. G., and Smith, M. A. 1998. Advanced lipid peroxidation end-products in Alexander's disease. Brain Res. 787:15–18.

Castellani, R. J., Perry, G., Siedlak, S. L., Nunomura, A., Shimohama, S., Zhang, J., Montine, T., Sayre, L. M., and Smith, M. A. 2002. Hydroxynonenal adducts indicate a role for lipid peroxidation in neocortical and brainstem Lewy bodies in humans. Neurosci. Lett. 319:25–28.

Chang, L. W., Lo, W. S., and Lin, P. 2005. *Trans*, *trans*-2,4-decadienal, a product found in cooking oil fumes, induces cell proliferation and cytokine production due to reactive oxygen species in human bronchial epithelial cells. Toxicol. Sci. 87:337–343.

Chellan, P., and Nagaraj, R. H. 2001. Early glycation products produce pentosidine cross-links on native proteins. Novel mechanism of pentosidine formation and propagation of glycation. J. Biol. Chem. 276:3895–3903.

Chen, H. J., and Chung, F. L. 1994. Formation of etheno adducts in reactions of enals via autoxidation. Chem Res Toxicol. 7:857–860.

Chen, H. J., Zhang, L., Cox, J., Cunningham, J. A., and Chung, F. L. 1998. DNA adducts of 2,3-epoxy-4-hydroxynonanal: detection of 7-(1′, 2′-dihydroxyheptyl)-3*H*-imidazo[2,1-i]purine and 1,*N*6-ethenoadenine by gas chromatography/negative ion chemical ionization/mass spectrometry. Chem. Res. Toxicol. 11:1474–1480.

Chung, F. L., Pan, J., Choudhury, S., Roy, R., Hu, W., and Tang, M. S. 2003. Formation of trans-4-hydroxy-2-nonenal- and other enal-derived cyclic DNA adducts from omega-3 and omega-6 polyunsaturated fatty acids and their roles in DNA repair and human p53 gene mutation. Mutat. Res. 531:25–36.

Chung, F. L., Young, R., and Hecht, S. S. 1984. Formation of cyclic 1,*N*2-propanodeoxyguanosine adducts in DNA upon reaction with acrolein or crotonaldehyde. Cancer Res. 44:990–995.

Cohn, J. A., Tsai, L., Friguet, B., and Szweda, L. I. 1996. Chemical characterization of a protein-4-hydroxy-2-nonenal cross-link: immunochemical detection in mitochondria exposed to oxidative stress. Arch. Biochem. Biophys. 328:158–164.

Cooke, M. S., Mistry, N., Ahmad, J., Waller, H., Langford, L., Bevan, R. J., Evans, M. D., Jones, G. D., Herbert, K. E., Griffiths, H. R., and Lunec, J. 2003. Deoxycytidine glyoxal: lesion induction and evidence of repair following vitamin C supplementation in vivo. Free Rad. Biol. Med. 34:218–225.

Dalle-Donne, I., Aldini, G., Carini, M., Colombo, R., Rossi, R., and Milzani, A. 2006. Protein carbonylation, cellular dysfunction, and disease progression. J. Cell Mol. Med. 10:389–406.

Del Rio, D., Stewart, A. J., and Pellegrini, N. 2005, A review of recent studies on malondialdehyde as toxic molecule and biological marker of oxidative stress. Nutr. Metab. Cardiovasc. Dis. 15:316–328.

Deng, Y., and Salomon, R. G. 2000. Total synthesis of oxidized phospholipids. 3. The (11*E*)-9-hydroxy-13-oxotridec-11-enoate ester of 2-lysophosphatidylcholine. J. Org. Chem. 65:6660–6665.

Doorn, J. A., Hurley, T. D., and Petersen, D. R. 2006. Inhibition of human mitochondrial aldehyde dehydrogenase by 4-hydroxynon-2-enal and 4-oxonon-2-enal. Chem. Res. Toxicol. 19:102–110.

Doorn, J. A., and Petersen, D. R. 2002. Covalent modification of amino acid nucleophiles by the lipid peroxidation products 4-hydroxy-2-nonenal and 4-oxo-2-nonenal. Chem. Res. Toxicol. 15:1445–1450.

Doorn, J. A., and Petersen, D. R. 2003. Covalent adduction of nucleophilic amino acids by 4-hydroxynonenal and 4-oxononenal. Chem. Biol. Interact. 143–144:93–100.

Doorn, J. A., Srivastava, S. K., and Petersen, D. R. 2003. Aldose reductase catalyzes reduction of the lipid peroxidation product 4-oxonon-2-enal. Chem. Res. Toxicol. 16:1418–1423.

Dozza, B., Smith, M. A., Perry, G., Tabaton, M., and Strocchi, P. 2004. Regulation of glycogen synthase kinase-3beta by products of lipid peroxidation in human neuroblastoma cells. J. Neurochem. 89:1224–1232.

Esterbauer, H., Ertl, A., and Scholz, N. 1976. The reaction of cysteine with α,β-unsaturated aldehydes. Tetrahedron 32:285–289.

Esterbauer, H., Schaur, R. J., and Zollner, H. 1991. Chemistry and biochemistry of 4-hydroxynonenal, malondialdehyde and related aldehydes. Free Rad. Biol. Med. 11:81–128.

Fenaille, F., Guy, P. A., and Tabet, J. C. 2003. Study of protein modification by 4-hydroxy-2-nonenal and other short chain aldehydes analyzed by electrospray ionization tandem mass spectrometry. J. Am. Soc. Mass Spectrom. 14:215–226.

Fenaille, F., Tabet, J. C., and Guy, P. A. 2004. Identification of 4-hydroxy-2-nonenal-modified peptides within unfractionated digests using matrix-assisted laser desorption/ionization time-of-flight mass spectrometry. Anal. Chem. 76:867–873.

Ferrali, M., Fulceri, R., Benedetti, A., and Comporti, M. 1980. Effects of carbonyl compounds (4-hydroxyalkenals) originating from the peroxidation of liver microsomal lipids on various microsomal enzyme activities of the liver. Res. Commun. Chem Path Pharm 30:99–112.

Ferrington, D. A., and Kapphahn, R. J. 2004. Catalytic site-specific inhibition of the 20S proteasome by 4-hydroxynonenal. FEBS Lett. 578:217–223.

Forman, H. J., Dickinson, D. A., and Iles, K. E. 2003. HNE-signaling pathways leading to its elimination. Mol. Aspects Med. 24:189–194.

Friguet, B., and Szweda, L. I. 1997. Inhibition of the multicatalytic proteinase (proteasome) by 4-hydroxy-2-nonenal cross-linked protein. FEBS Lett. 405:21–25.

Friguet, B., Stadtman, E. R., and Szweda, L. I. 1994. Modification of glucose-6-phosphate dehydrogenase by 4-hydroxynonenal. J. Biol. Chem. 269: 21639–21643.

Frye, E. B., Degenhardt, T. P., Thorpe, S. R., and Baynes, J. W. 1998. Role of the Maillard reaction in aging of tissue proteins. Advanced glycation end product-dependent increase in imidazolium cross-links in human lens proteins. J. Biol. Chem. 273:18714–18719.

Fu, M.-X., Requena, J. R., Jenkins, A. J., Lyons, T. J., Baynes, J. W., and Thorpe, S. R. 1996. The advanced glycation end product, N^{ε}-(carboxymethyl)-lysine, is a product of both lipid peroxidation and glycoxidation reactions. J. Biol. Chem. 271:9982–9986.

Furuhata, A., Ishii, T., Kumazawa, S., Yamada, T., Nakayama, T., and Uchida, K. 2003. N^{ε}-(3-methylpyridinium)lysine, a major antigenic adduct generated in acrolein-modified protein. J. Biol. Chem. 278:48658–48665.

Furuhata, A., Nakamura, M., Osawa, T., and Uchida, K. 2002. Thiolation of protein-bound carcinogenic aldehyde. An electrophilic acrolein-lysine adduct that covalently binds to thiols. J. Biol. Chem. 277:27919–27926.

Gardner, H. W. 1989. Oxygen radical chemistry of polyunsaturated fatty acids. Free Rad. Biol. Med. 7:65–86.

Gardner, H. W., and Crawford, C. G. 1981. Degradation of linoleic acid hydroperoxides by a cysteine ferric chloride catalyst as a model for similar biochemical reactions. III. A novel product, trans-12,13-epoxy-11-oxo-trans-9-octadecenoic acid, from 13-L-(*S*)-hydroperoxy-*cis*-9, trans-11-octadecadienoic acid. Biochim. Biophys. Acta 665:126–133.

Gardner, H. W., and Kleiman, R. 1981. Degradation of linoleic acid hydroperoxides by a cysteine. $FeCl_3$ catalyst as a model for similar biochemical reactions. II. Specificity in formation of fatty acid epoxides. Biochim. Biophys. Acta 665:113–125.

Glomb, M. A., and Lang, G. 2001. Isolation and characterization of glyoxal-arginine modifications. J. Agric. Food Chem. 49:1493–1501.

Glomb, M. A., and Monnier, V. M. 1995. Mechanism of protein modification by glyoxal and glycolaldehyde, reactive intermediates of the Maillard reaction. J. Biol. Chem. 270:10017–10026.

Glomb, M. A., and Pfahler, C. 2001. Amides are novel protein modifications formed by physiological sugars. J. Biol. Chem. 276:41638–41647.

Grace, J. M., MacDonald, T. L., Roberts, R. J., and Kinter, M. 1996. Determination of site-specific modifications of glucose-6-phosphate dehydrogenase by 4-hydroxy-2-nonenal using matrix assisted laser desorption time-of-flight mass spectrometry. Free Rad. Res. 25:23–29.

Grune, T., and Davies, K. J. 2003. The proteasomal system and HNE-modified proteins. Mol. Aspects Med. 24:195–204.

Gu, X., Meer, S. G., Miyagi, M., Rayborn, M. E., Hollyfield, J. G., Crabb, J. W., and Salomon, R. G. 2003. Carboxyethylpyrrole protein adducts and autoantibodies, biomarkers for age-related macular degeneration. J. Biol. Chem. 278:42027–42035.

Gugiu, B. G., and Salomon, R. G. 2003. Total syntheses of bioactive oxidized ethanolamine phospholipids. Org. Lett. 5:2797–2799.

Hansen, E., Even, Y., and Geneviere, A. M. 2004. The alpha, beta, gamma, delta-unsaturated aldehyde 2-trans-4-trans-decadienal disturbs DNA replication and mitotic events in early sea urchin embryos. Toxicol. Sci. 81:190–197.

Hao, Q., and Maret, W. 2006. Aldehydes release zinc from proteins. A pathway from oxidative stress/lipid peroxidation to cellular functions of zinc. FEBS J. 273:4300–4310.

Hashimoto, M., Sibata, T., Wasada, H., Toyokuni, S., and Uchida, K. 2003. Structural basis of protein-bound endogenous aldehydes. Chemical and immunochemical characterizations of configurational isomers of a 4-hydroxy-2-nonenal-histidine adduct. J. Biol. Chem. 278:5044–5051.

Haynes, R. L., Szweda, L., Pickin, K., Welker, M. E., and Townsend, A. J. 2000. Structure–activity relationships for growth inhibition and induction of apoptosis by 4-hydroxy-2-nonenal in raw 264.7 cells. Mol. Pharmacol. 58:788–794.

Herbst, U., Toborek, M., Kaiser, S., Mattson, M. P., and Hennig, B. 1999. 4-Hydroxynonenal induces dysfunction and apoptosis of cultured endothelial cells. J. Cell Physiol. 181:295–303.

Hidalgo, F. J., and Zamora, R. 1993. Fluorescent pyrrole products from carbonyl-amine reactions. J. Biol. Chem. 268:16190–16197.

Hidalgo, F. J., Zamora, R., and Vioque, E. 1992. Syntheses and reactions of methyl (*Z*)-9,10-epoxy-13-oxo-(*E*)-11-octadecenoate and methyl (*E*)-9,10-epoxy-13-oxo-(*E*)-11-octadecenoate. Chem. Phys. Lipids 60:225–233.

Hjelle, J. J., and Grubbs, J. H. 1982. Petersen DR. Inhibition of mitochondrial aldehyde dehydrogenase by malondialdehyde. Toxicol. Lett. 14:35–43.

Hyun, D. H., Lee, M. H., Halliwell, B., and Jenner, P. 2002. Proteasomal dysfunction induced by 4-hydroxy-2,3-*trans*-nonenal, an end-product of lipid peroxidation: a mechanism contributing to neurodegeneration? J. Neurochem. 83:360–370.

Ichihashi, K., Osawa, T., Toyokuni, S., and Uchida, K. 2001. Endogenous formation of protein adducts with carcinogenic aldehydes: implications for oxidative stress. J. Biol. Chem. 276:23903–23913.

Ishii, T., Tatsuda, E., Kumazawa, S., Nakayama, T., and Uchida, K. 2003. Molecular basis of enzyme inactivation by an endogenous electrophile 4-hydroxy-2-nonenal: identification of modification sites in glyceraldehyde-3-phosphate dehydrogenase. Biochemistry 42:3474–3480.

Isom, A. L., Barnes, S., Wilson, L., Kirk, M., Coward, L., and Darley-Usmar, V. 2004. Modification of cytochrome c by 4-hydroxy-2-nonenal: evidence for histidine, lysine, and arginine-aldehyde adducts. J. Am. Soc. Mass. Spectrom. 15:1136–1147.

Itakura, K., Furuhata, A., Shibata, N., Kobayashi, M., and Uchida, K. 2003. Maillard reaction-like lysine modification by a lipid peroxidation product: immunochemical detection of protein-bound 2-hydroxyheptanal in vivo. Biochem. Biophys. Res. Commun. 308:452–457.

Itakura, K., Osawa, T., and Uchida, K. 1998. Structure of a fluorescent compound formed from 4-hydroxy-2-nonenal and N^{α}-hippuryllysine: A model for fluorophores derived from protein modification by lipid peroxidation. J. Org. Chem. 63:185–187.

Itakura, K., and Uchida, K. 2001. Evidence that malondialdehyde-derived aminoenamine is not a fluorescent age pigment. Chem. Res. Toxicol. 14:473–475.

Itakura, K., and Uchida, K. 2003. Reaction of *N*(alpha)-hippuryllysine with 2-hydroxyheptanal: a model for lysine-directed protein modifications by lipid peroxidation. Chem. Phys. Lipids. 124:81–88.

Itakura, K., Uchida, K., and Osawa, T. 1996. A novel fluorescent malondialdehyde-lysine adduct. Chem. Phys. Lipids 84:75–79.

Iyer, R. S., Kobierski, M. E., and Salomon, R. G. 1994. Generation of pyrroles in the reaction of levuglandin E2 with proteins. J. Org. Chem. 59:6038–6043.

Ji, C., Amarnath, V., Pietenpol, J. A., and Marnett, L. J. 2001. 4-hydroxynonenal induces apoptosis via caspase-3 activation and cytochrome *c* release. Chem. Res. Toxicol. 14:1090–1096.

Ji, C., Kozak, K. R., and Marnett, L. J. 2001. IkappaB kinase, a molecular target for inhibition by 4-hydroxy-2-nonenal. J. Biol. Chem. 276:18223–18228.

Jian, W., Lee, S. H., Arora, J. S., Silva Elipe, M. V., and Blair, I. A. 2005a. Unexpected formation of etheno-2′-deoxyguanosine adducts from 5(*S*)-hydroperoxyeicosatetraenoic acid: evidence for a *bis*-hydroperoxide intermediate. Chem. Res. Toxicol. 18:599–610.

Jian, W., Arora, J. S., Oe, T., Shuvaev, V. V., and Blair, I. A. 2005b. Induction of endothelial cell apoptosis by lipid hydroperoxide-derived bifunctional electrophiles. Free Rad. Biol. Med. 39:1162–1176.

Jirousek, M. R., Murthi, K. K., and Salomon, R. G. 1990. Electrophilic levuglandin E2-protein adducts bind glycine: a model for protein crosslinking. Prostaglandins 40:187–203.

Kamido, H., Kuksis, A., Marai, L., and Myher, J. J. 1995. Lipid ester-bound aldehydes among copper-catalyzed peroxidation products of human plasma lipoproteins. J. Lipid Res. 36:1876–1886.

Kasai, H., Iwamoto-Tanaka, N., and Fukada, S. 1998. DNA modifications by the mutagen glyoxal: adduction to G and C, deamination of C and GC and GA cross-linking. Carcinogenesis 19:1459–1465.

Kato, H., Kaneko, S., Okitani, A., Ito, M., and Hayase, F. 1986. Modification of lysine residues to alkyl-substituted pyridiniums on exposure of proteins to vaporized hexanal. Agric. Biol. Chem. 50:1223–1228.

Kawai, K., Matsuno, K., and Kasai, H. 2006. Detection of 4-oxo-2-hexenal, a novel mutagenic product of lipid peroxidation, in human diet and cooking vapor. Mutat. Res. 603:186–192.

Kawai, Y., Furuhata, A., Toyokuni, S., Aratani, Y., and Uchida, K. 2003. Formation of acrolein-derived 2′-deoxyadenosine adduct in an iron-induced carcinogenesis model. J. Biol. Chem. 278:50346–50354.

Kawai, Y., Takeda, S., and Terao, J. 2007. Lipidomic analysis for lipid peroxidation-derived aldehydes using gas chromatography–mass spectrometry. Chem. Res. Toxicol. 20:99–107.

Keller, J. N., Hanni, K. B., and Markesbery, W. R. 1999. 4-hydroxynonenal increases neuronal susceptibility to oxidative stress. J. Neurosci. Res. 58:823–830.

Keller, J. N., and Mattson, M. P. 1998. Roles of lipid peroxidation in modulation of cellular signaling pathways, cell dysfunction, and death in the nervous system. Rev. Neurosci. 9:105–116.

Kern, W., and Spiteller, G. 1996. Synthesis and properties of natural occurring α-hydroxyaldehydes. Tetrahedron 52:4347–4362.

Kikugawa, K., and Beppu, M. 1987. Involvement of lipid oxidation products in the formation of fluorescent and cross-linked proteins. Chem. Phys. Lipids 44:277–296.

Kozekov, I. D., Nechev, L. V., Sanchez, A., Harris, C. M., Lloyd, R. S., and Harris, T. M. 2001. Interchain cross-linking of DNA mediated by the principal adduct of acrolein. Chem. Res. Toxicol. 4:1482–1485.

Kruman, I., Bruce-Keller, A. J., Bredesen, D., Waeg, G., and Mattson, M. P. 1997. Evidence that 4-hydroxynonenal mediates oxidative stress-induced neuronal apoptosis. J. Neurosci. 17:5089–5100.

Kumagai, T., Matsukawa, N., Kaneko, Y., Kusumi, Y., Mitsumata, M., and Uchida, K. 2004. A lipid peroxidation-derived inflammatory mediator: identification of 4-hydroxy-2-nonenal as a potential inducer of cyclooxygenase-2 in macrophages. J. Biol. Chem. 279:48389–48396.

Kurtz, A. J., and Lloyd, R. S. 2003. 1,*N*2-deoxyguanosine adducts of acrolein, crotonaldehyde, and trans-4-hydroxynonenal cross-link to peptides via Schiff base linkage. J. Biol. Chem. 278:5970–5976.

Laurora, S., Tamagno, E., Briatore, F., Bardini, P., Pizzimenti, S., Toaldo, C., Reffo, P., Costelli, P., Dianzani, M. U., Danni, O., and Barrera, G. 2005. 4-Hydroxynonenal modulation of p53 family gene expression in the SK-N-BE neuroblastoma cell line. Free Rad. Biol. Med. 38:215–225.

Le Curieux, F., Pluskota, D., Munter, T., Sjoholm, R., and Kronberg, L. 2000. Identification of fluorescent 2′-deoxyadenosine adducts formed in reactions of conjugates of malonaldehyde and acetaldehyde, and of malonaldehyde and formaldehyde. Chem. Res. Toxicol. 13:1228–1234.

Lee, S. H., and Blair, I. A. 2000. Characterization of 4-oxo-2-nonenal as a novel product of lipid peroxidation. Chem. Res. Toxicol. 13:698–702.

Lee, S. H., Oe, T., and Blair, I. A. 2001. Vitamin C-induced decomposition of lipid hydroperoxides to endogenous genotoxins. Science 292:2083–2086.

Lee, S. H., Oe, T., and Blair, I. A. 2002. 4,5-Epoxy-2(*E*)-decenal-induced formation of 1,*N*(6)-etheno-2′-deoxyadenosine and 1,*N*(2)-etheno-2′-deoxyguanosine adducts. Chem. Res. Toxicol. 15:300–304.

Lee, S. H., Silva Elipe, M. V., Arora, J. S., and Blair, I. A. 2005. Dioxododecenoic acid: a lipid hydroperoxide-derived bifunctional electrophile responsible for etheno DNA adduct formation. Chem. Res. Toxicol. 18:566–578.

Leonarduzzi, G., Robbesyn, F., and Poli, G. 2004. Signaling kinases modulated by 4-hydroxynonenal. Free Rad. Biol. Med. 37:1694–1702.

Lim, P., Sadre-Bazzaz, K., Shurter, J., Sarasin, A., and Termini, J. 2003. DNA damage and mutations induced by arachidonic acid peroxidation. Biochemistry 42:15036–15044.

Lin, D. 2007. Modification and cross-linking of proteins by lipoxidation derived electrophiles: chemical and biological consequences. Ph.D. Thesis, Case Western Reserve University, Cleveland.

Lin, D., Lee, H.-G., Liu, Q., Perry, G., Smith, M. A., and Sayre, L. M. 2005. 4-Oxo-2-nonenal is both more neurotoxic and more protein reactive than 4-hydroxy-2-nonenal. Chem. Res. Toxicol. 18:1219–1231.

Liu, Z., Minkler, P. E., and Sayre, L. M. 2003. Mass spectroscopic characterization of protein modification by 4-hydroxy-2-(*E*)-nonenal and 4-oxo-2-(*E*)-nonenal. Chem. Res. Toxicol. 16:901–911.

Liu, Z., and Sayre, L. M. 2003. Model studies on the modification of proteins by lipoxidation-derived 2-hydroxyaldehydes. Chem. Res. Toxicol. 16:232–241.

Liu-Snyder, P., McNally, H., Shi, R., and Borgens, R. B. 2006. Acrolein-mediated mechanisms of neuronal death. J. Neurosci. Res. 84:209–218.

Loidl-Stahlhofen, A., and Spiteller, G. 1994. alpha-Hydroxyaldehydes, products of lipid peroxidation. Biochim. Biophys. Acta. 1211:156–160.

Lopachin, R. M., Barber, D. S., Geohagen, B. C., Gavin, T., He, D., and Das, S. 2007. Structure–toxicity analysis of type-2 alkenes: in vitro neurotoxicity. Toxicol. Sci. 95:136–146.

Loureiro, A. P., de Arruda Campos, I. P., Gomes, O. F., di Mascio, P., and Medeiros, M. H. 2004. Structural characterization of diastereoisomeric ethano adducts derived from the reaction of 2′-deoxyguanosine with *trans, trans*-2,4-decadienal. Chem. Res. Toxicol. 17:641–649.

Loureiro, A. P., Di Mascio, P., Gomes, O. F., and Medeiros, M. H. 2000. *Trans*,-*trans*-2,4-decadienal-induced 1,*N*(2)-etheno-2′-deoxyguanosine adduct formation. Chem. Res. Toxicol. 13:601–609.

Lovell, M. A., and Markesbery, W. R. 2006. Amyloid beta peptide, 4-hydroxynonenal and apoptosis. Curr. Alzheimer Res. 3:359–364.

Lu, C., Chan, S. L., Fu, W., and Mattson, M. P. 2002. The lipid peroxidation product 4-hydroxynonenal facilitates opening of voltage-dependent Ca2+ channels in neurons by increasing protein tyrosine phosphorylation. J. Biol. Chem. 277:24368–24375.

Maekawa, M., Kawai, K., Takahashi, Y., Nakamura, H., Watanabe, T., Sawa, R., Hachisuka, K., and Kasai, H. 2006. Identification of 4-oxo-2-hexenal and other direct mutagens formed in model lipid peroxidation reactions as dGuo adducts. Chem. Res. Toxicol. 19:130–138.

Malecki, A., Garrido, R., Mattson, M. P., Hennig, B., and Toborek, M. 2000. 4-Hydroxynonenal induces oxidative stress and death of cultured spinal cord neurons. J. Neurochem. 74:2278–2287.

Mao, H., Reddy, G. R., Marnett, L. J., and Stone, M. P. 1999. Solution structure of an oligodeoxynucleotide containing the malondialdehyde deoxyguanosine adduct *N*2-(3-oxo-1-propenyl)-dG (ring-opened M1G) positioned in a (CpG)3 frameshift hotspot of the *Salmonella typhimurium* hisD3052 gene. Biochemistry 38:13491–13501.

Marnett, L. J., Basu, A. K., O'Hara, S. M., Weller, P. E., Maqsudur Rahman, A. F. M., and Oliver, J. P. 1986. Reaction of malondialdehyde with guanine nucleosides: formation of adducts containing oxadiazabicyclononene residues in the base-pairing region. J. Am. Chem. Soc. 108:1348–1350.

Marnett, L. J., Riggins, J. N., and West, J. D. 2003. Endogenous generation of reactive oxidants and electrophiles and their reactions with DNA and protein. J. Clin. Invest. 111:583–593.

Mitchell, D. Y., and Petersen, D. R. 1988. Inhibition of rat liver aldehyde dehydrogenases by acrolein. Drug Metab. Dispos. 16:37–42.

Mitchell, D. Y., and Petersen, D. R. 1991. Inhibition of rat hepatic mitochondrial aldehyde dehydrogenase-mediated acetaldehyde oxidation by trans-4-hydroxy-2-nonenal. Hepatology 13:728–734.

Mlakar, A., and Spiteller, G. 1994. Reinvestigation of lipid peroxidation of linolenic acid. Biochim. Biophys. Acta. 1214:209–220.
Mlakar, A., and Spiteller, G. 1996. Previously unknown aldehydic lipid peroxidation compounds of arachidonic acid. Chem. Phys. Lipids 79:47–53.
Montine, K. S., Kim, P. J., Olson, S. J., Markesbery, W. R., and Montine, T. J. 1997a. 4-Hydroxy-2-nonenal pyrrole adducts in human neurodegenerative disease. J. Neuropathol. Exp. Neurol. 56:866–871.
Montine, K. S., Olson, S. J., Amarnath, V., Whetsell, W. O. Jr, Graham, D. G., and Montine, T. J. 1997b. Immunohistochemical detection of 4-hydroxy-2-nonenal adducts in Alzheimer's disease is associated with inheritance of APOE4. Am. J. Pathol. 150:437–443.
Montine, T. J., Huang, D. Y., Valentine, W. M., Amarnath, V., Saunders, A., Weisgraber, K. H., Graham, D. G., and Strittmatter, W. J. 1996. Crosslinking of apolipoprotein E by products of lipid peroxidation. J. Neuropathol. Exp. Neurol. 55:202–210.
Mukai, F. H., and Goldstein, B. D. 1976. Mutagenicity of malonaldehyde, a decomposition product of peroxidized polyunsaturated fatty acids. Science 191:868–869.
Murthi, K. K., Friedman, L. R., Oleinick, N. L., and Salomon, R. G. 1993. Formation of DNA–protein cross-links in mammalian cells by levuglandin E2. Biochemistry 32:4090–4097.
Murthi, K. K., Salomon, R. G., and Sternlicht, H. 1990. Levuglandin E2 inhibits mitosis and microtubule assembly. Prostaglandins 39:611–622.
Nadkarni, D. V., and Sayre, L. M. 1995. Structural definition of early lysine and histidine adduction chemistry of 4-hydroxynonenal. Chem. Res. Toxicol. 8:284–291.
Nair, V., Offerman, R. J., Turner, G. A., Pryor, A. N., and Baenziger, N. C. 1988. Fluorescent 1,4-dihydropyridines: the malondialdehyde connection. Tetrahedron 44:2793–2803.
O'Brien, P. J., Siraki, A. G., and Shangari, N. 2005. Aldehyde sources, metabolism, molecular toxicity mechanisms, and possible effects on human health. Crit. Rev. Toxicol. 35:609–662.
Oe, T., Arora, J. S., Lee, S. H., and Blair, I. A. 2003a. A novel lipid hydroperoxide-derived cyclic covalent modification to histone H4. J. Biol. Chem. 278:42098–42105.
Oe, T., Lee, S. H., Silva Elipe, M. V., Arison, B. H., and Blair, I. A. 2003b. A novel lipid hydroperoxide-derived modification to arginine. Chem. Res. Toxicol. 16:1598–1605.
Okada, K., Wangpoengtrakul, C., Osawa, T., Toyokuni, S., Tanaka, K., and Uchida, K. 1999. 4-Hydroxy-2-nonenal-mediated impairment of intracellular proteolysis during oxidative stress. Identification of proteasomes as target molecules. J. Biol. Chem. 274:23787–23793.
O'Neil, J., Hoppe, G., Sayre, L. M., and Hoff, H. F. 1997. Inactivation of cathepsin B by oxidized LDL involves complex formation induced by binding of putative reactive sites exposed at low pH to thiols on the enzyme. Free Rad. Biol. Med. 23:215–225.
Orioli, M., Aldini, G., Beretta, G., Facino, R. M., and Carini, M. 2005. LC-ESI-MS/MS determination of 4-hydroxy-trans-2-nonenal Michael adducts with cysteine and histidine-containing peptides as early markers of oxidative stress in excitable tissues. J. Chromatogr. B Analyt. Technol. Biomed. Life Sci. 827:109–118.
Pan, J., and Chung, F. L. 2002. Formation of cyclic deoxyguanosine adducts from omega-3 and omega-6 polyunsaturated fatty acids under oxidative conditions. Chem. Res. Toxicol. 15:367–372.

Pawlowicz, A. J., Munter, T., Klika, K. D., and Kronberg, L. 2006. Reaction of acrolein with 2′-deoxyadenosine and 9-ethyladenine – formation of cyclic adducts. Bioorg. Chem. 34:39–48.

Pollack, M., Oe, T., Lee, S. H., Silva Elipe, M. V., Arison, B. H., and Blair, I. A. 2003. Characterization of 2′-deoxycytidine adducts derived from 4-oxo-2-nonenal, a novel lipid peroxidation product. Chem. Res. Toxicol. 16:893–900.

Requena, J. R., Fu, M. X., Ahmed, M. U., Jenkins, A. J., Lyons, T. J., Baynes, J. W., and Thorpe, S. R. 1997. Quantification of malondialdehyde and 4-hydroxynonenal adducts to lysine residues in native and oxidized human low-density lipoprotein. Biochem. J. 322:317–325.

Rindgen, D., Lee, S. H., Nakajima, M., and Blair, I. A. 2000. Formation of a substituted 1,*N*(6)-etheno-2′-deoxyadenosine adduct by lipid hydroperoxide-mediated generation of 4-oxo-2-nonenal. Chem. Res. Toxicol. 13:846–852.

Salomon, R. G. 2005. Levuglandins and isolevuglandins: stealthy toxins of oxidative injury. Antioxid. Redox. Signal 7:185–201.

Salomon, R. G., Kaur, K., Podrez, E., Hoff, H. F., Krushinsky, A. V., and Sayre, L. M. 2000. HNE-derived 2-pentylpyrroles are generated during oxidation of LDL, are more prevalent in blood plasma from patients with renal disease or atherosclerosis, and are present in atherosclerotic plaques. Chem. Res. Toxicol. 13:557–564.

Sayre, L. M., Arora, P. K., Iyer, R. S., and Salomon, R. G. 1993. Pyrrole formation from 4-hydroxynonenal and primary amines. Chem. Res. Toxicol. 6:19–22.

Sayre, L. M., Lin, D., Yuan, Q., Zhu, X., and Tang, X. 2006. Protein adducts generated from products of lipid oxidation: focus on HNE and ONE. Drug Metab. Rev. 38:651–675.

Sayre, L. M., Sha, W., Xu, G., Kaur, K., Nadkarni, D., Subbanagounder, G., and Salomon, R. G. 1996. Immunochemical evidence supporting 2-pentylpyrrole formation on proteins exposed to 4-hydroxy-2-nonenal. Chem. Res. Toxicol. 9:1194–1201.

Sayre, L. M., Smith, M. A., and Perry, G. 2001. Chemistry and biochemistry of oxidative stress in neurodegenerative disease. Curr. Med. Chem. 8:721–738.

Sayre, L. M., Zelasko, D. A., Harris, P. L., Perry, G., Salomon, R. G., and Smith, M. A. 1997. 4-Hydroxynonenal-derived advanced lipid peroxidation end products are increased in Alzheimer's disease. J. Neurochem. 68:2092–2097.

Sevilla, C. L., Mahle, N. H., Eliezer, N., Uzieblo, A., O'Hara, S. M., Nokubo, M., Miller, R., Rouzer, C. A., and Marnett, L. J. 1997. Development of monoclonal antibodies to the malondialdehyde-deoxyguanosine adduct, pyrimidopurinone. Chem. Res. Toxicol. 10:172–180.

Shapiro, R., and Hachmann, J. 1966. The reaction of guanine derivatives with 1,2-dicarbonyl compounds. Biochemistry 5:2799–2807.

Shibata, N., Yamada, S., Uchida, K., Hirano, A., Sakoda, S., Fujimura, H., Sasaki, S., Iwata, M., Toi, S., Kawaguchi, M., Yamamoto, T., and Kobayashi, M. 2004. Accumulation of protein-bound 4-hydroxy-2-hexenal in spinal cords from patients with sporadic amyotrophic lateral sclerosis. Brain Res. 1019:170–177.

Siems, W. G., Hapner, S. J., and van Kuijk, F. J. 1996. 4-Hydroxynonenal inhibits Na(+)-K(+)-ATPase. Free Rad. Biol. Med. 20:215–223.

Slatter, D. A., Avery, N. C., and Bailey, A. J. 2004. Identification of a new cross-link and unique histidine adduct from bovine serum albumin incubated with malondialdehyde. J. Biol. Chem. 279:61–69.

Slatter, D. A., Murray, M., and Bailey, A. J. 1998. Formation of a dihydropyridine derivative as a potential cross-link derived from malondialdehyde in physiological systems. FEBS Lett. 421:180–184.

Smith, R. A., Williamson, D. S., Cerny, R. L., and Cohen, S. M. 1990. Detection of 1,*N*6-propanodeoxyadenosine in acrolein-modified polydeoxyadenylic acid and DNA by 32P postlabeling. Cancer Res. 50:3005–3012.

Smith, S. A., Pestka, J. J., Gray, J. I., and Smith, D. M. 1999. Production and specificity of polyclonal antibodies to hexanal-lysine adducts. J. Agric. Food Chem. 47:1389–1395.

Sowell, J., Frei, B., and Stevens, J. F. 2004. Vitamin C conjugates of genotoxic lipid peroxidation products: structural characterization and detection in human plasma. Proc. Natl. Acad. Sci. U.S.A. 101:17964–17969.

Spiteller, P., Kern, W., Reiner, J., and Spiteller, G. 2001. Aldehydic lipid peroxidation products derived from linoleic acid. Biochim. Biophys. Acta 1531:188–208.

Srivastava, S., Watowich, S. J., Petrash, J. M., Srivastava, S. K., and Bhatnagar, A. 1999. Structural and kinetic determinants of aldehyde reduction by aldose reductase. Biochemistry 38:42–54.

Stapelfeldt, H., and Skibsted, L. H. 1996. Kinetics of formation of fluorescent products from hexanal and L-lysine in a two-phase system. Lipids 31:1125–1132.

Steinhilber, D. 1999. 5-Lipoxygenase: a target for antiinflammatory drugs revisited. Curr. Med. Chem. 6:71–85.

Tanel, A., and Averill-Bates, D. A. 2005. The aldehyde acrolein induces apoptosis via activation of the mitochondrial pathway. Biochim. Biophys. Acta 1743:255–267.

Tanito, M., Elliott, M. H., Kotake, Y., and Anderson, R. E. 2005. Protein modifications by 4-hydroxynonenal and 4-hydroxyhexenal in light-exposed rat retina. Invest. Ophthalmol. Vis. Sci. 46:3859–3868.

Tsai, L., Szweda, P. A., Vinogradova, O., and Szweda, L. I. 1998. Structural characterization and immunochemical detection of a fluorophore derived from 4-hydroxy-2-nonenal and lysine. Proc. Natl. Acad. Sci. U.S.A. 95:7975–7980.

Tuma, D. J. 2002. Role of malondialdehyde-acetaldehyde adducts in liver injury. Free Rad. Biol. Med. 32:303–308.

Uchida, K. 1999. Current status of acrolein as a lipid peroxidation product. Trends Cardiovasc. Med. 9:109–113.

Uchida, K. 2003. 4-Hydroxy-2-nonenal: a product and mediator of oxidative stress. Prog. Lipid Res. 42:318–343.

Uchida, K., Itakura, K., Kawakishi, S., Hiai, H., Toyokuni, S., and Stadtman, E. R. 1995. Characterization of epitopes recognized by 4-hydroxy-2-nonenal specific antibodies. Arch. Biochem. Biophys. 324:241–248.

Uchida, K., Kanematsu, M., Morimitsu, Y., Osawa, T., Noguchi, N., and Niki, E. 1998a. Acrolein is a product of lipid peroxidation reaction. Formation of free acrolein and its conjugate with lysine residues in oxidized low density lipoproteins. J. Biol. Chem. 273:16058–16066.

Uchida, K., Kanematsu, M., Sakai, K., Matsuda, T., Hattori, N., Mizuno, Y., Suzuki, D., Miyata, T., Noguchi, N., Niki, E., and Osawa, T. 1998b. Protein-bound acrolein: potential markers for oxidative stress. Proc. Natl. Acad. Sci. U. S.A. 95:4882–4887.

Uchida, K., Sakai, K., Tiakura, K., Osawa, T., and Toyokuni, S. 1997. Protein modification by lipid peroxidation products: formation of malondialdehyde-derived N^{ε}-(2-propenal)lysine in proteins. Arch. Biochem. Biophys. 346:45–52.

Uchida, K., and Stadtman, E. R. 1992. Modification of histidine residues in proteins by reaction with 4-hydroxynonenal. Proc. Natl. Acad. Sci. U.S.A. 89:4544–4548.

Uchida, K., and Stadtman, E. R. 1993. Covalent attachment of 4-hydroxynonenal to glyceraldehyde-3-phosphate dehydrogenase. J. Biol. Chem. 268:6388–6393.

Uchida, K., Szweda, L. I., Chae, H.-Z., and Stadtman, E. R. 1993. Immunochemical detection of 4-hydroxynonenal protein adducts in oxidized hepatocytes. Proc. Natl. Acad. Sci. U.S.A. 90:8742–8746.

VanderVeen, L. A., Hashim, M. F., Shyr, Y., and Marnett, L. J. 2003. Induction of frameshift and base pair substitution mutations by the major DNA adduct of the endogenous carcinogen malondialdehyde. Proc. Natl. Acad. Sci. U. S. A. 100:14247–14252.

Wataya, T., Nunomura, A., Smith, M. A., Siedlak, S. L., Harris, P. L., Shimohama, S., Szweda, L. I., Kaminski, M. A., Avila, J., Price, D. L., Cleveland, D. W., Sayre, L. M., and Perry, G. 2002. High molecular weight neurofilament proteins are physiological substrates of adduction by the lipid peroxidation product hydroxynonenal. J. Biol. Chem. 277:4644–4648.

Wells-Knecht, K. J., Brinkmann, E., and Baynes, J. W. 1995. Characterization of an imidazolium salt formed from glyoxal and *N*-alpha-hippuryllysine: a model for Maillard reaction crosslinks in proteins. J. Org. Chem. 60:6246–6247.

Werz, O., and Steinhilber, D. 2005. Development of 5-lipoxygenase inhibitors – lessons from cellular enzyme regulation. Biochem. Pharmacol. 70:327–333.

West, J. D., Ji, C., Duncan, S. T., Amarnath, V., Schneider, C., Rizzo, C. J., Brash, A. R., and Marnett, L. J. 2004. Induction of apoptosis in colorectal carcinoma cells treated with 4-hydroxy-2-nonenal and structurally related aldehydic products of lipid peroxidation. Chem. Res. Toxicol. 17:453–462.

West, J. D., and Marnett, L. J. 2005. Alterations in gene expression induced by the lipid peroxidation product, 4-hydroxy-2-nonenal. Chem. Res. Toxicol. 18:1642–1653.

Witz, G. 1989. Biological interactions of alpha,beta-unsaturated aldehydes. Free Rad. Biol. Med. 7:333–349.

Xu, D., Thiele, G. M., Kearley, M. L., Haugen, M. D., Klassen, L. W., Sorrell, M. F., and Tuma, D. J. 1997. Epitope characterization of malondialdehyde-acetaldehyde adducts using an enzyme-linked immunosorbent assay. Chem. Res. Toxicol. 10:978–986.

Xu, G., Liu, Y., Kansal, M. M., and Sayre, L. M. 1999. Rapid cross-linking of proteins by 4-ketoaldehydes and 4-hydroxy-2-alkenals does not arise from the lysine-derived monoalkylpyrroles. Chem. Res. Toxicol. 12:855–861.

Xu, G., Liu, Y., and Sayre, L. M. 1999. Independent synthesis, solution behavior, and studies on the mechanism of formation of a primary amine-derived fluorophore representing crosslinking of proteins by (*E*)-4-hydroxy-2-nonenal (HNE). J. Org. Chem. 64:5732–5745.

Xu, G., Liu, Y., and Sayre, L. M. 2000. Polyclonal antibodies to a fluorescent 4-hydroxy-2-nonenal (HNE)-derived lysine-lysine cross-link: characterization and application to HNE-treated protein and in vitro oxidized low-density lipoprotein. Chem. Res. Toxicol. 13:406–413.

Xu, G., and Sayre, L. M. 1998. Structural characterization of a 4-hydroxy-2-alkenal-derived fluorophore that contributes to lipoperoxidation-dependent protein cross-linking in aging and degenerative disease. Chem. Res. Toxicol. 11:247–251.

Yamada, S., Funada, T., Shibata, N., Kobayashi, M., Kawai, Y., Tatsuda, E., Furuhata, A., and Uchida, K. 2004. Protein-bound 4-hydroxy-2-hexenal as a marker of oxidized n-3 polyunsaturated fatty acids. J. Lipid Res. 45:626–634.

Yocum, A. K., Oe, T., Yergey, A. L., and Blair, I. A. 2005. Novel lipid hydroperoxide-derived hemoglobin histidine adducts as biomarkers of oxidative stress. J. Mass Spectrom. 40:754–764.

Yoritaka, A., Hattori, N., Uchida, K., Tanaka, M., Stadtman, E. R., and Mizuno, Y. 1996. Immunohistochemical detection of 4-hydroxynonenal protein adducts in Parkinsons disease. Proc. Natl. Acad. Sci. U. S. A. 93:2696–2701.

Yuan, Q. 2006. Modifications of biomolecules by lipoxidation derived aldehydes. Ph.D. Thesis, Case Western Reserve University.

Zamora, R., Alaiz, M., and Hidalgo, F. J. 1999. Modification of histidine residues by 4,5-epoxy-2-alkenals. Chem. Res. Toxicol. 12:654–660.

Zamora, R., Gallardo, E., Navarro, J. L., and Hidalgo, F. J. 2005. Strecker-type degradation of phenylalanine by methyl 9,10-epoxy-13-oxo-11-octadecenoate and methyl 12,13-epoxy-9-oxo-11-octadecenoate. J. Agric. Food Chem. 53:4583–4588.

Zamora, R., and Hidalgo, F. J. 1994. Modification of lysine amino groups by the lipid peroxidation product 4,5(*E*)-epoxy-2(*E*)-heptenal. Lipids 29:243–249.

Zamora, R., and Hidalgo, F. J. 2005. 2-Alkylpyrrole formation from 4,5-epoxy-2-alkenals. Chem. Res. Toxicol. 18:342–348.

Zhang, D., Dhillon, H. S., Mattson, M. P., Yurek, D. M., and Prasad, R. M. 1999. Immunohistochemical detection of the lipid peroxidation product 4-hydroxynonenal after experimental brain injury in the rat. Neurosci. Lett. 272:57–61.

Zhang, W.-H., Liu, J., Xu, G., Yuan, Q., and Sayre, L. M. 2003. Model studies on protein side chain modification by 4-oxo-2-nonenal Chem. Res. Toxicol. 16:512–523.

Zhu, X., and Sayre, L. M. 2007a. Mass spectrometric evidence for long-lived protein adducts of 4-oxo-2-nonenal. Redox. Rep. 12:45–49.

Zhu, X., and Sayre, L. M. 2007b. Long-lived 4-oxo-2-enal-derived apparent lysine Michael adducts are actually the isomeric 4-ketoamides. Chem. Res. Toxicol. 20:165–170.

9

Bioactivation and Protein Modification Reactions of Unsaturated Aldehydes

J. Cai[1], B.G. Hill[2,3,4], A. Bhatnagar[2,3,4], W.M. Pierce, Jr.[1] and R.A. Prough[2]
[1]*Departments of Pharmacology and Toxicology, University of Louisville School of Medicine, the University of Louisville, Louisville, KY 40292, USA*
[2]*Biochemistry and Molecular Biology, University of Louisville School of Medicine, the University of Louisville, Louisville, KY 40292, USA*
[3]*Division of Cardiology, Department of Medicine, University of Louisville School of Medicine, the University of Louisville, Louisville, KY 40292, USA*
[4]*Institute of Molecular Cardiology, University of Louisville School of Medicine, the University of Louisville, Louisville, KY 40292, USA*
e-mail: russ.prough@louisville.edu

Keywords: Biotransformation of α,β-Unsaturated Aldehydes · Protein Modification · Protein–GSH Adducts · Protein–Aldehyde Adducts · Acrolein · 4-Hydroxynonenal · Heart · Aorta · Endothelial Cells

9.1. Processes that Produce Aldehydes

Among the foreign compounds that have been shown to promote protein modification, aldehydes are notable due to their reactivity and prevalence in the environment and production in vivo. Humans are exposed to aldehydes from several exogenous and endogenous sources. Combustion processes from forest fires, open heating and cooking facilities, cigarette smoke, and energy production (coal-powered electrical plants) are prevalent sources of aldehydes. Furthermore, their use as chemicals to preserve organic materials like wood or their use as herbicide, fungicide, and germicide materials increases the likelihood of exogenous aldehyde exposure. Endogenously, the metabolism of biological and exogenous amines, alcohols, and lipids produces aldehydes. Although many of these processes are necessary metabolic pathways for energy production, other processes also produce aldehydes. These include unproductive lipid oxidation, infection, inflammation, chemically induced lipid peroxidation, or foreign compound metabolism involved in the detoxification of drugs or toxic chemicals. Some of these aldehydes are highly reactive, such as the α,β-unsaturated aldehydes, for example, 4-hydroxy-*trans*-2-nonenal (HNE) or acrolein, formed during lipid peroxidation or combustion. As the process

A.A. Elfarra (ed.), *Advances in Bioactivation Research*, DOI: 10.1007/978-0-387-77300-1_9,

of lipid peroxidation associated with oxidative stress becomes better understood, we note that some of the products formed may have biological functions as signaling molecules (Ruef et al. 1998; Ji, Kozak and Marnett 2004; Robino et al. 2001). Their properties require continued study to fully appreciate the effects these molecules have in biological systems. Several recent reviews thoroughly explore the possible role of endogenously generated aldehydes in mitogenic or proliferative processes, including those associated with aberrant glucose metabolism associated with diabetes and atherosclerosis (Ruef et al. 1998).

9.2. Metabolism of Aldehydes

Since there are a number of recent reviews on the metabolism of aldehydes, the focus in this article will not be directed toward the disposition of aldehydes by enzymatic oxidation or reduction reactions. However, our intent is to address how aldehydes form adducts with cellular nucleophiles in general, and with proteins in particular. A classic example of the adduction of thiols is the reaction catalyzed by glutathione S-transferases. These enzymes play important roles in metabolizing aldehydes and the reaction catalyzed by them is similar to the reactions that occur when aldehyde–protein adducts are formed spontaneously. Enzymatic pathways for aldehyde disposition have been recently reviewed by Conklin, Prough and Bhatnagar (2006).

In addition to oxidative, reductive, and conjugative metabolic transformations, aldehydes also participate in adduction reactions with several nucleophilic species in cells, including nucleic acids and proteins. Much of the toxicity of aldehydes may be linked with their ability to form adducts with proteins. Like metabolism, adduction of proteins is not static; it is a dynamic process. To examine the intracellular fate of protein–aldehyde adducts, we treated rat aortic smooth muscle (RASM) cells with reagent HNE. After removal of media containing HNE, fresh media was added and the cells were cultured in media without HNE. At appropriate times, the cells were collected, lysed, and protein adducts were quantified by

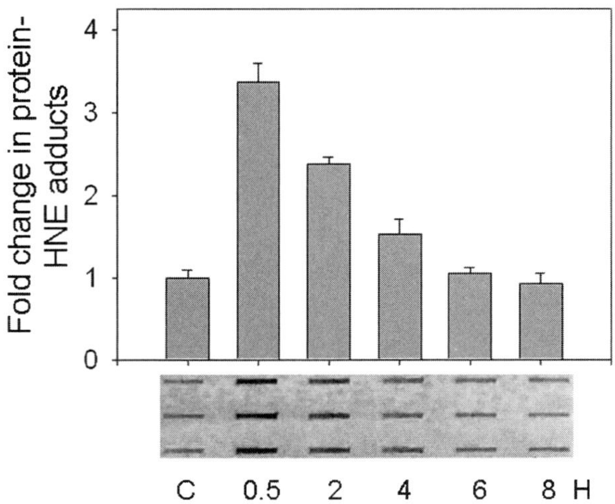

Figure 9.1 Removal of protein–HNE adducts in vascular cells. Anti-protein–HNE immunoblot analysis was performed on lysates from HNE-treated rat aortic smooth muscle (RASM) cells. RASM cells (5×10^5 cells ml^{-1}) were exposed to 50-μM HNE for 30 minutes. The medium was then removed and the cells were either collected or HNE-free growth medium was added to the cells for the indicated times. Cells were then lysed and protein–HNE adduct levels were assessed by slot immunoblotting with anti-protein–HNE antibodies. The figure is representative of at least three experiments. $n = 6$ per group.

immunoslot blotting using anti-protein–HNE antibodies. As shown in Figure 9.1, the level of anti-protein–HNE immune complexes increased more than three- to fourfold after 30 minutes of HNE treatment. The protein–HNE adducts disappeared during the next 8 hours in culture, until the level of protein–HNE complexes returned to the levels seen before treatment. These results clearly show that in exposed cells aldehydes rapidly form protein adducts and further that these adducts are removed from cells with time. The processes that allow adduct formation and the removal of protein–HNE adducts in these vascular cells are processes of importance in understanding aldehyde toxicity. Critical questions arise, such as, what are the reactions that form these adducts, are they reversible, and are they processed in the cell by proteolytic mechanisms? Studies are in progress in our laboratory to address the nature of these reactions and to identify the biochemical processes involved.

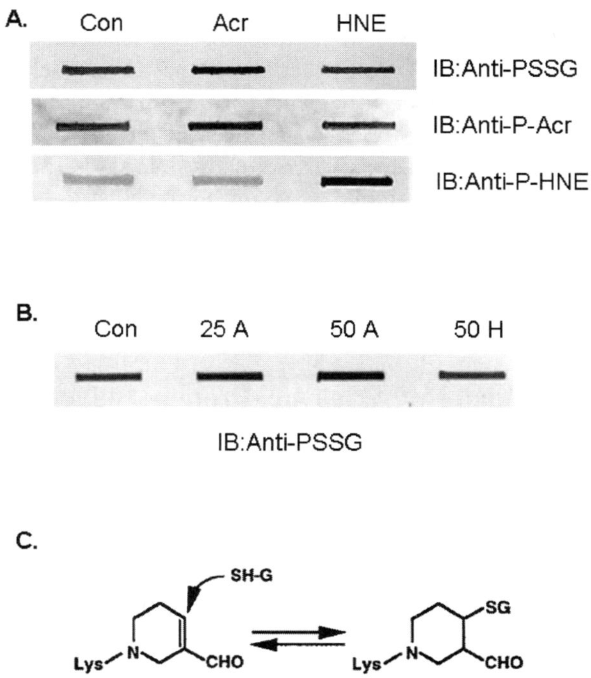

Figure 9.2 Complex protein adducts formed by the environmental pollutant and lipid peroxidation product, acrolein. Immunoblots of glutathiolated proteins and protein-bound acrolein or HNE. (**a**) Monkey kidney fibroblasts cells were exposed to vehicle, acrolein, or HNE for 30 minutes and protein modifications were assessed by immunoblotting with anti-protein glutathione (anti-PSSG), anti-protein acrolein (anti-P-Acr), or anti-protein HNE (anti-P-HNE) antibodies. Only acrolein increased the formation of protein–glutathione adducts. (**b**) Concentration-dependence of glutathiolation with acrolein. Acrolein at 25-μM (25 A) and 50-μM (50 A) concentrations increases protein glutathiolation; HNE (50 μM; 50 H) does not promote protein glutathiolation. (**c**) Potential mechanism for the formation of glutathiolated proteins due to protein–acrolein adducts. Acrolein can form a *bis*-adduct with lysine side chains (not shown) that condensates to form the N^{ε}-(3-formyl-3,4-dehydropiperidino)lysine (FDP-lysine) adduct. This adduct itself possesses α, β-unsaturation that can react with glutathione or can promote protein crosslinking reactions (scheme derived from the results of: Furuhata A. et al. 2002).

A subsequent series of experiments were performed to compare the effects of two different α,β-unsaturated aldehydes, acrolein and HNE, on the formation of protein–aldehyde and protein–glutathione adducts. Monkey kidney fibroblast (COS7) cells were exposed to either vehicle, acrolein or HNE, for 30 minutes and the protein modifications were assessed by immunoblotting with anti-protein glutathione, anti-protein acrolein, or anti-protein HNE antibodies. As shown in Figure 9.2a, row 2, acrolein formed protein adducts distinct from that observed in cells treated with HNE (row 3). Conversely, HNE formed protein adducts that were not recognized by anti-protein–acrolein antibodies. Of most interest, in row 1, acrolein treatment caused formation of protein–glutathione adducts, but HNE did not. This result clearly indicates that although both α,β-unsaturated aldehydes form protein adducts, only acrolein increases the formation of protein–glutathione modifications. Figure 9.2b shows the concentration dependence of acrolein-dependent protein glutathiolation reactions and the inability of HNE to enhance protein thiolation. We postulate that protein–acrolein–glutathione adducts are formed in reactions like that shown in Figure 9.2c. While these approaches allow us to study aspects of the kinetics of adduct formation and removal, they do not provide a method to clearly deduce the chemistry of these processes and explain why acrolein specifically increases the formation of glutathione-modified proteins. Our preliminary studies suggest that using mass spectrometric (MS) approaches to study these protein adducts offers considerable promise in understanding the processes of oxidative stress and the spectrum of products formed during oxidative stress or even normal metabolic processes.

9.3. The Chemistry of Aldehyde–Protein Adducts

Aldehydes owe their chemical reactivity to an activated carbonyl functional group with a proton attached to it. The separation of charge in this carbonyl allows the aldehyde functional group to interact readily with nucleophilic groups, such as amine groups, to form a reversible adduct commonly know as a Schiff base (Figure 9.3). The level of reactivity of aldehydes is determined by the electron deficiency at the carbonyl carbon caused by a variety of electron-withdrawing groups. The carbonyl carbon reacts with primary amine groups to form a hemiaminal intermediate, and after loss of water forms an aldimine Schiff base. As described by Klotz and coworkers studying the effect of aldimine formation with hemoglobin, many of these Schiff base intermediates were shown to be reversible, suggesting that their presence in proteins may be transient in nature (Zaugg, Walder and Klotz 1977).

For α,β-unsaturated aldehydes, electron withdrawal from the double bond by the conjugated carbonyl group decreases electron density at the β-carbon of the double bond, making the β-carbon very reactive with

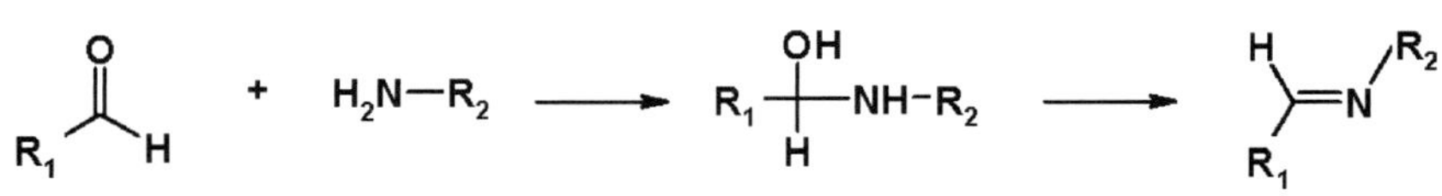

Figure 9.3 Schiff base formation.

Figure 9.4 Michael addition reaction.

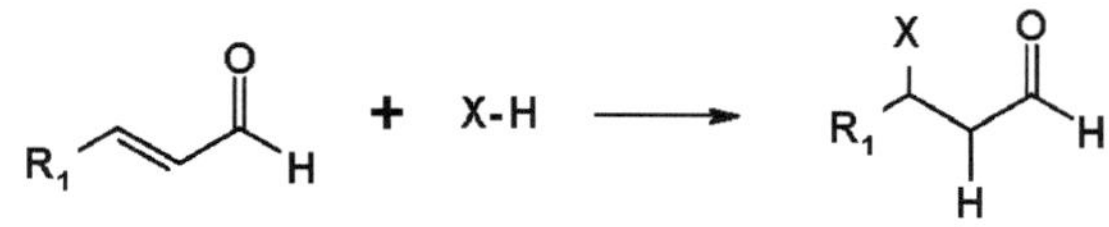

protein nucleophiles. The electrophilic β-carbon can react as a Michael acceptor with nucleophiles, such as the thiol group in cysteine (Cys), amine groups in lysine (Lys) and N-terminal α-amino acids, and the C3 of histidine imidazoles leading to the Michael addition reaction (Figure 9.4). Aldehydes that form Michael adducts are particularly reactive and can subsequently crosslink nucleic acids, proteins, and lipids. For many in this field, these crosslinked aldehyde products are thought to be an indicator of oxidative stress in general and important toxicological endpoints that are a phenotype of aldehyde toxicity.

In α,β-unsaturated aldehydes, the contribution of electrons from the double bond decreases the electron deficiency at the carbon in carbonyl groups, which makes the α,β-unsaturated aldehydes less reactive in Schiff base formation. In Michael addition products of α,β-unsaturated aldehydes, however, the double bond at α, β-carbon becomes saturated. The further reaction of Michael addition products with primary amine groups in proteins through Schiff base formation can result in further crosslinking of proteins. For example, acrolein causes crosslinking of proteins such as RNase (Burcham and Pyke 2006) and links glutathione (GSH) to proteins through putative lysine residues involved in formation of Michael addition products (Figure 9.2c). Thus, α,β-unsaturated aldehydes have multiple reactive functional groups available for protein adduct formation. In addition to the two basic reactions mentioned above, they also participate in more complex reactions to form other adducts.

9.3.1. Adducts Formed by Acrolein

Alkyl groups at the β-carbon decrease the reactivity of α,β-unsaturated aldehydes in Michael addition reactions by increasing electron density and causing steric hindrance at the β-carbon. Therefore acrolein, with no alkyl substitution at β-carbon, is by far the most reactive compound among the α,β-unsaturated aldehydes. Due to its high reactivity, acrolein readily forms covalent adducts with nucleophilic protein residues. As discussed in the Chapter 8, two types of such adducts, N^{ε}-(3-formyl-3,4-

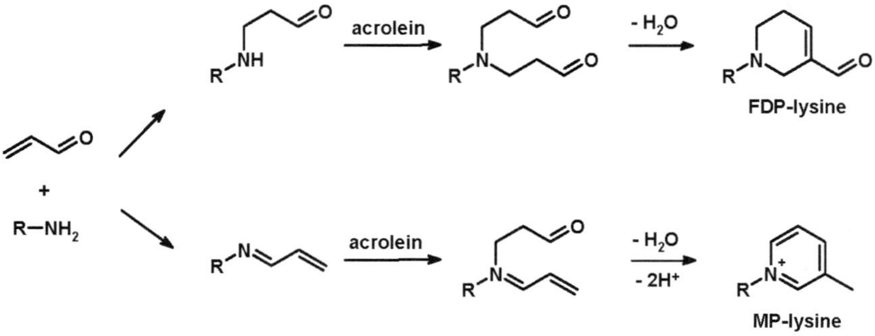

Figure 9.5 Proposed mechanism of MP-lysine and FDP-lysine formation.

dehydropiperidino)lysine (FDP-lysine) and N^{ε}-(3-methylpyridinium)-lysine (MP-lysine) have been identified by Uchida's group (Uchida et al. 1998a, 1998b; Furuhata et al. 2003; Figure 9.5).

FDP-lysine apparently is formed by the addition of two molecules of acrolein to the amino group at lysine by Michael addition, followed by cyclization and loss of water. The intermediates were not detected when N^{α}-acetyllysine was incubated with acrolein (Uchida et al. 1998a). An alternative mechanism might be involved in FDP-lysine formation. The possibility of an alternate mechanism is supported by the observation that a large excess of aldehyde over the amine is not necessary for the formation of FDP-lysine. Similar adducts can also form from other α,β-unsaturated aldehydes (Ichihashi et al. 2001). FDP-lysine is also a α,β-unsaturated aldehyde and it can react with glutathione to form a glutathione conjugate (Furuhata et al. 2002; Figure 9.2C).

Many pyridinium adducts, some that cause crosslinking of proteins, can form from α,β-unsaturated aldehydes through complex reactions (Alaiz and Barragan 1995; Baker et al. 1998; Ichihashi et al. 2001). Unlike many other adducts, the pyridinium adducts are highly stable. They carry a fixed positive charge and may have significant effect on protein function. MP-lysine adduct, a major antigenic adduct generated in acrolein-modified proteins (Furuhata et al. 2003), is one such adduct derived from acrolein. The mechanism of formation proposed by Furuhata et al. is shown in Figure 9.5. However, the mechanism of formation is still not clearly defined. However, existence of such adducts have been confirmed by nuclear magnetic resonance (NMR), and have been shown to be readily formed in acrolein-treated apolipoprotein AI (ApoAI) (Shao et al. 2005).

The possibility of complex adduction reactions between α,β-unsaturated aldehydes and proteins is supported by our data obtained using actin as a model protein. To examine its reactivity with α, β-unsaturated aldehydes, we

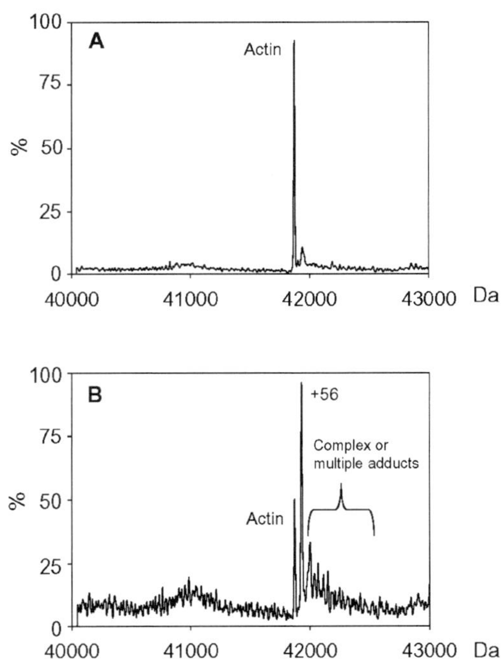

Figure 9.6 Detection of acrolein–actin adducts by electrospray ionization-mass spectrometry (ESI-MS). Deconvoluted spectra of actin: Actin was incubated with 100-mM DTT in 100-mM Tris, pH 7.5, for 1 hour at 37°C. Actin was then subjected to gel filtration on a Sephadex G25 column to remove DTT and to exchange buffer systems. The actin was then either analyzed by positive-mode ESI-MS (**a**) or incubated with 100-μM acrolein for 1 h at 37°C in 100-mM potassium phosphate buffer, pH 7.5. Excess acrolein was then removed by gel filtration and the modification state of actin was assessed by positive-mode ESI-MS (**b**).

first reduced actin with 100-mM dithiothreitol (DTT) in 100-mM Tris, pH 7.5, for 1 hat 37°C. Subsequently, the sample was desalted and DTT was removed by gel filtration. The actin was analyzed by electrospray ionization-mass spectrometry (ESI-MS) after incubation in the absence (Figure 9.6a) or presence (Figure 9.6b) of 100-μM acrolein for 1 hour at 37°C in 100-mM potassium phosphate buffer, pH 7.5. Excess acrolein was then removed by gel filtration and the modification state of actin was assessed by ESI-MS. Figure 9.6a and b show the deconvoluted mass spectra of actin and acrolein-modified actin, respectively. As seen in Figure 9.6b, one can observe a number of chemical species of actin in the spectrum suggesting that this single protein forms multiple protein–acrolein adducts, obviously with a variety of chemical modifications. The presence of intrachain cross-links cannot be determined without further analysis.

9.3.2. Adducts Formed by HNE

HNE has a hydroxyl group at C4. In Michael addition reactions of HNE, the aldehyde group can react with the hydroxyl group to form cyclic semiacetal as shown in Figure 9.7. The dihydrofuran adduct forms upon loss of water from the semiacetal (Liu, Minkler and Sayre 2003). This intermediate has the same mass as a Schiff base adduct, but it cannot be reduced by $NaBH_4$ as expected of a Schiff base. The Michael addition product of HNE has an aldehyde group. It can react with the ε-amino group of lysine side chains of proteins to form a Schiff base and subsequently cause crosslinking in proteins (Uchida and Stadtman 1993). However, Michael addition adducts exist predominantly in semiacetal form which prevents the further reaction of Schiff base formation.

When a Schiff base is formed before Michael addition, HNE can also form a 2-pentylpyrrole adduct as shown in Figure 9.8 (Sayre et al. 1993). The Schiff base can rearrange to form a γ-ketone, followed by cyclization to form an unstable semiaminal and loss of water to form 2-pentylpyrrole. Since Schiff base formation is not a favorable reaction for HNE, pyrrole adduct formation appears to be a minor pathway when compared with the Michael addition reaction. However, unlike other HNE adducts mentioned above, its formation is irreversible and it also removes positive charges carried by the parent lysine residues. Such adducts of HNE have been detected in human plasma and atherosclerotic plaques (Salomon et al.

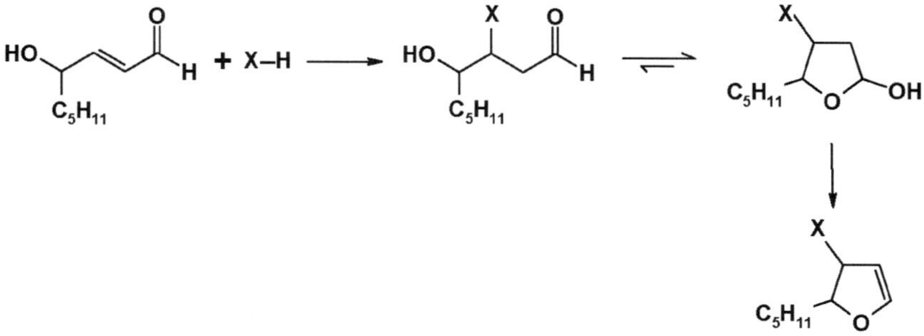

Figure 9.7 Cyclic semiacetal and dihydrofuran adducts from Michael addition adducts of HNE.

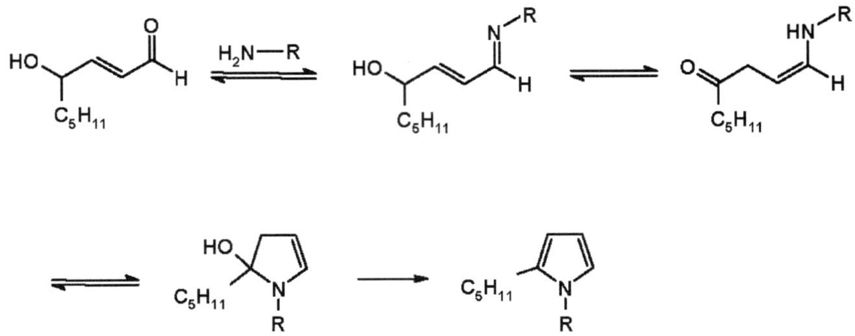

Figure 9.8 Formation of 2-pentylpyrrole adduct from HNE.

2000) and might be more relevant markers of permanent protein damage caused by HNE (Sayre et al. 1996).

9.3.3. Adducts Formed by 4-oxo-trans-2-nonenal

4-oxo-2-nonenal (ONE) has been identified as a common lipid peroxidation product, in addition to HNE (Lee and Blair 2000, Spiteller et al. 2001), and has much higher reactivity than HNE. Both α- and β-carbon can react with histidine (His) and Cys in Michael Addition reactions. The β-carbon is the more reactive position (Zhang et al. 2003). The reaction is irreversible and about 6–31 times faster than HNE (Lin et al. 2005.) However, ONE is less reactive than HNE toward the ϵ-amino group of lysine side chains through Michael addition. Instead it goes through a fast, but reversible reaction to form a Schiff base. Schiff base formation at lysine was found to be the fastest reaction of ONE with model compounds. Although this reaction might be transient and the products difficult to detect due to the reversibility of the reaction, the possible deleterious biological effects from this reaction should be considered (Lin et al. 2005).

The Michael Addition products of 4-oxononenals can further react through Schiff base formation, since they have two carbonyl groups. Under nonoxidative conditions, they can react with amine groups through Paal–Knorr condensation (Amarnath et al. 1995) to form pyrrole adducts as shown in Figure 9.9 (Xu and Sayre 1999, Zhang et al. 2003). Such

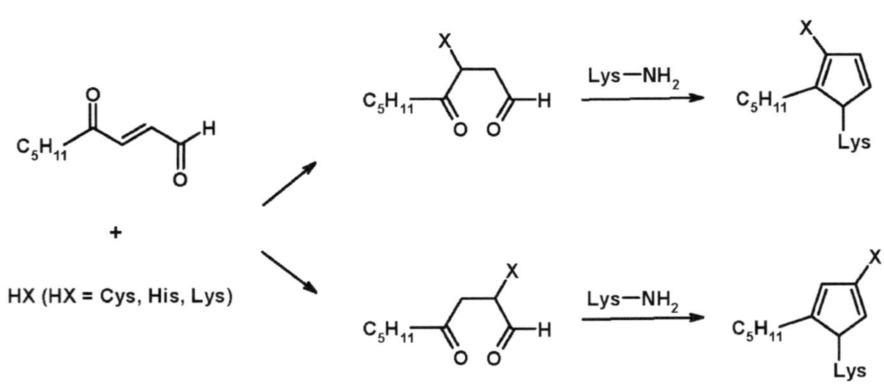

Figure 9.9 Formation of 2-pentylpyrrole adducts from ONE.

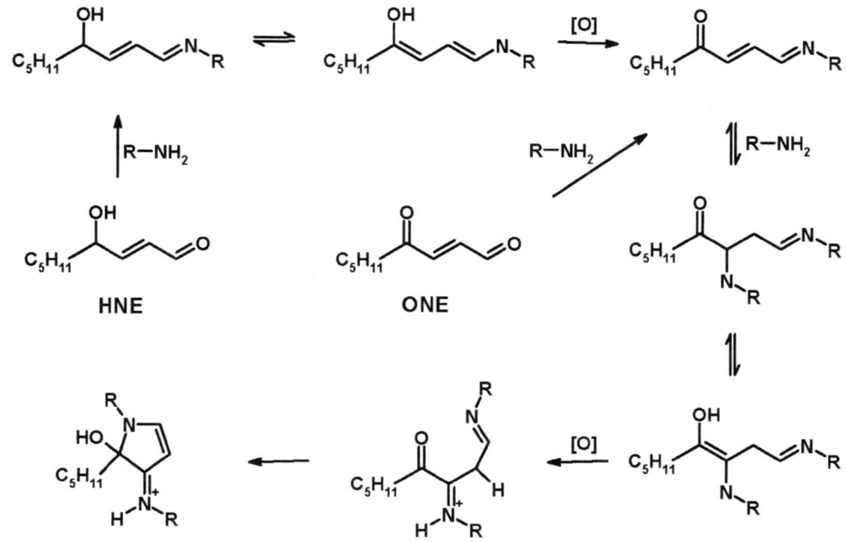

Figure 9.10 Formation of dihydropyrrole adducts from HNE and ONE.

intrachain crosslinking by ONE was found between histidine and lysine at a HAK motif of histone H4 (Oe et al. 2003b).

Under oxidative conditions, both HNE and ONE can react with two Lys residues through crosslinking reaction and oxidation to form a 2-alkyl-2-hydroxy-1,2-dihydropyrrol-3-one iminium adducts (Xu and Sayre 1998) as shown in Figure 9.10. This adduct is characterized by the emission of fluorescence at 430 nm when excited with light at 360 nm. The reaction for ONE is preceded by Schiff base formation at the aldehyde group, followed by Michael addition of another lysine, tautomerization, oxidation, and cyclization. Since Schiff base formation from HNE was very slow (not detected in kinetic studies with spectroscopy), HNE preferentially forms Michael addition products with the ε-amino group of lysine side chains (Lin et al. 2005). The decreased electron density at the carbonyl carbon enhances Schiff base formation. Formation of this adduct from HNE requires two steps and 4-electron oxidation instead of one step and 2-electron oxidation from ONE. The formation of this adduct is much slower for HNE than ONE (Xu and Sayre 1998).

Rapid crosslinking of proteins can occur with either HNE or ONE and lysine is normally involved in this crosslinking (Xu et al. 1999). Both nonoxidative and oxidative reactions can generate crosslinking adducts in proteins. However, the formation of pyrrole adducts from nonoxidative reactions are rare and the formation of the substituted 1,2-dihydropyrrol-3-one iminium adduct from oxidative reactions is enhanced particularly in the case of ONE (Zhang et al. 2003).

9.4. Reactivity of Nucleophilic Residues in Protein

The common nucleophilic residues in proteins include Cys, His, Lys, as well as the amino group at N-terminus. All these nucleophiles can participate in Michael addition, while only Lys and amino group at N-terminus can participate in Schiff base formation. Multiple reactions can occur with amino groups to form more complex products, such as FDP-lysine and MP-lysine. The nucleophilicity of the residues is determined by their polarizability and ionic state. The nucleophilicity of the sulfhydryl anion is much higher than amines. Therefore, Cys is much more reactive than His, Lys, and the N-terminal amino group. In order to be good nucleophiles, amines must exist in the free-base form. Amines with higher pKa will have lower percentage of amine free base at a given pH, which will decrease their reactivity in nucleophilic reactions. The average pKa values of these residues in protein can be estimated with model compounds that resemble amino acids chains (model pKa values). Some of these are listed in Table 9.1 (Nielsen and Vriend 2001).

The pKa value of the N-terminal amino group is much lower than that of Lys, and reactivity at the N-terminus can be much higher than Lys. A clear example is glycosylation of hemoglobin by glucose in which Schiff base formation is the first step of glycosylation. Higher levels of glycosylation occurs at N-terminus than at the ε-amino group of Lys. When hexanal was incubated with oxidized insulin β-chain, Schiff base formation was found predominantly at N-terminal Phe instead of Lys (Fenaille, Guy and Tabet 2003). Reactivity of HNE and ONE was evaluated with N-acetylated peptides containing one or more nucleophilic residues. Peptides were incubated with excess amount of HNE or ONE. Formation of adducts was monitored with spectrophotometry and confirmed by MS. The reactivity of residues was found to have the order of: Cys >> His > Lys (> arginine (Arg) for ONE) and the reactivity of ONE toward Cys was more than 100-fold higher than HNE (Doorn and Petersen 2002).

The guanidinium group in Arg is a strong base. Arg is mostly protonated at physiological pH. Delocalization of positive charge among the amino groups significantly decreases the reactivity of Arg in nucleophilic reactions. Only a very reactive aldehyde will react with Arg to form adducts. Formation of an imidazole adduct of ONE was reported by Blair's group (Oe et al. 2003a). The proposed mechanism of formation is shown in Figure 9.11. The amino group of guanidine reacts with aldehyde groups to form a carbinolamine intermediate. Then the secondary amine of guanidine reacts with β-carbon of ONE through an intramolecular Michael Addition to form a cyclic carbinolamine intermediate, and loss of water from the intermediate forms the imidazole adduct. Formation of HNE adducts with Arg has also been reported (Isom et al. 2004), and 2-pentylpyrrole was proposed to be the product. However, this has not been confirmed by NMR.

Table 9.1 Model pKa values of selected residues.

Residue type	Model pKa value
Arg	13.0
Lys	10.4
Cys	8.7
N-terminus	8.0

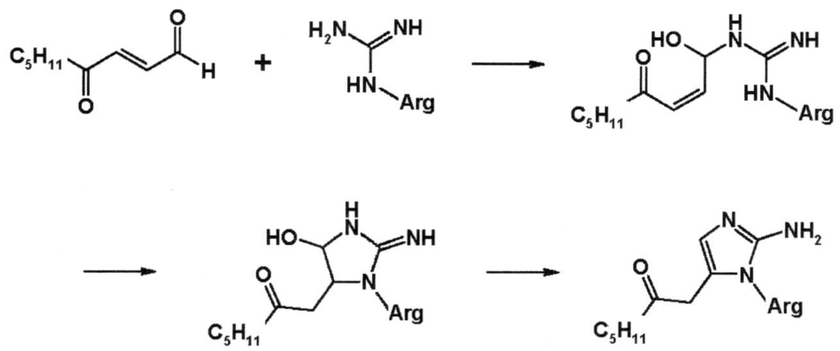

Figure 9.11 Formation of arginine adducts from ONE.

9.5. Effect of Neighboring Nucleophilic Amino Acid Residues

Reactivity of nucleophilic residues can be affected by other amino acid residues located nearby. The presence of an Arg on a Cys-containing peptide increased the reactivity of Cys toward HNE and ONE by a factor of 5–6 (Doorn and Petersen 2002). Formation of MP-lysine in peptide Ac-GEYAHKY is much higher than the peptides that His is replaced with Arg or Glu (Shao et al. 2005). When acrolein was incubated with apolipoprotein A-I, MP-lysine was formed preferentially at peptide sequences containing multiple lysine residues and only one of the Lys formed adduct with acrolein. Interestingly, FDP-lysine was not detected (Shao et al. 2005).

It is well known that the pKa and reactivity of amino acid side chains of proteins is greatly influenced by their microenvironment. Effect of environment on reactivity of residues with HNE was studied recently by Liebler's group (Szapacs et al. 2006). After incubation with HNE, human serum albumin (HSA) samples were reduced with $NaBH_4$, digested with trypsin, and analyzed by liquid chromatography (LC)/MS/MS. Ten Michael addition products at His and Lys were identified. The reactivity of different residues varied considerably. The kinetic study indicated the order of reactivity was $H_{242} > H_{510} > H_{67} > H_{367} > H_{247} \sim K_{233}$, which correlates well with the calculated pKa values of these residues (reactivity increases with decrease in pKa). The only exception was H_{367}, which has the second lowest pKa. Crystal structure of HSA indicates that it sits in a cleft and steric hindrance may limit its reactivity with HNE. The H_{242} residue sits in the hydrophobic binding cavity and has an unusually low pKa of 0.81; hence, its reactivity with HNE is much higher than that of any other residue. Finally, it should be noted that these reactivity considerations are for proteins in an essentially aqueous environment, so that membrane-incorporated protein reactivities would be expected to differ.

9.6. Reversibility of Aldehyde–Protein Adduction Reactions

Some reactions between aldehydes and amino acid residues in proteins are reversible. There is an optimal pH for Schiff base formation, depending on the reactants. Significant deviation from the optimal pH for Schiff base formation decreases the rates of formation and stability of the products. Schiff base formation of HNE and ONE with model compounds have been studied (Lin et al. 2005). Excess amounts of nucleophiles were used to react with HNE or ONE and the reactions were monitored by spectrophotometry. Michael addition of HNE with amines and Schiff base formation of ONE with amines were found to be reversible. The reversibility of adduct formation can complicate the detection of these adducts. For example, the thiol group in Cys is generally the most reactive nucleophile in proteins and acrolein is the most reactive α,β-unsaturated aldehyde. Acrolein adduct formation at Cys has not been reported to date and reversibility of reaction is the likely explanation because the thiol anion is an excellent leaving group. However, the effect caused by formation of reversible adducts in proteins should not be ignored. Adduct formation and its reversal are pH-dependent. This phenomenon may vary in different cellular microenvironments, may change the reactivity of proteins, and may even favor formation of species that serve as mediators or modulators of various biological responses.

9.7. Detection and Characterization of Aldehyde–Protein Adducts

Immunological assays have been widely used to monitor aldehyde–protein adduct formation. These have excellent sensitivity and specificity and are very useful in localizing adducts in tissues or cellular organelles. However, this technique cannot be used to establish final specific location of adducts in proteins or to elucidate structures of new adducts. For this, MS has emerged as a technique of choice. The basic MS techniques used in protein analysis have been reviewed recently (Domon and Aebersold 2006).

In qualitative studies, two types of data (MS and MS/MS) are usually acquired. In MS mode, MS spectra are dominated by peaks from intact peptides/proteins when soft-ionization techniques such as matrix-assisted laser desorption/ionization (MALDI) and ESI are used to ionize samples. Mixtures of peptides/proteins can be analyzed with this technique and intact molecular weight and charge state are the main information obtained from this technique. Sometimes limited fragmentation can occur during analysis. While this might provide structural information about the adduct, it might also lead to false identification or incorrect assignments. For example, in-source collision-induced dehydration of the Michael adduct of HNE could be incorrectly identified as a Schiff base adduct (Bolgar and Gaskell 1996).

In tandem MS/MS analyses, ions from samples of interest can be selected by the first mass analyzer (separated from other ions to avoid interference), the selected ion can be fragmented in a collision cell, and the fragment ions can be separated with a second mass analyzer and recorded to obtain MS/MS spectra (Figure 9.12). In other instruments (e.g., ion trap and Fourier transform (FT)-MS), ion selection, fragmentation, and separation often occurs within the trap, allowing the process to be repeated several times to generate higher-order tandem mass spectra. From MS/MS spectra of peptide/protein, sequences and specific location of modifications can be

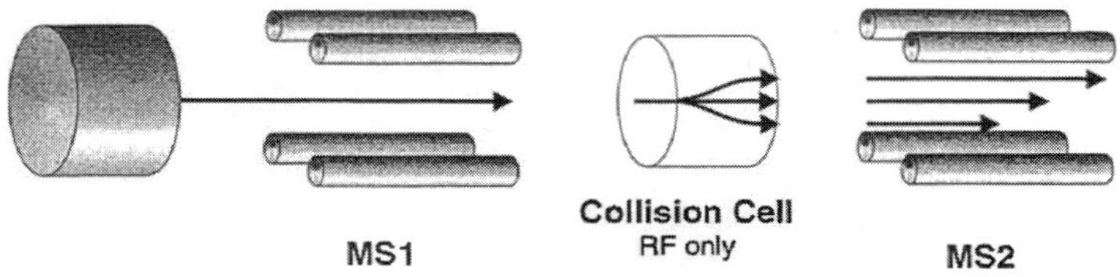

Linked Scan Type	MS1	CID	MS2	Result
Product ion scan	Static (on precursor ion of interest)	Collision	Scan	Discovers all product ions of a given precursor ion
Precursor ion scan	Scan	Collision	Static (on product ion of interest)	Discovers all precursor of a given product ion
Constant neutral loss scan	Scan	Collision	Scan (offset from MS1 by constant neutral loss mass)	Discovers all decompositions that lose same mass

Figure 9.12 Schematic depiction of use of tandem mass spectrometry experiments. The instrument configuration for MS/MS spectrometer (triple quadrupole) is shown in the *top panel*. The methods utilizing MS/MS mass spectrometry are shown in the *lower panel*: (**a**) product ion scanning; (**b**) precursor ion scanning; and (**c**) constant neutral loss scanning.

obtained. For unknown adducts from model compounds, MS/MS spectra can also provide useful information for structure elucidation.

9.7.1. Top-Down Approaches to Identify Protein Modifications Using MS

Two approaches, top-down and bottom-up, have been used to identify type and location of adducts or post-translational modifications in protein. In a top-down approach, the intact protein is fragmented by mass spectrometers. To obtain good efficiency in fragmentation, special fragmentation techniques are used. Application of top-down approach has historically been limited to small- or medium-sized proteins. With development of new techniques, such as high-resolution Fourier transformation ion cyclotron resonance MS, larger proteins can be analyzed by this approach (Han et al. 2006). Fragmentation of proteins will generate many fragments that could exist in a multiplicity of charge states. These factors make the MS/MS spectra from top-down experiment exceedingly complex. Capability of determination of charge states of peaks with large number of charges is essential for determining mass of fragments in these experiments. Therefore, mass spectrometers with very high sensitivity and mass resolution are required for these experiments. The advantage of this approach is that it has potential to determine the entire sequence of a protein (and adducts at any residue). It may also be useful for detecting unstable adducts in proteins.

9.7.2. Bottom-Up Approaches to Identify Protein Modification Using MS

Currently, most protein characterization studies are done with bottom-up approaches. In a bottom-up approach, either purified proteins or protein mixtures are first subjected to limited hydrolysis, usually using a purified and well-characterized endoprotease and then the peptides from partially digested proteins are analyzed by MS. In most cases, not all peptides are detected. Coverage might be increased by using a bank of proteases with different hydrolysis site specificities to digest proteins and/or by using different MS techniques to detect the peptides. However, coverage of the entire sequence is rare and adducts may not be detected if modification occurs on peptides undetected by the spectrometer. The most often used protease is trypsin. It cleaves protein at C-termini of Lys and Arg. Lys is one of the residues that reacts with aldehydes. Formation of adducts at Lys may prevent cleavage by trypsin. For example, trypsin does not cleave at Lys residues that form MP-lysine adducts (Shao et al. 2005). In these cases, other proteases such chymotrypsin, pepsin, or glutamic-C can be used to digest proteins.

9.7.3. Analysis of Unstable Aldehyde–Protein Adducts

Some protein adducts of aldehydes are not stable. These may be lost during digestion or during sample preparation before MS analysis. In sample preparation for MS analysis, low-pH solvents are often used. Schiff base formation is a reversible reaction and it can be fully reversible at low pH (Esterbauer, Schaur and Zollner 1991). To prevent loss of Schiff base adducts, protein samples can be reduced with $NaBH_4$ before MS analysis or digestion. The Michael addition product of HNE mainly exists as a semiacetal, and it can also be reduced with $NaBH_4$ to form 1,4-dihydroxy derivatives. Sometimes $Na(CN)BH_3$ is used to reduce Schiff bases to imines. It is a weaker reducing reagent compared with $NaBH_4$ and does not reduce carbonyl groups (Fenaille, Guy and Tabet 2003). In some cases, the use of sodium borodeuteride $NaBD_4$ is useful for simultaneous reduction and mass addition.

9.7.4. Techniques for Aldehyde–Protein Adduction Detection by MS

The type and location of adduct can be identified by a shift in the mass of peptides relative to the molecular weight of peptides from unmodified proteins. When multiple reactive residues exist in the same peptide, molecular weight alone is not enough to determine which residue forms the adduct. In these cases, specific sites of modification can be identified by MS/MS analysis. Some adducts introduce the same mass shifts in peptide spectra, and these may be distinguished by their pattern of fragmentation in MS/MS experiment or by their difference in chemical properties, such as reducibility by $NaBH_4$ or $Na(CN)BH_3$ or reactivity with 2,4-dinitrophenylhydrazine (DNPH).

The MS/MS data can be processed with special software, such as P-MOD (Hansen et al. 2005) and SALSA (Hansen et al. 2001), to reveal adducts at unknown locations. Other MS methods have also been used to selectively detect adducted peptides from peptide mixtures. A method to detect HNE adduct by MALDI-TOF was developed by Guy's group (Fenaille, Tabet and Guy 2004). In this method, the Michael addition adducts of HNE are derivatized with DNPH and analyzed by

MALDI-TOF with DNPH as matrix. When DNPH is used as the matrix, the hydrazone derivatives from Michael addition adducts of HNE have much better desorption/ionization efficiency while signals from unmodified peptides are suppressed.

Some additional MS/MS techniques can also be used to identify unknown location of modifications in proteins. Precursor ion scans and constant neutral loss scans are two of such techniques, both of them use the characteristic fragmentation of adducts to identify peptides with those adducts. In precursor ion scans (Figure 9.12), the instrument is set to identify which precursor ion (intact peptide with adduct) produces a specific product ion in MS/MS mode, which is a characteristic ion from an adduct. The Michael addition adducts of HNE at His, for example, produces an immonium ion of modified His at *m*/*z* 266. Precursor ion scans can be set to identify all peptides with a Michael addition adduct of HNE at His (precursors) that produce *m*/*z* 266 fragment in MS/MS, and MS/MS spectra from these precursors can be acquired to confirm the sequences and location of modification of the peptides (Bolgar and Gaskell 1996). In precursor ion scans, the selectivity of precursor ion identification is determined by the exclusiveness of formation of the fragment ion. All Michael addition adducts of HNE can produce a fragment ion at *m*/*z* 139 (dehydrated HNE). However, this fragment is not exclusively generated from HNE adducts. Using *m*/*z* 139 as fragment ion in precursor scan can result in identification of some precursor ions that do not have HNE adducts (Bolgar and Gaskell 1996). In constant neutral loss scans (Figure 9.12), intact peptides that can generate a fragment with known fixed difference in mass from the intact peptide are identified. This technique is useful for unstable adducts that can be easily lost in fragmentation. The Michael addition adduct of HNE can easily lose HNE (M-156) in fragmentation. It is possible to identify all Michael addition adducts of HNE by identifying peptides that have M-156 fragment in a constant neutral loss scan. However, there is difficulty in predetermining the appropriate fragmentation energy for different peptides and their different charge states (Bolgar and Gaskell 1996).

The sensitivity of precursor ion scanning and constant neutral loss scanning is relatively low. An alternative precursor detection method with a hybrid quadrupole-time of flight (Q-TOF) instrument was developed recently (Bateman et al. 2002). In this method, MS scans at alternating low and high collision energies are acquired. The spectra are compared to ascertain whether there are fragment ions in high-collision-energy spectrum that match with ions in low-collision-energy spectrum with a fixed mass difference. Once such precursor ions are identified, MS/MS spectra from these precursor ions are immediately acquired in a data-dependent acquisition mode. With this technique, better sensitivity and selectivity can be obtained because the Q-TOF instrument has excellent mass resolution and can identify constant neutral loss with higher mass accuracy.

9.7.5. Quantification of Protein and Adduct by MS

Mass spectrometry can also be used to measure protein adduct levels with high sensitivity and selectivity. Quantification is usually done by analyzing the digested samples by LC/MS. Adduct levels can be calculated from the peak areas of ion chromatogram specific to the peptide with adduct. To increase the specificity of adduct quantification, a technique called multiple ion monitoring can be used. In this technique, ions of adduct-containing peptides are selected and fragmented. The fragment ions specific to the peptides can be selectively detected. Adduct levels can be calculated from the peak areas of the ion chromatograms, and peak area ratios from different fragments can be used to confirm that the detected levels are indeed of the targeted adduct. Signals from different peptides vary significantly; therefore, an internal standard must be used in quantification. The best internal standard should have similar chemical and physical properties as the compounds to be quantified and stable isotope-labeled compounds are the best internal standards in MS quantification. For quantification of absolute amount, authentic compound to be quantified and internal standard are required.

The Michael addition adduct of α,β-unsaturated aldehydes with Cys residues in protein has a thioether bond. It can be reduced under strong reducing conditions (Uchida and Stadtman 1992). Methods based on this reduction have been established to detect protein adduct of HNE and 1,4-dihydroxy-*trans*-2-nonene (DHN), the reduced adduct of HNE, in plasma or whole-blood proteins as shown in Figure 9.13 (Veronneau, Comte and Des Rosiers 2002; Asselin et al. 2006). The HNE adduct was first reduced to the DHN adduct with $NaBD_4$, which introduced a deuterium to the DHN from HNE adduct to distinguish the DHN adduct. The proteins were then precipitated and reduced with Raney Ni at 55°C for 20 hours to release DHN. The released DHN was then extracted with ethyl acetate, derivatized with dimethyl-*tert*-butylsilyltrifluoroacetamide (MtBSTFA) to TBDMS, and analyzed by gas chromatography (GC)/MS with D_{11}-DHN as internal standard. This method provides very high sensitivity. It measures the total level of HNE adduct without identifying specific location of adduct in protein and has been used to measure HNE adduct as biomarker of HNE exposure (Asselin et al. 2006).

Some techniques have been developed to measure relative changes, instead of absolute amounts of protein. In these cases, the relative quantification can be accomplished by adding different tags to samples from different treatments. Authentic compounds are not needed and best results are obtained when tags with different isotope compositions are used.

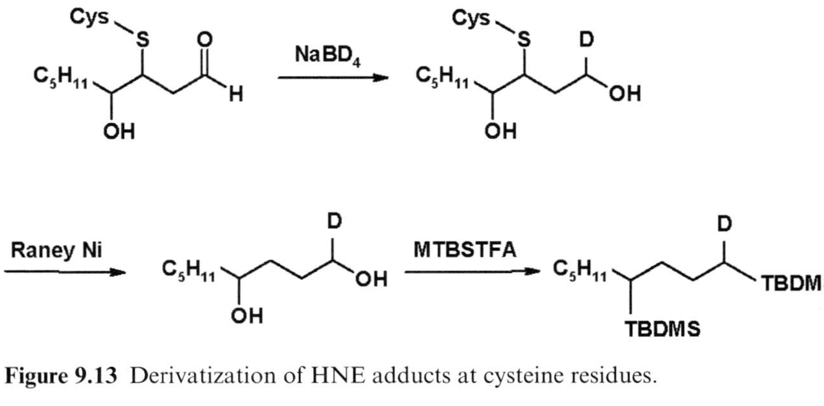

Figure 9.13 Derivatization of HNE adducts at cysteine residues.

Relative quantification of proteins is most often done after digestion of samples with protease. Chemical tags, such as phenylisocyanate (PIC), can be added to proteins before or after digestion. Labeling proteins with tags before digestion will limit the labeling to some of the peptides from proteins. With specially designed tags that include a moiety that is separable using chemical affinity techniques, the labeled peptides can be separated from unlabeled peptides. This simplifies subsequent detection and increases sensitivity by enriching the sample in labeled peptides. This approach has limited application in protein adduct quantification because the adduct can form on peptides without such targeted residues and adducts may form on the same targeted residues. These limitations can be avoided by adding tags to either N- or C-terminus of peptides after digestion. In most cases, all peptides can be labeled with tags (except, in some cases, peptides at N- or C-terminus of proteins). Therefore, relative changes of all proteins at any locations can be monitored, if the peptides are detected by MS analysis. Another advantage of this approach is multiple peptides from same protein can be detected. The agreement of relative changes from different peptides will make the detection of relative change of protein more reliable.

This approach has been used to study the kinetics of HNE adduct formation in HSA (Szapacs et al. 2006). Human serum albumin was incubated with HNE and samples at different time points were collected. The samples were reduced with $NaBH_4$ to stabilize HNE adducts and digested with trypsin. The N-termini of treated samples were labeled with $^{12}C_6$-PIC, referred as light tag, and mixed at 1:1 ratio (based on HSA amount) with a reference sample which was obtained from 24-hours incubation with HNE and prepared the same way except that it was labeled with $^{13}C_6$-PIC (heavy tag). The samples were then analyzed by LC/MS/MS and ion chromatograms of characteristic fragments of sample and reference peptides were extracted. The amount ratios (sample/reference) were obtained from the average of light/heavy ratios of three fragments from same peptide and rate constants of formation of these HNE adducts were calculated from the amount ratios. An alternative approach for labeling involves use of $H_2{}^{18}O$ for labeling the carboxy terminus (reviewed by Miyagi and Rao, 2007.)

9.8. Conclusions and Summary

The purpose of this chapter has been to describe the dynamic process of aldehyde–protein adduct formation and their characterization. Understanding how reactive aldehydes are formed during lipid peroxidation and oxidative stress and how much of these products are formed has challenged research in this area of biomedical sciences for decades. A major reason for the slow progress in understanding these processes has been the lack of clear chemical mechanisms as to how these events occur. Since aldehydes are increasingly shown to be important toxicological agents, new methods to study the chemistry and biochemistry of adduct formation by aldehydes with cellular nucleophiles are required. Mass spectrometry has increasingly become an enabling methodology in toxicology and medicine. The information reviewed in the preceding sections will focus researchers to implement these MS methods, in combination with other biochemical approaches, to study the formation and turnover of protein adducts with aldehydes and their role in aldehyde toxicity in cells and in vivo.

The application of these MS methods in several recent studies on the reactivity of aldehydes provides encouragement to future studies of how endogenous and exogenous aldehydes evoke their toxicity or how they alter cell signaling. For example, Szapacs et al. (2006) defined in chemical terms the reaction of HNE with HSA and provided a new direction toward establishing defined biomarkers of lipid peroxidation-dependent processes easily obtained from human blood. This approaches hold promise to provide useful biomarkers in the future. In a recent study, Petersen and coworkers (Sampey et al. 2007) have convincingly shown that HNE form covalent adducts with extracellular signal-regulated kinase (Erk-1/2) at residue histidine 178, a process that is linked to inhibition of function of this important kinase. Clearly, these methods provide promise as to our ability to understand the chemical basis of oxidative stress and lipid peroxidation, as well as approaches to develop important biomarkers of human diseases caused by oxidative stress and lipid peroxidation, such as inflammation, atherosclerosis, and diabetes.

Acknowledgements. Supported in part by PO1 ES11860 and ES12062. The authors wish to thank David Hoetker for his expert technical assistance with ESI-MS analyses. JC and BGH contributed jointly as first authors in the preparation of this article.

References

Alaiz, M., and Barragan, S. 1995. Changes induced in bovine serum albumin following interactions with the lipid peroxidation product *E*-2-octenal. Chem. Phys. Lipids. 77:217–223.

Amarnath, V., Amarnath, K., Valentine, W. M., Eng, M. A., and Graham, D. G. 1995. Intermediates in the Paal–Knorr synthesis of pyrroles. 4-Oxoaldehydes. Chem. Res. Toxicol. 8:234–238.

Asselin, C., Bouchard, B., Tardif, J. C., and Des Rosiers, C. 2006. Circulating 4-hydroxynonenal-protein thioether adducts assessed by gas chromatography-mass spectrometry are increased with disease progression and aging in spontaneously hypertensive rats. Free Rad. Biol. Med. 41:97–105.

Baker, A., Zidek, L., Wiesler, D., Chmelik, J., Pagel, M., and Novotny, M. V. 1998. Reaction of *N*-acetylglycyllysine methyl ester with 2-alkenals: an alternative model for covalent modification of proteins. Chem. Res. Toxicol. 11:730–740.

Bateman, R. H., Carruthers, R., Hoyes, J. B., Jones, C., Langridge, J. I., Millar, A., and Vissers, J. P. C. 2002. A novel precursor ion discovery method on a hybrid quadrupole orthogonal acceleration time-of-flight (Q-TOF) mass spectrometer for studying protein phosphorylation. J. Am. Soc. Mass Spectrom. 13:792–803.

Bolgar, M. S., and Gaskell, S. J. 1996. Determination of the sites of 4-hydroxy-2-nonenal adduction to protein by electrospray tandem mass spectrometry. Anal. Chem. 68:2325–2330.

Burcham, P. C., and Pyke, S. M. 2006. Hydralazine inhibits rapid acrolein-induced protein oligomerization: role of aldehyde scavenging and adduct trapping in cross-link blocking and cytoprotection. Mol. Pharmacol. 69:1056–1065.

Conklin, D. J., Prough, R. A., and Bhatnagar, A., 2006. Aldehyde metabolism in the cardiovascular system. Mol. Biosys. 2:1–16.

Domon, B., and Aebersold, R. 2006. Mass spectrometry and protein analysis. Science 312:212–217.

Doorn, J. A., and Petersen, D. R. 2002. Covalent modification of amino acid nucleophiles by the lipid peroxidation products 4-hydroxy-2-nonenal and 4-oxo-2-nonenal. Chem. Res. Toxicol. 15:1445–1450.

Esterbauer, H., Schaur, R. J., and Zollner, H. 1991. Chemistry and biochemistry of 4-hydroxynonenal, malonaldehyde and related aldehydes. Free Rad. Biol. Med. 11:81–128.

Fenaille, F., Guy, P. A., and Tabet, J. C. 2003. Study of protein modification by 4-hydroxy-2-nonenal and other short chain aldehydes analyzed by electrospray ionization tandem mass spectrometry. J. Am. Soc. Mass Spectrom. 14:215–226.

Fenaille, F., Tabet, J. C., and Guy, P. A. 2004. Identification of 4-hydroxy-2-nonenal-modified peptides within unfractionated digests using matrix-assisted laser desorption/ionization time-of-flight mass spectrometry. Anal. Chem. 76:867–873.

Furuhata, A., Ishii, T., Kumazawa, S., Yamada, T., Nakayama, T., and Uchida, K. 2003. N^{ε}-(3-methylpyridinium)lysine, a major antigenic adduct generated in acrolein-modified protein. J. Biol. Chem. 278:48658–48665.

Furuhata, A., Nakamura, M., Osawa, T., and Uchida, K. 2002. Thiolation of protein-bound carcinogenic aldehyde. An electrophilic acrolein–lysine adduct that covalently binds to thiols. J. Biol. Chem. 277:27919–27926.

Ichihashi, K., Osawa, T., Toyokuni, S., and Uchida, K. 2001. Endogenous formation of protein adducts with carcinogenic aldehydes: implications for oxidative stress. J. Biol. Chem. 276:23903–23913.

Isom, A. L., Barnes, S., Wilson, L., Kirk, M., Coward, L., and Darley-Usmar, V. 2004. Modification of cytochrome c by 4-hydroxy-2-nonenal: evidence for histidine, lysine, and arginine–aldehyde adducts. J. Am. Soc. Mass Spectrom. 15:1136–1147.

Han, X., Jin, M., Breuker, K., and McLafferty, F. W. 2006. Extending top-down mass spectrometry to proteins with masses greater than 200 kilodaltons. Science 314:109–112.

Hansen, B. T., Jones, J. A., Mason, D. E., and Liebler, D. C. 2001. SALSA: a pattern recognition algorithm to detect electrophile-adducted peptides by automated evaluation of CID spectra in LC-MS-MS analyses. Anal. Chem. 73:1676–1683.

Hansen, B. T., Davey, S. W., Ham, A. J., and Liebler, D. C. 2005. P-Mod: an algorithm and software to map modifications to peptide sequences using tandem MS data. J. Proteome Res. 4:358–368.

Ji, C., Kozak, K. R., and Marnett, L. J. 2004. IkappaB kinase, a molecular target for inhibition by 4-hydroxy-2-nonenal. J. Biol. Chem. 276:18233–18228.

Lee, S. H., and Blair, I. A. 2000. Characterization of 4-oxo-2-nonenal as a novel product of lipid peroxidation. Chem. Res. Toxicol. 13:698–702.

Lin, D., Lee, H. G., Liu, Q., Perry, G., Smith, M. A., and Sayre, L. M. 2005. 4-Oxo-2-nonenal is both more neurotoxic and more protein reactive than 4-hydroxy-2-nonenal. Chem. Res. Toxicol. 18:1219–1231.

Liu, Z., Minkler, P. E., and Sayre, L. M. 2003. Mass spectroscopic characterization of protein modification by 4-hydroxy-2-(*E*)-nonenal and 4-oxo-2-(*E*)-nonenal. Chem. Res. Toxicol. 16:901–911.

Miyagi, M., and Rao, K. C. S. 2007. Proteolytic ^{18}O-labeling strategies for quantitative proteomics. Mass Spectrom. Rev. 26:121–136.

Nielsen, J. E., and Vriend, G. 2001. Optimizing the hydrogen-bond network in Poisson–Boltzmann equation-based pK(a) calculations. Proteins 43:403–412.

Oe, T., Lee, S. H., Silva Elipe, M. V., Arison, B. H., and Blair, I. A. 2003a. A novel lipid hydroperoxide-derived modification to arginine. Chem. Res. Toxicol. 16:1598–1605.

Oe, T., Arora, J. S., Lee, S. H., and Blair, I. A. 2003b. A novel lipid hydroperoxide-derived cyclic covalent modification to histone H4. J. Biol. Chem. 278:42098–42105.

Robino, G., Zamara, E., Novo, E., Dianzani, M. U., Parola, M. 2001. 4-hydroxy-2,3-alkenals as signal molecules modulating proliferative and adaptative cell responses. Biofactors 15:103–106.

Ruef, J., Rao, G. N., Li, F., Bode, C., Patterson, C., Bhatnagar, A., and Runge, M. S. 1998. Induction of rat aortic smooth muscle cell growth by the lipid peroxidation product 4-hydroxy-2-nonenal. Circulation 97:1071–1078.

Salomon, R. G., Kaur, K., Podrez, E., Hoff, H. F., Krushinsky, A. V., and Sayre, L. M. 2000. HNE-derived 2-pentylpyrroles are generated during oxidation of LDL, are more prevalent in blood plasma from patients with renal disease or atherosclerosis, and are present in atherosclerotic plaques. Chem. Res. Toxicol. 13:557–564.

Sampey, B. P., Carbone, D. L., Doorn, J. A., Drechsel, D. A. and Peterson, D. R. 2007. 4-Hydroxy-2-nonenal adduction of extracelluar signal-regulated kinase (ERK) and the inhibition of hepatocyte Erk-Est-like Protein-1-activating Protein-1 signal transduction. Mol. Pharmacol. 71:871–883.

Sayre, L. M., Arora, P. K., Iyer, R. S., and Salomon, R. G. 1993. Pyrrole formation from 4-hydroxynonenal and primary amines. Chem. Res. Toxicol. 6:19–22.

Sayre, L. M., Sha, W., Xu, G., Kaur, K., Nadkarni, D., Subbanagounder, G., and Salomon, R. G. 1996. Immunochemical evidence supporting 2-pentylpyrrole formation on proteins exposed to 4-hydroxy-2-nonenal. Chem. Res. Toxicol. 9:1194–1201.

Shao, B., Fu, X., McDonald, T. O., Green, P. S., Uchida, K., O'Brien, K. D., Oram, J. F., and Heinecke, J. W. 2005. Acrolein impairs ATP binding cassette transporter A1-dependent cholesterol export from cells through site-specific modification of apolipoprotein A-I. J. Biol. Chem. 280:36386–36396.

Spiteller, P., Kern, W., Reiner, J., and Spiteller, G. 2001. Aldehydic lipid peroxidation products derived from linoleic acid. Biochim. Biophys. Acta 1531:188–208.

Szapacs, M. E., Riggins, J. N., Zimmerman, L. J., and Liebler, D. C. 2006. Covalent adduction of human serum albumin by 4-hydroxy-2-nonenal: kinetic analysis of competing alkylation reactions. Biochemistry 45:10521–10528.

Uchida, K., Kanematsu, M., Morimitsu, Y., Osawa, T., Noguchi, N., and Niki, E. 1998a. Acrolein is a product of lipid peroxidation reaction. Formation of free acrolein and its conjugate with lysine residues in oxidized low density lipoproteins. J. Biol. Chem. 273:16058–16066.

Uchida, K., Kanematsu, M., Sakai, K., Matsuda, T., Hattori, N., Mizuno, Y., Suzuki, D., Miyata, T., Noguchi, N., Niki, E., and Osawa, T. 1998b. Protein-bound acrolein: potential markers for oxidative stress. Proc. Natl. Acad. Sci. USA. 95:4882–4887.

Uchida, K., and Stadtman, E. R. 1992. Selective cleavage of thioether linkage in proteins modified with 4-hydroxynonenal. Proc. Natl. Acad. Sci. USA. 89:5611–5615.

Uchida, K., and Stadtman, E. R. 1993. Covalent attachment of 4-hydroxynonenal to glyceraldehyde-3-phosphate dehydrogenase. A possible involvement of intra- and intermolecular cross-linking reaction. J. Biol. Chem. 268:6388–6393.

Veronneau, M., Comte, B., and Des Rosiers, C. 2002. Quantitative gas chromatographic-mass spectrometric assay of 4-hydroxynonenal bound to thiol proteins in ischemic/reperfused rat hearts. Free Rad. Biol. Med. 33:1380–1388.

Xu, G., Liu, Y., Kansal, M. M., and Sayre, L. M. 1999. Rapid cross-linking of proteins by 4-ketoaldehydes and 4-hydroxy-2-alkenals does not arise from the lysine-derived monoalkylpyrroles. Chem. Res. Toxicol. 12:855–861.

Xu, G., and Sayre, L. M. 1998. Structural characterization of a 4-hydroxy-2-alkenal-derived fluorophore that contributes to lipoperoxidation-dependent protein cross-linking in aging and degenerative disease. Chem. Res. Toxicol. 11:247–251.

Xu, G., and Sayre, L. M. 1999. Structural elucidation of a 2:2 4-ketoaldehyde-amine adduct as a model for lysine-directed cross-linking of proteins by 4-ketoaldehydes. Chem. Res. Toxicol. 12:862–868.

Zaugg, R. H., Walder, J. A., and Klotz, I. M. 1977. Schiff base adducts of hemoglobin. Modifications that inhibit erythrocyte sickling. J. Biol. Chem. 252:8542–8548.

Zhang, W. H., Liu, J., Xu, G., Yuan, Q., and Sayre, L. M. 2003. Model studies on protein side chain modification by 4-oxo-2-nonenal. Chem. Res. Toxicol. 16:512–523.

Part II

Tissue-Specific Features and Risk Assessment Applications

10

Adaptive Responses and Signal Transduction Pathways in Chemically Induced Mitochondrial Dysfunction and Cell Death

Lawrence H. Lash
Department of Pharmacology, Wayne State University School of Medicine, Detroit, MI 48201, USA
e-mail: l.h.lash@wayne.edu

Keywords: Membrane Permeability Transition · Kidney Mitochondria · Liver Mitochondria · Heat Shock Proteins · Apoptosis · Caspases · Bioactivation · Reactive-Oxygen Species · Nitric Oxide

10.1. Introduction

The ability to adapt to physiological changes or pathological or chemical stresses is critical for growth, development, and survival. Adaptation can be seen at numerous levels, ranging from the organism (system), the tissue (organ), the cellular, the subcellular, and the molecular levels. One important site at which adaptation occurs is the mitochondrion. This cellular organelle is ultimately responsible for generating most of the ATP needed for cellular work in most tissues. Intuitively, one can view as an adaptation the ability of mitochondria to tightly regulate ATP production so that ATP supply matches cellular energy demands. Mitochondria are unique in possessing their own genome and transcription and translation mechanisms for protein synthesis. Although mitochondria have the capacity to synthesize proteins (13 polypeptides), most mitochondrial proteins are encoded by nuclear genes, which are synthesized as precursors and imported into mitochondria by virtue of possessing mitochondrial targeting sequences. Besides cellular ATP production, other functions of mitochondria include metabolite and ion transport, drug metabolism, and regulation of cell death pathways (Kroemer 2003; Green and Kroemer 2004; Danial and Korsmeyer 2004; Orrenius, Gogvadze and Zhivotovsky 2007; Schoolwerth and LaNoue 1985). Regulation of each of these pathways is critical to the ability of cells to respond to their environment and adapt to physiological changes and stresses. The integration

A.A. Elfarra (ed.), *Advances in Bioactivation Research*, DOI: 10.1007/978-0-387-77300-1_10,

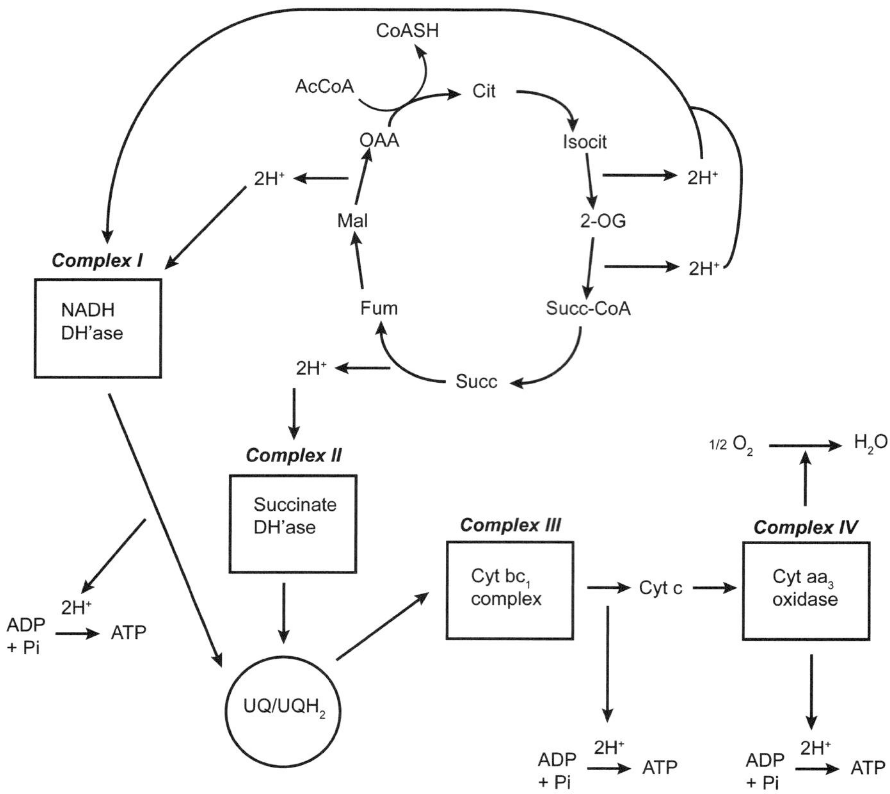

Figure 10.1 Scheme of intermediary metabolism and mitochondrial electron transport chain. This scheme summarizes how reducing equivalents are transferred, during the oxidation of carbohydrate substrates in the citric acid cycle, to the electron transport chain.
Abbreviations: AcCoA, acetyl-CoA; Cit, citrate; CoASH, coenzyme A; Cyt, cytochrome; DH'ase, dehydrogenase; Fum, fumarate; Isocit, isocitrate; Mal, malate; OAA, oxaloacetate; 2-OG, 2-oxoglutarate; Pi, inorganic phosphate; Succ, succinate; Succ-CoA, succinyl-CoA; UQ, oxidized ubiquinone; UQH_2, reduced ubiquinone.

of intermediary metabolism and the mitochondrial electron transport chain (ETC) is shown schematically in Figure 10.1.

Mitochondria are also an important target site in cells for reactive metabolites of drugs and other xenobiotics. There are several reasons for the mitochondria being the prominent targets: (1) mitochondria are the primary sites of cellular oxygen consumption and can be a significant source of reactive-oxygen species (ROS); (2) mitochondria contain a large number of enzymes and transporters with sulfhydryl groups that are only active in the reduced form (Lê-Quôc and Lê-Quôc 1985, 1989); this provides an extensive array of molecular targets for ROS and reactive electrophiles; (3) the mitochondrial genome may be more susceptible to reactive electrophiles because they lack the histone proteins found in the nuclear genome; and (4) mitochondria have lower activities and/or a less extensive array of detoxication enzymes than the cytoplasm. In spite of these factors and limitations, mitochondria still have an extensive capacity to modulate their structure and function to adapt to physiological and pathological changes.

The distribution, structure, and function of mitochondria in mammalian cells occur in distinct patterns that are characteristic for different cell types and tissues (Aw and Jones 1989). Thus, for example, mitochondria are localized adjacent to (Na^+–K^+)-ATPase-containing plasma membranes in transporting epithelia such as the renal proximal tubular and gastric parietal cells. Mitochondria are localized adjacent to contractile elements in skeletal, cardiac muscle, and other motile cells. Mitochondria are localized adjacent to synapses in neurons. These various spatial distributions are associated with specific molecular interactions between mitochondria and cytoskeletal elements and reflect the need for ATP production by the cellular structures that are associated with the mitochondria.

Substantial structural and functional heterogeneity also exist in mitochondria in various mammalian cells (Table 10.1). Early cytological studies revealed large variations in size and shape of mitochondria, ranging from large ovoid to small spherical particles and including thread-like forms as well as extensive, irregularly shaped reticula. Such differences in size and shape are easily visualized when comparing mitochondria from tissues with markedly different physiological functions, such as cardiac myocytes and hepatocytes. These variations are also observed in different cell types within a given tissue, such as those in the different cell populations comprising the mammalian nephron (Guder, Wagner and Wirthensohn 1986; Lash 1990). Moreover, structural and functional differences in mitochondria can even be observed within individual cells, such as exists between perinuclear and peripheral mitochondria in renal proximal tubular cells; the former are smaller and more spherical in shape than the latter.

In terms of adaptation, the ability of mitochondria to change their structure and shape in response to physiological or pathological conditions

Table 10.1 Structural and functional heterogeneity in mammalian mitochondria.

Property	Characteristics
Morphology	
Size	Small (<0.1-μm diameter) to large (>10-μm length)
Shape	Spherical to ovoid; thread-like; reticular
Appearance	Plate-like to tube-like cristae
Localization	
	Uniform throughout cell
	Perinuclear
	Adjacent to plasma membrane Na^+ pump in transport epithelia
	Adjacent to contractile elements in skeletal muscle and other motile cells
Biochemical	
	Quantitative and qualitative differences in ETC components
	Qualitative differences in specific enzyme content (e.g., bile acid synthesis in liver; vitamin D synthesis in renal proximal tubule)
	Tissue-specific isozymic forms of membrane transporters

Summary of basic structural and functional heterogeneity of mitochondria in mammalian cells. *Abbreviations*: ETC, electron transport chain.

is called "plasticity" (Aw and Jones 1989). In this regard, mitochondria are viewed as dynamic organelles that can change their morphology, composition, and consequently, their function, in response to specific signals. These signals include nutritional variation (e.g., starvation, high-protein diets), changes in work load (e.g., aerobic activity, different developmental stages), and changes in oxygen availability (e.g., hypoxia). Responses to these signals include parallel changes in ETC enzymes in skeletal muscle mitochondria after changes in aerobic activity, increased urea cycle enzymes in high-protein diets, increased ETC enzymes in liver and kidney mitochondria with increased protein load or potassium depletion, decreased ETC enzymes in chronic hypoxia, increased ETC enzymes in regenerating tissues, and changes in activities and ratios of ETC and other enzymes at different developmental stages.

Overall, these changes in mitochondrial enzymes are typically reversible and serve to match ATP production to energy needs of the tissue. Similar types of adaptive responses as described for physiological changes also occur with exposure to chemical toxicants. The main difference is that for exposure to chemical toxicants, responses are only reversible if the exposure levels are relatively low. In that case, sufficient activities of detoxication enzymes and regenerative mechanisms are present to return the mitochondria to normal function. It is only when chemical exposure levels are relatively high and/or detoxication or regenerative mechanisms are deficient (such as in certain genetic disorders or nutritional deficiencies) do the changes in mitochondrial function become permanent, often leading to cell death.

Some of the key processes that are used to produce mitochondrial adaptations include (1) control of the supply of oxidizable substrates and precursors (e.g., pyruvate, glutamate, fatty acyl carnitine, ADP, inorganic phosphate) and the elimination of products (e.g., ATP, carnitine) through regulation of membrane transporters; (2) regulation of electrical ($\Delta\psi$) and chemical (ΔpH) components of the electrochemical proton gradient (Δp) by control of electron flow through the ETC; (3) regulation of the supply of NADH by control of dehydrogenase activities; and (4) control of redox status through the glutathione (GSH)/glutathione disulfide (GSSG), thioredoxin (Trx)/thioredoxin reductase (Trd), glutaredoxin (Grx), superoxide dismutase (SOD), and peroxiredoxin III (PrxIII) systems.

The focus of this chapter is to present information of the processes involved in mitochondrial adaptation in response to physiological, pathological, and toxicological stresses. The chapter is divided into four main sections. The first section will discuss the role of redox status in mitochondrial function and adaptation. The second section will discuss the mitochondrial membrane permeability transition (MPT) and its function in mediating cell death. The third section will discuss some key sensors and signaling processes or mediators of mitochondrial adaptation. Finally, the last section will briefly discuss four examples of physiological or pathological stresses that are associated with alterations in mitochondrial function. The importance of bioactivation processes, particularly those that result in generation of reactive species, will be emphasized where appropriate.

10.2. Role of Redox Status in Determining Mitochondrial Function and Adaptation

Two central points that make regulation of redox status so important in the control of mitochondrial function and adaptation are that, as mentioned above, mitochondria are the primary sites within the cell for oxygen consumption and they contain a large array of enzymes and membrane transporters that are susceptible to oxidative inactivation. Although mitochondrial respiration is tightly coupled to ADP phosphorylation and reduction of molecular oxygen to water under normal, physiological conditions, approximately 1%–2% of the molecular oxygen consumed is thought to be converted to superoxide anion radicals (Orrenius, Gogvadze and Zhivotovsky 2007). Increased levels of superoxide anion can be released at two specific points in the ETC, at complex I and complex III (cf. Figure 10.1). Besides the ETC, other mitochondrial sources of ROS include oxidases such as monoamine oxidase, which generate hydrogen peroxide, and cytochrome P450, which can become uncoupled and release superoxide anion.

Reactive-oxygen species that are generated by mitochondria can produce damage to various cellular macromolecules, including nucleic acids, phospholipids, and proteins. The polyunsaturated fatty acid residues of phospholipids are particularly susceptible to oxidation. This occurs by generation of hydroxyl radicals via the Fenton reaction. Oxidative damage to DNA can cause modification of both purine and pyrimidine bases or the deoxyribose backbone, single- or double-strand breaks, or crosslinking of DNA to other molecules. Such changes can be mutagenic and/or carcinogenic. Oxidative damage to proteins can occur at many sites, including oxidation of sulfhydryl groups of cysteinyl residues, formation of oxidative adducts on certain amino acid residues, protein–protein crosslinking, and protein fragmentation. Direct oxidation of certain amino acid residues, such as lysines, arginines, prolines, and threonines, can lead to formation of protein carbonyls, which can dramatically alter protein tertiary structure. Such alterations often result in unfolding, promotion of protein–protein interactions, a loss of function, and enhanced proteolytic degradation.

In mitochondria, specific targets include mitochondrial DNA, iron–sulfur proteins, other mitochondrial enzymes such as aconitase (Cooper, Bruschi and Anders 2002; James et al. 2002), and various dehydrogenases. Because of the multiplicity of molecular targets for ROS in mitochondria, a variety of adaptive responses exist. For example, Lee et al. (2000) studied responses of MRC-5 cells, a human lung fibroblast cell line, to various treatments that induce an oxidative stress. They observed that mitochondria from such oxidatively stressed cells compensate for the decline in respiratory function by increasing the copy number of mitochondrial DNA and mitochondrial mass. More commonly, excess formation of ROS in mitochondria has been associated with the mitochondrial MPT and apoptosis (Cai and Jones 1998).

In addition to ROS, recent attention has also focused on the potential regulatory roles for reactive-nitrogen species (RNS), which are generated from nitric oxide (NO) produced in mitochondria (Giulivi, Poderoso and Boveris 1998; Tatoyan and Giulivi 1998). Both NO and peroxynitrite ($ONOO^-$) are associated with mitochondrial damage by causing DNA damage, cytochrome *c* release, and apoptosis (Ghafourifar et al. 1999; Li, Trudel and Wogan 2002). Giulivi and colleagues (Giulivi, Poderoso and Boveris 1998; Tatoyan and Giulivi 1998) showed that most of the mitochondrial nitric oxide synthase (mtNOS) is localized in the inner mitochondrial membrane, is constitutive, and requires flavin mononucleotide, calcium ions, calmodulin, and tetrahydrobiopterin as cofactors. Nitric oxide directly inhibits cytochrome oxidase (Barone, Darley-Usmar and Brookes 2003; Borutaite, Budriunaite and Brown 2000; Brookes et al. 2003), thereby inhibiting mitochondrial respiration (Bellamy, Griffiths and Garthwaite 2002; Beltrán et al. 2002).

Besides direct reactions with cellular molecules, effects of NO may also be mediated by formation of *S*-nitrosoglutathione (GSNO) (Ji et al. 1999; Sandau, Callsen and Brüne 1999; Sarkela et al. 2001; Wong and Fukuto, 1999). Figure 10.2 illustrates reactions by which NO reacts with GSH to form GSNO and those by which NO can be generated from GSNO, showing how GSNO can then function as an NO donor. The normally high concentration of GSH in mitochondrial matrix (~5 mM) and the presence of a constitutively expressed NOS in the organelle suggest that formation of GSNO plays an important physiological role. Nitric oxide can also modulate cell injury and growth. Delineation of the function of NO, however, is quite complex. While NO is antiapoptotic in some cell types by processes such as inhibition of caspases (Li et al. 1999; Mannick et al. 2001) or inhibition of Bcl-2 cleavage (Kim et al. 1998), NO is proapoptotic in other cell types. For example, NO promotes apoptosis in human mononuclear cell lines by nitrosylation of cytochrome *c*, which induces its release from mitochondria (Schonhoff, Gaston and Mannick 2003). Nitric oxide inhibits c-Jun DNA binding, by formation of GSNO and glutathiony- lation of c-Jun (Klatt, Molina and Lamas 1999), and can regulate the expression levels of several zinc-finger transcription

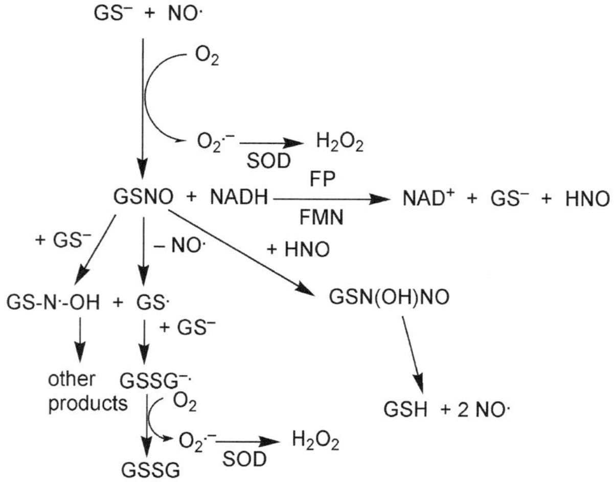

Figure 10.2 Reactions of glutathione (GSH) with nitric oxide (NO) to form *S*-nitrosoglutathione (GSNO). GSH, as the thiolate, reacts with NO in the presence of O_2 and forms GSNO. GSNO can release NO (function of GSNO as an NO donor) or it may react in the presence of the thiolate to form a species that can glutathionylate protein sulfhydryl groups. GSNO acts as an NO donor by two reactions, the first of which is mediated by a flavoprotein (FP) containing FMN. The HNO generated from the first reaction can react with another molecule of GSNO to form an intermediate that decomposes to GSH and NO. *Abbreviations*: FMN, flavin mononucleotide; SOD, superoxide dismutase.

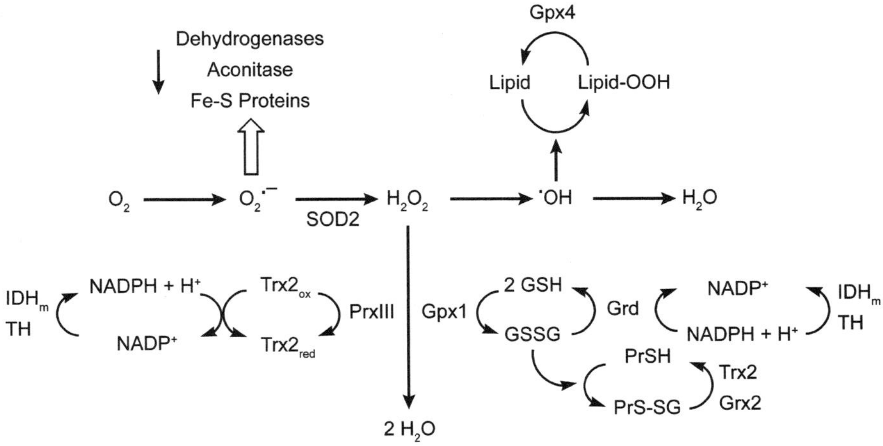

Figure 10.3 Antioxidant enzyme systems in mitochondria. Although the majority of molecular oxygen is fully reduced to water, a minor portion (~1%–2%) is partially reduced to superoxide anion even under physiological conditions. This fraction may increase under conditions of pathological or toxicological stress. If the various antioxidant systems are inadequate or inhibited, consequences can include inhibition of mitochondrial enzymes, particularly in the electron transport chain, and lipid peroxidation.
Abbreviations: Gpx1/4, glutathione peroxidase 1/4; Grd, glutathione disulfide reductase; Grx2, glutaredoxin 2; GSH, glutathione; GSSG, glutathione disulfide; IDH_m, mitochondrial isocitrate dehydrogenase; PrSH, protein containing reduced sulfhydryl group(s); PrS-SG, protein containing mixed disulfide(s) with GSH; PrxIII, peroxiredoxin III; SOD2, mitochondrial Mn-superoxide dismutase; TH, transhydrogenase; Trx2, thioredoxin 2.

factors (Kröncke et al. 2002). Thus, multiple signaling mechanisms are elicited in response to formation of NO and other RNS.

The tight regulation of mitochondrial redox balance is evident from the broad spectrum of antioxidant enzymes that are present (Figure 10.3). A supply of reducing equivalents and the battery of antioxidant enzymes help maintain the levels of ROS at very low concentrations. There are five major antioxidant systems or enzymes that are involved in regulation of ROS levels, the GSH–GSH peroxidase (Gpx)–GSSG reductase (Grd) system, the Trx–Trd system, Grx, PrxIII, and Mn-SOD (SOD2).

The Trx–Trd system has been shown to play a critical role in maintenance of the mitochondrial $\Delta\psi$ and to interact with specific components of the ETC (Damdimopoulos et al. 2002). Moreover, overexpression of Trx2 in HEK-293 cells (Damdimopoulos et al. 2002) or HeLa cells (Hansen, Zhang and Jones 2006) protects from oxidant-induced mitochondrial dysfunction and cell death. In contrast, cells containing a dominant-negative, active-site mutation in Trx2 (Hansen, Zhang and Jones 2006) or B-cells that are Trx2-deficient (Tanaka et al. 2002) are markedly more sensitive to ROS-induced mitochondrial dysfunction and apoptosis.

Unlike the cytoplasmic GSH pool, the mitochondrial GSH pool cannot be directly increased by increases in synthesis, because the enzymes for GSH synthesis are only found in the cytoplasm (Griffith and Meister 1985; McKernan, Woods and Lash 1991). Instead, the mitochondrial GSH pool is determined by transport of cytoplasmic GSH (Lash 2006). Taking into account that the GSH molecule is an anion at physiological pH and the existence of the $\Delta\psi$ across the mitochondrial inner membrane, we suggested that one or more of the carriers for anionic intermediary metabolites is (are) involved in transport of cytoplasmic GSH into the mitochondrial matrix (McKernan, Woods and Lash 1991; Chen and Lash 1998; Chen, Putt and Lash 2000). Indeed, we demonstrated that most, if not all, of the transport of GSH into mitochondria of rat renal cortex is mediated by two electroneutral, anionic metabolite carriers, the dicarboxylate carrier (DIC; *Slc25a10*) and the 2-oxoglutarate carrier (OGC; *Slc25a11*) (Figure 10.4). The DIC exchanges dicarboxylates, such as malate, for inorganic phosphate, whereas the OGC exchanges 2-oxoglutarate for other dicarboxylates.

Because the DIC and OGC are both involved in transport of citric acid cycle intermediates, their function in GSH transport indicates that alterations in mitochondrial GSH status will alter that of citric acid cycle intermediates, amino acids, and the malate–aspartate shuttle, which will in turn alter respiratory function. Indeed, overexpression of either the DIC or OGC in NRK-52E cells, a rat renal proximal tubular cell line, markedly protects from oxidant-induced mitochondrial dysfunction and apoptosis (Lash, Putt and Matherly 2002; Xu et al. 2006). Conversely, overexpression of mutant DIC or OGC carriers with markedly reduced transport function in the NRK-52E cells increased susceptibility to oxidant-induced apoptosis (Lash, Putt and Matherly 2002; Xu et al. 2006).

The function of the various aforementioned systems in regulation of mitochondrial redox status has traditionally been viewed as functioning to maintain an appropriate balance between oxidants and reductants (Sies 1985). In light of the accumulation of data on redox signaling pathways

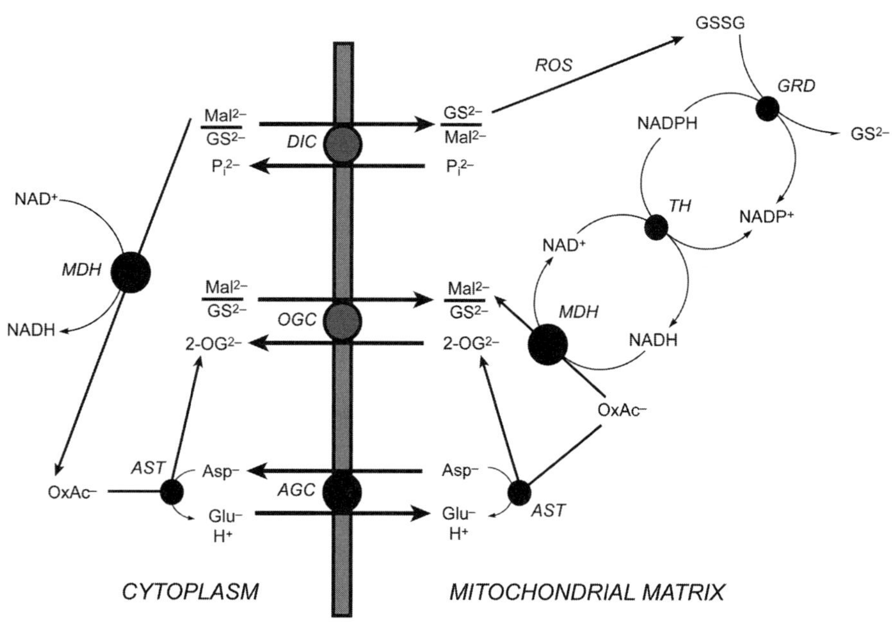

Figure 10.4 Pathways of mitochondrial GSH transport. Scheme illustrating how GSH transport by either the DIC or OGC interfaces with the malate–aspartate shuttle and other pathways of metabolism of citric acid cycle intermediates.

Abbreviations: AGC, glutamate–aspartate exchanger; AST, aspartate transaminase; DIC, dicarboxylate carrier; GRD, glutathione disulfide reductase; MDH, malic dehydrogenase; 2-OG, 2-oxoglutarate; OGC, 2-oxoglutarate carrier; $OxAC^{-}$, oxaloacetate; ROS, reactive-oxygen species.

and the lack of significant therapeutic benefits in intervention trials with free-radical scavengers and antioxidants, Jones (2006) has redefined mitochondrial oxidative stress. Rather than the traditional or classic definition of mitochondrial oxidative stress as an imbalance between oxidants and reductants in favor of the former, Jones proposes a disruption of mitochondrial redox circuitry as a consequence of exposure to ROS and other oxidants that can be generated by bioactivation reactions. He describes mitochondria as possessing two types of redox circuits: (1) high-flux pathways that regulate ATP production; and (2) low-flux pathways that use sulfur switches of proteins for metabolic regulation and regulation of the mitochondrial ETC. Furthermore, he proposes that superoxide anions provide a link between the two pathways. The hypothesis is that superoxide anions, rather than being merely by-products of electron transfer, are generated by the mitochondrial ETC to serve as a positive signal to coordinate energy metabolism. Electron mediators, such as free Fe^{3+}, redox cycling agents, and free-radical scavengers, are then proposed to cause oxidative stress by disrupting the normal superoxide anion signal. When viewed in this manner, the array of redox enzymes and redox couples could then respond in exquisitely sensitive ways to environmental signals, thereby facilitating adaptation of mitochondrial function.

10.3. Mitochondrial MPT and Cell Death

Mitochondria play a key role in cell death induced by pathological conditions, such as ischemia, or exposure to toxic chemicals that are generated by bioactivation reactions. The long-standing dogma had been that cells die by necrosis in an unregulated manner when cellular structure collapses and there is a generalized lysis of organelle and plasma membranes. Necrosis was often associated with the death of a large number of cells that triggered the release of macrophages and phagocytes. In contrast, apoptosis was considered a programmed mechanism whereby a series of ATP-dependent processes occur that culminate in the death of individual cells. Recently, however, it has become clear that the mechanisms behind how cells die is not that simple (Chiarugi 2005). Cell death occurs by a broad spectrum of mechanisms that range from apoptotic-like to necrotic-like. Moreover, both types of mechanisms can occur by both ATP-dependent and ATP-independent processes. Both apoptotic and necrotic pathways have common upstream mediators and chemicophysical agents can trigger either apoptosis or necrosis, depending on the intensity of the exposure. A key component in many of the apoptotic and necrotic forms of cell death induced by diverse agents is the MPT (Lemasters et al. 1998), suggesting that mitochondria act as universal stress sensors (Kroemer 2003).

Mitochondria from liver, kidney, and several other tissues undergo a ‘permeability transition’ whereby the inner membrane becomes permeable to ions and other molecules of low-to-moderate molecular weight. The MPT can be readily reversible under certain conditions and occurs when Ca^{2+} loading is followed or preceded by addition of a second agent, referred to as an “inducing agent” or calcium-releasing agent. The chemical diversity of MPT inducing agents is illustrated in Table 10.2. Despite

Table 10.2 Some agents that induce the mitochondrial permeability transition.

Fatty acids and lipids	NAD(P)H oxidants	ANT inhibitors
L-carnitine Long-chain acyl carnitines Long-chain acyl-CoA	Acetoacetate *tert*-butylhydroperoxide, H_2O_2, oxaloacetate	Atractyloside Carboxyatractyloside
Heavy and transition metals	**Organic sulfhydryl reagents**	**Other chemicals**
Cd^{2+}, Cu^{2+}, Fe^{3+}, Hg^{2+}, organic mercurials, Pb^{2+}, Zn^{2+}	Arsenite Diamide Iodoacetate, iodoacetamide, Mersalyl phenylarsine oxide	Phosphate, pyrophosphate Dopamine, 6-OH-dopamine Phosphoenolpyruvate Pyridoxal phosphate Nitrofurantoin Cyanide Allantoin

this diversity, it is thought that inducing agents act through a common mechanism. Perturbation of a phospholipid acylation– deacylation cycle is seen as a central event leading to the MPT. Calcium ions are hypothesized to increase activity of this cycle by stimulating the mitochondrial phospholipase A_2. The inducing agent is thought to inhibit phospholipid reacylation through various direct or indirect mechanisms. As a result, phospholipase A_2 reaction products (e.g., arachidonic acid) accumulate and increase membrane permeability.

The structure of the permeability pore (Figure 10.5) includes dimers of the voltage-dependent anion channel (VDAC) and the adenine nucleotide translocase (ANT), which span the outer and inner mitochondrial membranes, cyclophilin D (CyD) bound to the ANT subunit on the inner face of the inner membrane, Ca^{2+} ions bound to the CyD molecule, the mitochondrial or peripheral benzodiazepine receptor (mBzR), which spans the outer mitochondrial membrane and associates with VDAC, and hexokinase (HK), which associates with VDAC at the outer surface of the outer mitochondrial membrane. The acidic phospholipid cardiolipin (CL), which is unique to the inner mitochondrial membrane, binds cytochrome *c* via electrostatic and hydrophobic interactions and prevents its release from mitochondria. Upon oxidation of CL, cytochrome *c* binding is decreased, thereby facilitating its release from mitochondria. A notable characteristic of the permeability transition is that it is completely blocked by the immunosuppressive peptide cyclosporin A (CsA). The permeability transition can occur both with and without matrix swelling.

Several mechanisms are currently proposed to explain the role of opening of the MPT in inducing cell death by either necrosis (oncosis) or apoptosis. In many cases, opening of the MPT is associated with osmotic swelling of the mitochondrial matrix, rupture of the outer mitochondrial membrane, and release of intermembrane space proteins, including cytochrome *c* (Orrenius, Gogvadze and Zhivotovsky 2007). For many years,

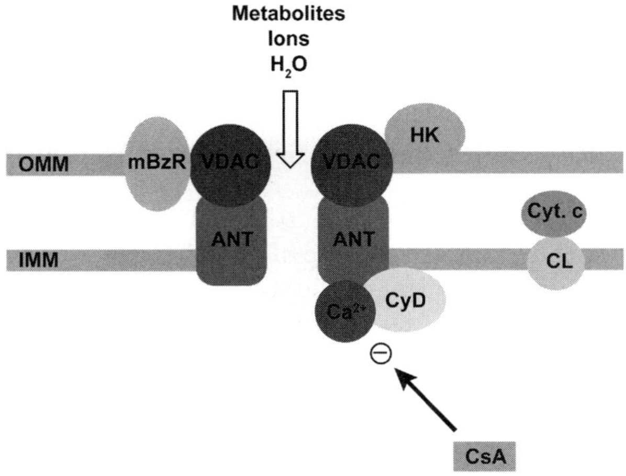

Figure 10.5 Structure of the mitochondrial permeability pore. The pore is comprised of dimers of the VDAC on the OMM that is associated with dimers of the ANT on the IMM. CyD associates with the inner surface of the IMM and binds Ca^{2+} ions and the mBzR spans the OMM and associates with one subunit of VDAC. The phospholipid CL in the IMM binds cytochrome *c* (Cyt. c) on the outer surface of the IMM, promoting its retention in the mitochondria. Additionally, HK associates with a subunit of VDAC on the outer surface of the OMM.
Abbreviations: ANT, adenine nucleotide translocase; CL, cardiolipin; CyD, cyclophilin D; Cyt. C, cytochrome c; HK, hexokinase; IMM, inner mitochondrial membrane; mBzR, mitochondrial or peripheral benzodiazepine receptor; OMM, outer mitochondrial membrane; VDAC, voltage-dependent anion channel.

the MPT was regarded as the primary mechanism for permeabilization of the outer mitochondrial membrane. A scheme summarizing the sequence of events by which the MPT leads to alterations in mitochondrial function is shown in Figure 10.6. While this 'classic' mechanism is certainly relevant under conditions of mitochondrial Ca^{2+} overload that are associated with a severe oxidative stress, it became clear that other mechanisms and patterns of MPT occur. For example, transient pore opening may also occur whereby a small fraction of mitochondrial matrix proteins in a fraction of mitochondria are released. In this case, no large-amplitude swelling occurs and the overall $\Delta\psi$ of the mitochondrial population is maintained. This pattern of MPT would likely occur as a reversible adaptation to changing physiological conditions or to a mild exposure to a toxicant or pathological condition.

Other recent studies have brought the importance of the MPT as a key prerequisite for apoptosis into question (Baines et al. 2005; Li et al. 2004; Nakagawa et al. 2005). Studies with either CyD-overexpressing or CyD-deficient cells showed that the MPT does not always accompany

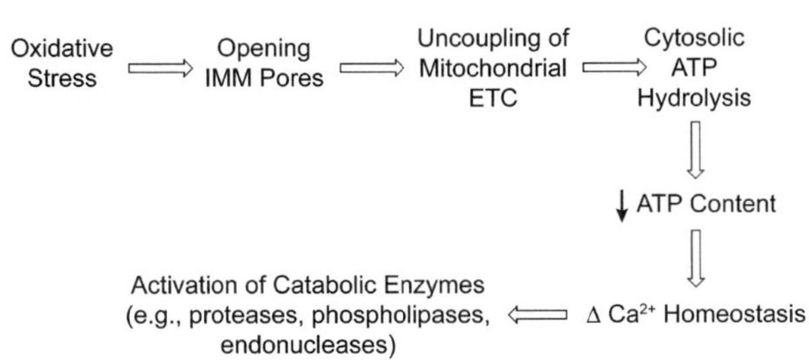

Figure 10.6 Sequence of events in the classical view of the mitochondrial membrane permeabilization.
Abbreviations: ETC, electron transport chain; IMM, inner mitochondrial membrane.

apoptosis. Moreover, these studies also suggested that CyD-dependent MPT can be involved in necrotic, but not apoptotic, cell death.

10.4. Mitochondrial Sensors and Mediators of Adaptation

This section will discuss some of the major signaling pathways involved in the response of mitochondria to chemical and pathological stresses. A common feature of many of these stresses is the involvement of ROS and oxidative stress. At the cellular level, oxidant injury elicits a wide spectrum of responses, many of which are initiated at the level of mitochondria. Whatever the observed response and whatever the causative agent or disease state, it reflects a balance between diverse signaling pathways that exhibit a large degree of cross-talk (Martindale and Holbrook 2002). While these pathways are by no means completely understood, it is clear that the existence of so many diverse signals implies both a redundancy of function and an exquisite ability of cells to respond to challenges. The examples that are discussed in the following subsections are by no means a complete set of mediators, but represent those that have been most closely associated with mitochondria.

10.4.1. Bcl-2 Family Proteins

An important group of proteins that is involved in mediating many of the responses of mitochondria to environmental stresses is the Bcl-2 family (reviewed in Danial and Korsmeyer (2004) and Orrenius, Gogvadze and Zhivotovsky (2007)). This family consists of more than 30 proteins, which are divided into three subgroups: (1) Bcl-2-like survival factors; (2) Bax-like death factors; and (3) BH3-only death factors. The first indications that members of this family of proteins were involved at the level of mitochondria in controlling apoptosis came in the late-1990s, when it was shown that Bcl-2 could prevent the efflux of cytochrome *c* and thereby prevent apoptosis. Bax was then shown to stimulate cytochrome *c* release and promote apoptosis by binding to Bcl-2. Thus, the ratio of Bcl-2 to Bax is seen as functioning as 'a rheostat that sets the threshold of susceptibility to apoptosis for the intrinsic pathway' (Danial and Korsmeyer 2004). The intrinsic pathway refers to the pathway for induction of apoptosis that is initiated in the mitochondria.

Besides Bcl-2, Bcl-X_L is also an antiapoptotic member of the Bcl-2 family. Like Bcl-2, Bcl-X_L serves an antiapoptotic function by binding and sequestering BH3-only molecules, which prevents their activation. Members of the family that include Bax, Bak, and tBid act as proapoptotic signals. Bax and Bak can undergo oligomerization and insert into the outer mitochondrial membrane, leading to permeabilization (Figure 10.7). Besides cytochrome *c*, three other proteins have been identified as being released from mitochondria: apoptosis-inducing factor (AIF), endonuclease G, and HtrA2/Omi. Apoptosis-inducing factor translocates to the nucleus, where it causes chromatin condensation and generates

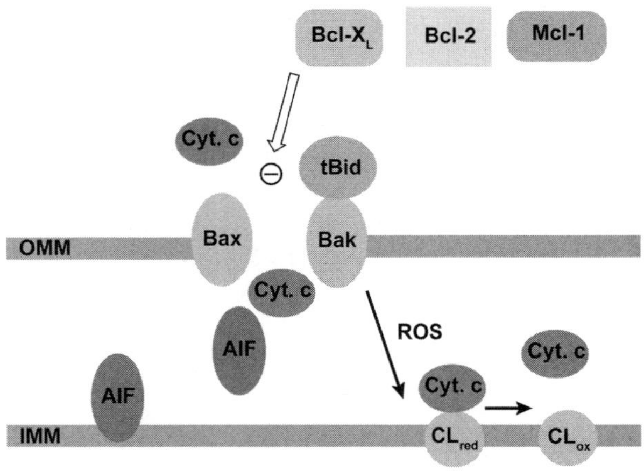

Figure 10.7 Bax- and Bak-dependent mitochondrial membrane permeabilization. In addition to the classic mechanism involving the mitochondrial MPT, the OMM may become permeabilized by the action of three BH3-only proteins, Bax, Bak, and tBid; the first two are intrinsic proteins of the OMM whereas tBid binds externally to Bax or Bak. Creation of a pore is associated with AIF. Interaction of AIF with Bax/Bak leads to ROS-dependent oxidation of CL on the inner mitochondrial membrane (IMM). CL, which in its reduced form binds cytochrome *c*, releases it upon oxidation. Permeabilization of the OMM is inhibited by three Bcl-2 family proteins, Bcl-2, Bcl-X_L, and Mcl-1.
Abbreviations: AIF, apoptosis-inducing factor; CL, cardiolipin; MPT, membrane permeability transition; OMM, outer mitochondrial membrane; ROS, reactive-oxygen species.

high-molecular-weight chromatin fragments in a CyD-dependent manner. Endonuclease G translocates to the nucleus where it produces DNA-strand breaks. HtrA2/Omi is a serine protease that accumulates in the cytoplasm and degrades several antiapoptotic proteins.

10.4.2. Heat Shock Proteins

Heat shock proteins (HSPs) are a group of conserved proteins induced in prokaryotes and eukaryotes by numerous types of cellular stresses, including oxidative stress and formation of reactive species generated by bioactivation reactions. Heat shock proteins are classified according to their apparent molecular weight, their intracellular location, their primary inducer(s), and their functions. For example, the Hsp70 family are proteins found in the cytoplasm (Hsp72, Hsp73), the endoplasmic reticulum (grp78), or the mitochondria (Hsp60, Hsp70). These HSPs act as molecular chaperones and play a role in protein folding, refolding, transport, and translocation (Polla et al. 1996). Small HSPs (Hsp25/27; Hsp25 is found in rodents and Hsp27 is the human homologue) are found primarily in the cytoplasm.

One of the earliest studies implicating HSPs in the mitochondrial response to injury from reactive metabolites was that of Bruschi et al. (1993). These investigators showed that Hsp60 and a protein identified as one of the members of the Hsp70 family (originally called "mortalin") were early molecular targets of *S*-(1,1,2,2-tetrafluoroethyl)-L-cysteine (TFEC)-induced nephrotoxicity. Both of these proteins are found in renal mitochondria. These authors suggested that part of the mechanism of TFEC-induced nephrotoxicity is mediated by adduction of Hsp60 and Hsp70 family members in renal proximal tubular mitochondria, thereby decreasing the ability of the renal proximal tubular cell to degrade damaged or otherwise abnormal proteins. In a subsequent study (Bruschi, Lindsay and Crabb 1998), these investigators demonstrated recognition and binding of abnormal proteins generated by adducts formed from reactive metabolites of TFEC with mitochondrial Hsp60 and Hsp70.

In another study, murine hepatocytes were used to investigate the cellular responses to mitochondrial toxicity caused by exposure to TFEC (Ho et al. 2006). Using complementary DNA (cDNA) microarray analysis and reverse transcriptase-polymerase chain reaction (RT-PCR), they showed that the mRNA for several cytoplasmic HSPs, including Hsp25 and Hsp70, were strongly upregulated within the first few hours after treatment. Interestingly, none of the upregulated HSPs were mitochondrial in origin despite the well-documented intramitochondrial toxicity of TFEC. The authors suggested that early damage to mitochondria transmits signals to the cytoplasm that lead to the compensatory, genomic response. It was noted, however, that there is some evidence that two pools of Hsp25/27 may exist, one in the cytoplasm and one in mitochondria.

Most studies of HSPs and mitochondria, however, have identified these proteins as being responsible for protection against oxidative stress and chemically induced mitochondrial dysfunction. Polla et al. (1996) showed that Hsp70 protects human premonocytic U937 cells from hydrogen peroxide-induced alterations in mitochondrial $\Delta\psi$ and cristae structure. Induction of Bcl-2 expression was also found, showing linkage between HSPs and the intrinsic pathway for apoptosis.

A large number of studies have demonstrated protective functions of the small HSP Hsp25/27. Hsp25/27 exists as oligomers and undergoes reversible phosphorylation and dephosphorylation reactions. Increased expression and/or phosphorylation of Hsp25/27 has been associated with suppression of oxidant-induced MPT (He and Lemasters 2003), decreased apoptosis induced by diverse toxicants and physicochemical agents, including *S*-(1,2-dichlorovinyl)-L-cysteine (DCVC) (de Graauw et al. 2005; Lash et al. 2005a), hydrogen peroxide (Lee et al. 2004; Vertii et al. 2006; Zheng et al. 2006), arachidonic acid (Zheng et al. 2006), and Cs irradiation (Lee et al. 2005).

Hsp25/27 has also been shown to produce other effects besides those involving mitochondria. For example, Hsp27 promotes the ubiquitination and proteasomal degradation of the cell-cycle regulatory protein $p27^{Kip1}$ in human U937 cells, thereby enhancing S-phase re-entry (Parcellier et al. 2006). In LLC-PK_1 cells, a porcine proximal tubule-derived cell line, DCVC-induced upregulation of Hsp27 was associated with preservation of cytoskeleton organization, thereby suppressing renal cell apoptosis (de Graauw et al. 2005). Hsp25 expression in L929 mouse fibroblasts was induced by hydrogen peroxide and reduced DNA fragmentation (Lee et al. 2004). Hsp25/27 also interacts with other signaling pathways, including the phosphatidylinositol 3-kinase (PI-3 K)–Akt (protein kinase B; PKB) (Rane et al. 2003; Zheng et al. 2006), protein kinase Cδ (PKCδ)

(Lee et al. 2005), and mitogen-activated protein kinase (MAPK) (Lee et al. 2004; Zheng et al. 2006) pathways.

From this discussion on Hsp25/27, it is clear that the protective effects of these proteins are universal, being identified in cells from multiple tissues and species, and involves both mitochondrial and extramitochondrial processes. It is also apparent that there is significant cross-talk between Hsp25/27 and multiple signaling pathways, indicating that there is exquisite regulation of these responses.

10.4.3. Protein Kinases: PKB (Akt), PKC-α, PKC-ε, PKD

Protein kinases are involved in the phosphorylation of a diverse array of protein targets, leading to their inhibition or activation. In terms of regulation of mitochondrial function, four protein kinases have been identified as having a pivotal role. Several protein kinase isoforms exist, but the effects of each one differs; whereas some isoforms have been shown to promote ROS- or toxicant-induced mitochondrial dysfunction and cell death, some are protective and promote repair and regeneration of cells.

Protein Kinase B (or Akt) is a serine/threonine kinase that is activated in a PI-3 K-dependent manner. Products of PI-3 K result in translocation to the plasma membrane, where Akt is phosphorylated. Such activation has been associated with increases in cell proliferation, growth, differentiation, and survival (Li and Zhu 2002; Storz and Toker 2002). As reviewed by Shaik, Fifer, and Nowak (2007); the protective role of Akt against apoptosis initiated by mitochondrial damage is well established. Akt activation inhibits cytochrome *c* release and activation of caspase-3 and caspase-9, and several proapoptotic (e.g., Bad, Bax, and caspase-9) and antiapoptotic (e.g., Bcl-X_L and Bcl-2) proteins are downstream targets of Akt. Consistent with these earlier results, Akt activation was shown to protect WRL-68 human liver cells from hydrogen peroxide-induced apoptosis (Tapodi et al. 2005). The protection was associated with inhibition of poly(ADP-ribose)polymerase (PARP), which challenges the dogma that cytoprotection by PARP inhibitors is associated exclusively with preservation of pyridine nucleotides.

In a similar vein, Akt activation protected rabbit renal proximal tubules from DCVC-induced inhibition of mitochondrial respiration, decreases in ATP levels, and necrosis (Shaik, Fifer and Nowak 2007). Both pharmacological inhibition of Akt activation and overexpression of a dominant-negative, inactive Akt exacerbated DCVC-induced necrosis. In contrast, there was no effect of Akt activation on DCVC-induced apoptosis. This lack of protection against apoptosis and data suggesting the Akt activation prevents the MPT, are consistent with the hypothesis that the MPT is associated with necrotic, rather than apoptotic, cell death.

Protein kinase C is a family of serine/threonine protein kinases that exists as several isoforms, each of which regulates distinct functions. In one study, Nowak (2003) showed, without specifying the isoform involved, that PKC activation promoted recovery of mitochondrial function and active Na^+ transport in *tert*-butyl hydroperoxide- and DCVC-treated rabbit proximal tubular cells whereas inhibition of PKC activity decreased the repair of cellular functions after *tert*-butyl hydroperoxide treatment. In contrast with that study, other work from Nowak and colleagues (Nowak 2002; Nowak, Bakajsova and Clifton 2004; Liu, Godwin and Nowak 2004) showed that both PKC-α and PKC-ε inhibit recovery of oxidative phosphorylation and active Na^+ transport in rabbit renal proximal tubules after toxicant exposure. These effects were seen with exposure to DCVC, cisplatin, and *tert*-butyl hydroperoxide, indicating the broad applicability of the findings. Mechanisms by which these inhibitory effects occur include the phosphorylation of the β-subunit of the F_1F_0-ATPase by PKC-α.

Protein Kinase D is a ubiquitously expressed, serine/threonine kinase and a member of the calcium–calmodulin-dependent kinase superfamily. Storz, Döppler, and Toker (2005) studied the role of PKD in the response of HeLa cells to agents that produce mitochondrial ROS (hydrogen peroxide, rotenone, and diphenyleneiodonium). In each case, they found that mitochondrial ROS activated PKD, which in turn activated the NF-κB transcription factor, leading to induction of SOD2. This PKD-mediated upregulation of SOD2 resulted in increased survival of the cells.

10.4.4. MAPK Pathway

One signaling pathway that has received considerable attention with respect to renal repair and regeneration after chemical- or ischemia-induced acute renal failure is the MAPK pathway (Tian, Zhang and Cohen 2000). Several in vivo and in vitro models of proliferative or toxic renal injury are associated with changes in MAPK regulation. The MAPK system consists of a specific MAPK, its upstream activator, which is also a group of kinases called MAPK kinase or MKK, and a further upstream activator, which is a group of kinases called MAPK kinase kinase or MKKK. MAPKs are broadly divided into three families on the basis of sequence similarities (i.e., extracellular signal-regulated kinase (ERK), c-Jun NH_2-terminal kinase (JNK), and p38 MAPK), upstream activators, and substrate specificity. Although the classical paradigm of discrete stimuli for each MAPK family exists, there is significant cross-talk between the families.

Mitogen-activated protein kinases are activated by ROS in renal epithelial cells (Ramachandiran et al. 2002), and cell survival (i.e., recovery) from ischemic renal injury has been associated in some cases with activation of both ERK and JNK (Di Mari, Davis and Safirstein 1999). Effectors of MAPKs have also been identified as being activated in response to renal injury. For example, transcription of the growth arrest and DNA-damage inducible transcript 153 (*gadd*153) mRNA in LLC-PK_1 cells is increased by DCVC and other nephrotoxic cysteine S-conjugates (Chen et al. 1992), and activation of p53 (Healy et al. 1998; Dmitrieva, Michea and Burg 2001) and p21 and regulation of the cell cycle (Megyesi et al. 2002) are involved in the response to renal injury as well.

In contrast to the above results, several investigators have found that activation of the ERK1/2 pathway is associated with oxidant-induced decreases in mitochondrial function and enhancement of toxicant-induced apoptosis in renal proximal tubules (Nowak 2002; Nowak et al. 2006; Sinha et al. 2004; Zhuang et al. 2007). These apoptosis-promoting and mitochondrial recovery-inhibiting effects occur in opposition to the activation of Akt (Sinha et al. 2004; Zhuang et al. 2007). As an illustration of the cell type-specificity of ERK1/2 action, Ambrose et al. (2006) showed that dephosphorylation of ERK1/2 increased apoptosis in renal cell carcinoma cells but not in normal human renal epithelial cells. This result suggests a potentially novel therapeutic approach for the treatment of renal cell carcinoma, which is highly refractory to antineoplastic agents. Lee et al. (2004) also found that ERK1/2 activation promoted hydrogen peroxide-induced cell death in murine L929 cells.

In the traditional view of the role of members of the MAPK pathway in cellular responses to toxicants and other stresses, ERK and JNK are viewed as acting in opposing manners to influence cell survival during stress (Martindale and Holbrook 2002). As indicated above, this view is oversimplified. Similarly, conflicting results have also been obtained about the influence of p38 MAPK in cell survival in different cell types. In a recent review on the role of ERK in promotion of cell death, Zhuang and Schnellmann (2006) explain that some of the apparently contradictory results are due to tissue-specific actions of ERK activation, leading in some cases to promotion of cell survival and in others to promotion of cell death. Activation of ERK1/2 by phosphorylation can occur at several steps in various signaling pathways. Points of action that have been identified include increased recruitment of tumor necrosis factor-α (TNF-α) to plasma membrane receptors, increased cleavage of caspase-8, recruitment of Bax to the mitochondria, and increased release of cytochrome *c* from mitochondria.

The complexity of these response mechanisms is further highlighted by interactions identified between small HSPs, PKC, Akt, and members of the MAPK pathway (Lee et al. 2004, 2005; Vertii et al. 2006; Zheng et al. 2006). Again, as noted above for the pathways that regulate mitochondrial redox status, there are complex interactions (cross-talk) between signaling pathways and varying degrees of functional redundancy, which allows for exquisitely sensitive responses of cells to environmental stresses. For many drugs and xenobiotics, the initial step that activates these signaling pathways is a bioactivation reaction, many occurring within mitochondria. Viewed in this manner, mitochondrial bioactivation of potentially toxic chemicals is the initiating step in a myriad of pathways that enable cells to adapt to environmental stresses.

10.4.5. Nuclear Factor-Kappa B Pathway

The transcription factor nuclear factor-kappa B (NF-κB) is predominantly localized in the cytoplasm in the absence of an inducing agent. There are five members of the NF-κB/Rel family of proteins: (1) p50/NF-κB1, (2) p65/RelA, (3) p52/NF-κB2, (4) RelB, and (5) c-Rel. The most commonly studied form of NF-κB is a heterodimer of the p50 and p65 subunits (see Ghosh, May and Kopp (1998) for an overview). In unstimulated conditions, NF-κB is complexed in the cytoplasm with members of the IκB family (IκBα, IκBβ, and IκBε isoforms), which inhibit the action of the NF-κB transcription factors. Upon stimulation of cells with agents such as

TNF-α or ROS, IκB kinase (IKK) is activated and phosphorylates IκBα or IκBβ. The phosphorylated IκB is then readily ubiquitinated and undergoes proteasomal degradation. This releases NF-κB to translocate to the nucleus, where it binds to target sequences in the regulatory region of genes that encode various proteins, such as cytokines, cytokine receptors, antiapoptotic proteins, and cell-cycle regulators. In this manner, NF-κB activation serves an early, protective role in the adaptive response of cells to toxic chemicals.

Cogswell et al. (2003) demonstrated that NF-κB and IκBα are localized in mitochondria of rat liver and human U937 cells. They demonstrated that stimulation of cells with TNF-α led to phosphorylation of IκBα and its subsequent non-proteasome-dependent degradation. This response was associated with a reduction of the transcription of mitochondrial genes encoding cytochrome oxidase III subunit and cytochrome *b* mRNAs. This negative effect on mitochondrial gene transcription implies that function of the mitochondrial ETC will be compromised, leading to decreased production of ATP. Because other studies have shown NF-κB to activate transcription of antiapoptotic genes such as Bcl-X_L, further studies are needed to reconcile this NF-κB-dependent inhibition of ETC function and ATP generation. This example again highlights the complexity of mitochondrial adaptive responses.

10.4.6. Epidermal Growth Factor

Epidermal growth factor (EGF) is a potent mitogen for renal proximal tubular cells and is synthesized within the kidneys (Humes et al. 1989; Norman et al. 1987; Nowak and Schnellmann 1995; Rall et al. 1985). EGF acts at the plasma membrane by binding to the EGF receptor. Nowak et al. (1999) studied the role of EGF on repair of cellular functions in rabbit renal proximal tubules exposed to the nephrotoxicant DCVC. As shown in many other studies by these and other authors, DCVC potently inhibited mitochondrial respiration. Presumably as a secondary effect due to ATP depletion, (Na^++K^+)-ATPase activity and Na^+-dependent glucose uptake were also inhibited by DCVC. Addition of EGF to incubation media did not directly reverse the inhibitory effects of DCVC. Rather, EGF promoted the recovery of mitochondrial function and (Na^++K^+)-ATPase activity, but not Na^+-dependent glucose uptake, after DCVC bioactivation was completed and the remaining cells could recover. The action of EGF on the plasma membrane with subsequent recovery of mitochondrial function suggests that pathways must be activated to transmit a signal from the cell surface to the mitochondria. These pathways are likely many of those discussed above, including protein kinases, the MAPK pathway, and HSPs.

10.4.7. Peroxisome Proliferator-Activated Receptor γ Cofactor-1α and Mitochondrial Biogenesis

Peroxisome proliferator-activated receptor γ cofactor-1α (PGC-1α) is a transcription coactivator that interacts with a broad range of transcription factors and elicits a variety of biological responses, including adaptive thermogenesis, mitochondrial biogenesis, regulation of glucose and fatty acid metabolism, fiber-type switching in skeletal muscle, and cardiac development (Liang and Ward 2006). A transcription coactivator is a protein or protein complex that increases the probability of gene transcription by interacting with transcription factors. It does not, by itself, bind to a specific DNA sequence. PGC-1α is a 92-kDa protein, has two putative nuclear localization sequences, and is localized in the nucleus. It is highly expressed in tissues with abundant mitochondria and active oxidative phosphorylation, such as brown adipose tissue, heart, brain, and kidney. There are three known members of the PGC-1 family (PGC-1α, PGC-1β, and PGC-1-related coactivator), although the greater interest and most studies have been done on PGC-1α, because of its powerful effects on regulation of energy metabolism in both normal and many disease states.

Rasbach and Schnellmann (2007a,b) studied the effect of PGC-1α overexpression on repair and recovery of mitochondrial function in rabbit renal proximal tubules treated with oxidants (hydrogen peroxide, *tert*-butyl hydroperoxide). Their studies showed that a 10-fold overexpression of PGC-1α increased mitochondrial number by 52%, respiratory activity by 27%, and mitochondrial marker proteins by 30%. Moreover, treatment of rabbit renal proximal tubules with a sublethal dose of *tert*-butyl hydroperoxide initially caused a marked decrease in mitochondrial function; however, this was followed over a period of 4 days by recovery of mitochondrial function. The increase in PGC-1α expression during the recovery period was shown to be associated with the sequential activation of Src, p38 MAPK, and the EGF receptor. Even in control renal proximal tubular cells, overexpression of PGC-1α increases basal and uncoupled cellular respiration, cellular ATP content, and mitochondrial number (Rasbach and Schnellmann 2007b). Thus, PGC-1α appears to have a fundamental role in regulation of mitochondrial function and biogenesis under both physiological and toxicological conditions.

10.5. Physiological, Pathological and Toxicological States Affecting Mitochondrial Function

Although several examples of reactive metabolites of chemicals and disease states have been mentioned in the sections above, the focus of those sections was primarily on the signaling pathways that mediate and the mechanisms involved in the adaptive responses of mitochondria. This final section will focus on four specific examples and will highlight how normal homeostatic mechanisms in mitochondria are altered under the specified conditions. The first example, "aging", can be considered as a physiological response in which mitochondria and cellular energetics are central to the response. Diabetic nephropathy and chronic kidney disease and compensatory renal hypertrophy are pathological examples in which mitochondria again play key roles in how affected tissues respond to environmental changes. Finally, the example of cysteine S-conjugate-induced nephrotoxicity will be considered further. This is an example of a class of chemicals for whom mitochondria are an early and prominent intracellular target; bioactivation plays a determining role in their mitochondrial and cellular toxicity.

From these brief considerations of physiological, pathological, and bioactivation-dependent mitochondrial adaptation, it should be clear that regardless of the inducing agent or condition, many of the responses of mitochondria are the same. Thus, in analogy with the so-called "heat shock response", in which a very broad range of conditions and chemicals can produce the response, here too, adaptive responses of mitochondria can be induced by a similarly broad range of conditions and chemicals. This emphasizes the fundamental nature of mitochondrial adaptation. When these adaptive responses go to extremes because of genetic or nutritional deficiencies, for example, a pathological state develops. A broad range of diseases have been associated with mitochondrial dysfunction (Pieczenik and Neustadt 2007), again emphasizing the fundamental nature of mitochondria in tissue function.

10.5.1. Aging

Decreases in the efficiency of mitochondrial function with time are seen as a central component of the aging process and are part of the free-radical theory of aging (Cadenas and Davies 2000). Evidence in support of this theory exists at the cellular level as well, and in species ranging from *Drosophila* to humans (Sohal and Brunk 1992). Thus, whereas the release of partially reduced oxygen species from the ETC may occur at a frequency of 1%–2% in normal mitochondria from young adults, this frequency is suggested to increase with age. One factor that may be important in this process is a decrease in the expression of antioxidant enzymes in mitochondria. Thus, for example, Rohrbach et al. (2006) reported decreased expression and activity of Trd2 in aging skeletal and cardiac muscle. One consequence of this is an increased susceptibility to apoptotic stimuli.

There are complex changes in signaling pathways that mediate the age-dependent changes in mitochondrial function. Among the components of the signaling pathways that impact mitochondrial function and have been linked to longevity is the 66-kDa isoform of the growth factor adapter Shc ($p66^{Shc}$) (Hajnóczky and Hoek 2007; Pinton et al. 2007). $p66^{Shc}$ is a cytoplasmic protein that, upon induction of oxidative conditions, is phosphorylated by PKC-β; this phosphorylation, along with recognition by the prolyl isomerase Pin1, promotes mitochondrial accumulation of $p66^{Shc}$, which then alters mitochondrial Ca^{2+} responses and three-dimensional structure, finally resulting in apoptosis.

10.5.2. Diabetic Nephropathy and Chronic Kidney Disease

Hyperglycemia that results from various modes of uncontrolled glucose regulation provides causal links between diabetes and many of the complications that arise. Mitochondrial function and cellular energetics are central to the altered glucose regulation (Brownlee 2001; Rolo and Palmeira 2006). Four major pathways are thought to be involved in mediating the pathological effects of chronic hyperglycemia (Figure 10.8). Each of the four pathways is in turn further stimulated by increases in mitochondrial ROS. In their review, Rolo and Palmeira (2006) describe the hyperglycemia-induced overproduction of ROS by mitochondria as the trigger

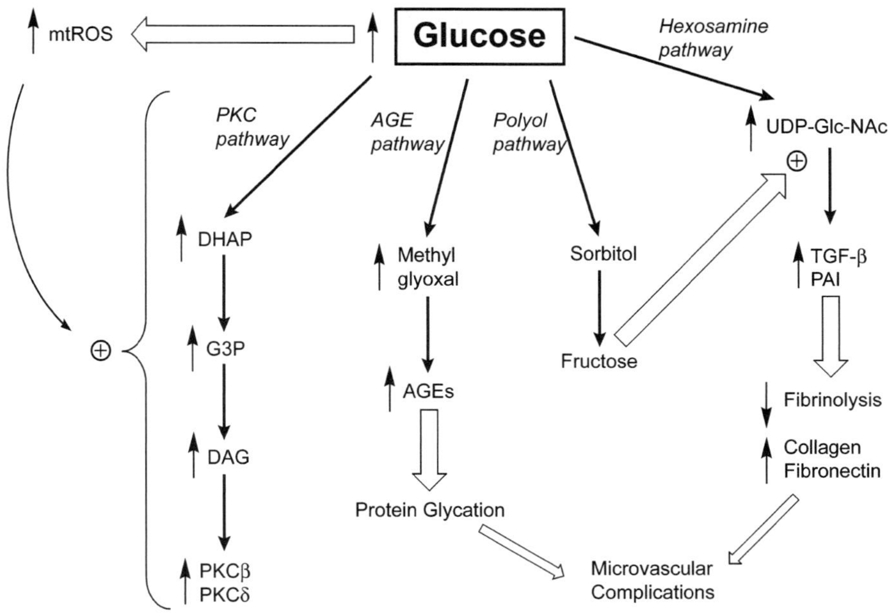

Figure 10.8 Biochemical pathways leading from hyperglycemia to cell damage in diabetes. This scheme summarizes some of the key pathways that ultimately mediate much of the damage associated with chronic hyperglycemia in either type 1 or type 2 diabetes. Superimposed on the four major pathways is the stimulation of mitochondrial ROS formation, which enhances each pathway.
Abbreviations: AGE, advanced glycation end-products; DAG, diacylglycerol; DHAP, dihydroxyacetone phosphate; G3P, glyceraldehydes-3-phosphate; mtROS, mitochondrial reactive-oxygen species; PAI, plasminogen activator inhibitor; PKC, protein kinase C; TGF-β, transforming growth factor-β.

for each of these four pathways. The prevailing hypothesis for how this occurs is that hyperglycemia induces an increase in the electron donors NADH and $FADH_2$, which increase flux through the ETC. The increase in the ATP/ADP ratio and hyperpolarization of the mitochondrial inner membrane would result in inhibition of electron transport at complex III, resulting in an increased ratio of reduced to oxidized ubiquinone. As illustrated in Figure 10.1, this can result in significant formation and release of superoxide anions. Mitochondrial thiol-disulfide redox status also plays a key role. For example, Ghosh et al. (2005) demonstrated the importance of depletion of the mitochondrial GSH pool in cardiomyocyte apoptosis in diabetic rats. In contrast, depletion of the cytoplasmic GSH pool was not associated with apoptosis or the diabetic state.

Impairment of mitochondrial function is thus viewed as being intrinsically related to the diabetic state (Rolo and Palmeira 2006). Several studies indicate that the alterations in mitochondrial energetics precede the onset of glucose intolerance, suggesting that mitochondrial dysfunction plays a key role in diabetes progression. The early adaptive response of mitochondria to the diabetic state is concluded to likely reflect changes in gene expression induced by hyperglycemia. This is viewed as a mechanism for cellular adaptation to glucose toxicity.

Besides the tubular epithelial cell oxidative stress that occurs in diabetic nephropathy, other forms of chronic renal insufficiency leading to chronic renal disease are associated with oxidative stress as well (Shah et al. 2007). As with many of the changes that occur with diabetic nephropathy, changes that occur in other forms of chronic kidney disease can be viewed, at least in the early stages, as reversible adaptations. As the disease progresses, however, the changes produce permanent alterations in cellular and mitochondrial function.

10.5.3. Compensatory Renal Cellular Hypertrophy

In all mammalian species, reductions in functional renal mass are rapidly followed by a series of compensatory physiological, morphological, and biochemical changes (Fine 1986; Shirley and Walter 1991). Such reductions can occur as a result of aging, various forms of renal disease, or uninephrectomy. The compensatory response is primarily a cellular hypertrophy rather than hyperplasia, and occurs predominantly in the proximal tubules. The acute phase of the compensatory response in rodents is complete within 7–10 days. Characteristics of the hypertrophic response include increases in cellular protein content, brush-border and basolateral membrane surface area, overall cell size, cellular energy metabolism, and activities of specific enzymes over and above overall cellular protein content.

At the level of the proximal tubular epithelial cell and intact kidney, the hypertrophic response leads to changes that have significant toxicological impact. For example, GSH content, activity and expression of γ-glutamylcysteine synthetase, the rate-limiting enzyme in GSH synthesis, activities of several GSH-dependent enzymes, transcription of certain metallothionein genes, and activity and/or expression of several ion and metabolite transporters, including the $(Na^{+}+K^{+})$-stimulated ATPase, are markedly increased as a consequence of compensatory renal cellular hypertrophy (Epstein, Charney and Silva 1978; Jacobson et al. 1980; Lash and Zalups 1994; Lash et al. 2005b; Salehmoghaddam et al. 1985; Zalups and Lash 1990; Zalups, Fraser and Koropatnick 1995). The increased workload imposed by changes in transport and metabolism led to the hypothesis that this resulted in increased energy demands on proximal tubular cells with consequent increases in rates of mitochondrial electron transport (Harris, Chan and Schrier 1988; Shapiro et al. 1994).

To validate this hypothesis of a hypermetabolic state in proximal tubular cells from remnant kidneys of uninephrectomized rats, we isolated mitochondria from remnant kidneys of uninephrectomized rats and from kidneys of control rats and compared their respiratory function and selected enzyme and transport activities (Lash et al. 2001). Rates of state 3 respiration with succinate as respiratory substrate were increased by approximately 70% when normalized to protein content in mitochondria from remnant kidneys as compared to those in mitochondria from control kidneys. Additionally, activities of malic dehydrogenase and succinate:cytochrome *c* oxidoreductase were increased by 382% and 138%, respectively, as a consequence of compensatory renal cellular hypertrophy. Besides this evidence of a hypermetabolic state, increases were also observed in both basal and toxicant-stimulated lipid peroxidation and in rates of GSH uptake into mitochondria. These findings suggest that besides compensating for increased need of ATP, mitochondria also upregulate GSH transport in response to an increase in basal oxidant levels.

10.5.4. Cysteine Conjugate-Induced Nephrotoxicity

As a final example of mitochondrial adaptation and responses to environmental changes, the impact of cysteine conjugate bioactivation will be briefly reviewed. The classic view of GSH conjugation is that this reaction serves to detoxify reactive electrophiles, which are processed to the corresponding cysteine conjugates, then N-acetylated (to form the corresponding mercapturate) and excreted in the urine. For certain classes of GSH S-transferase substrates, however, this pathway represents a bioactivation rather than a detoxification mechanism. The cysteine conjugate formed, although it can be metabolized by the "classic" route to a mercapturate, is also a potential substrate for one of two bioactivation enzymes, the cysteine conjugate β-lyase (β-lyase; EC 4.4.1.13) or the flavin-containing monooxygenase (FMO; EC 1.14.13.8) (Figure 10.9). Because of the tissue distribution of the various membrane transporters and enzymes involved in the disposition of metabolites of this pathway, acute toxicity is observed almost exclusively in the renal proximal tubules (Lash, Parker and Scott 2000; Lash et al. 2000).

One of the most frequently studied chemicals, whose metabolism by the GSH conjugation pathway produces a nephrotoxic cysteine conjugate, is trichloroethylene. While the precise role and importance of the cysteine conjugate DCVC in producing nephrotoxicity (particularly in humans) from exposure to trichloroethylene remain controversial, the critical

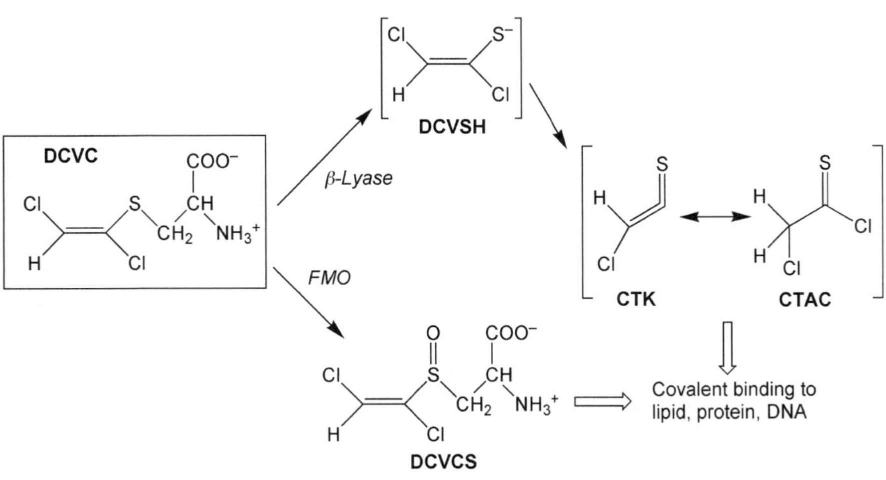

Figure 10.9 Bioactivation of DCVC to produce reactive metabolites. This scheme shows the formation of reactive metabolites derived from bioactivation of DCVC, the cysteine conjugate of the environmental contaminant trichloroethylene, as catalyzed by either the cysteine conjugate β-lyase (β-lyase) or FMO. Note that for FMO-dependent bioactivation, the initial metabolite is the sulfoxide, which, like the thiol metabolite (*S*-1,2-dichlorovinylthiol; DCVSH) of the β-lyase reaction, rearranges to form either the CTK or the CTAC. These latter two metabolites can form covalent adducts with cellular macromolecules, including lipids, protein, and DNA.
Abbreviations: CTK, chlorothioketene; DCVC, *S*-(1,2-dichlorovinyl)-L-cysteine; FMO, flavin-containing monooxygenase; CTAC, chlorothionoacetyl chloride.

importance of bioactivation to reactive intermediates and mitochondrial dysfunction in the early effects of DCVC in the target cell are clear and indisputable.

After identification of DCVC as the toxic by-product of trichloroethylene-extracted soybean meal in cattle (McKinney et al. 1959), subsequent work showed that DCVC could be formed enzymatically in tissue of various animal species (Anderson and Schultze 1965; Bhattacharya and Schultze 1967). Although the predominant cellular target of DCVC is now known to be the renal proximal tubular cell (Lash, Parker and Scott 2000), early studies on its intracellular toxicity used isolated liver mitochondria and showed that it produced potent inhibition of mitochondrial function in a metabolism-dependent manner (Parker 1965; Stonard 1973; Stonard and Parker 1971). Functional liver mitochondria are easier to obtain in adequate amounts than those from the kidney. Although many of the effects observed in hepatic mitochondria also occur in renal mitochondria, the liver is not an in vivo target organ for trichloroethylene via the GSH conjugation pathway.

Metabolic and functional effects of DCVC in renal mitochondria may be divided into primary and secondary effects. In both cases, all effects have been demonstrated to be dependent on bioactivation in that inhibition of metabolism prevents the deleterious effects associated with DCVC exposure. Primary effects may be defined as those resulting directly from formation of the reactive thiol, thioketene, and chlorothionoacetyl chloride metabolites, and include the following: GSH oxidation (Lash and Anders 1987), direct inhibition of mitochondrial enzymes such as dehydrogenases that contain critical sulfhydryl groups (Bruschi, Lindsay and Crabb 1998; Bruschi et al. 1993; Cooper et al. 2002; James et al. 2002; Lash and Anders 1987; Lock and Schnellmann 1990; van de Water et al. 1995), and binding of reactive species derived from DCVC metabolism to mitochondrial proteins, lipids, and DNA (Banki and Anders 1989; Hayden and Stevens 1990; Hayden et al. 1991, 1992).

Secondary effects of cysteine conjugate metabolites are defined as those resulting from changes in redox status, as a consequence of covalent adducts formed between conjugate metabolites and macromolecules, or as a consequence of inhibition of specific enzymes. These include induction of the MPT (Brown et al. 1996), alterations in mitochondrial calcium ion homeostasis (Chen, Jones and Stevens 1994; Lash and Anders 1986; Vamvakas et al. 1990, 1992; van de Water et al. 1993, 1994), inhibition of mitochondrial respiration (Lash and Anders 1986, 1987; Lash et al. 2003; Schnellmann, Cross and Lock 1989; Wallin et al. 1987), and activation of mitochondrial HSPs (Bruschi, Lindsay and Crabb 1998; Bruschi et al. 1993; Ho et al. 2006). Through all these diverse effects, renal mitochondria alter their function in response to the toxic insult. At relatively low levels of toxicant, responses are reversible and may be considered as adaptive. At higher levels of toxicant, the various regulatory processes that control mitochondrial redox status and $\Delta\psi$ lose their capacity to return mitochondria to normal function, and cell death usually occurs.

10.6. Summary and Conclusions

Mitochondria respond in numerous ways to environmental signals and stresses (both physiological and toxicological/pathological). An important stress includes bioactivation of drugs and other xenobiotics to generate reactive intermediates and ROS. The ultimate goal is for the mitochondria to regulate ATP production so that it matches energy needs. A complex and diverse array of processes exist in mitochondria to alter activities of the ETC and other enzymes. Regulation of redox status occurs through processes involving the GSH-GSSG-Gpx-Grd, Trx2-Trd2, Grx, or PrxIII systems. These are critical components of a redox circuit that enables mitochondria to maintain activities of key proteins. Superoxide anion formation in mitochondria may function as a mediator by which mitochondria sense redox status.

A primary response of mitochondria to a broad range of toxic chemicals, pathological conditions, and metabolites of endogenous chemicals is induction of the MPT. The MPT may occur by either an intrinsic pathway or through activation of proapoptotic Bcl-2 family proteins. Increasing evidence suggests that rather than being solely involved in initiating apoptosis, the MPT may actually be more central to initiation of necrotic cell death. A variety of signaling pathways also operate in mitochondria, and are central to the adaptive and toxic responses of the organelle. These pathways include those involving HSPs (both those of the Hsp60 and Hsp70 families and the small HSPs), Bcl-2 family proteins, several classes of protein kinases (PKB or Akt, PKC isoforms, PKD), MAPKs, NF-κB, EGF and EGF receptor, and PGC-1α. There exists a high degree of cross-talk between the pathways and functional redundancy. These features make the systems that regulate mitochondrial function exquisitely sensitive to environmental stimuli and stresses.

Four examples of physiological and pathological conditions and bioactivation-dependent mitochondrial adaptation were briefly discussed to highlight the fundamental nature of the responses of mitochondria. These responses include upregulation of ETC protein expression in the face of increased need for ATP, upregulation of GSH transport and metabolism in the face of an increased basal oxidative stress, as well as alterations in redox status, binding of reactive species to DNA, protein, and lipids, and alterations in integrated mitochondrial functions, such as respiration and calcium ion homeostasis.

References

Ambrose, M., Ryan, A., O'Sullivan, G. C., Dunne, C., and Barry, O. P. 2006. Induction of apoptosis in renal cell carcinoma by reactive oxygen species: Involvement of extracellular signal-regulated kinase 1/2, p38δ/γ, cyclo-oxygenase-2 down-regulation, and translocation of apoptosis-inducing factor. Mol. Pharmacol. 69:1879–1890.

Anderson, P. M., and Schultze, M. O. 1965. Cleavage of *S*-(1,2-dichlorovinyl)-L-cysteine by an enzyme of bovine origin. Arch. Biochem. Biophys. 111:593–602.

Aw, T. Y., and Jones, D. P. 1989. Nutrient supply and mitochondrial function. Annu. Rev. Nutr. 9:229–251.

Baines, C. P., Kaiser, R. A., Purcell, N. H., Blair, N. S., Osinska, H., Hambleton, M. A., Brunskill, E. W., Sayen, M. R., Gottlieb, R. A., Dorn II, G. W., Robbins, J., and Molkentin, J. D. 2005. Loss of cyclophilin D reveals a critical role for mitochondrial permeability transition in cell death. Nature 434:658–662.

Banki, K., and Anders, M. W. 1989. Inhibition of rat kidney mitochondrial DNA, RNA and protein synthesis by halogenated cysteine S-conjugates. Carcinogenesis 10:767–772.

Barone, M. C., Darley-Usmar, V. M., and Brookes, P. S. 2003. Reversible inhibition of cytochrome *c* oxidase by peroxynitrite proceeds through ascorbate-dependent generation of nitric oxide. J. Biol. Chem. 278:27520–27524.

Bellamy, T. C., Griffiths, C., and Garthwaite, J. 2002. Differential sensitivity of guanylyl cyclase and mitochondrial respiration to nitric oxide measured using clamped concentrations. J. Biol. Chem. 277:31801–31807.

Beltrán, B., Quintero, M., Garcia-Zaragozá. E., O'Connor, E., Esplugues, J. V., and Moncada, S. 2002. Inhibition of mitochondrial respiration by endogenous nitric oxide: A critical step in Fas signaling. Proc. Natl. Acad. Sci. U.S.A. 99:8892–8897.

Bhattacharya, R. K., and Schultze, M. O. 1967. Enzymes from bovine and turkey kidneys which cleave *S*-(1,2-dichlorovinyl)-L-cysteine. Comp. Biochem. Physiol. 22:723–735.

Borutaite, V., Budriunaite, A., and Brown, G. C. 2000. Reversal of nitric oxide-, peroxynitrite- and *S*-nitrosothiol-induced inhibition of mitochondrial respiration or complex I activity by light and thiols. Biochim. Biophys. Acta 1459:405–412.

Brookes, P. S., Kraus, D. W., Shiva, S., Doeller, J. E., Barone, M. C., Patel, R. P., Lancaster, Jr., J. R., and Darley-Usmar, V. 2003. Control of mitochondrial respiration by NO, effects of low oxygen and respiratory state. J. Biol. Chem. 278:31603–31609.

Brown, P. C., Sokolove, P. M., McCann, D. J., Stevens, J. L., and Jones, T. W. 1996. Induction of a permeability transition in rat kidney mitochondria by pentachlorobutadienyl cysteine: A β-lyase-independent process. Arch. Biochem. Biophys. 331:223–231.

Brownlee, M. 2001. Biochemistry and molecular cell biology of diabetic complications. Nature 414:813–820.

Bruschi, S. A., Lindsay, J. G., and Crabb, J. W. 1998. Mitochondrial stress protein recognition of inactivated dehydrogenases during mammalian cell death. Proc. Natl. Acad. Sci. U.S.A. 95:13413–13418.

Bruschi, S. A., West, K. A., Crabb, J. W., Gupta, R. S., and Stevens, J. L. 1993. Mitochondrial HSP60 (P1 protein) and a HSP70-like protein (mortalin) are major targets for modification during *S*-(1,1,2,2-tetrafluoroethyl)-L-cysteine-induced nephrotoxicity. J. Biol. Chem. 268:23157–23161.

Cadenas, E., and Davies, K. J. A. 2000. Mitochondrial free radical generation, oxidative stress, and aging. Free Rad. Biol. Med. 29:222–230.

Cai, J., and Jones, D. P. 1998. Superoxide in apoptosis: Mitochondrial generation triggered by cytochrome *c* loss. J. Biol. Chem. 273:11401–11404.

Chen, Q., Jones, T. W., and Stevens, J. L. 1994. Early cellular events couple covalent binding of reactive metabolites to cell killing by nephrotoxic cysteine conjugates. J. Cell. Physiol. 161:293–302.

Chen, Z., and Lash, L. H. 1998. Evidence for mitochondrial uptake of glutathione by dicarboxylate and 2-oxoglutarate carriers. J. Pharmacol. Exp. Ther. 285:608–618.

Chen, Z., Putt, D. A., and Lash, L. H. 2000. Enrichment and functional reconstitution of glutathione transport activity from rabbit kidney mitochondria: Further evidence for the role of the dicarboxylate and

2-oxoglutarate carriers in mitochondrial glutathione transport. Arch. Biochem. Biophys. 373:193–202.

Chen, Q., Yu, K., Holbrook, N. J., and Stevens, J. L. 1992. Activation of the growth arrest and DNA damage-inducible gene *gadd* 153 by nephrotoxic cysteine conjugates and dithiothreitol. J. Biol. Chem. 267:8207–8212.

Chiarugi, A. 2005. "Simple but not simpler": Toward a unified picture of energy requirements in cell death. FASEB J. 19:1783–1788.

Cogswell, P. C., Kashatus, D. F., Keifer, J. A., Guttridge, D. C., Reuther, J. Y., Bristow, C., Roy, S., Nicholson, D. W., and Baldwin Jr., A. S. 2003. NF-κB and IκBα are found in the mitochondria: Evidence for regulation of mitochondrial gene expression by NF-κB. J. Biol. Chem. 278:2963–2968.

Cooper, A. J. L., Bruschi, S. A., and Anders, M. W. 2002. Toxic, halogenated cysteine S-conjugates and targeting of mitochondrial enzymes of energy metabolism. Biochem. Pharmacol. 64:553–564.

Damdimopoulos, A. E., Miranda-Vizuete, A., Pelto-Huikko, M., Gustafsson, J.-A., and Spyrou, G. 2002. Human mitochondrial thioredoxin: Involvement in mitochondrial membrane potential and cell death. J. Biol. Chem. 277:33249–33257.

Danial, N. N., and Korsmeyer, S. J. 2004. Cell death: Critical control points. Cell 116:205–219.

de Graauw, M., Tijdens, I., Cramer, R., Corless, S., Timms, J. F., and van de Water, B. 2005. Heat shock protein 27 is the major differentially phosphorylated protein involved in renal epithelial cellular stress response and controls focal adhesion organization and apoptosis. J. Biol. Chem. 280:29885–29898.

Di Mari, J. F., Davis, R., and Safirstein, R. L. 1999. MAPK activation determines renal epithelial cell survival during oxidative injury. Am. J. Physiol. 277:F195–F203.

Dmitrieva, N., Michea, L., and Burg, M. 2001. p53 Protects renal inner medullary cells from hypertonic stress by restricting DNA replication. Am. J. Physiol. 281:F522–F530.

Epstein, F. H., Charney, A. N., and Silva, P. 1978. Factors influencing the increase in Na–K-ATPase in compensatory renal hypertrophy. Yale J. Biol. Med. 51:365–372.

Fine, L. 1986. The biology of renal hypertrophy. Kidney Int. 29:619–634.

Ghafourifar, P., Schenk, U., Klein, S. D., and Richter, C. 1999. Mitochondrial nitric-oxide synthase stimulation causes cytochrome *c* release from isolated mitochondria: Evidence for intramitochondrial peroxynitrite formation. J. Biol. Chem. 274:31185–31188.

Ghosh, S., May, M., and Kopp, E. 1998. NF-κB and Rel proteins: Evolutionarily conserved mediators of immune responses. Annu. Rev. Immunol. 16:225–260.

Ghosh, S., Pulinilkunnil, T., Yuen, G., Kewalramani, G., An, D., Qi, D., Abrahani, A., and Rodrigues, B. 2005. Cardiomyocyte apoptosis induced by short-term diabetes requires mitochondrial GSH depletion. Am. J. Physiol. 289:H768–H776.

Giulivi, C., Poderoso, J. J., and Boveris, A. 1998. Production of nitric oxide by mitochondria. J. Biol. Chem. 273:11038–11043.

Green, D. R., and Kroemer, G. 2004. The pathophysiology of mitochondrial cell death. Science 305:626–629.

Griffith, O. W., and Meister, A. 1985. Origin and turnover of mitochondrial glutathione. Proc. Natl. Acad. Sci. U.S.A. 82:4668–4672.

Guder, W. G., Wagner, S., and Wirthensohn, G. 1986. Metabolic fuels along the nephron: Pathways and intracellular mechanisms of interaction. Kidney Int. 29:41–45.

Hajnóczky, G., and Hoek, J. B. 2007. Mitochondrial longevity pathways. Science 315:607–609.

Hansen, J. M., Zhang, H., and Jones, D. P. 2006. Mitochondrial thioredoxin-2 has a key role in determining tumor necrosis factor-α-induced reactive oxygen species generation, NF-κB activation, and apoptosis. Toxicol. Sci. 91:643–650.

Harris, D. C. H., Chan, L., and Schrier, R. W. 1988. Remnant kidney hypermetabolism and progression of chronic renal failure. Am. J. Physiol. 254:F267–F276.

Hayden, P. J., and Stevens, J. L. 1990. Cysteine conjugate toxicity, metabolism, and binding to macromolecules in isolated rat kidney mitochondria. Mol. Pharmacol. 37:468–476.

Hayden, P. J., Ichimura, T., McCann, D. J., Pohl, L. R., and Stevens, J. L. 1991. Detection of cysteine conjugate metabolite adduct formation with specific mitochondrial proteins using antibodies raised against halothane metabolite adducts. J. Biol. Chem. 266:18415–18418.

Hayden, P. J., Welsh, C. J., Yang, Y., Schaefer, W. H., Ward, A. J. I., and Stevens, J. L. 1992. Formation of mitochondrial phospholipid adducts by nephrotoxic cysteine conjugate metabolites. Chem. Res. Toxicol. 5:231–237.

He, L., and Lemasters, J. J. 2003. Heat shock suppresses the permeability transition in rat liver mitochondria. J. Biol. Chem. 278:16755–16760.

Healy, E., Dempsey, M., Lally, C., and Ryan, M. P. 1998. Apoptosis and necrosis: Mechanisms of cell death induced by cyclosporin A in a renal proximal tubular cell line. Kidney Int. 54:1955–1966.

Ho, H. K., Jia, Y., Coe, K. J., Gao, Q., Doneanu, C. E., Hu, Z., Bammler, T. K., Beyer, R. P., Fausto, N., Bruschi, S. A., and Nelson, S. D. 2006. Cytosolic heat shock proteins and heme oxygenase-1 are preferentially induced in response to specific and localized intramitochondrial damage by tetrafluoroethylcysteine. Biochem. Pharmacol. 72:80–90.

Humes, H. D., Cieslinski, D. A., Coimbra, T. M., Messana, J. M., and Galvao, C. 1989. Epidermal growth factor enhances renal tubule cell regeneration and repair and accelerates the recovery of renal function in postischemic acute renal failure. J. Clin. Invest. 84:1757–1761.

Jacobson, M. P., Rodriguez, H. J., Hogan, W. C., and Klahr, S. 1980. Mechanism of activation of renal Na^{+}–K^{+}-ATPase in the rat: Effects of reduction of renal mass. Am. J. Physiol. 239:F281–F288.

James, E. A., Gygi, S. P., Adams, M. L., Pierce, R. H., Fausto, N., Aebersold, R. H., Nelson, S. D., and Bruschi, S. A. 2002. Mitochondrial aconitase modification, functional inhibition, and evidence for a supramolecular complex of the TCA cycle by the renal toxicant *S*-(1,1,2,2-tetrafluoroethyl)-L-cysteine. Biochemistry 41:6789–6797.

Ji, Y., Akerboom, T. P., Sies, H., and Thomas, J. A. 1999. S-Nitrosylation and S-glutathionylation of protein sulfhydryls by *S*-nitrosoglutathione. Arch. Biochem. Biophys. 362:67–78.

Jones, D. P. 2006. Disruption of mitochondrial redox circuitry in oxidative stress. Chem. Biol. Interact. 163:38–53.

Kim, Y.- M., Kim, T.- H., Seol, D.- W., Talanian, R. V., and Billiar, T. R. 1998. Nitric oxide suppression of apoptosis occurs in association with an inhibition of Bcl-2 cleavage and cytochrome *c* release. J. Biol. Chem. 273:31437–31441.

Klatt, P., Molina. E. P., and Lamas, S. 1999. Nitric oxide inhibits c-Jun DNA binding by specifically targeted S-glutathionylation. J. Biol. Chem. 274:15857–15864.

Kroemer, G. 2003. Mitochondrial control of apoptosis: An introduction. Biochem. Biophys. Res. Commun. 304:433–435.

Kröncke, K.- D., Klotz, L.- O., Suschek, C. V., and Sies, H. 2002. Comparing nitrosative versus oxidative stress towards zinc finger-dependent transcription factors: Unique role for NO. J. Biol. Chem. 277:13294–13301.

Lash, L. H. 1990. Susceptibility to toxic injury in different nephron cell populations. Toxicol. Lett. 53:97–104.

Lash, L. H. 2006. Mitochondrial glutathione transport: Physiological, pathological and toxicological implications. Chem. Biol. Interact. 163:54–67.

Lash, L. H., and Anders, M. W. 1986. Cytotoxicity of *S*-(1,2-dichlorovinyl)glutathione and *S*-(1,2-dichlorovinyl)-L-cysteine in isolated rat kidney cells. J. Biol. Chem. 261:13076–13081.

Lash, L. H., and Anders, M. W. 1987. Mechanism of *S*-(1,2-dichlorovinyl)-L-cysteine- and *S*-(1,2-dichlorovinyl)-L-homocysteine-induced renal mitochondrial toxicity. Mol. Pharmacol. 32:549–556.

Lash, L. H., and Zalups, R. K. 1994. Activities of enzymes involved in renal cellular glutathione metabolism after uninephrectomy in the rat. Arch. Biochem. Biophys. 209:129–138.

Lash, L. H., Fisher, J. W., Lipscomb, J. C., and Parker, J. C. 2000. Metabolism of trichloroethylene. Environ. Health Perspect. 108(Suppl. 2):177–200.

Lash, L. H., Hueni, S. E., Putt, D. A., and Zalups, R. K. 2005b. Role of organic anion and amino acid carriers in transport of inorganic mercury in rat renal basolateral membrane vesicles: Influence of compensatory renal growth. Toxicol. Sci. 88:630–644.

Lash, L. H., Parker, J. C., and Scott, C. S. 2000. Modes of action of trichloroethylene for kidney tumorigenesis. Environ. Health Perspect. 108(Suppl. 2):225–240.

Lash, L. H., Putt, D. A., Horky III, S. J., and Zalups, R. K. 2001. Functional and toxicological characteristics of isolated renal mitochondria: Impact of compensatory renal growth. Biochem. Pharmacol. 62:383–395.

Lash, L. H., Putt, D. A., Hueni, S. E., and Horwitz, B. P. 2005a. Molecular markers of trichloroethylene-induced toxicity in human kidney cells. Toxicol. Appl. Pharmacol. 206:157–168.

Lash, L. H., Putt, D. A., Hueni, S. E., Krause, R. J., and Elfarra, A. A. 2003. Roles of necrosis, apoptosis, and mitochondrial dysfunction in *S*-(1,2-dichlorovinyl)-L-cysteine sulfoxide-induced cytotoxicity in primary cultures of human renal proximal tubular cells. J. Pharmacol. Exp. Ther. 305:1163–1172.

Lash, L. H., Putt, D. A., and Matherly, L. H. 2002. Protection of NRK-52E cells, a rat renal proximal tubular cell line, from chemical induced apoptosis by overexpression of a mitochondrial glutathione transporter. J. Pharmacol. Exp. Ther. 303:476–486.

Lee, Y.- J., Cho, H.- N., Jeoung, D.- I., Soh, J.- W., Cho., C. K., Bae, S., Chung, H.- Y., Lee, S.-J., and Lee, Y.-S. 2004. HSP25 overexpression attenuates oxidative stress-induced apoptosis: Roles of ERK1/2 signaling and manganese superoxide dismutase. Free Rad. Biol. Med. 36:429–444.

Lee, Y.- J., Lee, D.- H., Cho, C.- K., Bae, S., Jhon, G.- J., Lee, S.- J., Soh, J.-W., and Lee, Y.-S. 2005. HSP25 inhibits protein kinase Cδ-mediated cell death through direct interaction. J. Biol. Chem. 280:18108–18119.

Lemasters, J. J., Nieminen, A.- L., Qian, T., Trost, L. C., Elmore, S. P., Nishimura, Y., Crowe, R. A., Cascio, W. E., Bradham, C. A., Brenner, D. A., and Herman, B. 1998. The mitochondrial permeability transition in cell death: A common mechanism in necrosis, apoptosis and autophagy. Biochim. Biophys. Acta 1366:177–196.

Lee, H.- C., Yin, P.- H., Lu, C.- Y., Chi, C.-W., and Wei, Y.-H. 2000. Increase of mitochondria and mitochondrial DNA in response to oxidative stress in human cells. Biochem. J. 348:425–432.

Lê-Quôc, K., and Lê-Quôc, D. 1985. Crucial role of sulfhydryl groups in the mitochondrial inner membrane structure. J. Biol. Chem. 260:7422–7428.

Lê-Quôc, D., and Lê-Quôc, K. 1989. Relationships between the NAD(P) redox state, fatty acid oxidation, and inner membrane permeability in rat liver mitochondria. Arch. Biochem. Biophys. 273:466–478.

Li, J., Bombeck, C. A., Yang, S., Kim, Y.-M., and Billiar, T. R. 1999. Nitric oxide suppresses apoptosis via interrupting caspase activation and mitochondrial dysfunction in cultured hepatocytes. J. Biol. Chem. 274:17325–17333.

Li, C.- Q., Trudel, L. J., and Wogan, G. N. 2002. Nitric oxide-induced genotoxicity, mitochondrial damage, and apoptosis in human lymphoblastoid cells expressing wild-type and mutant p53. Proc. Natl. Acad. Sci. U.S.A. 99:10364–10369.

Li, Y., Johnson, N., Capano, M., Edwards, M., and Crompton, M. 2004. Cyclophilin-D promotes the mitochondrial permeability transition but has opposite effects on apoptosis and necrosis. Biochem. J. 383:101–109.

Li, Q., and Zhu, G. D. 2002. Targeting serine/threonine protein kinase B/Akt and cell-cycle checkpoint kinases for treating cancer. Curr. Top. Med. Chem. 2:939–971.

Liang, H., and Ward, W. F. 2006. PGC-1α: A key regulator of energy metabolism. Adv. Physiol. Educ. 30:145–151.

Liu, X., Godwin, M. L., and Nowak, G. 2004. Protein kinase C-α inhibits the repair of oxidative phosphorylation after *S*-(1,2-dichlorovinyl)-L-cysteine injury in renal cells. Am. J. Physiol. 287:F64–F73.

Lock, E. A., and Schnellmann, R. G. 1990. The effect of haloalkene cysteine conjugates on rat renal glutathione reductase and lipoyl dehydrogenase activities. Toxicol. Appl. Pharmacol. 104:180–190.

Mannick, J. B., Schonhoff, C., Papeta, N., Ghafourifar, P., Szibor, M., Fang, K., and Gaston, B. 2001. S-Nitrosylation of mitochondrial caspases. J. Cell Biol. 154:1111–1116.

Martindale, J. L., and Holbrook, N. J. 2002. Cellular response to oxidative stress: Signaling for suicide and survival. J. Cell. Physiol. 192:1–15.

McKernan, T. B., Woods, E. B., and Lash, L. H. 1991. Uptake of glutathione by renal cortical mitochondria. Arch. Biochem. Biophys. 288:653–663.

McKinney, L. L., Picken Jr., J. C., Weakley, F. B., Eldridge, A. C., Campbell, R. E., Cowan, J. C., and Biester, H. E. 1959. Possible toxic factor of trichloroethylene-extracted soybean oil meal. J. Am. Chem. Soc. 81:909–915.

Megyesi, J., Andrade, L., Vieira, Jr., J. M., Safirstein, R. L., and Price, P. M. 2002. Coordination of the cell cycle is an important determinant of the syndrome of acute renal failure. Am. J. Physiol. 283:F810–F816.

Nakagawa, T., Shimizu, S., Watanabe, T., Yamaguchi, O., Otsu, K., Yamagata, H., Inohara, H., Kubo, T., and Tsujimoto, Y. 2005. Cyclophilin D-dependent mitochondrial permeability transition regulates some necrotic but not apoptotic cell death. Nature 434:652–658.

Norman, J., Badie-Desfooly, B., Nord, E. P., Kurtz, I., Schlosser, J., Chaudhari, A., and Fine, L. G. 1987. EGF-induced mitogenesis in proximal tubular cells: Potentiation by angiotensin II. Am. J. Physiol. 253:F299–F309.

Nowak, G. 2002. Protein kinase C-α and ERK1/2 mediate mitochondrial dysfunction, decreases in active Na^+ transport, and cisplatin-induced apoptosis in renal cells. J. Biol. Chem. 277:43377–43388.

Nowak, G. 2003. Protein kinase C mediates repair of mitochondrial and transport functions after toxicant-induced injury in renal cells. J. Pharmacol. Exp. Ther. 306:157–165.

Nowak, G., Bakajsova, D., and Clifton, G. L. 2004. Protein kinase C-ε modulates mitochondrial function and active Na^+ transport after oxidant injury in renal cell. Am. J. Physiol. 286:F307–F316.

Nowak, G., Clifton, G. L., Godwin, M. L., and Bakajsova, D. 2006. Activation of ERK1/2 pathway mediates oxidant-induced decreases in mitochondrial function in renal cells. Am. J. Physiol. 291:F840–F855.

Nowak, G., Keasler, K. B., McKeller, D. E., and Schnellmann, R. G. 1999. Differential effects of EGF on repair of cellular functions after dichlorovinyl-L-cysteine-induced injury. Am. J. Physiol. 276:F228–F236.

Nowak, G., and Schnellmann, R. G. 1995. Integrative effects of EGF on metabolism and proliferation in renal proximal tubular cells. Am. J. Physiol. 269:C1317–C1325.

Orrenius, S., Gogvadze, V., and Zhivotovsky, B. 2007. Mitochondrial oxidative stress: Implications for cell death. Annu. Rev. Pharmacol. Toxicol. 47:143–183.

Parcellier, A., Brunet, M., Schmitt, E., Col. E., Didelot, C., Hammann, A., Nakayama, K., Nakayama, K. I., Khochbin, S., Solary, E., and Garrido, C. 2006. HSP27 favors ubiquitination and proteasomal degradation of $p27^{Kip1}$ and helps S-phase re-entry in stressed cells. FASEB J. 20:E281–E293.

Parker, V. H. 1965. A biochemical study of the toxicity of S-dichlorovinyl-L-cysteine. Food Cosmet. Toxicol. 3:75–84.

Pieczenik, S. R., and Neustadt, J. 2007. Mitochondrial dysfunction and molecular pathways of disease. Exp. Mol. Pathol. 83:84–92.

Pinton, P., Rimessi, A., Marchi, S., Orsini, F., Migliaccio, E., Giorgio, M., Contursi, C., Minucci, S., Mantovani, F., Wieckowski, M. R., Del Sal, G., Pelicci, P. G., and Rizzuto, R. 2007. Protein kinase Cβ and prolyl isomerase 1 regulate mitochondrial effects of the life-span determinant $p66^{Shc}$. Science 315:659–663.

Polla, B. S., Kantengwa, S., François, D., Salvioli, S., Franceschi, C., Marsac, C., and Cossarizza, A. 1996. Mitochondria are selective targets for the protective effects of heat shock against oxidative injury. Proc. Natl. Acad. Sci. U.S.A. 93:6458–6463.

Rall, L. B., Scott, J., Bell, G. I., Crawford, R. J., Penschow, J. D., Niall, H. D., and Coghlan, J. P. 1985. Mouse prepro-epidermal growth factor synthesis by the kidney and other tissues. Nature 313:228–231.

Ramachandiran, S., Huang, Q., Dong, J., Lau, S. S., and Monks, T. J. 2002. Mitogen-activated protein kinases contribute to reactive oxygen species-induced cell death in renal proximal tubule epithelial cells. Chem. Res. Toxicol. 15:1635–1642.

Rane, M. J., Pan, Y., Singh, S., Powell, D. W., Wu, R., Cummins, T., Chen, Q., McLeish, K. R., and Klein, J. B. 2003. Heat shock protein 27 controls apoptosis by regulating Akt activation. J. Biol. Chem. 278:27828–27835.

Rasbach, K. A., and Schnellmann, R. G. 2007a. Signaling of mitochondrial biogenesis following oxidant injury. J. Biol. Chem. 282:2355–2362.

Rasbach, K. A., and Schnellmann, R. G. 2007b. PGC-1α over-expression promotes recovery from mitochondrial dysfunction and cell injury. Biochem. Biophys. Res. Commun. 355:734–739.

Rohrbach, S., Gruenler, S., Teschner, M., and Holtz, J. 2006. The thioredoxin system in aging muscle: Key role of mitochondrial thioredoxin reductase in the protective effects of caloric restriction? Am. J. Physiol. 291: R927–R935.

Rolo, A. P., and Palmeira, C. M. 2006. Diabetes and mitochondrial function: Role of hyperglycemia and oxidative stress. Toxicol. Appl. Pharmacol. 212:167–178.

Salehmoghaddam, S., Bradley, T., Mikhail, N., Badie-Dezfooly, B., Nord, E. P., Trizna, W., Kheyfets, R., and Fine, L. G. 1985. Hypertrophy of basolateral Na–K pump activity in the proximal tubule of the remnant kidney. Lab. Invest. 53:443–452.

Sandau, K. B., Callsen, D., and Brüne, B. 1999. Protection against nitric oxide-induced apoptosis in rat mesangial cells demands mitogen-activated protein kinases and reduced glutathione. Mol. Pharmacol. 56:744–751.

Sarkela, T. M., Berthiaume, J., Elfering, S., Gybina, A. A., and Giulivi, C. 2001. The modulation of oxygen radical production by nitric oxide in mitochondria. J. Biol. Chem. 276:6945–6949.

Schnellmann, R. G., Cross, T. J., and Lock, E. A. 1989. Pentachlorobutadienyl-L-cysteine uncouples oxidative phosphorylation by dissipating the proton gradient. Toxicol. Appl. Pharmacol. 100:498–505.

Schonhoff, C. M., Gaston, B., and Mannick, J. B. 2003. Nitrosylation of cytochrome *c* during apoptosis. J. Biol. Chem. 278:18265–18270.
Schoolwerth, A. C., and LaNoue, K. F. 1985. Transport of metabolic substrates in renal mitochondria. Annu. Rev. Physiol. 47:143–171.
Shah, S. V., Baliga, R., Rajapurkar, M., and Fonseca, V. A. 2007. Oxidants in kidney disease. J. Am. Soc. Nephrol. 18:16–28.
Shaik, Z. P., Fifer, E. K., and Nowak, G. 2007. Protein kinase B/Akt modulates nephrotoxicant-induced necrosis in renal cells. Am. J. Physiol. 292:F292–F303.
Shapiro, J. I., Elkins, N., Reiss, O. K., Suleymanlar, G., Jin, H., Schrier, R. W., and Chan, L. 1994. Energy metabolism following reduction of renal mass. Kidney Int. 45(Suppl.):S100–S105.
Shirley, D. G., and Walter, S. J. 1991. Acute and chronic changes in renal function following unilateral nephrectomy. Kidney Int. 40:62–68.
Sies, H. 1985. Oxidative stress: Introductory remarks. In: Oxidative Stress, ed. H. Sies, pp. 1–8. London: Academic Press.
Sinha, D., Bannergee, S., Schwartz, J. H., Lieberthal, W., and Levine, J. S. 2004. Inhibition of ligand-independent ERK1/2 activity in kidney proximal tubular cells deprived of soluble survival factors up-regulates Akt and prevents apoptosis. J. Biol. Chem. 279:10962–10972.
Sohal, R. S., and Brunk, U. T. 1992. Mitochondrial production of pro-oxidants and cellular senescence. Mut. Res. 275:295–304.
Stonard, M. D. 1973. Further studies on the site and mechanism of action of *S*-(1,2-dichlorovinyl)-L-cysteine and *S*-(1,2-dichlorovinyl)-3-mercaptopropionic acid in rat liver. Biochem. Pharmacol. 22:1329–1335.
Stonard, M. D., and Parker, V. H. 1971. The metabolism of *S*-(1,2-dichlorovinyl)-L-cysteine by rat liver mitochondria. Biochem. Pharmacol. 20:2429–2437.
Storz, P., Döppler, H., and Toker, A. 2005. Protein kinase D mediates mitochondrion-to-nucleus signaling and detoxification from mitochondrial reactive oxygen species. Mol. Cell. Biol. 25:8520–8530.
Storz, P., and Toker, A. 2002. 3'-Phosphoinositide-dependent kinase-1 (PDK-1) in PI 3-kinase signaling. Front. Biosci. 7:D886–D902.
Tanaka, T., Hosoi, F., Yamaguchi-Iwai, Y., Nakamura, H., Masutani, H., Ueda, S., Nishiyama, A., Takeda, S., Wada, H., Spyrou, G., and Yodoi, J. 2002. Thioredoxin-2 (Trx-2) is an essential gene regulating mitochondria-dependent apoptosis. EMBO J. 21:1695–1703.
Tapodi, A., Debreceni, B., Hanto, K., Bognar, Z., Wittmann, I., Gallyas Jr., F., Varbiro, G., and Sumegi, B. 2005. Pivotal role of Akt activation in mitochondrial protection and cell survival by poly(ADP-ribose)polymerase-1 inhibition in oxidative stress. J. Biol. Chem. 280:35767–35775.
Tatoyan, A., and Giulivi, C. 1998. Purification and characterization of a nitric-oxide synthase from rat liver mitochondria. J. Biol. Chem. 273:11044–11048.
Tian, W., Zhang, Z., and Cohen, D. M. 2000. MAPK signaling and the kidney. Am. J. Physiol. 279:F593–F604.
Vamvakas, S., Bittner, D., Dekant, W., and Anders, M. W. 1992. Events that precede and that follow *S*-(1,2-dichlorovinyl)-L-cysteine-induced release of mitochondrial Ca^{2+} and their association with cytotoxicity to renal cells. Biochem. Pharmacol. 44:1131–1138.
Vamvakas, S., Sharma, V. K., Sheu, S.-S., and Anders, M. W. 1990. Perturbations of intracellular calcium distribution in kidney cells by nephrotoxic haloalkenyl cysteine S-conjugates. Mol. Pharmacol. 38:455–461.
van de Water, B., Zietbey, J. P., de Bront, H. J. G. M., Mulder, G. J., and Nagelkerke, J. F. 1993. The relationship between intracellular Ca^{2+} and the mitochondrial membrane potential in isolated proximal tubular cells from rat kidney exposed to the nephrotoxin 1,2-dichlorovinyl-cysteine. Biochem. Pharmacol. 45:2259–2267.

van de Water, B., Zoeteweij, J. P., de Bont, H. J. G. M., Mulder, G. J., and Nagelkerke, J. F. 1994. Role of mitochondrial Ca^{2+} in the oxidative stress-induced dissipation of the mitochondrial membrane potential: Studies in isolated proximal tubular cells using the nephrotoxin 1,2-dichlorovinyl-L-cysteine. J. Biol. Chem. 269:14546–14552.

van de Water, B., Zoeteweij, J. P., de Bont, H. J. G. M., and Nagelkerke, J. F. 1995. Inhibition of succinate:ubiquinone reductase and decrease of ubiquinol in nephrotoxic cysteine S-conjugate-induced oxidative cell injury. Mol. Pharmacol. 48:928–937.

Vertii, A., Hakim, C., Kotlyarov, A., and Gaestel, M. 2006. Analysis of properties of small heat shock protein Hsp25 in MAPK-activated protein kinase 2 (MK2)-deficient cells: MK2-dependent insolubilization of Hsp25 oligomers correlates with susceptibility to stress. J. Biol. Chem. 281:26966–26975.

Wallin, A., Jones, T.W., Vercesi, A.E., Cotgreave, I., Ormstad, K., and Orrenius, S. 1987. Toxicity of S-pentachlorobutadienyl-L-cysteine studied with isolated rat renal cortical mitochondria. Arch. Biochem. Biophys. 258:365–372.

Wong, P. S.-Y., and Fukuto, J. M. 1999. Reaction of organic nitrate esters and S-nitrosothiols with reduced flavins: A possible mechanism of bioactivation. Drug Metab. Dispos. 27:502–509.

Xu, F., Putt, D. A., Matherly, L. H., and Lash, L. H. 2006. Modulation of expression of rat mitochondrial 2-oxoglutarate carrier in NRK-52E cells alters mitochondrial transport and accumulation of glutathione and susceptibility to chemically induced apoptosis. J. Pharmacol. Exp. Ther. 316:1175–1186.

Zalups, R. K., Fraser, J., and Koropatnick, J. 1995. Enhanced transcription of metallothionein genes in rat kidney: Effect of uninephrectomy and compensatory renal growth. Am. J. Physiol. 268:F643–F650.

Zalups, R. K., and Lash, L. H. 1990. Effects of uninephrectomy and mercuric chloride on renal glutathione homeostasis. J. Pharmacol. Exp. Ther. 254:962–970.

Zheng, C., Lin, Z., Zhao, Z. J., Yang, Y., Niu, H., and Shen, X. 2006. MAPK-activated protein kinase-2 (MK2)-mediated formation and phosphorylation-regulated dissociation of the signal complex consisting of p38, MK2, Akt, and Hsp27. J. Biol. Chem. 281:37215–37226.

Zhuang, S., and Schnellmann, R. G. 2006. A death-promoting role for extracellular signal-regulated kinase. J. Pharmacol. Exp. Ther. 319:991–997.

Zhuang, S., Yan, Y., Daubert, R. A., Han, J., and Schnellmann, R. G. 2007. ERK promotes hydrogen peroxide-induced apoptosis through caspase-3 activation and inhibition of Akt in renal epithelial cells. Am. J. Physiol. 292:F440–F447.

11

Hepatic Bioactivation and Drug-Induced Liver Injury

Raymond A. Kemper[1] and George Lai[2]
[1]Department of Toxicology and Safety Assessment;
[2]Department of Drug Discovery Support; Boehringer Ingelheim Pharmaceuticals, Ridgefield, CT 06877–0368, USA
e-mail: rkemper@rdg.boehringer-ingelheim.com

Keywords: Idiosyncratic Toxicity · Hapten Hypothesis · P450 · Phase I and Phase II Reactions · Acylglucuronides · Quinones · Epoxides · Hydroxylamines and Nitroso Compounds · Acetyl Halides · Michael Acceptors · Free Radicals · Reactive-Oxygen Species · Glutathione

11.1. Introduction

Adverse reactions to drugs are responsible for approximately 50% of the cases of acute liver failure in the United States. While the majority of these cases (74%) are related to accidental or intentional overdose with acetaminophen (Ostapowicz et al. 2002), approximately 10% of the cases of acute liver failure reported each year are due to drug-related idiosyncratic hepatotoxicity (Kaplowitz 2005; Lee 2003). In general, the incidence of drug-induced liver injury (DILI) is very low; on the order of 1:1000 to 1:100 000 for most drugs. However, difficult diagnosis and poor reporting practices are problematic, and it is likely that the true incidence of DILI is higher than current estimates based on clinical reports. The liver has a large functional reserve and a remarkable regenerative capacity, both of which may complicate clinical diagnosis. DILI is the most frequent reason for regulatory action by the FDA (Navarro and Senior 2006). Such actions include withdrawal from the market (e.g., troglitazone, bromfenac), black box warnings and other labeling actions (e.g., nevirapine), restriction of use (e.g., trovafloxacin), and refusal to approve (e.g., ximelagatran). A representative selection of drugs causing DILI and their associated regulatory actions is presented in Table 11.1. Although DILI may only occur in a relatively small population of patients, it can result in removal of an otherwise beneficial drug from the market, depriving patients of a much-needed therapy.

A.A. Elfarra (ed.), *Advances in Bioactivation Research*, DOI: 10.1007/978-0-387-77300-1_11,

Table 11.1 Drugs with regulatory actions based on hepatotoxicity.

Drug	Regulatory action
Acitretin	Black box warning
Benoxaprofen	Withdrawn (1982)
Bosentan	Black box warning
Bromfenac	Withdrawn (1998)
Dacarbazine	Black box warning
Dantrolene	Black box warning
Felbamate	Black box warning
Flutamide	Black box warning
Gemtuzamab	Black box warning
Iproniazid	Withdrawn (1958)
Isoniazid	Black box warning
Ketoconazole	Black box warning
Naltrexone	Black box warning
Nefazodone	Withdrawn (2004)
Nevirapine	Black box warning
Pemoline	Black box warning
Tolcapone	Black box warning
Tricrynafen	Withdrawn (1980)
Troglitazone	Withdrawn (2000)
Trovafloxacin	Black box warning
Valproic acid	Black box warning
Ximelagatran	Failure to approve
Zalcitabine	Black box warning
Zidovudine	Black box warning

Source: Compiled from Walgren et al. (2005) and Gunawan and Kaplowitz (2004).

Clinically, DILI may be characterized as hepatocellular, cholestatic, or mixed type, depending on the initial pattern of biomarkers observed (Navarro and Senior 2006). The hallmark of hepatocellular liver injury is an early elevation of serum transaminases, primarily alanine aminotransferase (ALT), which is released into the systemic circulation following necrosis of hepatic parenchymal cells. In general, ALT levels exceeding three times the upper limit of normal are considered indicative of clinically significant hepatocellular-type liver injury. Cholestatic liver injury is characterized by initial elevations of serum alkaline phosphatase (AP) and serum bilirubin. AP is localized primarily in the biliary epithelium, and elevations in this enzyme are frequently associated with damage to the biliary tract. Similarly, increases in serum bilirubin may reflect deficits in hepatobiliary function. Frequently, the clinical picture of DILI presents features of both hepatocellular and cholestatic injury, leading to classification as a mixed-type injury. It has recently been proposed that significant concurrent increases in indicators of both hepatic injury (e.g., ALT) and hepatic function (e.g., total or conjugated bilirubin) are predictive of the potential for serious DILI, an observation originally noted by Dr. Hyman Zimmerman and commonly referred to as “Hy’s law” (Lewis 2006).

In addition to classification based on clinical pathology, DILI may be further classified as predictable (type A reactions) or idiosyncratic (type B reactions). Predictable DILI is generally dose-related and there is a clear temporal relationship between the start of drug therapy and the onset of liver damage. Furthermore, predictable DILI generally occurs by mechanisms common to most mammals, and as the name implies, is frequently detected in nonclinical safety assessment in laboratory animals. Acetaminophen and cyclosporine are examples of drugs that cause predictable hepatotoxicity. Idiosyncratic DILI may be very rare (1:10 000–1:100 000) and is by nature essentially unpredictable. Idiosyncratic DILI is usually not dose-related, at least in the commonly understood sense, and the temporal relationship between initiation of drug treatment and manifestation of disease is frequently obscure. Idiosyncratic hepatotoxicity has been further subdivided into metabolic idiosyncracy, which is thought to be related to polymorphic expression of drug-metabolizing enzymes, and allergic idiosyncracy, which is proposed to involve loss of immune tolerance to drug–protein adducts (Castell and Castell 2006). Allergic hepatotoxicity may be accompanied by other signs of allergic reaction, including skin rash, eosinophilia, and fever. The distinction between metabolic and allergic idiosyncracy has been criticized as an oversimplification (Boelsterli 2003), since both enzyme and/or transporter polymorphisms and immune factors likely contribute to development of toxicity.

Development of DILI is a complex, multifactorial process that may be attributed to the interplay between three major determinants: characteristics of the drug or treatment regimen, characteristics of the patient, and environmental factors (Boelsterli 2003). Characteristics of the drug and treatment regimen that impact the pathogenesis of DILI include the chemical structure, the dosage, and the duration of treatment. The chemical structure of a drug is clearly of paramount importance in determining whether or not treatment may result in DILI. As the focus of this volume indicates, DILI frequently involves drugs containing chemically reactive functional groups, or more commonly, inert moieties that may be converted to reactive ones via metabolism (i.e., bioactivation). The influence of the dose and dose rate is clearly illustrated by the common hepatotoxicant acetaminophen, which is efficiently detoxified by sulfonation and glucuronidation at therapeutic doses, but undergoes significant bioactivation following overdose, resulting in dose-related hepatocellular necrosis. Less clear is the relationship between the dose and the incidence of idiosyncrastic hepatotoxicity. However, it has been generally recognized that drugs associated with idiosyncratic toxicity tend to be administered at relatively high daily doses, while drugs that are administered at very low doses ($\leq$10 mg day^{-1}) are rarely associated with idiosyncratic DILI (Uetrecht 2001; Knowles, Uetrecht and Shear 2000). Similarly, the duration of treatment has a significant influence on the development of DILI, particularly for idiosyncratic hepatotoxicity, which may not become manifest for weeks to months after initiation of drug therapy (Kaplowitz 2005).

The second major determinant of DILI is related to the characteristics of the individual patient, and includes genetic and physiological factors and the presence of underlying disease. Polymorphisms in drug-metabolizing enzymes or drug transporters are thought to play a significant role in development of idiosyncratic DILI. Such effects might include overexpression of an enzyme responsible for bioactivation of a drug (i.e., gene duplication for CYP2D6), deficiency in expression or activity of detoxifying enzymes such as glutathione S-transferases (GSTs), or deficiency in the activity of a critical transporter, leading to abnormal accumulation of a drug within a particular cellular compartment. In general, elderly patients appear to be more susceptible to DILI compared to younger patients and females tend to be somewhat more susceptible than males (Lee 2003; Kaplowitz 2005). The presence of an underlying disease state may also be an important factor in development of DILI. A question that has stimulated much debate in the scientific community is whether or not pre-existing liver disease increases susceptibility to drug-related liver injury. In general, the presence of pre-existing liver disease does not, as a rule, appear to predispose individuals to development of DILI (Lee 2003). However, in some cases, such as concurrent HIV and hepatitis C infection, affected individuals are more susceptible to development of hepatotoxicity from highly active antiretroviral drug therapy than are their healthy counterparts (Pol, Vallet-Pichard and Fontaine 2002; Clark et al. 2002). There is considerable evidence to suggest that mediators of inflammation may play an important role in DILI (Roth et al. 1997), which suggests that patients suffering from inflammatory disorders may be more susceptible than other individuals.

Numerous environmental factors may also contribute to development of drug-related hepatotoxicity. These include things such as diet, alcohol consumption and concurrent use of other drugs, herbal remedies, and nutraceuticals. The composition and adequacy of the diet has a marked influence on the physiological state of the individual. For example, components of normal foods may act as inducers or inhibitors of drug-metabolizing enzymes, resulting in alterations in the balance between bioactivation and detoxication. On the other hand, nutritional deficiencies may lead to depletion of cofactors necessary for detoxification of drugs and reactive metabolites such as glutathione, predisposing an individual to development of DILI (Whitcomb and Block 1994). Excessive chronic consumption of ethanol is another frequently cited risk factor for development of DILI. Chronic alcohol consumption can lead to induction of CYP2E1, which is active in the bioactivation of numerous low-molecular-weight compounds, including acetaminophen. Both of these factors may render the individual more susceptible to acetaminophen hepatotoxicity (Schmidt, Dalhoff and Poulsen 2002; Whitcomb and Block 1994). The relationship between enzyme induction and bioactivation is discussed in detail in Chapter 4 of this volume, while the role of CYP2E1 in bioactivation reactions is addressed in detail in Chapter 6. Finally, the use of herbal remedies and nutritional supplements has increased markedly in recent years. Since these substances, often complex mixtures, are not subject to regulation by the FDA, their health effects and interactions with pharmaceutical agents are often not well characterized. For example, herbals may increase susceptibility to coadministered drugs by depletion of cofactors or inactivation of critical enzymes in detoxification pathways (Fau et al. 1997; Berardinis et al. 2000).

11.2. Mechanisms of Drug-Induced Liver Injury

On a cellular level, hepatotoxicity may involve a variety of different mechanisms, including disruption of bile acid synthesis and excretion, upregulation of cellular adhesion molecules leading to recruitment and activation of polymorphonuclear leukocytes (PMNs), generation of reactive-oxygen and -nitrogen species leading to oxidative stress and fibrosis, and induction of the mitochondrial permeability transition leading to both necrotic and apoptotic cell death (Jaeschke et al. 2002; Lee 2003). Development of clinical DILI is a complex multi-factorial process, and several global hypotheses have been advanced to explain the pathogenesis of adverse hepatic drug reactions. These include the hapten hypothesis, the danger hypothesis (Matzinger 1994; Pirmohamed et al. 2002), and the pharmacological interaction with immune receptor (p-i) hypothesis (Pichler 2005). Not surprisingly, no single mechanism can account for all of the clinical and experimental observations related to adverse drug reactions, and it is likely that most DILI results from a combination of immunologic and nonimmunologic mechanisms. Potential mechanisms of idiosyncratic hepatotoxicity are the subject of several recent reviews (e.g. Boelsterli 2003; Castell and Castell 2006; Kaplowitz 2005). The interested reader is referred to these reviews for an in depth treatment of this subject.

11.3. Enzymology of Hepatic Bioactivation

Regardless of which mechanism or combination of mechanisms is called upon to explain the hepatotoxicity of a given drug, the formation of reactive metabolites often plays a critical role in DILI. The liver contains the highest concentration of drug-metabolizing enzymes and is the principle site of drug metabolism, particularly following oral administration. The central role of the liver in drug metabolism and its anatomical location with respect to the gastrointestinal tract are major determinants in the high prevalence of drug-related liver injury related to bioactivation.

Drug metabolism reactions are generally divided into two major types. Phase I reactions are functionalization reactions in which a polar functional group is added to a lipophilic moiety or a nonpolar blocking group is removed, unmasking a polar functional group. Addition of a polar functionality increases the water solubility of the molecule to some extent, facilitating renal excretion. Perhaps more importantly, phase I functionalization provides a metabolic handle for further metabolism by phase II drug-metabolizing enzymes. Phase II reactions are biosynthetic conjugation reactions in which a highly polar, usually charged functional group is added to an existing polar functional group. Conjugation results in a large increase in water solubility and in many cases converts the molecule into a good substrate for various efflux transporters. While the net effect of combined phase I/phase II metabolism is to accelerate removal of the drug from the body, both phase I and phase II reactions can result in formation of reactive intermediates that may participate in adverse drug reactions.

11.3.1. Phase I Reactions

The great majority of phase I drug metabolism reactions are catalyzed by the cytochrome P-450 (CYP) superfamily of mixed-function oxidases. These enzymes catalyze a wide variety of reactions including aliphatic and aromatic hydroxylation, heteroatom dealkylation and oxidation, aliphatic desaturation, epoxide formation, and other minor oxidative reactions (Testa 1995; Guengerich 1996). Under certain conditions, CYPs can also catalyze reductive reactions, such as the reductive dehalogenation of carbon tetrachloride, which results in generation of the highly reactive trichloromethyl radical. CYPs have been implicated in bioactivation of numerous drugs, natural products, solvents, and other industrial chemicals. The major isoforms of CYP involved in human drug metabolism include CYP3A4, the most abundant form in human liver, CYP2C9, CYP2C19, CYP2D6, and CYP1A2 (Lewis 2004). In addition, CYP1A1, CYP2A6, CYP2B6, and CYP2E1 are involved in drug metabolism in humans, though to a lesser extent. Most CYP isoforms have been associated with the formation of reactive metabolites. Furthermore, multiple CYP isozymes may be involved in bioactivation of the same substrate. For example, bioactivation of acetaminophen to the reactive species *N*-acetyl-*p*-benzoquinonimine (NAPQI) is catalyzed by at least three isoforms, CYP2E1, CYP3A4, and CYP1A2 (Bessems and Vermeulen 2001). Where known, the involvement of various CYP isoforms in specific bioactivation reactions will be highlighted throughout this chapter.

Although the majority of phase I bioactivation reactions are carried out by CYPs, other phase I enzyme systems may also play a role in hepatic bioactivation of drugs. Such systems include the flavin-containing monooxygenases (FMOs), NAD(P)H:quinone oxidoreductases (NQOs), amine oxidases, alcohol dehydrogenases, and various peroxidases. The FMOs constitute a second NADPH-dependent microsomal monooxygenase system and are particularly active in the oxidation of heteroatoms in xenobiotics. At least five isoforms of FMO are expressed in humans, of which FMO3 is quantitatively the most important in human liver. FMOs are known to be involved in bioactivation of several drugs including ketoconazole, which has been reported to be hepatotoxic in humans (Lake-Bakaar, Scheuer and Sherlock 1987). Bioactivation of ketoconazole by FMOs appears to be initiated by N-oxidation of *N*-deacetylketoconazole, leading ultimately to formation of a reactive dialdehyde (Rodriquez and Acosta 1997). Other examples of bioactivation reactions catalyzed by FMOs include sulfoxidation of 1,1,2-trichlorovinylcysteine (Ripp et al. 1997) and metabolism of thiacetazone to reactive sulfenic and carbodiimide metabolites (Qian and Ortiz de Montellano 2006). NAD(P)H:quinone oxidoreductases catalyze the two-electron reduction of quinones to hydroquinones. Whether this represents a detoxification or a bioactivation reaction depends on the chemical stability of the resulting hydroquinone. Unstable hydroquinones can autooxidize resulting in generation of reactive-oxygen species and, consequently, toxicity. Reduction of benzoquinones and aromatic nitro compounds results in formation of potent alkylating and DNA crosslinking agents. NQOs are involved in bioactivation of nitroquinolones, naphthoquinones, aziridinylbenzoquinones, and dinitropyrenes (Ross et al. 2000). Monoamine oxidase (MAO) and semicarbazine-sensitive amine oxidase (SSAO) catalyze oxidative deamination of secondary and tertiary amines resulting in formation of aldehydes and H_2O_2. Amine oxidase-mediated bioactivation of drugs and other xenobiotics is comparatively rare. However, MAO and SSAO are thought to be involved in bioactivation of 1-methyl-4-phenyl-1,2,5,6-tetrahydropyridine (Benedetti 2001) and 3-aminopropene (Haenen et al. 1988), respectively. Like the amine oxidases, bioactivation of pharmaceuticals by alcohol dehydrogenases is relatively uncommon. One example is the bioactivation of the HIV reverse transcriptase inhibitor abacavir. Metabolic activation was catalyzed by human liver cytosol preparations and purified human alcohol dehydrogenase (ADH) isoforms and was characterized in vitro by covalent binding to cytosolic proteins or added serum albumin (Walsh, Reese and Thurmond 2002). Another example of ADH-mediated bioactivation is oxidation of the industrial chemical allyl alcohol to the hepatotoxin acrolein (Atzori, Dore and Congiu 1989). Peroxidases are involved in numerous biosynthetic reactions such as synthesis of prostaglandins, leukotrienes, and thromboxanes. Peroxidases such as prostaglandin H synthase can also catalyze bioactivation of drugs and other xenobiotics, utilizing organic peroxides such as prostaglandin G2 as an oxygen source (Vogel 2000). Examples include oxidation of acetaminophen to NAPQI in renal medulla and N-hydroxylation of procainamide in macrophages, ultimately resulting in formation of nitrosoprocainamide. As the cited examples suggest, bioactivation by peroxidases tends to be more important in extrahepatic tissues with low CYP activity (e.g., neutrophils).

11.3.2. Phase II Reactions

Although phase II reactions are generally associated with detoxification, phase II conjugating enzymes can catalyze bioactivation reactions as well. Formation of reactive metabolites may be catalyzed by UDP-glucuronosyltransferases, sulfatases, N-acetyltransferases (NATs), and GSTs. As will be discussed in more detail in a later section, an important pathway for bioactivation of many acidic nonsteroidal anti-inflammatory drugs (NSAIDs) involves formation of reactive acylglucuronides (Baily and Dickenson 2003; Grillo et al. 2003). These metabolites are subject to transacylation reactions with protein nucleophiles, as well as ring opening, followed by Schiff's base formation with lysine residues in proteins. As with CYPs, multiple isoforms of glucuronosyltransferase (UDPGT) are expressed in mammals, and may play a role in bioactivation of carboxylic acid-containing drugs. Isoforms thought to play a significant role in bioactivation of carboxylate drugs include UGT1A1, UGT1A9, and UGT2B7 (Zhou et al. 2005).

Sulfotransferases (SULTs) catalyze the sulfonation of aromatic and aliphatic alcohols, diols, and aromatic amines and hydroxylamines (Glatt 2000; Glatt et al. 2001). Sulfate anion is a good leaving group, and a number of sulfates decompose to form reactive cationic intermediates that can bind to tissue nucleophiles including proteins and DNA (Glatt 2000). Examples of SULT-mediated bioactivation include sulfonation of the hydroxylamine of acetylaminofluorene, which subsequently decomposes to form a highly reactive nitrenium–carbonium ion resonance pair, and 1′-hydroxysafrole, the sulfate of which undergoes heterolytic cleavage to yield a reactive carbonium ion (Glatt 1997). The substrate specificities of various SULT isoforms are overlapping and complex, and reactive sulfate formation from a given substrate may be catalyzed by several isoforms with different efficiencies. SULT1A1, SULT1A2, and SULT2A1 have high hepatic expression levels (Glatt et al. 2001), suggesting that these isoforms may play a significant role in hepatic bioactivation of xenobiotics.

N-acetyltransferases catalyze addition of an acetyl group to primary aliphatic and aromatic amines and hydrazines. N-acetyltransferase-mediated acetylation of isoniazid is the initial step in metabolism of this drug to a reactive species (Nelson et al. 1976). Treatment with isoniazid is associated with a relatively high incidence of liver injury in humans, and administration of acetylisoniazid resulted in covalent binding of the acetyl moiety to hepatic proteins and hepatotoxicity in rats (Timbrell et al. 1980). N-acetyltransferases also catalyze acetylation of aromatic hydroxylamines, thought to be an essential step in conversion of polycyclic aromatic amines to mutagenic nitrenium and carbonium ions.

Conjugation of electrophilic compounds with glutathione (GSH) is generally viewed as a detoxification reaction and a hepatoprotective phenomenon. However, in some cases, such as conjugation of bifunctional electrophiles, conversion to reactive species may result (Anders 2004). For example, conjugation of 1,2-dibromoethane results in formation of a reactive episulfonium ion that binds covalently to DNA bases. Indeed, the major DNA adduct resulting from exposure to the carcinogen, 1,2-dibromoethane, was *S*-2-N^7-guanylethylglutathione (Inskeep et al. 1986).

11.4. Structural Alerts for Hepatic Bioactivation

With few exceptions, reactive metabolites are electrophiles; molecules containing one or more centers of low electron density. Electrophilic reactive metabolites with delocalized centers of low electron density are referred to as soft electrophiles and electrophilic reactive metabolites with highly localized centers of low electron density are referred to as hard electrophiles. Soft electrophiles tend to react with endogenous soft nucleophiles, such as thiol residues in glutathione or proteins, while hard nucleophiles tend to react with hard nucleophiles such as the side-chain amino group of lysine residues in proteins. While reaction of electrophiles with glutathione provides some degree of protection to the host, formation of covalent adducts with cellular macromolecules, such as proteins, peptides, and nucleic acids is thought to be a critical step in mechanisms of hepatotoxicity. In addition to formation of covalent adducts some redox active metabolites such as quinones can also oxidize proteins and lipids, thereby initiating oxidative stress. The interaction of reactive metabolites with cellular components has been associated with a wide variety of toxicities, including cellular necrosis, hypersensitivity, carcinogenicity, and teratogenicity (Nelson 1982).

Although many compounds can form reactive metabolites to some extent, there are "favored" moieties that frequently undergo bioactivation

Table 11.2 Examples of reactive metabolites associated with hepatotoxicity.

Structural alerts	Reactive metabolites	Examples
Alkenes/alkynes/benzenes/ heteroaromatics	Epoxides/arene oxides	Thalidomide Carbamazepine Ticrynaphen Cephaloridine Tenidap Aflatoxin B_1 Benzo[a]pyrene Furosemide
Michael acceptor precursors	Quinones/quinone imines/ quinone methides	Acetaminophen Amodiaquine Diclofenac Prinomide Tacrine Trimethoprim Troglitazone Valproic acid
Alkyl halides	Acetyl chlorides	Halothane
Aromatic amines/ nitroaromatics	Hydroxylamines/nitrosos	Sulfamethoxazole Procainamide Misonidazole
Hydrazines	Carbon cations	Isoniazid
Free-radical sources	Free radicals	Carbon tetrachloride Halothane Quinones
Carboxylic acids	Acyl glucuronides/acyl-CoA thioesters	Benoxaprofen Bromfenac Tolmetin Ibufenac Zomepirac Diclofenac Ibuprofen Trovafloxacin Valproic acid Clofibric acid

and cause hepatotoxicity (Table 11.2). The presence of such functional groups within a compound suggests the potential for metabolic bioactivation and as such, serves as a 'structural alert' for toxicity. Compounds may present multiple structural alerts, one or more of which may be toxicologically relevant. A brief review of common structural alerts and their role in hepatotoxicity is presented in the following section. The reader is also referred to Chapters 1 and 2 in this volume for more detailed information on structure–activity relationships in bioactivation.

11.4.1. Epoxidation of Alkenes and Aromatic Rings

Through a common metabolic pathway, epoxidation of unsaturated carbon–carbon bonds may result in formation of potentially toxic epoxides from a range of structurally distinct compounds (Figure 11.1). The

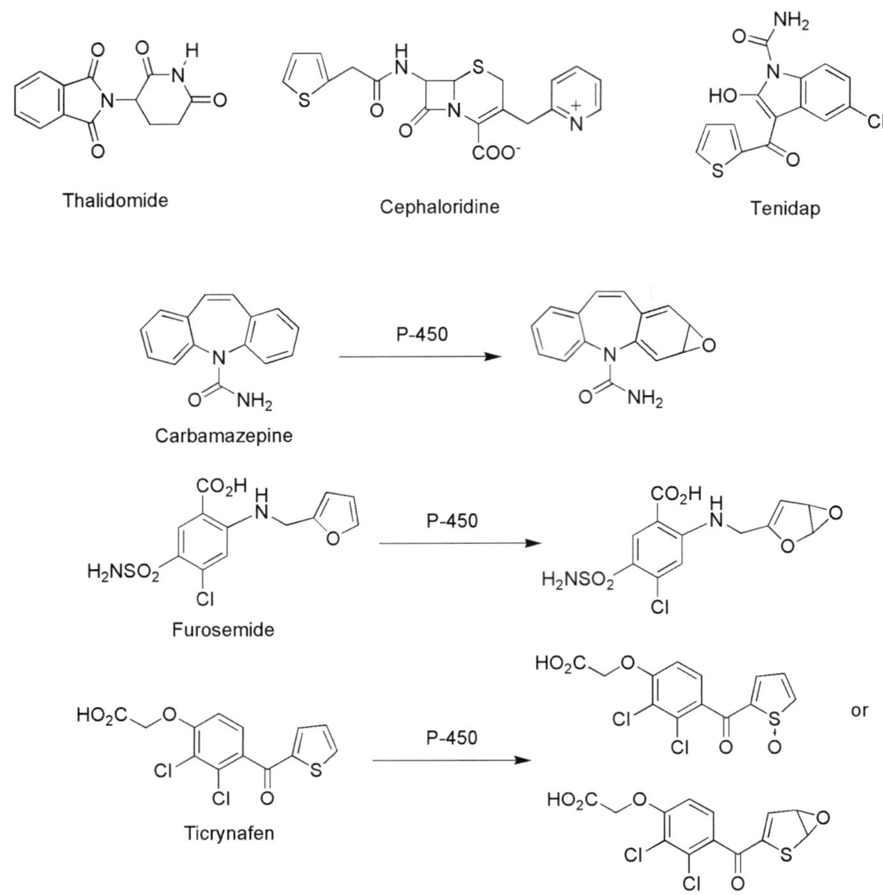

Figure 11.1 Examples of compounds associated with reactive arene oxide metabolites.

reactivity of epoxides is the result of two major factors: the electrophilicity of the epoxide carbon atoms and the high degree of strain associated with the three-membered heterocyclic ring. The 8,9-epoxide of aflatoxin B1 is one of the most potent hepatocarcinogens known (Guengerich et al. 1998). Epoxidation of aflatoxin B1 is catalyzed primarily by CYP3A4 and CYP1A2, but may also be catalyzed by peroxidases such as prostaglandin H synthase (Gallagher et al. 1994; Battista and Marnett 1985). Epoxides formed on benzenoid aromatics are often referred to as arene oxides. Perhaps the most thoroughly characterized example of arene oxide formation is the epoxidation of the environmental carcinogen benzo[a]pyrene, the 7,8-epoxy-9,10-diol of which is most strongly associated with nucleic acid binding and carcinogenicity. Epoxidation of benzene rings in pharmaceutical agents is less common than with environmental compounds, although there is evidence that thalidomide can be metabolized to an arene oxide, an intermediate that has been implicated in its cytotoxicity and teratogenicity (Gordon et al. 1981). Although the exact biological effects of the epoxide metabolite(s) of thalidomide in humans are not fully understood, reactive metabolites appear to be associated with glutathione depletion and oxidative stress in animal models (Hansena, Carneyb and Harris 1999). Since the revival of this compound as an anti-cancer agent, there have been reports of rare but severe hepatotoxicity in the clinic (Fowler and Imrie 2001; Hanje et al. 2006). However, the potential role of reactive metabolites in thalidomide-induced hepatotoxicity is still unclear. Carbamazepine can form a reactive arene oxide (carbamazepine-10,11-epoxide) which has been shown to covalently bind to cellular proteins and has been associated with idiosyncratic hypersensitive reactions, including hepatotoxicity, agranulocytosis, and skin rash (Park, Pirmohamed and Kitteringham 1998). Several CYP isoforms have been implicated in bioactivation of carbamazepine, and CYPs 2B6 and 3A4 are likely the major contributors to the formation of reactive metabolites (Pearce, Vakkalagadda and Leeder 2002). CYP2C8 was also shown to have a minor role in carbamazepine epoxidation (Kerr et al. 1994). The reactive epoxide metabolite generated from the furan moiety of furosemide has been implicated in the toxicity of this compound, including hepatotoxicity in both humans and mice. The role of the reactive epoxide in the hepatotoxicity of furosemide has been demonstrated by studies in which both liver damage and covalent binding in mice could be decreased by inhibiting epoxide formation (Mitchell et al. 1976; Walker and McElligott 1981). Although early studies established that epoxidation of furosemide was induced by phenobarbital but not 3-methylcholanthrene (Wirth, Bettis and Nelson 1976), studies aimed at identification of the specific CYP isoforms involved in this reaction have not been published. Epoxidation may play a role in the hepatotoxicity of thiophene-containing drugs, several of which have been associated with idiosyncratic reactions involving liver and kidney. Examples include ticrynafen (removed from the market post approval for liver toxicity) and tenidap (withdrawn post new drug application (NDA) submission for both liver and kidney toxicity). Reactive oxidative metabolites of the thiophene nucleus have been implicated in the mechanism of toxicity of these compounds. However, it is unclear whether a thiophene epoxide or a thiophene sulfoxide metabolite is the ultimate toxic species (Bonierbale et al. 1999). In the case of tienilic acid (ticrynafen), it has been suggested that CYP2C9 was primarily responsible for covalent binding, followed by CYP2C19 and CYP2C8 (Jean et al. 1996). This compound also caused mechanism-based inactivation of recombinantly expressed CYP2C9.

Some epoxides and arene oxides, such as the 4,5-epoxide of benzo[a]-pyrene, are detoxified to corresponding diols by epoxide hydrolases. Epoxide hydrolases can be membrane-bound or cytosolic, each form having a distinct substrate specificity. These enzymes are found in organs involved in elimination of xenobiotics along with cytochromes P450. It is thought that one of major functions of epoxide hydrolases is detoxification of highly reactive epoxides and arene oxides that are generated as intermediates during cytochrome P450-mediated metabolism. Epoxides and arene oxides that are resistant to epoxide hydrolase activity, such as benzo[a]-pyrene-7,8-dihydrodiol-9,10-epoxide are generally more toxic.

11.4.2. Michael Acceptors

α,β-Unsaturated carbonyls and imines are reactive electrophilic species that can form covalent adducts with biologically important nucleophiles via 1,4-

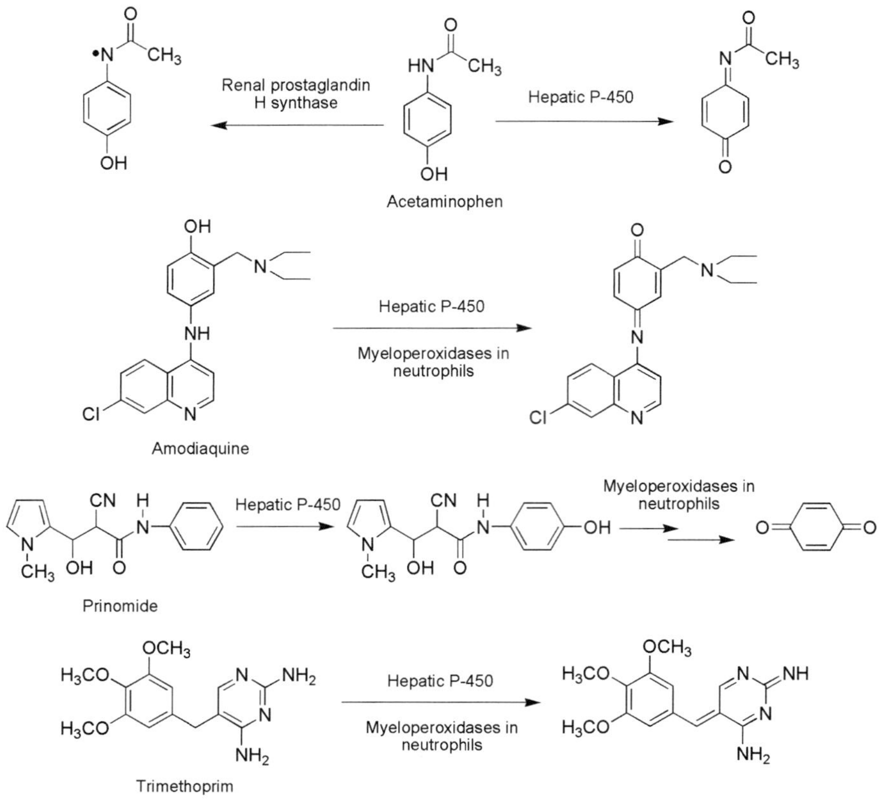

Figure 11.2 Examples of bioactivation to Michael acceptors.

or 1,2- Michael addition reactions (Figure 11.2). Since the electron density of these conjugated systems is delocalized over three carbons and the heteroatom, Michael acceptors are considered soft electrophiles. Soft nucleophiles, such as glutathione or the reduced sulfhydryl groups of proteins, are referred to as Michael donors. Acetaminophen and amodiaquine are examples of compounds containing a *para*-substituted acetanilide core that can be biotransformed into reactive Michael acceptors. The antimalarial drug amodiaquine can be bioactivated to a reactive quinone imine species by both cytochromes P450 in liver and myeloperoxidases in neutrophils. This reactive metabolite is thought to be responsible for the idiosyncratic hepatotoxicity and agranulocytosis associated with amodiaquine therapy (Park, Pirmohamed and Kitteringham 1998). The NSAID diclofenac has been associated with relatively high incidence of hepatotoxicity. Through cytochrome P450-mediated metabolism, diclofenac forms reactive quinone imines and arene oxides, both of which can be trapped by glutathione (Poon et al. 2001; Yan et al. 2005). As with many other NSAIDs, diclofenac also contains a carboxylic acid group that forms a reactive acyl glucuronide via UDP-glucuronosyltransferase-mediated conjugation (described later). The combination of these reactive metabolites may act synergistically to cause the observed hepatotoxicity of NSAIDs (Nelson 2001; Figure 11.3). Quinones and quinone methides are also reactive Michael acceptors that may contribute to adverse reactions of several drugs, such as prinomide,

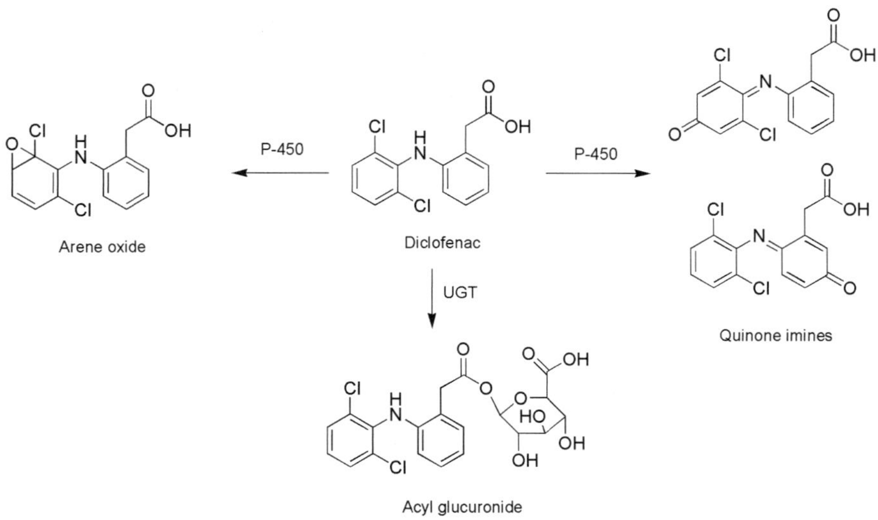

Figure 11.3 Multiple bioactivation pathways leading to reactive metabolites of diclofenac.

trimethoprim (Parrish et al. 1997; Lai, Zahid and Uetrecht 1999), and troglitazone (Kassahun et al. 2001). In addition to formation of adducts with nucleophiles, quinones may also undergo a single-electron reduction to semiquinone free radicals and produce oxidative stress in liver and other tissues. Redox cycling of quinones is discussed in more detail in a later section of this chapter and is the primary subject of Chapter 7 of this volume.

11.4.3. Acetyl Halides

The inhalational anesthetic halothane induces a rare, but potentially severe hepatitis in humans by an immune-mediated mechanism. Halothane is metabolized by human CYP2E1 to a reactive trifluoroacetyl chloride, which binds covalently to proteins by nucleophilic substitution with the chloride ion as the leaving group. Autoantibodies against the trifluoroacetyl antigen and endogenous antigens on microsomal proteins have been detected in the serum of patients who developed hypersensitivity against halothane. Interestingly, a structural analogue of halothane, isoflurane is metabolized to essentially the same reactive metabolite but to a much lesser extent, and the risk of hepatotoxicity has been shown to be significantly reduced relative to halothane (Pohl et al. 1988; Njoku et al. 1997; Figure 11.4). These data clearly implicate the acyl chloride moiety in the mechanism of anesthetic-induced idiosyncratic hepatotoxicity.

11.4.4. Hydroxylamines and Nitroso Compounds

The use of sulfonamide-containing antibiotics has been linked to a relatively high incidence (~0.1%) of idiosyncratic reactions including hepatotoxicity (Cribb et al. 1996a). Sulfamethoxazole, the most commonly used sulfonamide, is metabolized by CYP2C9 to the corresponding hydroxylamine, which is further oxidized to reactive nitroso metabolite (Figure 11.5). The nitroso metabolite can covalently bind to sulfhydryl-containing proteins by

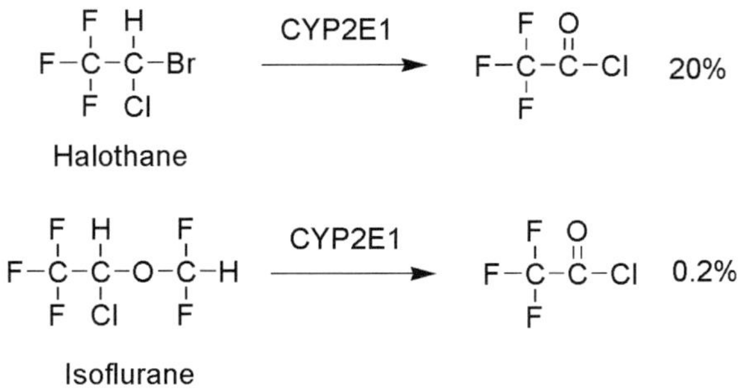

Figure 11.4 Bioactivation of inhalational anesthetics to reactive acetyl chlorides.

forming sufinamides, which have been implicated in both direct and immune-mediated toxicity (Cribb et al. 1996b). Other aromatic amines, such as procainamide, are also metabolized to reactive nitroso metabolites. Bioactivation of some aromatic amines involves a two-step pathway in which the parent amine is metabolized to the corresponding hydroxylamine, followed by conjugation of the hydroxylamine by sulfate or acetate. These conjugates are often unstable and may readily decompose to form reactive nitrenium ions, which can bind to nucleophilic groups in macromolecules. If one of the carbon atoms adjacent to the nitrenium nitrogen is unsubstituted, a carbonium–nitrenium resonance pair may occur, leading to formation of both nitrogen-centered and carbon-centered covalent adducts, both of which may contribute to carcinogenicity and toxicity of aromatic amines such as acetylaminofluorene (Guengerich 2002). Hydroxylamine and nitroso intermediates can also be generated from nitroaromatics by reductive metabolism. For example, the antitumor agent misonidazole is known to be reduced to hydroxylamine and nitroso intermediates, which contribute to its selective cytotoxicity toward hypoxic cells (Varghese and Whitmore 1985; Djuric 1989).

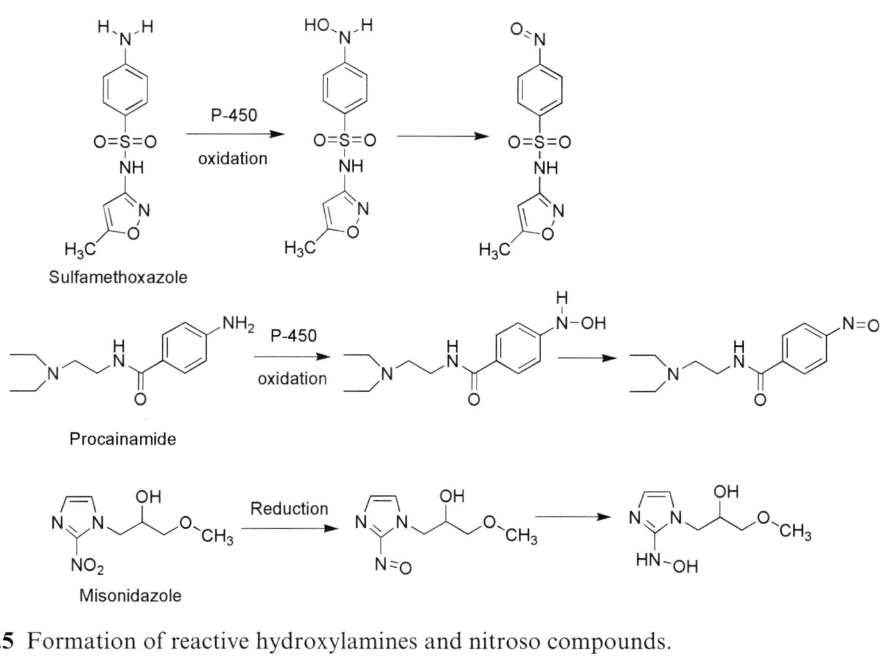

Figure 11.5 Formation of reactive hydroxylamines and nitroso compounds.

11.4.5. Carbocations

Hydrazines are bioactivated by cytochromes P450 or flavin-containing monooxygenases to highly reactive carbocations via diazonium intermediates. Isoniazid, used widely for treatment of tuberculosis, has been associated with severe liver toxicity in a relatively high proportion of patients. In a process catalyzed by NATs and CYP2E1, the drug is initially acetylated and then further bioactivated to the reactive acylating carbocation (Figure11.6). The reactive metabolite modifies proteins both in vitro and in vivo and is thought to be responsible for hepatotoxicity (Nelson et al. 1976). Isoniazid is mostly acetylated by the highly polymorphic NAT2. Since N-acetylation is the initial step leading to the reactive carbocation, it might be expected that fast acetylators would be more vulnerable to isoniazid hepatotoxicity. Some early clinical observations support this hypothesis (Yamamoto, Suou and Hirayama 1986). However, further acetylation of acetylhydrazine to diacetylhydrazine is a detoxification process and can compete with the oxidative formation of the reactive carbocation. Recent clinical studies suggest that the slow acetylators may actually be more susceptible to isoniazid-induced hepatotoxicity (Huang et al. 2002).

11.4.6. Free Radicals

Some chemical structures may be metabolized to relatively stable free radicals. Carbon tetrachloride, a common halogenated solvent, is a well-known hepatotoxin. It is bioactivated to a trichloromethyl free radical by cytochrome P450-mediated reductive dehalogenation. The carbon- centered free radical can initiate lipid peroxidation and lead to cellular membrane damage. Although the specific isoform(s) responsible for this reaction have not been identified, the rate of the reaction was increased by induction with phenobarbital but not 3-methylcholanthrene (Frank, Haussmann and Remmer 1982), suggesting minimal involvement by CYP1A isoforms. The inhalational anesthetic halothane can also be

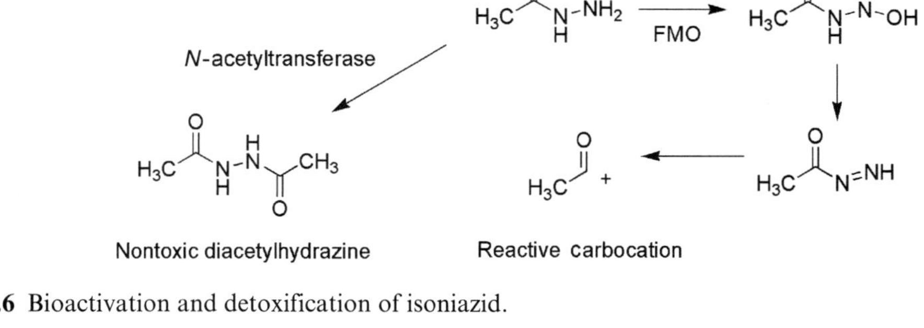

Figure 11.6 Bioactivation and detoxification of isoniazid.

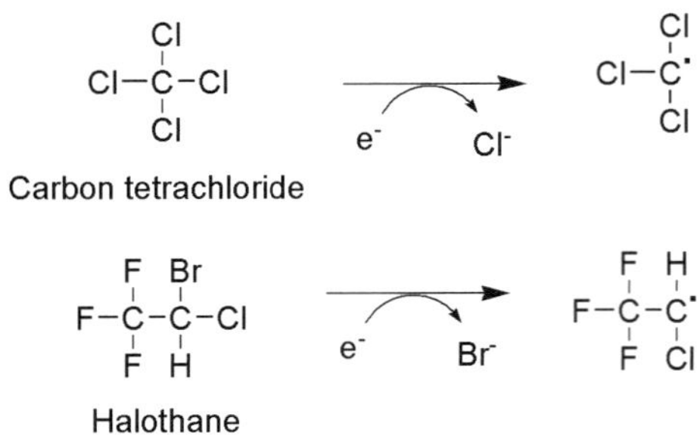

Figure 11.7 Formation of free radicals of carbon tetrachloride and halothane.

converted by reductive dehalogenation to a free radical (Figure 11.7), a reaction that has been associated with halothane-induced hepatotoxicity in rats (Cheeseman et al. 1985; De Groot and Sies 1989). It is unclear if this mechanism is also operative in human halothane-induced hepatotoxicity.

Quinones may undergo one-electron or two-electron reduction to semiquinone radicals or hydroquinones, respectively. Under aerobic conditions most semiquinone radicals are reoxidized back to quinones generating superoxide anion during the process (Figure 11.8). The resultant superoxide anions may undergo enzymatic or spontaneous dismutation to form hydrogen peroxide, which may ultimately generate hydroxyl free radicals via Fenton chemistry. Hydroxyl radicals are extremely reactive and can damage cellular membranes by initiation of lipid peroxidation leading to cell death. Hydroxyl radicals also bind to nucleobases and the sugar moieties in DNA, resulting in mutations and strand breaks (Martinez et al. 2003). Usually, cellular defensive systems, such as GSH or catalase are able to protect the cell from the quinone-induced oxidative stress. However, when these systems are compromised due to depletion of GSH or alkylation of cellular enzymes, uncontrolled oxidative stress can lead to hepatotoxicity (O'Brien 1991).

11.4.7. Acyl Glucuronides and Acyl-CoA thioesters

Covalent binding to proteins has been demonstrated for numerous acyl glucuronides both in *vitro* and in vivo. Acyl glucuronides are formed by glucuronidation of carboxylic acid-containing compounds. Glucuronidation is normally associated with rapid clearance and detoxification of xenobiotics. However, covalent modification of protein, as a consequence of the

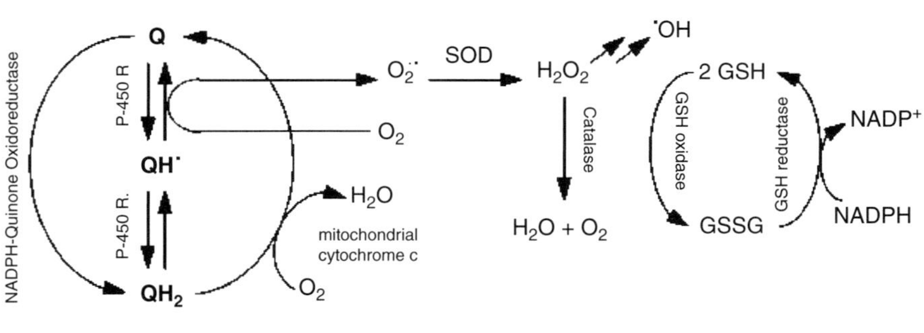

Figure 11.8 Quinone-induced free radical formation and oxidative stress.
Abbreviations: GSH, glutathione; GSSG, oxidized glutathione; Q, quinone; QH, semiquinone; QH_2, hydroquinone; P450 R, cytochrome P450 reductase; SOD, –superoxide dismutase.

formation of these acyl glucuronides, is thought to contribute to some severe adverse reactions, including general anaphylactic reactions, various hematological toxicities, and hepatotoxicity (Benet et al. 1993; Boelsterli, Zimmerman and Kretz-Rommel 1995; Spahn-Langguth, Dahms and Hermening 1996). Carboxylic acids can also form acyl-CoA thioesters (Figure 11.9). Since the CoA moiety is a good leaving group, these thioesters may also contribute to the covalent binding associated with carboxylic acids (Boelsterli 2002). Although the 1-*O*-acyl glucuronides of both zomepirac and tolmetin are among the most reactive glucuronide conjugates characterized to date, they can also be metabolized to reactive acyl-CoA thioesters, and recent studies suggest that these reactive acyl-CoA intermediates play a role in covalent modification of hepatic protein both in vitro and in vivo (Olsen et al. 2005, 2007).

A number of carboxylic acid-containing drugs, primarily NSAIDs, have been associated with reactive conjugate formation (Table 11.2), and several carboxylic acid-containing NSAIDs have been withdrawn from the market due to an unacceptably high incidence of severe adverse drug reactions including hepatotoxicity. These include benoxaprofen, bromfenac, tolmetin, ibufenac, and zomepirac (Bakke et al. 1995; FDA 2000), all of which are metabolized to acyl glucuronides in humans. Some carboxylic NSAIDs exhibit a lower incidence of toxicity. Ibuprofen is generally considered to be the safest NSAID with very rare incidences of

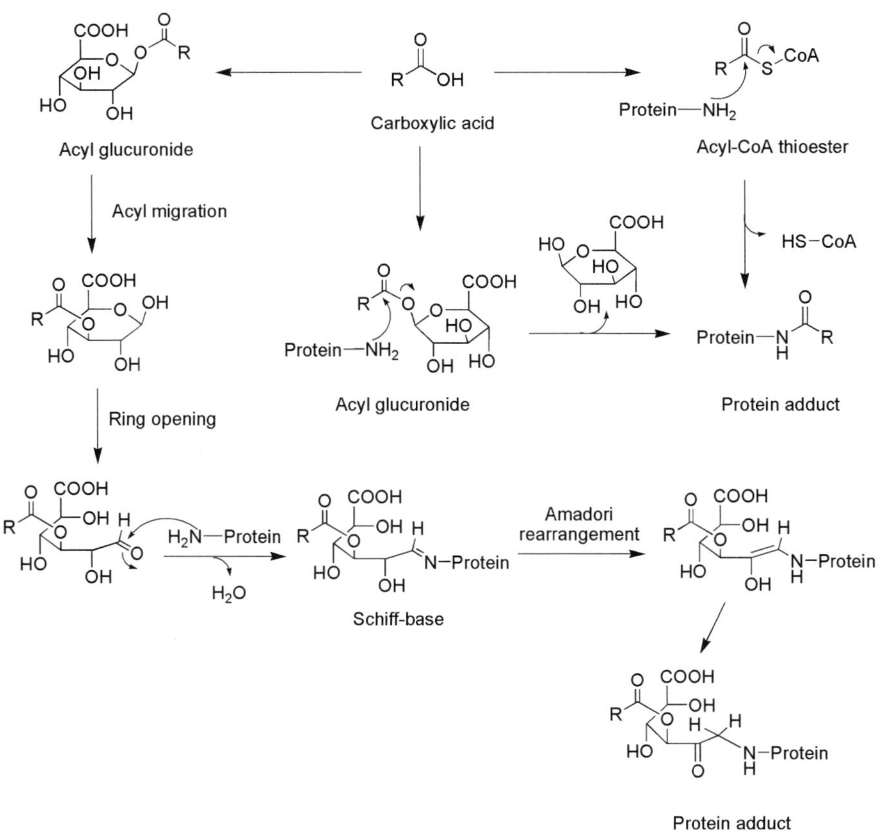

Figure 11.9 Bioactivation of carboxylic acids via glucuronidation and acyl-CoA conjugation.

hepatotoxicity and anaphylaxis (Boelsterli, Zimmerman and Kretz-Rommel 1995; van Puijenbroek et al. 2002). However, ibuprofen use can lead to hepatotoxicity in patients with chronic hepatitis C (Riley and Smith 1998), lending credence to the idea that underlying liver disease may increase susceptibility to some types of DILI. While formation of acyl glucuronides and consequent hepatotoxicity appears to be a class effect of NSAIDs, this mechanism is also operative in other classes of drugs. Trovafloxacin is a recent example of a non-NSAID carboxylic acid-containing drug that causes idiosyncratic hepatotoxicity and leukopenia. This has led to restricted use of this drug (FDA 2000a).

11.5. Molecular Targets of Reactive Metabolites in Liver

The early studies of Mitchell and colleagues (Mitchell et al. 1973a, 1973b) highlighted the critical role of covalent binding to the hepatotoxicity of compounds such as acetaminophen and bromobenzene. Similarly, the pioneering studies of Elizabeth and James Miller on the genotoxic and carcinogenic mechanism of polycyclic aromatic amines and other hepatocarcinogens demonstrated the fundamental importance of covalent binding to DNA in chemical carcinogenesis. Over the past several decades, the hepatotoxicity of numerous drugs and environmental chemicals has been found to be associated with bioactivation and covalent binding to hepatic proteins, and this has led to the general hypothesis that covalent binding of reactive metabolites to critical proteins is often a prerequisite for development of target organ toxicity. On the other hand, some studies have demonstrated that target organ toxicity can be attenuated by pharmacological or other intervention without a corresponding decrease in overall covalent binding, and such results have called the covalent binding hypothesis into question. Early studies relied heavily on the use of radiolabeled test compounds for detection and study of covalent binding. While these studies provide definitive evidence for covalent modification of proteins, they lack specificity and only supply information on the extent of overall binding. More recent studies using immunological techniques and mass spectrometry have started to identify individual target molecules for reactive metabolites of specific drugs. Such studies suggest that toxicity may correlate more closely with covalent modification of specific target proteins than with overall covalent binding, providing a rationale for the seemingly contradictory results of earlier studies. In this section we discuss identification of specific targets for reactive intermediates of selected drugs in the liver and present evidence linking modification of these targets with the observed toxicity. The analgesic drug acetaminophen and the NSAID diclofenac were chosen to illustrate these principles since these are two of the most extensively characterized hepatotoxic drugs in the public literature.

11.5.1. Acetaminophen

Perhaps the most thoroughly studied example of drug-induced hepatotoxicity related to bioactivation and covalent binding is that of the common analgesic and antipyretic drug acetaminophen (APAP). APAP is responsible for approximately 74% of all cases of drug-induced liver failure, largely related to accidental overdose or suicide attempts. Overdose of APAP is associated with centrilobular necrosis, and is characterized by massive elevations in serum transaminase levels. A series of pivotal mechanistic studies conducted at the National Institutes of Health (Jollow et al. 1973; Mitchell et al. 1973a, 1973b) demonstrated that the time course and severity of APAP hepatotoxicity correlated with covalent binding of ^{14}C-APAP to hepatic proteins, and that electrophile scavengers such as *N*-acetylcysteine (Mucomyst®), which decrease covalent binding, also protect against hepatotoxicity. In these studies, the protective effect of CYP inhibitors and the aggravating effect of CYP inducers on APAP-mediated hepatotoxicity clearly demonstrated the critical role of bioactivation in toxicity.

Despite intensive efforts by numerous laboratories, the molecular mechanisms of APAP-induced hepatotoxicity are still incompletely understood. While it is generally agreed that depletion of hepatic GSH is a prerequisite for development of hepatotoxicity, there is still much debate as to whether the critical initiating event in APAP toxicity is covalent binding of the reactive metabolite NAPQI to critical target proteins or oxidative stress. A critical role for covalent binding to hepatic proteins is supported by immunohistochemical studies, which demonstrated that patterns of APAP–cysteine adduct formation in the liver of treated mice tracked with histopathological evidence of toxicity with respect to localization, severity, dose–response, and time course (Roberts et al. 1991). Originally, it was thought that the overall accumulation of nonspecific covalent adducts eventually led to compromised cellular function resulting in necrotic cell death. However, the observation of similar levels of covalent binding with the nontoxic APAP isomer 3-hydroxyacetanelide suggested that binding to specific targets, rather than overall covalent binding was a key feature of APAP-induced hepatotoxicity (Bessems and Vermeulen 2001). Numerous cellular proteins have now been found to be specific targets for APAP covalent binding (James, Mayeux and Hinson 2003). Proteins targeted by APAP are found in a variety of subcellular compartments including the endoplasmic reticulum, mitochondria, nucleus, and cytosol. Among the proteins for which APAP adducts have been identified, several are enzymes involved in cellular bioenergetics. The activities of several of these enzymes are decreased following formation of APAP adducts, and enzyme inhibition is thought to play a role in some aspects of APAP-induced hepatotoxicity. For example, covalent binding of NAPQI to glyceraldehyde-3-phosphate dehydrogenase (GAPDH) in vitro has been found to decrease the activity of this enzyme by more than 80% (Dietze et al. 1997). Inhibition of this enzyme is the result of binding of NAPQI to Cys-149 in the active site of GAPDH, and may contribute to the decrease in ATP production observed following administration of APAP to mice (Tirmenstein and Nelson 1990). Another enzyme targeted by NAPQI is 10-formyl-tetrahydrofolate dehydrogenase, which converts formaldehyde to CO_2. The activity of this enzyme was decreased by approximately 20% in mice treated with APAP (Pumford, Martin and Hinson 1997). Glutamate dehydrogenase, which is responsible for metabolism of glutamate to α-ketoglutarate and NH_3, was also inhibited by about 25% in

APAP-treated mice. Zhou et al. (1996) have demonstrated covalent binding of NAPQI to endoplasmic reticulum proteins calreticulin and protein disulfide isomerase, both of which play a role in intracellular calcium homeostasis. These authors postulated that interference with the function of these proteins may be related to the increase in intracellular Ca^{2+} observed following treatment of mice with APAP (Corcoran, Wong and Neese 1987, 1988). Another common target of covalent binding for APAP is the so-called acetaminophen binding protein (ABP), also known as selenium binding protein (Pumford, Martin and Hinson 1992; Hoivik et al. 1996). ABP is a 58-kDa cytosolic protein whose physiological function is currently unknown. The toxicological significance of covalent modification of ABP by APAP is unclear. However, after binding to NAPQI or other electrophiles such as bromobenzene oxide, ABP translocates to the nucleus, and has thus been suggested to play a role in cellular signaling and defense against electrophiles (Bessems and Vermeulen 2001). In addition to mitochondrial, microsomal, and cytosolic proteins, NAPQI has also been found to bind to the nuclear proteins laminin A (Khairallah et al. 1995) and ribonucleotide reductase (Brunborg, Holme and Hongslo 1995). The latter target may be related to the genotoxic effects observed in rats and mice following massive doses of APAP (Hongslo et al. 1994)

Although covalent binding of NAPQI to target proteins and inhibition of their function likely contributes to the overall toxicity of APAP, covalent binding alone is unlikely to account for the myriad biochemical effects leading to hepatotoxicity. In most cases, the degree of inhibition observed is modest (20–25%), and in others, the mechanistic connection of covalent binding to hepatotoxicity is tenuous (e.g., ABP). In addition to reaction with protein nucleophiles, NAPQI is also capable of inducing oxidative stress, and this is thought to be a major contributing mechanism to APAP-induced hepatotoxicity (James, Mayeux and Hinson 2003).

11.5.2. Diclofenac

A number of NSAIDs have been associated with hepatotoxicity in humans and this has resulted in withdrawal of several NSAIDs from the market (e.g., bromphenac, benoxaprofen). Diclofenac is an NSAID that has been associated with a rare but potentially severe hepatitis that on rare occasions has progressed to fulminant liver failure. Clinically, diclofenac hepatotoxicity is characterized by increases in serum transaminases, γ-?glutamyltransferase (GGT) and AP, jaundice, hepatomegaly, nausea, and anorexia. Diclofenac hepatotoxicity is idiosyncratic in nature, with an incidence in the range of 3.6 in 100 000 patients and an 8% case–fatality rate (Aithal et al. 2004).

Evidence for the role of bioactivation in the toxicity of diclofenac comes?from in vitro studies, which demonstrated that cytotoxicity of the drug in rat hepatocytes was time- and dose-dependent, decreased by CYP?inhibition, and exacerbated by CYP induction (Schmitz et al. 1992, Kretz-Rommel and Boelsterli 1993, Jumira-Romet, Crawford and Huang 1994). The mechanism of cytotoxicity in hepatocytes appears to involve uncoupling of oxidative phosphorylation, resulting in compromised ATP synthesis (Ponsoda et al. 1995; Masubuchi et al. 2000). Covalent binding of diclofenac in rat hepatocytes was shown to occur in a time- and concentration-dependent manner, and was sensitive to UDPGT inhibitors, such as 7,7,7-triphenylheptyl-UDP and borneol (Kretz-Rommel and Boelsterli 1993). These authors also demonstrated that cytotoxicity of diclofenac was attenuated by CYP inhibitors, but that total covalent binding remained unchanged, indicating that covalent binding was mediated largely if not solely by acyl glucuronide formation. Thus these studies demonstrated divergent mechanisms for direct acute toxicity and covalent adduct formation by diclofenac. In a subsequent study (Kretz-Rommel and ?Boelsterli 1994), it was shown that the glucuronide moiety was retained in covalent adducts to microsomal proteins, suggesting that covalent binding involved ring opening and Schiff's base formation. A mechanistic role for covalent adduct formation, and therefore acyl glucuronide formation, was indicated by experiments in which splenocytes from mice immunized with a diclofenac–keyhole limpet hemocyanin (KLH) conjugate in which the diclofenac moiety was adducted to KHL via an acyl linkage were toxic to mouse hepatocytes treated with the parent drug. Cytotoxicity involved both T-cell and non-T-cell-mediated mechanisms (Kretz- ?Rommel and Boelsterli 1995). Collectively, these studies suggest that bioactivation is intimately involved in hepatotoxicity of diclofenac, and provide evidence that both direct cytotoxic and immune-mediated effects may play a role in the overall mechanism of toxicity.

Specific protein targets for diclofenac metabolites have been investigated by several research groups. Using a primary rat hepatocyte model, Kretz-Rommel and Boelsterli (1993) demonstrated that ^{14}C-diclofenac bound with high specific activity to proteins in the endoplasmic reticulum and plasma membrane, and that the extent of covalent binding shifted from the microsomal fraction to the plasma membrane fraction over time. Little adduct formation was observed in the cytosolic fraction, and the mitochondrial fraction was not examined. The major target of diclofenac in microsomal and plasma membrane fractions was a protein with a molecular weight of 60 kDa. Immunochemical analysis confirmed the presence of the 60-kDa protein adduct and revealed the presence of a second adduct with an apparent molecular weight of 50 kDa. As demonstrated previously, adduct formation was dependent on UDPGT activity and was insensitive to inhibitors of CYP2C. At higher drug concentrations, additional adducts were identified at 80 kDa and 126 kDa. Finally, in vivo administration of diclofenac (30 mg kg^{-1}) to rats for 4 days resulted in detection of the 60 kDa and 80 kDa adducts in the livers of treated rats. Although the targets proteins were not identified, these experiments demonstrated that binding of diclofenac metabolites to hepatocellular proteins was relatively selective.

Selective adduct formation was also demonstrated in mice treated with diclofenac using immunochemical techniques (Pumford et al. 1993). In this study, target proteins with molecular weights of 50, 70, 110, and 140 kDa were detected. The 110-kDa protein was subsequently identified as dipeptidyl peptidase IV (DPP), also known as CD26, and its activity was found to be modestly inhibited by diclofenac treatment (Hargus et al. 1995). The 200-kDa protein detected with anti-diclofenac antibodies is thought to be a dimeric form of DPP. This protein is localized to the outer hepatocyte membrane on the canalicular surface. Although the function of DPP in hepatocytes is not known, its presence on the outer cell surface suggests that it might play a role in immune-mediated hepatotoxicity by serving as a neoantigen. Interestingly, sulindac, another NSAID associated with idiosyncratic hepatotoxicity, also forms adducts to DPP, whereas the nontoxic NSAID ibuprofen does not (Wade et al. 1997). Diclofenac decreases the?functioning of other cannilicular membrane proteins, including Mg^{2+}-ATPase, leucine aminopeptidase, and GGT following in vivo administration to rats (Sallustio and Holbrook 2001). Relative enrichment of Mg^{2+}-ATPase and leucine aminopeptidase in the cannilicular membrane was unchanged, suggesting an in situ decrease in activity, while the relative enrichment of GGT was decreased, suggesting redistribution of this enzyme away from the cannilicular membrane. Consistent with this hypothesis was the observation that diclofenac glucuronide formed adducts upon incubation with GGT in vitro, but adduct formation had no effect on enzyme activity.

Another specific target of diclofenac covalent binding in rats is CYP2C11, which catalyzes bioactivation of the drug in this species ?(Masubuchi et al. 2001). Covalent binding of diclofenac to CYP2C11 appears to involve the intermediacy of an epoxide species since neither 5′- nor 4′-hydroxydiclofenac, precursors of reactive benzoquinonimines, were active. Interestingly, the human homologue CYP2C9 is not inactivated by diclofenac, suggesting that covalent binding to CYPs is a rodent-specific phenomenon (Tang 2003).

Both metabolic and immunological factors have been implicated in?diclofenac-mediated hepatotoxicity in humans. Genetic polymorphisms in drug-metabolizing enzymes may play a role in diclofenac hepatotoxicity in humans. Polymorphisms in UGT2B7, CYP2C8, and ABCC2 (MRP2) are associated with enhanced susceptibility to diclofenac hepatotoxicity. The functional consequences of enzyme polymorphism are unclear, as studies on the function of allelic variants have given mixed results (Daly et al. 2007). Other genetic polymorphisms (i.e., cytokines) may also play a role in individual susceptibility to diclofenac-induced hepatotoxicity. Patients suffering from diclofenac-induced hepatotoxicity expressed hepatic protein adducts recognized by antiserum to a diclofenac–KLH conjugate. Serum from patients treated with diclofenac with (7/7) or without (12/20) associated hepatotoxicity contained antibodies to diclofenac–liver protein adducts. Polymorphisms in IL-10 (low formation) and IL-4 (high formation) were more frequent in patients with diclofenac-associated hepatotoxicity than in untreated controls or in patients receiving diclofenac without associated hepatotoxicity. The combination of high IL-4 and low IL-10 could result in a more extensive immune response, potentially contributing to development of diclofenac-induced hepatotoxicity (Aithal et al. 2004).

Taken together, these data serve to highlight the complex, multifactorial mechanism(s) of diclofenac hepatotoxicity. Reactive metabolites from both phase I and phase II pathways appear to play a key role in the etiology of the disorder. There is evidence for both a metabolic and an immunological component, and susceptibility appears to be modulated by genetic polymorphisms?in drug-metabolizing enzymes and various cytokines.

Nevertheless, despite years of intensive research, our understanding of the mechanisms of diclofenac hepatotoxicity is far from complete.

11.6. Methods for Assessment of Reactive Metabolites

In the pharmaceutical industry, formation of reactive metabolites is one of the major concerns during the process of optimization of drug candidates, in large part due to the mechanistic link with idiosyncratic toxicity. Identification of the pathway leading to reactive metabolites is considered as one of the key studies for understanding the mechanism of hepatotoxicity associated with a compound of interest. To this end, several in vitro methods have been developed for detecting the formation of reactive metabolites.

Many electrophilic reactive metabolites, particularly soft electrophiles, can be trapped in vitro by conjugation with glutathione, an endogenous thiol that participates in detoxification of electrophilic reactive metabolites by forming conjugates with its nucleophilic sulfhydryl group. Conjugation with GSH may be mediated by GSTs or may occur nonenzymatically. Glutathione conjugates formed in the liver in vivo may be excreted intact in bile, or converted to mercapturic acids (*N*-acetylcysteine conjugates) and excreted in urine. A simple in vitro assay for detection of reactive metabolite formation involves addition of glutathione to liver microsomal incubations containing the test compound to trap reactive intermediates. Incubating the test compounds in freshly isolated hepatocytes can also provide assessment of glutathione conjugate formation in a more physiologically relevant test system. To detect glutathione conjugates, mass spectrometry is the preferred tool, and the constant neutral loss of 129 amu corresponding to the γ-glutamyl group can be used to give relatively selective detection for glutathione conjugates (Evans et al. 2004). In negative scan mode, the precursor of m/z 143 and 272 can also help reveal the presence of glutathione conjugates (Dieckhaus et al. 2005). Electrophilic reactive metabolites with more centralized areas of positive charge (hard electrophiles) may not be trapped effectively by glutathione, but can be trapped with cyanide ion, a hard nucleophile (Hoag et al. 1987). To facilitate detection of cyanide adduct by mass spectrometry, a mixture of $^{12}C^{14}N$ and $^{13}C^{15}N$ can be used as the trapping agent to produce a characteristic isotope pattern (Kalgutkar et al. 2002). The results from trapping studies are essentially qualitative, and may provide important information on bioactivation pathway and possible structure of the reactive species. More definitive and quantitative assessment requires covalent binding studies using radiolabeled test compounds. More recently, semiquantitative methods for detection of glutathione conjugates that do not rely on availability of authentic standards have been developed (Gan et al. 2005; Soglia et al. 2006). These approaches may potentially serve as higher-throughput surrogate for the extent of reactive metabolite generation. However, good correlations with covalent binding have yet to be established.

The reactivity of acyl glucuronides with protein nucleophiles is correlated with their chemical stability, which can be assessed by comparison of pseudo first-order degradation half-life values of the 1-*O*-acyl glucuronides and rate of acyl migration in a simple buffer system. This approach allows a rank-ordering of acylglucuronides based on their stability, providing a preliminary assessment of their potential for covalent adduct formation (Benet et al. 1993; Bolze et al. 2002). The angiotensin II receptor antagonist telmisartan is primarily metabolized to a very stable 1-*O*-acyl glucuronide with a degradation half-life of 26 h. Its high stability was further confirmed by its very low extent of covalent binding to human serum albumin in contrast to the more reactive acyl glucuronide of diclofenac (Ebner et al. 1999).

Mechanism-based enzyme inactivation can also serve as a surrogate marker for the formation of reactive metabolites. Reactive metabolites generated by drug-metabolizing enzymes (e.g., cytochromes P450) can covalently modify the apoprotein or the heme moiety of the enzyme. In some cases, this modification leads to irreversible inactivation of the enzyme (for details see Chapter 5). Notable examples include troglitazone-mediated CYP3A4 inactivation (Lim et al. 2005) and ticrynafen-mediated CYP2C9 inactivation (Lopez-Garcia, Dansette and Mansuy 1994). Enzyme kinetic studies offer a quantitative in vitro approach to assess enzyme inactivation. In this approach, the test compound is incubated with an enzyme source (usually microsomes) for varying lengths of time after which the residual enzyme activity is measured using selective probe substrates. Loss of CYP enzyme activity that is time-, concentration-, NADPH-dependent and demonstrates saturation kinetics indicates potential mechanism-based inactivation of the enzyme (Silverman 1988). The apparent inactivation may be due to formation of reactive species that bind irreversibly to the enzyme apoprotein. However, CYP enzyme inactivation can also occur through metabolite complex formation with the heme, and not all reactive metabolites lead to enzyme inactivation (De Montellano and Correia 1995). Overall, mechanism-based enzyme inactivation studies can indicate the propensity of a test compound to be metabolized to reactive intermediates and provide useful information on the potential kinetic interactions with coadministrated substrates for the same enzyme. However, although enzyme inactivation may suggest the formation of reactive metabolites, additional experiments are required to definitively demonstrate this mechanism.

Covalent binding is a more definitive method to address the formation of reactive metabolites. In drug development, the use of radiolabeled tracers can provide an early assessment of the propensity of a drug candidate to undergo covalent binding to cellular macromolecules (Pohl and Branchflower 1981; Baillie and Kassahun 2001). Covalent binding of a reactive metabolite to proteins can also be detected by immunological methods. However, this is a very time-consuming approach requiring generation of antibodies to the reactive metabolite bound to protein. Covalent binding studies can be performed both in vitro and in vivo. An advantage of the in vitro approach is that human tissue can be used (e.g., human liver microsomes). Covalent binding studies clearly demonstrate a direct consequence of formation of a reactive metabolite, that is, binding to a protein. Hepatocytes provide both the activating enzymes and also possible detoxification pathways (further metabolism and protective thiols), as well as the molecular targets of reactive metabolites.

In vivo studies provide the most physiologically relevant test for reactive metabolite formation; as such studies permit the observation covalent binding and toxicity in whole animals. However, differences in the activating enzymes (e.g., cytochromes P450) between species may limit the utility of data generated in intact animals for the prediction of covalent binding potential in humans. Therefore, in vivo results in animals should be compared to in vitro findings in order to relate to possible outcomes in humans. In a procedure developed at Merck Co. (Evans et al. 2004), rats are administered a standard dose of the test article with a specified level of radioactivity and the extent of covalent binding of ^{14}C in liver extracts is measured. Covalent adducts of drug-related material (total radioactivity) bound to liver protein of greater than 50 pmol mg^{-1} protein are considered a high risk. This cutoff value was assigned based on covalent binding analysis of some model hepatotoxins and incorporating a 20-fold safety margin (Evans et al. 2004). In view of the difficulties in extrapolating between in vitro and in vivo, it is usually not possible to quantitatively predict in vivo consequences from in vitro data. These different approaches complement each other, providing corroborating data. In short, the approach of assessing covalent binding in drug discovery and development can help characterize the risk associated with chemical insults of potential drug candidates mediated by reactive intermediates.

11.7. Conclusions

Drug-related hepatotoxicity continues to be a significant cause for failure of new pharmaceutical agents in clinical trials and post-launch. Despite years of intensive research, we are only beginning to scratch the surface with respect to our mechanistic understanding of DILI. In vitro and preclinical screening approaches such as glutathione trapping and assessment of covalent binding provide a means for drug discovery scientists to minimize the potential for formation of reactive metabolites. Though the ultimate impact of these approaches on late-stage attrition remains to be seen, the general opinion is that by minimizing bioactivation potential, we will also minimize the risk of many drug-related adverse reactions, particularly idiosyncratic toxicity. Powerful technologies, such as "omics", promise new insight into mechanisms of hepatotoxicity and the role played by reactive metabolites. It is to be hoped that increased mechanistic understanding offered by such technologies will stimulate development of improved pre-clinical screening and testing methodologies, dramatically improving the safety of new drugs entering the market.

References

Aithal, G. P., Ramsay, L., Daly, A. K., Sonchit, N., Leathart, J. B. S., Alexander,? G., Kenna, J. G., Caldwell, J., and Day, C.P. 2004. Hepatic adducts, circulating antibodies and cytokine polymorphism in patients with diclofenac hepatotoxicity. Hepatology 39:1430–1440.

Anders, M. W. 2004. Glutathione-dependent bioactivation of haloalkanes and haloalkenes. Drug Metab. Rev. 36:583–594.

Atzori, L., Dore, M., and Congiu, L. 1989. Aspects of allyl alcohol toxicity. Drug Metab. Drug Interact. 7:295–319.

Baily, M. J., and Dickinson, R. G. 2003. Acyl glucuronide reactivity in perspective: Biological consequences. Chem. Biol. Interact. 145:117–137.

Baillie, T.A., and Kassahun, K. 2001. Biological reactive intermediates in drug discovery and development: a perspective from the pharmaceutical industry. Adv. Exp. Med. Biol. 500:45–51.

Bakke, O. M., Manocchia, M., de Abayo, F., Kaitin, K. I., and Lasagna, L. 1995. Drug safety discontinuations in the United Kingdom, the United States, and Spain from 1974 through 1993: A regulatory perspective. Clin. Pharmacol. Ther. 58:108–117.

Battista, J. R., and Marnett, L. J. 1985. Prostaglandin H synthase-dependent epoxidation of aflatoxin B1. Carcinogenesis 6:1227–1229.

Benedetti, M. S. 2001. Biotransformation of xenobiotics by amine oxidases. Fund. Clin. Pharmacol. 15: 75–84.

Benet, L. Z., Spahn-Langguth, H., Iwakawa, S., Volland, C., Mizuma, T., Mayer, S., Mutschler, E., and Lin, E. T. 1993. Predictability of the covalent binding of acidic drugs in man. Life Sci. 53:PL141–146.

Berardinis, V. E., Moulis, C., Maurice, M., Beaune, P., Pessayre, D., Pompon, D., and Loeper, J. 2000. Human microsomal epoxide hydrolase is the target of germander-induced autoantibodies on the surface of human hepatocytes. Mol. Pharmacol. 58:542–551.

Bessems, J. G. M., and Vermeulen, N. P. E. 2001. Paracetamol (acetaminophen)-induced toxicity: Molecular and biochemical mechanisms, analogues and protective approaches. Crit. Rev. Toxicol. 31:55–138.

Boelsterli, U. A., Zimmerman, H. J., and Kretz-Rommel, A. 1995. Idiosyncratic liver toxicity of nonsteroidal antiinflammatory drugs: molecular mechanisms and pathology. Crit. Rev. Toxicol. 25:207–235.

Boelsterli, U. A. 2002. Xenobiotic acyl glucuronides and acyl CoA thioesters as protein-reactive metabolites with the potential to cause idiosyncratic drug reactions. Curr. Drug Metab. 3:439–450.

Boelsterli, U. A. 2003. Idiosyncratic drug hepatotoxicity revisited: New insights from mechanistic toxicology. Toxicol. Mech. Meth. 13:3–20.

Bolze, S., Bromet, N., Gay-Feutry, C., Massiere, F., Boulieu, R., and Hulot, T. 2002. Development of an in vitro screening model for the biosynthesis of acyl glucuronide metabolites and the assessment of their reactivity toward human serum albumin. Drug Metab. Dispos. 30:404–413.

Bonierbale, E., Valadon, P., Pous, C., Desfosses, B., Dansette, P.M., and Mansuy, D. 1999. Opposite behaviors of reactive metabolites of tienilic acid and its isomer toward liver proteins: Use of specific anti-tienilic acid-- protein addduct antibodies and the possible relationship with different hepatotoxic effects of the two compounds. Chem. Res. Toxicol. 12:286–296.

Brunborg, G., Holme, J. A., and Hongslo, J. K. 1995. Inhibitory effects of paracetamol on DNA repair in mammalian cells. Mutat. Res. 342:157–170.

Castell, J. V., and Castell, M. 2006. Allergic hepatitis induced by drugs. Curr. Opin. Allergy Clin. Immunol. 6:258–265.

Cheeseman, K. H., Albano, E. F., Tomasi, A., and Slater, T. F. 1985. Biochemical studies on the metabolic activation of halogenated alkanes. Environ. Health Perspect. 64:85–101.

Clark, C. J., Creighton, S., Portmann, B., Taylor, C., Wendon, J. A., and Cramp,? M. E. 2002. Acute liver failure associated with antiretroviral treatment for HIV: A report of six cases. J. Hepatol. 36:295–310.

Corcoran, G. B., Wong, B. K., and Neese, B. L. 1987. Early sustained rise in total liver calcium during acetaminophen hepatotoxicity in mice. Res. Commun. Chem. Pathol. Pharmacol. 58:291–305.

Corcoran, G. B., Bauer, J. A., and Lau, T. A. 1988. Immediate rise in intracellular calcium and glycogen phosphorylase activity upon acetaminophen covalent binding leading to hepatotoxicity in mice. Toxicology 50:157–167.

Cribb, A. E., Lee, B. L., Trepanier, L. A., and Spielberg, S. P. 1996a. Adverse reactions to sulphonamide and sulphonamide-trimethoprim antimicrobials: clinical syndromes and pathogenesis. Adverse Drug React. Toxicol. Rev. 15:9–50.

Cribb, A. E., Nuss, C. E., Alberts, D. W., Lamphere, D. B., Grant, D. M., ? Grossman, S. J., and Spielberg, S. P. 1996b. Covalent binding of sulfamethoxazole reactive metabolites to human and rat liver subcellular fractions assessed by immunochemical detection. Chem. Res. Toxicol. 9:500–507.

Daly, A. K., Aithal, G. P., Leathart, J. B. S., Swainsbury, R. A., Dang, T. S., and Day, C. P. 2007. Genetic susceptibility to diclofenac-induced hepatotoxicity: contribution of UGT2B7, CYP2C8 and ABCC2 genotypes. Gastroenterology 132:272–281.

De Groot, H., and Sies, H. 1989. Cytochrome P-450, reductive metabolism, and cell injury. Drug Metab. Rev. 20:275–284.

De Montellano, P. R., and Correia, M. A. 1995. Inhibition of cytochrome P450 enzymes. In Cytochrome P450: Structure, Mechanism, and Biochemistry. 2 nd Edn. pp. 308–333.New York: Plenum Press.

Dieckhaus, C. M., Fernandez-Metzler, C. L., King, R., Krolikowski, P. H., and Baillie, T. A. 2005. Negative ion tandem mass spectrometry for the detection of glutathione conjugates. Chem. Res. Toxicol. 18:630–638.

Dietze, E. C., Schäfer, A., Omichinski, J. G., and Nelson, S. D. 1997. Inactivation of glyceraldehyde-3-phosphate dehydrogenase by a reactive metabolite of acetaminophen and mass spectral characterization of an arylated active site peptide. Chem. Res. Toxicol. 10:1097–1103.

Djuric, Z. 1989. Reductive metabolism and DNA binding of misonidazole. Toxicol. Appl. Pharmacol. 101:47–54.

Ebner, T., Heinzel, G., Prox, A., Beschke, K., and Wachsmuth, H. 1999. Disposition and chemical stability of telmisartan 1-*O*-acylglucuronide. Drug Metab. Dispos. 27:1143–1149.

Evans, D. C., Watt, A. P., Nicoll-Griffith, D. A., and Baillie, T. A. 2004. Drug–protein adducts: an industry perspective on minimizing the potential for drug bioactivation in drug discovery and development. Chem. Res. Toxicol. 17:3–16.

Fau, D., Lekehal, M., Farrell, G., Moreau, A., Moulis, C., Feldman, G. Haouzi,? D., and Pesayre, D. 1997. Diterpenoids from germander, an herbal medicine, induce apoptosis in isolated rat hepatocytes. Gastroenterology 113:1334–1346.

FDA. 2000. Clinical White Paper. CDER-PhRMA-AASLD Conference on Drug-induced Hepatotoxicity pp. 1–13.

Fowler, R., and Imrie, K. 2001. Thalidomide-associated hepatitis: a case report. Am. J. Hematol. 66:300–302.

Frank, H., Haussmann, H. J., and Remmer, H.1982. Metabolic activation of carbon tetrachloride: induction of cytochrome P-450 with phenobarbital or 3-methylcholanthrene and its effect on covalent binding. Chem. Biol. Interact. 40:193–208.

Gallagher, E.P., Wienkers, L.C., Stapleton, P.L., Kunze, K.L., and Eaton, D.L. 1994. Role of human microsomal and human complementary DNA-expressed cytochromes P4501A2 and P4503A4 in the bioactivation of aflatoxin B1. Cancer Res. 54:101–108.

Gan, J., Harper, T. W., Hsueh, M. M., Qu, Q., Humphreys, W. G. 2005. Dansyl glutathione as a trapping agent for the quantitative estimation and identification of reactive metabolites. Chem. Res. Toxicol. 18:896–903.
Glatt, H. 1997. Bioactivation of mutagens via sulfation. FASEB J. 11:314–321.
Glatt, H. 2000. Sulfotransferases in the bioactivation of xenobiotics. Chem. Biol. Interact. 129:141–170.
Glatt, H., Boeing, H., Engelke, C. E. H., Ma, L., Kuhlow, A., Pabel, U., Pomplun,? D., Teubner, W., and Meinl, W. 2001. Human cytosolic sulfotransferases: genetics, characteristics, toxicological aspects. Mutat. Res. 482:27–40.
Gordon, G. B., Spielberg, S. P., Blake, D. A., and Balasubramanian, V. 1981. Thalidomide teratogenesis: Evidence for a toxic arene oxide metabolite. Proc. Natl. Acad. Sci. USA 78:2545–2548.
Grillo, M. P., Hua, F., Knutson, C. G., Ware, J. A., and Li, C. 2003. Mechanistic studies on the bioactivation of dichlofenac: Identification of dichlofenac-*S*-acyl-glutathione in vitro in incubations with rat and human hepatocytes. Chem. Res. Toxicol. 16:1410–1417.
Guengerich, F.P. 1996. The chemistry of cytochrome P450 reactions. In: Cytochrome P450: Metabolic and toxicological aspects. C. Ioannides ed, pp. 55–74. CRC Press, Boca Raton.
Guengerich, F. P., Johnson, W. W., Shimada, T., Ueng, Y. F., Yamazaki, H., and Langouet, S. 1998. Activation and detoxication of aflatoxin B_1. Mutat. Res. 402:121–128.
Guengerich, F. P. 2002. *N*-hydroxyarylamines. Drug Metab. Rev. 34:607–623.
Haenen, G. R. M., Vermeulen, N. P. E., Tai Tin Tsoni, J. N. L., Regetti, H. M. N., Timmerman, H., and Bast, A. 1988. Activation of the microsomal glutathione S-?transferase and reduction of the glutathione dependent protection against lipid?peroxidation by acrolein. Biochem. Pharmacol. 37:1933–1938.
Hanje, A. J., Shamp, J. L., Thomas, F. B., and Meis, G. M. 2006. Thalidomide-induced severe hepatotoxicity. Pharmacotherapy 26:1018–1022.
Hansena, J. M., Carneyb, E. W., and Harris C. 1999. Differential alteration by thalidomide of the glutathione content of rat vs. rabbit conceptuses in vitro. Reprod. Toxicol. 13:547–554.
Hargus, S. J., Martin, B. M., George, J. W., and Pohl, L. R. 1995. Covalent modification of rat liver dipeptidyl peptidase IV (CD26) bu the nonsteroidal anti-inflammatory drug diclofenac. Chem. Res. Toxicol. 8: 993–996.
Hoag, M. K., Trevor, A. J., Kalir, A., Castagnoli, N. Jr. 1987. Phencyclidine iminium ion. NADPH-dependent metabolism, covalent binding to macromolecules, and inactivation of cytochrome(s) P-450. Drug Metab. Dispos. 15:485–490.
Hoivik, D. J., Manautou, J. E., Tveit, A., Mankowski, D. C., Khairallah, E. A. and Cohen, S. D. 1996. Evidence suggesting that the 58-kDa acetaminophen binding protein is a preferential target for acetaminophen electrophile. Fund. Appl. Toxicol. 32:79–86.
Hongslo, J. K., Smith, C. V., Brunborg, G., Soderlund, E. J. and Holme, J. A. 1994. Genotoxicity of paracetamol in mice and rats. Mutagenesis 9: 93–100.
Huang, Y. S., Chern, H. D., Su, W. J., Wu, J. C., Lai, S. L., Yang, S. Y., ?Chang,?? F.??Y., and Lee, S. D. 2002. Polymorphism of the *N*-acetyltransferase 2 gene as a susceptibility risk factor for antituberculosis drug-induced hepatitis. Hepatology 35:883–889.
Inskeep, P. B., Koga, N., Cmarik, J. L., and Guengerich, F. P. 1986. Covalent binding of 1,2-dihaloalkanes to DNA and stability of the major DNA adduct, S42-(*N*7-guanyl)ethyl] glutathione. Cancer Res. 46:2839–2844.
James, L. P., Mayeux, P. R. and Hinson, J. A. 2003. Acetaminophen-induced hepatotoxicity. Drug Metab. Dispos. 31:1499–1506.

Jaeschke, H., Gores, G. J., Cederbaum, A. I., Hinson, J. A., Pessayre, D., and Lemasters, J. J. 2002. Mechanisms of hepatotoxicity. Tox. Sci. 65:166–176.

Jean, P., Lopez-Garcia, P., Dansette, P., Mansuy, D., and Goldstein, J.L. 1996. Oxidation of tienilic acid by human yeast-expressed cytochromes P-450 2C8, 2C9, 2C18, and 2C19. Evidence that this drug is a mechanism-based inhibitor specific for cytochrome P-450 2C9. Eur. J. Biochem. 241: 797–804.

Jollow, D. J.,Mitchell, J. R., Potter, W. Z., Davis, D. C., Gillette, J. R. and Brodie,??B. B. 1973. Acetaminophen-induced hepatic necrosis. II. Role of covalent binding in vivo. J. Pharmacol. Exp. Ther. 187:195–202.

Jumira-Romet, M., Crawford, K. and Huang, H. S. 1994. Comparative cytotoxicity of non-steroidal anti-inflammatory drugs in primary cultures of rat hepatocytes. Toxicol. in Vitro 8:55–66.

Kalgutkar, A. S., Dalvie, D. K., O'Donnell, J. P., Taylor, T. J., Sahakian, D. C. 2002. On the diversity of oxidative bioactivation reactions on nitrogen- ?containing xenobiotics. Curr. Drug Metab. 3:379–424.

Kaplowitz, N. 2005. Idiosyncratic drug hepatotoxicity. Nature Rev. Drug Discov. 4:489–499.

Kassahun, K., Pearson, P. G., Tang, W., McIntosh, I., Leung, K., Elmore, C., Dean, D., Wang, R., Doss, G., Baillie, T. A. 2001. Studies on the metabolism of troglitazone to reactive intermediates in vitro and in vivo. Evidence for novel biotransformation pathways involving quinone methide formation and thiazolidinedione ring scission. Chem. Res. Toxicol. 14:62–70.

Kerr, B. M., Thummel, K. E., Wurden, C. J., Klein, S. M., Kroetz, D. L., Gonzalez, F. J., and Levy, R. H. 1994. Human liver carbamazepine metabolism: Role of CYP3A4 and CYP2C8 in 10,11-epoxide formation. Biochem. Pharmacol. 47:1969–1979.

Khairallah, E. A., Bruno, M. K., Hong, M. and Cohen, S. D. 1995. Cellular consequences of protein adduct formation (abstract). Toxicologist 15:86.

Knowles, S. R., Uetrecht, J., and Shear, N.H. 2000. Idiosyncratic drug reactions: the reactive metabolite syndromes. Lancet 356:1587–1591.

Kretz-Rommel, A., and Boelsterli, U. A. 1993. Diclofenac covalent binding is dependent on acyl glucuronide formation and is inversely related to P450-mediated acute cell injury in cultured rat hepatocytes. Toxicol. Appl. Pharmacol. 120:155–161.

Kretz-Rommel, A., and Boelsterli, U. A. 1994. Mechanism of covalent adduct formation of diclofenac to rat hepatic microsomal proteins: Retention of the glucuronic acid moiety. Drug Metab. Dispos. 22:956–961.

Kretz-Rommel, A., and Boelsterli, U. A. 1995. Cytotoxic activity of T-cells and non T-cells from diclofenac-immunized mice against cultured syngeneic hepatocytes exposed to diclofenac. Hepatology 22:213–222.

Lai, W. G., Zahid, N., and Uetrecht, J. P. 1999. Metabolism of trimethoprim to a reactive iminoquinone methide by activated human neutrophils and hepatic microsomes. J. Pharmacol. Exp. Ther. 291:292–299.

Lake-Bakaar, G., Scheuer, P. J., and Sherlock, S. 1987 Hepatic reactions associated with ketoconazole in the United Kingdom. Br. Med. J. 294: 419–422.

Lee, W. M. 2003. Drug-induced hepatotoxicity. N. Eng. J. Med. 349:474–485.

Lewis, D. F. V. 2004. 57 Varieties: the human cytochromes P450. Pharmacogenomics 5:305–318.

Lewis, J. H. 2006. 'Hy's law', the 'Rezulin rule' and other predictors of severe drug-induced hepatotoxicity: putting risk–benefit into perspective. Pharmacoepidemiol. Drug Saf. 15: 221–229.

Lim, H. K., Duczak, Jr., N., Brougham, L., Elliot, M., Patel, K., and Chan, K. 2005. Automated screening with confirmation of mechanism-based inactivation

of CYP3A4, CYP2C9, CYP2C19, CYP2D6, and CYP1A2 in pooled human liver microsomes. Drug Metab. Dispos. 33:1211–1219.
Lopez-Garcia, M. P., Dansette, P. M., and Mansuy, D. 1994. Thiophene derivatives as new mechanism-based inhibitors of cytochromes P-450: inactivation of yeast-expressed human liver cytochrome P-450 2C9 by tienilic acid. Biochemistry 33:166–175.
Masubuchi, Y., Yamada, S., and Horie, T. 2000. Possible mechanism of hepatocyte injury induced by diphenylamine and its structurally related nonsteroidal anti-inflammatory drugs. J. Pharmacol. Exp. Ther. 292: 982–987.
Martinez, G. R., Loureiro, A. P. M., Marques, S. A., Miyamoto, S., Yamaguchi, L. F., Onuki, J., Almeida, E. A., Garcia, C. M. C., Barbosa, L. F., Medeiros, M. H. G., and Di Mascio, P. 2003. Oxidative and alkylating damage in DNA. Mutat. Res. 544:115–127.
Matzinger, P. 1994. Tolerance, danger and the extended family. Annual Rev. Immunol. 12:991–1045.
Navarro, V. J., and Senior, J. R. 2006. Drug-related hepatotoxicity. N. Eng. J. Med. 354:731–739.
Mitchell, J. R., Jollow, D .J., Potter, W. Z., Davis, D. C., Gillette, J. R., and Brodie,??B. B. 1973a. Acetaminophen-induced hepatic necrosis. I. Role of drug metabolism. J. Pharmacol. Exp. Ther. 187:185–194.
Mitchell, J. R., Jollow, D. J., Potter, W. Z., Davis, D. C., Gillette, J. R., and Brodie,??B. B. 1973b. Acetaminophen-induced hepatic necrosis. IV. Protective role of glutathione. J. Pharmacol. Exp. Ther. 187:211–217.
Mitchell, J. R., Nelson, W. L., Potter, W. Z., Sasame, H. A., and Jollow, D. J. 1976. Metabolic activation of furosemide to chemically reactive, hepatotoxic metabolite. J. Pharmacol. Exp. Ther. 199:41–52.
Nelson, S. D. 1982. Metabolic activation and drug toxicity. J. Med. Chem. 25:753–765.
Nelson, S. D. 2001. Structure toxicity relationships – how useful are they in predicting toxicities of new drugs. Adv. Exp. Med. Biol. 500:33–43.
Nelson, S. D., Mitchell, J. R., Timbrell, J. A., Snodgrass, W. R., and Corcoran, G. B. 3rd 1976. Isoniazid and iproniazid: activation of metabolites to toxic intermediates in man and rat. Science 193:901–903.
Njoku, D., Laster, M. J., Gong, D. H., Eger, E. I., 2 nd, Reed, G. F., and Martin, J. L. 1997. Biotransformation of halothane, enflurane, isoflurane, and desfurane to trifluoroacetylated liver proteins: association between protein acylation and hepatic injury. Anesth. Analg. 84:173–178.
O'Brien, P .J. 1991. Molecular mechanisms of quinone cytotoxicity. Chem. Biol. Interact. 80:1–41.
Olsen, J., Li, C., Bjørnsdottir, I., Sidenius, U., Hansen, S. H., and Benet, L. Z. 2005. In vitro and in vivo studies on acyl-coenzyme A-dependent bioactivation of zomepirac in rats. Chem. Res. Toxicol. 18:1729–1736.
Olsen, J., Li, C., Skonberg, C., Bjørnsdottir, I., Sidenius, U., Benet L. Z., and Hansen, S. H. 2007. Studies on the metabolism of tolmetin to the chemically reactive acyl-coenzyme A thioester intermediate in rats. Drug Metab. Dispos. 35:758–764.
Ostapowicz, G., Fontana, R. J., Schiodt, F. V., Larson, A., Davern, T. J., Han, S. H. B., McCashland, T. M., Shakil, O., Hay, E., Hynan, L., Crippen, J. S., Blei, A. T., Samuel, G., Reisch, J., Lee, W. M. and the U.S. Acute Liver Failure Study Group. 2002. Results of a prospective study of acute liver failure at 17 tertiary care centers in the United States. Ann. Intern. Med. 137:947–954.
Park, B. K., Pirmohamed, M., and Kitteringham, N. R. 1998. Role of drug disposition in drug hypersensitivity: a chemical, molecular, and clinical perspective. Chem. Res. Toxicol. 11:969–988.

Parrish, D. D., Schlosser, M. J., Kapeghian, J. C., and Traina, V. M. 1997. Activation of CGS 12094 (prinomide metabolite) to 1,4-benzoquinone by myeloperoxidase: implications for human idiosyncratic agranulocytosis. Fundam. Appl. Toxicol. 35:197–204.

Pearce, R. E., Vakkalagadda, G. R., and Leeder, J. S. 2002. Pathways of carbamazepine bioactivation in vitro I. Characterization of human cytochromes P450 responsible for the formation of 2- and 3-hydroxylated metabolites. Drug Metab. Dispos. 30:1170–1179.

Pichler, W. J. 2005. Direct T-cell stimulation by drugs – bypassing the innate immune system. Toxicol. 209: 95-100.

Pirmohamed, M., Nasibitt, D. J., Gordon, F., and Park, B. K. 2002. The danger hypothesis – potential role in idiosyncratic drug reactions. Toxicol. 181-182: 55–63.

Pohl, L. R., and Branchflower, R. V. 1981. Covalent binding of electrophilic metabolites to macromolecules. Meth. Enzymol. 77:43–50.

Pohl, L. R., Satoh, H., Christ, D. D., and Kenna, J. G. 1988. The immunologic and metabolic basis of drug hypersensitivities. Annu. Rev. Pharmacol. Toxicol. 28:367–387.

Pol, S., Vallet-Pichard, A., and Fontaine, H. 2002. Hepatatis C and human immune deficiency coinfection in the era of highly active retroviral therapy. J.Viral. Hepat. 9:1–8.

Ponsada, X., Bort, R., Jover, R., Gómez-Lechón, M. J., and Castell, J. V. 1995. Molecular mechanism of diclofenac hepatotoxicity: Association of cell injury with oxidative metabolism and decrease in ATP levels. Toxicol. In Vitro. 9:439–444.

Poon, G. K., Chen, Q., Teffera, Y., Ngui, J. S., Griffin, P. R., Braun, M. P., Doss, G. A., Freeden, C., Stearns, R. A., Evans, D. C., Baillie, T. A., and Tang, W. 2001. Bioactivation of diclofenac via benzoquinone imine intermediates – identification of urinary mercapturic acid derivatives in rats and humans. Drug Metab. Dispos. 29:1608–1613.

Pumford, N. R., Martin, B. M., and Hinson, J.A.1992. A metabolite of acetaminophen covalently binds to the 56 kDa selenium binding protein. Biophys. Biochem. Res. Comm. 182:1348–1355.

Pumford, N. R., Myers, T. G., Davila. J. C., Highet, R. J., and Pohl, L. R. 1993. Immunochemical detection of liver protein adducts of the nonsteroidal anti-inflammatory drug diclofenac. Chem. Res. Toxicol. 6:147–150.

Qian, L., and Ortiz de Montellano, P. R. 2006. Oxidative activation of thiacetazone by the *Mycobacterium tuberculosis* flavin monooxygenase EtaA and human FMO1 and FMO3. Chem. Res. Toxicol. 19:443–449.

Riley, T. R., 3rd, and Smith, J. P.1998. Ibuprofen-induced hepatotoxicity in patients with chronic hepatitis C: a case series. Am. J. Gastroenterol. 93:1563–1565.

Ripp, S. L., Overby, L. H., Philpot, R. M., and Elfarra, A. A.1997. Oxidation of cysteine S-conjugates by rabbit liver microsomes and cDNA-expressed flavin-containing monooxygenases: studies with *S*-(1,2-dichlorovinyl)-L-cysteine, *S*-(1,2,2-trichlorovinyl)-L-cysteine, *S*-allyl-L-cysteine, and *S*-benzyl-L-cysteine. Mol. Pharmacol. 51:507–515.

Roberts, D. W., Bucci, T. J., Benson, R. W., Warbritton, A. R., McRae, T. A., Pumford, N. R., and Hinson, J. A. 1991. Immunohistochemical localization and quantification of the 3-(cysteine-S-yl)-acetaminophen protein adduct in acetaminophen hepatotoxicity. Am. J. Pathol. 138:359–371.

Rodriquez, J. R., and Acosta, D. 1997. Metabolism of ketoconazole and deacetylated ketoconazole by rat hepatic microsomes and flavin-containing monooxygenases. Drug Metab. Dispos. 25:772–777.

Ross, D., Kepa, J. K., Winski, S. L., Beall, H. D., Anwar, A., and Siegel, D. 2000. NAD(P)H:quinone oxidoreductase 1 (NQO1): Chemoprotection, bioactivation, gene regulation and genetic polymorphisms. Chem. Biol. Interact. 129:77–97.
Roth, R. A., Harkema, J. R., Pestka, J. P., and Ganey, P. E. 1997. Is exposure to bacterial endotoxin a determinant of susceptibility to intoxication from xenobiotic agents Toxciol. Appl. Pharmacol. 147:300–311.
Sallustio, B., and Holbrook, F. L. 2001. In vivo perturbation of rat hepatocyte canalicular membrane function by diclofenac. Drug Metab. Dispos. 29:1535–1538.
Schmidt, L. E., Dalhoff, K., and Poulsen, H. E. 2002. Acute versus chronic alcohol consumption in acetaminophen-induced hepatotoxicity. Hepatology 35:876–882.
Schmitz, G., Stauffert, I., Sippel, H., Lepper H., and Estler, C.-J. 1992. Toxicity of diclofenac to isolated hepatocytes. J. Hepatol. 14:408–409.
Silverman, R. B. 1988. Mechanism-Based Enzyme Inactivation: Chemistry and Enzymology. Vol. I. pp.3–30. Boca Raton: CRC Press, Inc.
Soglia, J. R., Contillo, L. G., Kalgutkar, A. S., Zhao, S., Hop, C. E., Boyd, J. G., and Cole, M. J. 2006. A semiquantitative method for the determination of reactive metabolite conjugate levels in vitro utilizing liquid chromatography – tandem mass spectrometry and novel quaternary ammonium glutathione analogues. Chem. Res. Toxicol. 19:480–490.
Spahn-Langguth, H., Dahms, M., and Hermening, A. 1996. Acyl glucuronides: covalent binding and its potential relevance. Adv. Exp. Med. Biol. 387:313–328.
Testa, B. 1995. The metabolism of drugs and other xenobiotics. Biochemistry of redox reactions. London: Academic Press.
Timbrell, J. A., Mitchell, J. R., Snodgrass, W. R., and Nelson S. 1980. Isoniazid hepatotoxicity: the relationship between covalent binding and metabolism in vivo. J. Pharmacol. Exp. Ther. 213:364–369.
Tirmenstein, M. A., and Nelson, S. D. 1990. Acetaminophen-induced oxidation of protein thiols: contribution of impaired thiol metabolilzing enzymes to the breakdown of adenine nucleotides. J. Biol. Chem. 265:3059–3065.
Uetrecht, J. 2001. Prediction of a new drug's potential to cause idiosyncratic reactions. Curr. Opin. Drug Discov. Devel. 4:55–59.
van Puijenbroek, E. P., Egberts, A. C., Meyboom, R. H., and Leufkens, H. G. 2002. Different risks for NSAID-induced anaphylaxis. Ann. Pharmacother. 36:24–29.
Varghese, A. J., and Whitmore, G. F. 1985. Properties of 2-hydroxylaminoimidazoles and their implications for the biological effects of 2-nitroimidazoles. Chem. Biol. Interact. 56:269–287.
Vogel, C. 2000. Prostaglandin H synthetases and their importance in chemical toxicity. Curr. Drug Metab. 1:391–404.
Wade, L. T., Kenna, J. G., and Caldwell, J. 1997. Immunochemical identification of mouse hepatic protein adducts derived from the nonsteroidal anti-inflammatory drugs diclofenac, sulindac and ibuprofen. Chem. Res. Toxicol. 10: 546–555.
Walker, R. M., and McElligott, T. F. 1981. Furosemide induced hepatotoxicity. J. Pathol. 135:301–314.
Walsh, J. S., Reese, M. J., and Thurmond, L. M. 2002. The metabolic activation of abacavir by human liver cytosol and expressed human alcohol dehydrogenase isozymes. Chem. Biol. Interact. 142:135–154.
Whitcomb, D. C., and Block, D. G. 1994. Association of acetaminophen hepatotoxicity with fasting and ethanol use. J. Am. Med. Assoc. 272:1845–1850.

Wirth, P. J., Bettis, C. J., and Nelson, W.L. 1976. Microsomal metabolism of furosemide. Evidence for the nature of the reactive intermediate involved in covalent binding. Mol. Pharmacol. 12:759–768.

Yamamoto, T., Suou, T., and Hirayama, C. 1986. Elevated serum aminotransferase induced by isoniazid in relation to isoniazid acetylator phenotype. Hepatology 6:295–298.

Yan, Z., Li, J., Huebert, N., Caldwell, G. W., Du, Y., and Zhong, H. 2005. Detection of a novel reactive metabolite of diclofenac: evidence for CYP2C9-mediated bioactivation via arene oxides. Drug Metab. Dispos. 33:706–713.

Zhou, S., Duan, W., Huang, M., and Chen, Y.-Z. 2005. Drug bioactivation, covalent binding to target proteins and toxicity relevance. Drug Metab. Rev. 37:41–213.

12

Role of Cysteine S-Conjugate β-Lyases in the Bioactivation of Renal Toxicants

Arthur J.L. Cooper and John T. Pinto
Department of Biochemistry and Molecular Biology, New York Medical College, Valhalla, NY 10595, USA
e-mail: arthur_cooper@nymc.edu

Keywords: Cysteine S-conjugates · Cysteine S-conjugate β-lyases · Mercapturate Pathway · β-elimination · Pyridoxal 5′-phosphate Enzymes · Pyruvate · Sulfur-containing Elimination Fragment

12.1. Introduction

Halogenated alkenes (e.g., trichloroethylene, tetrachloroethylene, tetrafluoroethylene, and hexachloro-1:3-butadiene) are among several hundred potentially dangerous toxicants listed as present in Superfund sites in the US (http://www.atsdr.cdc.gov/cxcx3.html). Part of the US population is exposed to haloalkenes from such sites and in the workplace (Wu and Schaum 2000), and possibly through "recreational" abuse (Marjot and McLeod 1989). Haloalkenes are nephrotoxic in experimental animals (Dekant, Vamvakas and Anders 1994). In humans, heavy exposure to trichloroethylene is associated with an increased risk of kidney cancer (Brauch et al. 2004). The cysteine S-conjugate formed from trichloroethylene, namely S-(1,2-dichlorovinyl)-L-cysteine (DCVC)[1], induces expression of the proto-oncogenes c-*fos* and c-*myc* in LLC-PK_1 cells (a pig kidney cell line) (Vamvakas and Köster 1993).

[1] Abbreviations used: AlaAT, alanine aminotransferase; AGAT II, alanine-glyoxylate aminotransferase isoenzyme II; AspAT, aspartate aminotransferase; AOA, aminooxyacetate; $BCAT_c$, cytosolic branched-chain amino acid aminotransferase; $BCAT_m$, mitochondrial branched-chain amino acid aminotransferase; BCDHC, branched-chain α-keto acid dehydrogenase complex; BTC, S-(2-benzothiazolyl)-L-cysteine; cyt, cytosolic; DCVC, S-(1,2-dichlorovinyl)-L-cysteine; GST, glutathione *S*-transferase; GTK, glutamine transaminase K; KAT I, kynurenine aminotransferase isoenzyme I; KGDHC, α-ketoglutarate dehydrogenase complex; mit, mitochondrial; PCBC, *S*-(1,2,3,4,4-pentachloro-1,3-butadienyl)-L-cysteine; PDHC, pyruvate dehydrogenase complex; PLP, pyridoxal 5′-phosphate; PMP, pyridoxamine 5′-phosphate; TCA cycle, tricarboxylic acid cycle; TFEC, S-(1,1,2,2-tetrafluoroethyl)-L-cysteine.

A.A. Elfarra (ed.), *Advances in Bioactivation Research*, DOI: 10.1007/978-0-387-77300-1_12,

The nephrotoxicity of halogenated alkenes is due at least in part to their conversion to the corresponding cysteine S-conjugate followed by the action of cysteine S-conjugate β-lyases. In this review, we describe the cysteine S-conjugate β-lyase bioactivation pathway and identify enzymes known to catalyze β-lyase reactions with nephrotoxic halogenated cysteine S-conjugates. We discuss mechanisms whereby reactive fragments generated from these conjugates by the action of cysteine S-conjugate β-lyases modify proteins, including enzymes of energy metabolism and heat shock proteins. We also provide examples of electrophilic xenobiotics other than haloalkenes that may also be bioactivated by mechanisms that involve cysteine S-conjugate β-lyases.

12.2. The Mercapturate Pathway

A large number of reactive electrophiles, whether generated endogenously or ingested, are converted to mercapturates. The mercapturate pathway may be depicted as X (electrophile) → GSX (glutathione S-conjugate) → L-cysteinylglycine S-conjugate → L-cysteine S-conjugate → *N*-acetyl-L-cysteine S-conjugate (mercapturate) (Figure 12.1). (For reviews see, for example, Chasseaud 1976; Stevens and Jones 1989; Cooper and Tate 1997). Mercapturates are often more polar and water soluble than the parent electrophile and are readily excreted. Excretion of the mercapturate represents a detoxification process. However, as discussed below, the mercapturate pathway may on occasion act as a bioactivation pathway if the cysteine S-conjugate is converted by cysteine S-conjugate β-lyases to a reactive sulfur-containing fragment.

The first step in the mercapturate pathway is attack of glutathione thiolate (GS^-) on the electrophile generating the corresponding glutathione S-conjugate. Glutathione S-conjugate formation may occur spontaneously, but in most cases it is catalyzed (or accelerated) by members of a superfamily of glutathione S-transferases (GSTs). Cytosolic GSTs are classified into several classes (A (alpha), M (mu), P (pi), T (theta), Z (zeta), O (omega), and S (sigma)) according to their isoelectric point, substrate and inhibitor properties, antibody recognition, and N-terminal amino acid sequences. Glutathione S-transferases may also be broadly classified on the basis of their cellular location, namely microsomal, mitochondrial, and cytosolic (Hayes, Flanagan and Jowsey 2005). Glutathione S-transferases catalyze three types of reactions (Anders 2004). For example, haloalkenes and dichloroacetylene undergo GST-catalyzed vinylic substitution (S_NV) reactions, which may be either an addition reaction (e.g., with tetrafluoroethylene (Eq. 12.1), dichloroacetylene (Eq. 12.2)), or an addition–elimination reaction (e.g., with trichloroethylene (Eq. 12.3)). Glutathione S-transferases also catalyze reactions with epoxide moieties (e.g., in the conversion of leukotriene A_4 to leukotriene C_4). Glutathione S-conjugate formation with haloalkenes is catalyzed by both microsomal (MGST1) and cytosolic GSTs in ratios that depend to some extent on the structure of the haloalkene (Anders 2004; Wolf et al. 1984; Wallin et al. 1988; McLellan, Wolf and Hayes 1989; Oesch and Wolf

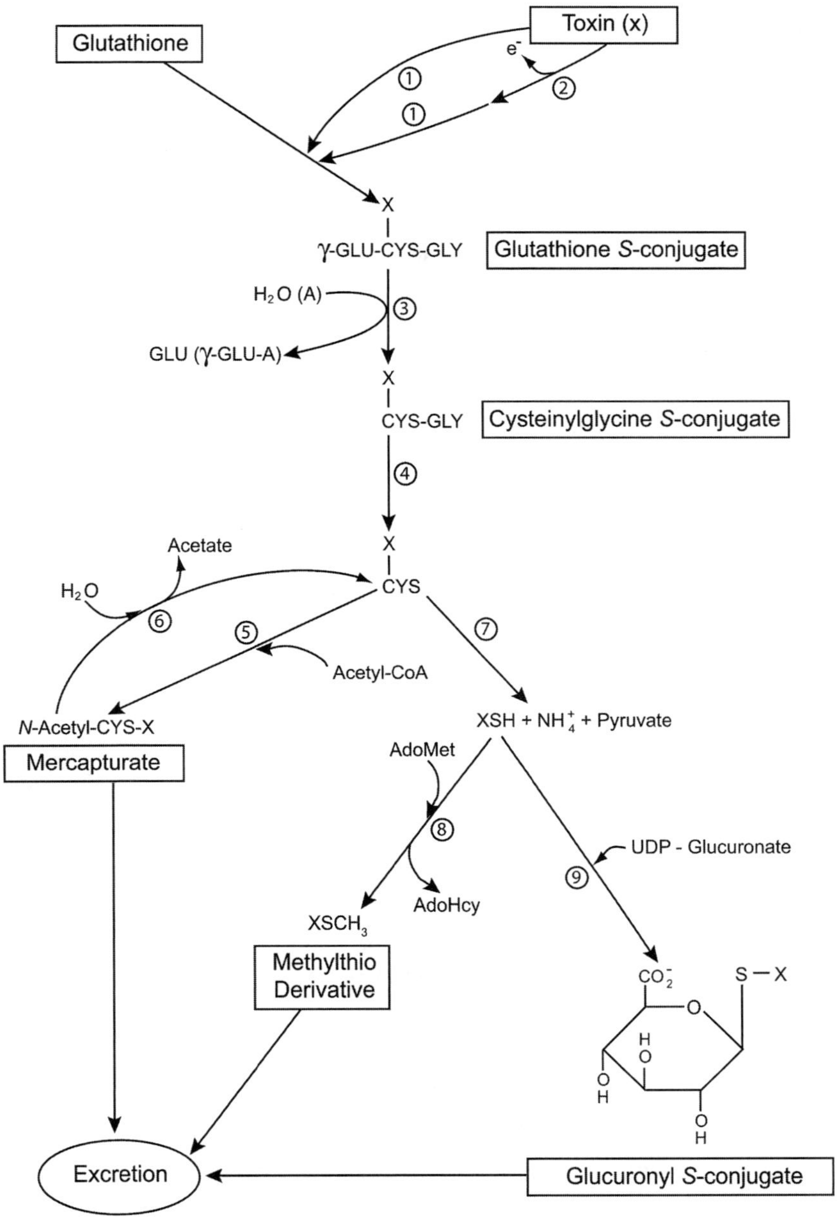

Figure 12.1 Detoxification via the mercapturate pathway and associated side reactions. If the potential toxin contains an electrophilic center it may react directly with GS^- (reaction 1). In that case the GSTs may be regarded as phase I detoxifying enzymes. Alternatively, the toxin may be oxidized via the P450 system prior to the GST-catalyzed reaction to generate a metabolite with an electrophilic center. In that case the glutathione S-transferases may be regarded as phase II detoxifying enzymes and glutathione S-conjugate formation will require two steps (reaction 2 followed by reaction 1). Urinary metabolites of the methylthio compound may also include a sulfoxide, a sulfone and sulfate (not shown). Enzymes: (1) glutathione S-transferases, (2) oxidases that generate an electrophilic center for attack by GS^-; (3) γ-glutamyltransferase (= γ-glutamyl transpeptidase); (4) aminopeptidase M/cysteinylglycinase; (5) *N*-acetyltransferases; (6) aminoacylases; (7) cysteine S-conjugate β-lyases; (8) thiomethyltransferase; (9) UDP-glucuronosyltransferases. *Abbreviations*: AdoHcy, *S*-adenosyl-L-homocysteine; AdoMet, *S*-adenosyl-L-methionine; A, amino acid or dipeptide acceptor for the γ-glutamyltransferase reaction; γ-GLU-A, γ-glutamyl amino acid (or γ-glutamyldipeptide).

1989; Hargus et al. 1991; Cummings, Parker and Lash 2000; Jolivette and Anders 2002, 2003).

$$F_2C{=}CF_2 + GS^- + H^+ \rightarrow F_2C(H)CF_2SG \quad (12.1)$$

$$ClC{\equiv}CCl + GS^- + H^+ \rightarrow ClC(H){=}C(Cl)SG \quad (12.2)$$

$$Cl(H)C{=}CCl_2 + GS^- \rightarrow ClC(H){=}C(Cl)SG + Cl^- \quad (12.3)$$

Conversion of the glutathione S-conjugate to the L-cysteinylglycine S-conjugate, L-cysteinyl S-conjugate, and mercapturate is catalyzed by the consecutive action of γ-glutamyltransferase, aminopeptidase M/cysteinylglycinase, and an N-acetyltransferase, respectively (Figure 12.1).

12.3. Nephrotoxic Haloalkene Glutathione- and Cysteine S-Conjugates

Trichloroethylene induces (1) aplastic anemia in cattle and (2) kidney damage in all animal species tested, including cattle (Lock et al. 1996). Depending on the structure, halogenated alkenes may be metabolized by cytochrome P450 isoenzymes (especially CYP2E1) and/or by glutathione S-conjugation. The ratio of the two activities varies markedly among the various halogenated alkenes. For example, hexachloro-1:3-butadiene (Wallin et al. 1988) and tetrafluoroethylene (Odum and Green 1984) are metabolized exclusively in rats via glutathione S-conjugation. However, trichloroethylene and tetrachloroethylene are metabolized mainly by cytochrome P450s. Only a small portion (<1%) is metabolized by glutathione S-conjugation (e.g., Koob and Dekant 1991). Nevertheless, although the cytochrome P450 pathway generates toxic species from trichloroethylene and tetrachloroethylene (Bull et al. 2002), a major contributor to the overall toxicity of trichloroethylene and tetrachloroethylene is the corresponding cysteine S-conjugate despite the fact that the glutathione S-conjugation pathway is quantitatively minor (Dekant 2003).

The glutathione S-conjugate, cysteinylglycine S-conjugate, cysteine S-conjugate, and *N*-acetylcysteine S-conjugate (mercapturate) derived from halogenated alkenes are all nephrotoxic/hepatotoxic, and in many cases nephrocarcinogenic/hepatocarcinogenic in experimental animals (e.g., Dekant 2003; Anders 2004; Koob and Dekant 1991; Anders and Dekant 1994, 1998). The mercapturates derived from the halogenated alkenes are toxic because they can be hydrolyzed back to the corresponding cysteine S-conjugate by aminoacylases (e.g., Uttamsingh et al. 2000). As noted above, the nephrotoxicity of halogenated cysteine S-conjugates is due at least in part to the action of cysteine S-conjugate β-lyases. Thus, the mercapturate pathway enzymes together with cysteine S-conjugate β-lyases contribute to the bioactivation of halogenated alkenes. (For reviews see, for example, Cooper 1998; Dekant 2003; 2004; Dekant, Vamvakas and Anders 1994.) The reactive fragments generated from haloalkene cysteine S-conjugates by the action of cysteine S-conjugate β-lyases are especially cytotoxic in experimental animals to the proximal renal tubules, in particular to the S3 region and, to a lesser extent, the S2 region (e.g., Jones et al. 1988).

12.4. The Cysteine S-Conjugate β-Lyase Reaction

In 1965, Colucci and Buyske showed that benzothiazole-2-sulfonamide is converted in rats, rabbits, and dogs, not only to the corresponding mercapturate but also to 2-mercaptobenzothiazine in which the sulfur of the mercaptan moiety is derived from glutathione (GSH). Work from Schultze and colleagues suggested that the toxicity of DCVC is associated with a "C-S" lyase reaction. Experiments with labeled DCVC showed the formation of a reactive sulfur-containing species that adds to macromolecules, including proteins and nucleic acids (e.g., Anderson and Schultze 1965; Bhattacharya and Schultze 1967, 1972). It was known for many years that several electrophilic xenobiotics (e.g., phenacetin, acetaminophen, *N*-hydroxy-2-acetylaminofluorene) are thiomethylated in vivo. It was initially assumed that thiomethylation involves formation of a sulfonium compound derived from methionine followed by decomposition of the sulfonium compound to homoserine lactone plus methylthio compound. However, Chatfield and Hunter (1973) showed that the conversion of 2-acetamido-4-chloromethylthiazole to 2-acetamido-4-methylthiomethylthiazole in rats involves the mercapturate pathway.

The mechanism for the thiomethylation reactions was elucidated by the work of Tateishi and colleagues (1978a,b). When bromazepam was administered to rats, the corresponding mercapturate and 6′-methylthiobromazepam were identified in the bile (Tateishi, Suzuki and Shimizu 1978a). The authors also showed that the thioether bond of the cysteine S-conjugates of 2,4-dinitrobenzene and bromobenzene was readily cleaved by an enzyme present in rat liver cytosol. Incubation of the purified enzyme with *S*-(2,4-dinitrophenyl)cysteine resulted in the formation of pyruvate, ammonium, and 2,4-dinitrobenzenethiol. Incubation of the thiol product with a microsomal thiomethyltransferase and *S*-adenosylmethionine resulted in formation of the corresponding methylthio compound (Tateishi, Suzuki and Shimizu 1978a). Tateishi, Suzuki and Shimizu (1978a,b) coined the term "cysteine conjugate β-lyase" to describe an enzyme that catalyzes β-elimination from a cysteine S-conjugate. The net cysteine S-conjugate β-lyase-catalyzed reaction is shown in Eq. 12.4.

$$XSCH_2CH(NH_3^+)CO_2^- + H_2O \rightarrow CH_3C(O)CO_2^- + NH_4^+ + XSH \quad (12.4)$$

The actual products of the enzyme-catalyzed reaction are XSH and aminoacrylate ($CH_2{=}C(NH_3{}^+)CO_2{}^-$). The latter product undergoes nonenzymatic tautomerization to the α-imino acid ($CH_3C({=}NH_2{}^+)CO_2{}^-$) and subsequent hydrolysis to pyruvate ($CH_3C(O)CO_2{}^-$) and ammonium. When the eliminated sulfur-containing fragment (XSH) is stable (i.e., does not contain electrophilic moieties that cause XSH to be converted to an extremely reactive electrophile), the -SH group may be (1) methylated as in the case of the sulfur-containing fragment derived from *S*-(2,4-dinitrophenyl)cysteine (Tateishi, Suzuki and Shimizu 1978a; Figure 12.1, reaction 8), or (2) glucuronidated as in the case of 2-benzothiazole derived from benzothiazolyl-L-cysteine (BTC) (Elfarra and Hwang 1990; Figure 12.1, reaction 9). Mercapturates, methylthio derivatives, and S-glucuronates are readily excreted.

12.5. Identification of Cysteine S-Conjugate β-Lyases

Although Tateishi, Suzuki, and Shimizu (1978b) obtained a highly purified preparation of a cysteine S-conjugate β-lyase from rat liver they did not identify it. Subsequently, kynureninase (Stevens 1985) and glutamine transaminase K (GTK) (Stevens, Robbins and Byrd 1986) were identified as major cysteine S-conjugate β-lyases of rat liver and kidney cytosol, respectively. Over the last 20 years many more cysteine S-conjugate β-lyases have been identified (Table 12.1). All are pyridoxal 5′-phosphate

Table 12.1 Mammalian PLP-dependent enzymes with L-cysteine S-conjugate β-lyase activity.[a,b]

	β-Lyase substrates			Syncatalytic inactivation	Competing transamination	Approximate specific activity (U mg^{-1}[c])
	DCVC	TFEC	BTC			
Enzyme (cytosolic)						
Kynureninase (R)	+	ND	+	+	ND	0.25
GTK/KAT I (R)[d]	+	+	–	–	+	0.6–6.4
cytAspAT (R)	+	+	±	+	–	0.04–0.16
AlaAT (P)	+	+	+	+	–	0.004–0.06
$BCAT_c$ (H)	+	+	+	+	–	0.3–0.5
Cystathionine γ-lyase (R)	–	+	–	–	–	0.05–0.1
Enzyme (mitochondrial)						
mitAspAT (R)	+	+	+	+	+	0.8–2.3
$BCAT_m$ (H)	+	+	–	+	–	0.2–0.5
AGAT II (R)	+	+	+	+	+	0.2
GABA aminotransferase (P)	ND	+	ND	ND	ND	0.016
High-M_r β-lyase (R)	+	+	+	–	+	1.0–1.2

[a]This table is an update of that of Cooper and Pinto (2006). For original references see Cooper and Pinto (2006). A unit of enzyme activity is defined as the amount of enzyme that catalyzes the formation of 1 μmol of pyruvate per min (usually at 37°C, but temperature was not specified in all cases). ND, not determined. Species abbreviations: R, rat; P, pig; H, human.
[b]AGAT II and cystathionine γ-lyase are homotetramers with M_r values of ~210 000 and ~17 600, respectively. The high-M_r β-lyase of rat kidney and liver homogenates has a M_r >200 000. All other enzymes listed are homodimers with M_r values for the intact holoenzyme of ~90 000 – 110 000.
[c]Activity with DCVC and/or TFEC.
[d]Human liver contains a KAT with strong cysteine S-conjugate β-lyase activity. A cysteine S-conjugate β-lyase has been highly purified from human kidney. The lyase activity co-purifies with GTK. The human GTK, unlike the rat enzyme, has activity with BTC. In the rat, some GTK activity is also present in mitochondria.

(PLP)-containing enzymes and include (1) the cytosolic enzymes kynureninase, GTK, cytosolic aspartate aminotransferase (cytAspAT), alanine aminotransferase (AlaAT), and cytosolic branched-chain aminotransferase ($BCAT_c$), and (2) the mitochondrial enzymes mitochondrial aspartate aminotransferase (mitAspAT), mitochondrial branched-chain aminotransferase ($BCAT_m$), alanine-glyoxylate aminotransferase isozyme II (AGAT II), and GABA aminotransferase (Cooper and Pinto 2006). In addition, high-M_r β-lyases occur in both cytosolic and mitochondrial fractions of rat kidney and, to a lesser extent, rat liver. High-M_r forms in rat kidney cytosol and mitochondria contain GTK and mitAspAT, respectively (manuscript in preparation).

Most cysteine S-conjugate β-lyases identified thus far are aminotransferases (Table 12.1), and a transamination reaction may therefore compete with the β-elimination reaction. When transamination competes with the β-lyase reaction, an α-keto acid substrate (or PLP) must be present in the reaction mixture to maintain the β-elimination reaction. A half-transamination reaction will convert the PLP coenzyme to its pyridoxamine 5′-phosphate (PMP) form, which cannot catalyze a β-lyase reaction. The α-keto acid substrate forms a Schiff base with PMP that is converted to the corresponding amino acid and PLP. The PLP form of the enzyme can then catalyze another round of the β-lyase reaction (Stevens, Robbins and Byrd 1986; Cooper 1998).

Table 12.1 indicates that cysteine S-conjugate β-lyases exhibit some degree of substrate specificity toward the commonly used β-lyase substrates (DCVC, TFEC, BTC). For example, DCVC and TFEC are β-lyase substrates of rat kidney GTK, whereas BTC is not. Curiously, however, BTC has been reported to be a substrate of human kidney GTK (Lash et al. 1990). On the other hand, all three cysteine S-conjugates are substrates of rat mitAspAT. S-(1,1,2,2-Tetrafluoroethyl)-L-cysteine (TFEC), but not DCVC, is a β-lyase substrate of γ-cystathionase. Table 12.1 also indicates that many of the cysteine S-conjugate β-lyases are prone to syncatalytic (i.e., self) inactivation. For example, rat liver mitAspAT-catalyzed β-elimination with TFEC leads to inactivation on average after about 2700 turnover events (Cooper et al. 2002). Inactivation of human $BCAT_m$ and $BCAT_c$, in the presence of TFEC, occurs on average after about 200 and 45 turnover events, respectively (Cooper et al. 2003). Thus, factors such as the presence or absence of α-keto acids in the assay mixture, length of incubation time, the nature of cysteine S-conjugate used as substrate, and organ distribution of a given PLP-dependent enzyme, together with variable K_m values and pH optima will affect the apparent level of cysteine S-conjugate β-lyase activity measured in crude tissue homogenates.

12.6. Nephrotoxicity of Haloalkene Cysteine S-Conjugates

Although GSTs are present in most tissues, the liver is the major organ contributing to the formation of glutathione S-conjugates (Anders 2004). As noted above, the conversion of the glutathione S-conjugate to the corresponding cysteine S-conjugate is catalyzed by the sequential action of γ-glutamyltransferase and aminopeptidase M/cysteinylglycinase (Figure 12.1). These ectoenzymes are present in epithelial tissues such as bile duct, intestine, renal tubules, and choroid plexus. The cysteine S-conjugates are taken up in the kidneys by glomerular filtration or more importantly by active uptake (Anders 2004). Both Na^+-dependent and Na^+-independent transporters have been implicated in the renal uptake of DCVC (e.g., Lash and Anders 1989; Schaeffer and Stevens 1987a, b; Anders 2004). Most of these studies have focused on uptake of DCVC across the basolateral (peritubular) membrane of the renal proximal cells (Wright et al. 1998). Wright et al. (1998) showed that DCVC is taken up by a Na^+-dependent uptake system in isolated renal brush-border membrane vesicles. Several neutral amino acids, but especially phenylalanine, cysteine, and leucine, compete with uptake of DCVC across the luminal membrane in this system (Wright et al. 1998).

Acivicin, a selective inhibitor of γ-glutamyltransferase, protects renal tubule cells against S-(1,2-dichlorovinyl)glutathione-induced toxicity (Elfarra, Jakobson and Anders 1986; Lash and Anders 1986). On the other hand, it has been reported that acivicin does not protect rats against the nephrotoxicity of hexachloro-1:3-butadiene (Davis 1988). However, others have shown that S-(1,2,3,4,4-pentachloro-1,3-butadienyl)-L-cysteine (PCBC; the cysteine S-conjugate of hexachloro-1:3-butadiene) is cytotoxic to LLC-PK_1 cells (Blackmore et al. 2002). Aminooxyacetate (AOA), a general inhibitor of PLP enzymes, protects against DCVC-induced toxicity (e.g., Lash et al. 1986; Beuter et al. 1989; Chen et al. 1990; Chen, Jones and Stevens 1994; Blackmore et al. 2002) and PCBC-induced toxicity (Blackmore et al. 2002) in LLC-PK_1 cells. AOA partially protects against DCVC-induced toxicity in isolated rat kidney proximal tubules (Lash and Anders 1986), but apparently not in isolated human renal proximal tubule cells (Cummings and Lash 2000). α-Keto acids stimulate the toxicity of DCVC toward rat renal cells (Elfarra, Lash and Anders 1987). Exacerbation of toxicity by α-keto acids suggests involvement of aminotransferases in the bioactivation process. Taken together, despite an occasional study to the contrary, the literature strongly supports important roles for γ-glutamyltransferase and cysteine S-conjugate β-lyases in promoting the nephrotoxicity of halogenated alkenes. However, it appears that human renal tissue is less susceptible than that of rat to damage from haloalkene cysteine S-conjugates, presumably as a result of lower specific activities of cysteine S-conjugate β-lyases in human renal tissue and allometric scaling (see discussion by Anders 2005).

Although the evidence is strong that cysteine S-conjugate β-lyases contribute to the nephrotoxicity of DCVC and other halogenated cysteine S-conjugates, other studies support additional mechanisms for bioactivation. DCVC can be oxidized by a flavin-containing monooxygenase to DCVC sulfoxide (Park et al. 1992), which may be even more nephrotoxic than DCVC itself (Lash et al. 1994, 2003). Moreover, the mercapturates derived from both trichloroethylene and tetrachloroethylene are both bioactivated to their sulfoxide forms by a cytochrome P450 (CYP3A) (Werner, Birner and Dekant 1996). One possibility for the toxicity of DCVC sulfoxide is that cysteine S-conjugate β-lyases catalyze the elimination of a reactive sulfenic acid [RS(O)H], which forms a covalent adduct to macromolecules. However, AOA is not protective against the nephrotoxicity of DCVC sulfoxide in rats and only partially protects against DCVC (Lash et al. 1994). Thus, sulfoxidation of DCVC is a bioactivation event in addition to, and probably distinct from, the β-lyase pathway (Lash et al. 1994). DCVC sulfoxide was shown to react with GSH generating the glutathione S-conjugate, *S*-[1-chloro-2- (*S*-glutathionyl)vinyl]-L-cysteine sulfoxide, which was isolated from the bile of rats given DCVC sulfoxide (Sausen and Elfarra 1991). It has been suggested that the nephrotoxicity of DCVC sulfoxide is related in part to oxidative stress, possibly as a result of depleted mitochondrial GSH stores (Lash et al. 1994, 2003). The β-lyase pathway may result in greater bioactivation of DCVC than does the oxidation pathway in rat proximal tubules, whereas the converse may be true for human proximal tubules (Cummings and Lash 2000). Thus, although this review focuses on bioactivation of haloalkene cysteine S-conjugates via cysteine S-conjugate β-lyases, it is important to note that other bioactivation pathways exist. Moreover, species and sex differences in the mechanisms by which certain haloalkene cysteine S-conjugates are bioactivated must also be considered when evaluating the nephrotoxicity of halogenated cysteine S-conjugates.

Cysteine S-conjugates derived from bromine-containing fluoroalkenes are more mutagenic than those lacking bromine. The mutagenicity of these cysteine S-conjugates may be associated with the formation of a reactive 2,2-difluoro-3-halothiirane following a β-lyase reaction (Anders 2004).

12.7. β-Lyase-Catalyzed Generation of Reactive Fragments from Nephrotoxic Halogenated Cysteine S-Conjugates

Active-site-generated aminoacrylate can cause syncatalytic inactivation of enzymes that catalyze β-elimination reactions with amino acids containing a good leaving group in the β-position. For example, pig heart cytAspAT is syncatalytically inactivated by β-chloro-L-alanine (Morino and Okamoto 1973) and L-serine O-sulfate (Ueno, Likos and Metzler 1982). Thiosulfate protects this enzyme against aminoacrylate generated from both L-serine O-sulfate and L-cysteine sulfinic acid (Cavallini et al. 1973). Michael addition of thiosulfate to the double bond yields cysteine sulfonic acid. Thus, thiosulfate competes with cytAspAT for interaction with aminoacrylate (Cavallini et al. 1973). Historically, it is interesting to note that the "C-S" lyase purified by Anderson and Schultze (1965) was rapidly inactivated by products of the reaction with DCVC. Moreover, protection was afforded in part by GSH (Anderson and Schultze 1965). Possibly, the "C-S" lyase was inactivated in part by aminoacrylate and in part by a reactive sulfur-containing fragment (see below). In that case, GSH may have protected against inactivation by competing with a susceptible enzyme moiety for Michael addition to aminoacrylate.

Initially, it was suggested that inactivation of pig heart cytAspAT by aminoacrylate, generated from β-lyase reactions, is due to modification of an active-site lysine moiety (Morino and Okamoto 1973). Ueno and colleagues (1982), however, showed that aminoacrylate adds to the PLP coenzyme, resulting in the formation of a pyruvate-PLP aldol condensation product, which could also result in inactivation. Thus, the nephrotoxicity of halogenated cysteine S-conjugates could theoretically be due to the syncatalytic inactivation of key PLP enzymes by aminoacrylate either reacting with susceptible protein moieties or by direct attack on the aldehyde group of PLP. However, toxicity through these mechanisms may be limited to special cases because cysteine S-conjugates that undergo β-elimination are not generally toxic if the eliminated sulfur-containing fragment is unreactive (i.e., does not contain highly electronegative substituents), despite the fact that aminoacrylate will be produced. An example of a relatively nontoxic cysteine S-conjugate that undergoes enzyme-catalyzed β-elimination in vivo is BTC. As noted above, a sulfur-containing elimination fragment is glucuronidated and excreted in rats treated with BTC (Elfarra and Hwang 1990). Possibly, the aminoacrylate is scavenged by endogenous small-M_r nucleophiles (e.g., GSH), or syncatalytic loss of activity of PLP-containing enzymes is relatively slow.

On the other hand, if the eliminated sulfur-containing fragment is reactive (i.e., contains highly electronegative substituents, as is the case with cysteine S-conjugates derived from halogenated alkenes) the parent cysteine S-conjugate may be toxic, especially to the kidneys. The cysteine S-conjugate β-lyase reaction with DCVC (**1**) gives rise to pyruvate (**2**), ammonium and a sulfur-containing fragment that has the theoretical structure 1,2-dichloroethylenethiolate (**3**) (Figure 12.2). However, 1,2-dichloroethylenethiolate is extremely unstable and may tautomerize to chlorothioacetyl chloride ($ClC(=S)CH_2Cl$) (not shown) or spontaneously lose Cl^- to form the highly reactive chlorothioketene (**4**) (Anders 2004; and references cited therein). The chlorothioketene reacts with a variety of nucleophiles (Nu:) to generate a thioacylated adduct (**5**). In biological systems the nucleophile can be macromolecules, such as nucleic acids (Müller et al. 1998) and proteins (Eyre et al. 1995). This chemistry provides an explanation for the previous finding of Anderson and Schultze (1965), who as alluded to above, showed covalent incorporation of a sulfur-containing fragment from DCVC into macromolecules via the action of "C-S" lyases.

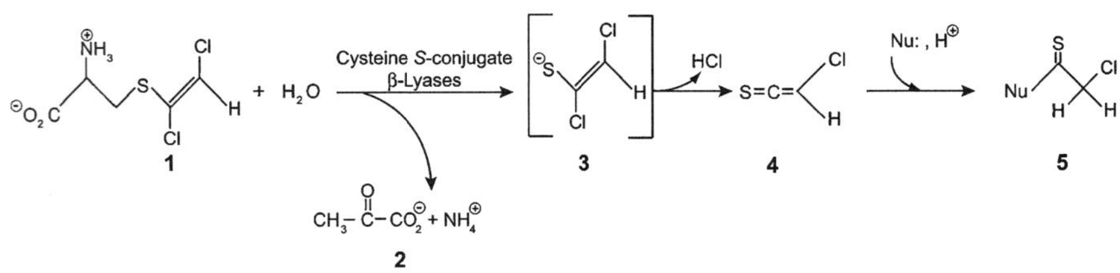

Figure 12.2 Bioactivation of DCVC by cysteine S-conjugate β-lyases. DCVC (**1**) is converted to pyruvate (**2**), ammonium, and a sulfur-containing fragment that has the theoretical structure 1,2-dichloroethylenethiolate (**3**). 1,2-Dichloroethylenethiolate is unstable and loses HCl to form the highly reactive chlorothioketene (**4**). The thioketene reacts with tissue nucleophiles (Nu:) to generate thioacylated products (**5**). Based in part on Anders (2004).

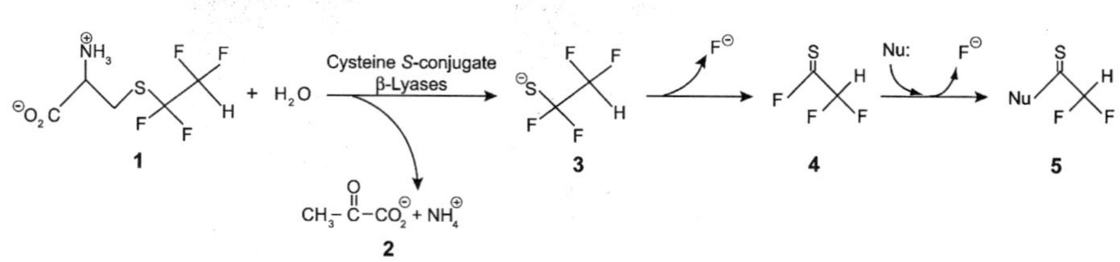

Figure 12.3 Bioactivation of TFEC by cysteine S-conjugate β-lyases. TFEC (**1**) is converted to pyruvate (**2**), ammonium, and a sulfur-containing fragment that has the structure 1,1,2,2-tetrafluoroethanethiolate (**3**). 1,1,2,2-Tetrafluoroethanethiolate (**3**) is unstable and loses F^- to form difluorothioacetyl fluoride (**4**). Difluorothioacetyl fluoride reacts with tissue nucleophiles (Nu:) to generate thioacylated products (**5**). Based in part on Anders (2004). Note that **3** may also react by a separate pathway. Thus, addition of **3** to a lysine residue in a protein may result in loss of H_2S and modification of the ε-amino group by replacement of an H with $-CF_2CF_2(H)$ (see Figure 12.4).

Cysteine S-conjugate β-lyase-catalyzed bioactivation of TFEC is shown in Figure 12.3. The β-lyase reaction with TFEC (**1**) results in the formation of pyruvate (**2**), ammonium and 1,1,2,2-tetrafluoroethanethiolate (**3**). 1,1,2,2-Tetrafluoroethanethiolate is very reactive, losing F^- to generate difluorothioacetyl fluoride (**4**), which thioacylates nucleophiles. ^{35}S-Labeling studies performed in vivo show that phosphatidylethanolamine is a major nucleophile thioacylated in mitochondria by the action of cysteine S-conjugate β-lyases on TFEC (Hayden et al. 1992). The ε-amino group of protein lysyl moieties are also especially vulnerable to thioacylation by **4** (Hayden and Stevens 1990; Harris, Dekant and Anders 1992; Fisher et al. 1993; Hayden et al. 1991).

Rat liver mitAspAT is syncatalytically inactivated by TFEC following fewer β-lyase turnover events than with β-chloroalanine (Cooper et al. 2002). This finding was ascribed to the fact that only one reactive fragment is generated from β-chloroalanine (i.e., aminoacrylate) whereas two reactive fragments are generated from TFEC, namely aminoacrylate and 1,1,2,2-tetrafluoroethanethiolate ($^-SCF_2CF_2H$). We have recently begun to investigate the mechanism by which rat liver mitAspAT is syncatalytically inactivated by TFEC. Mass spectrometric analysis showed that two active-site lysyl moieties are modified by addition of a fragment that results in a net gain of 100 amus for each lysyl moiety. The finding is consistent with a $-CF_2CF_2H$ linkage to the ε-amino group of a lysyl residue. This linkage apparently results from direct attack of the ε-amino group of a lysine residue on tetrafluoroethanethiolate with loss of hydrogen sulfide. This type of addition has not been described previously, and may have been obscured in studies with ^{35}S-labeled TFEC as a result of loss of radiolabel as H_2S. Interestingly, another lysyl moiety distal from the active site is modified by 96 amus, which is consistent with thioacylation. Finally, one cysteine residue was noted to be modified by 87 amus consistent with Michael addition of a cysteine thiolate to aminoacrylate generating a lanthionine moiety.[2] Mechanisms whereby fragments derived from a β-lyase reaction on TFEC form covalent adducts with proteins are shown in Figure 12.4.

[2] The mass spectral data have been presented at a national meeting (Villar et al. 2007).

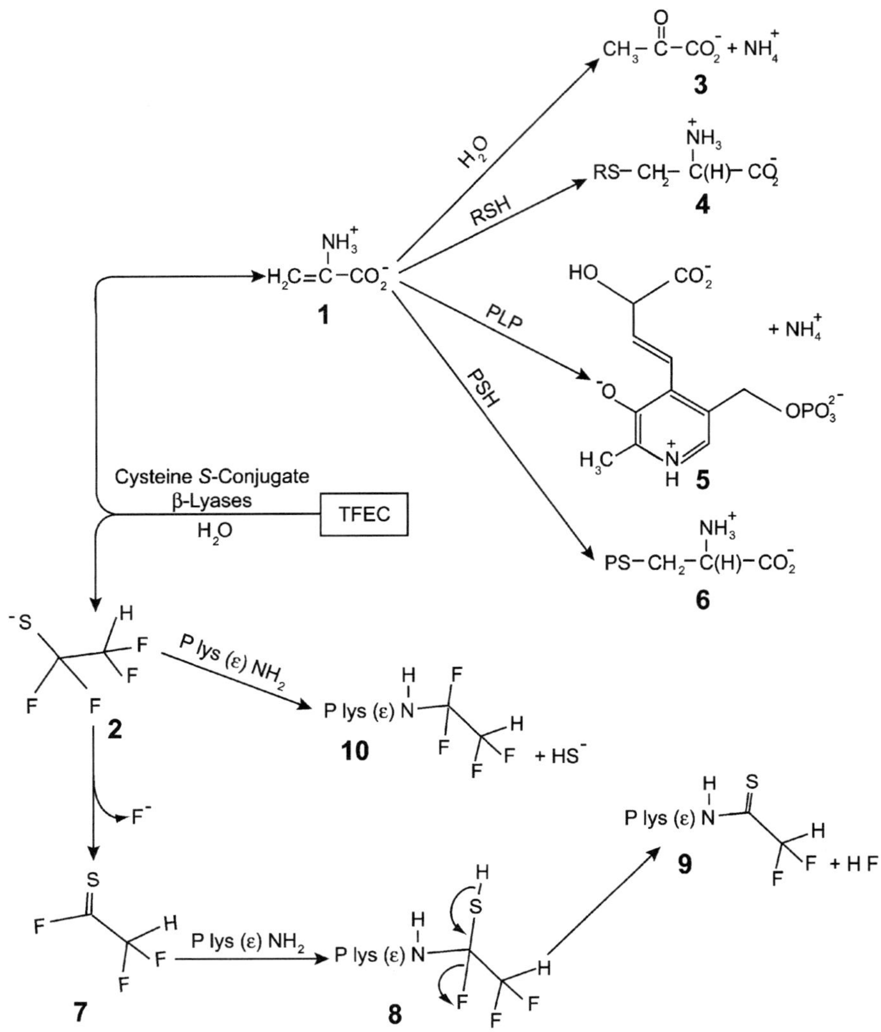

Figure 12.4 Protein modifications resulting from the β-lyase reaction on TFEC. The initial products of the β-lyase reaction are aminoacrylate (**1**) and 1,1,2,2-tetrafluoroethanethiolate (**2**). Aminoacrylate tautomerizes and hydrolyzes to pyruvate (**3**) and ammonium. However, in the presence of suitable nucleophiles such as RSH (e.g., GSH, thiosulfate), the aminoacrylate can be trapped as a "new" cysteine S-conjugate (**4**). It is also possible that aminoacrylate generated from TFEC will react with PLP at the active site of a susceptible enzyme to form the pyruvate-PLP aldol product (**5**). Michael addition of the sulfhydryl of a protein cysteinyl residue (PSH) to aminoacrylate will result in the formation of a protein-bound lanthionine residue [$PSCH_2CH(NH_3^+)CO_2^-$, **6**]. 1,1,2,2-Tetrafluoroethanethiolate (**2**) loses F^- to generate difluorothioacetyl fluoride (**7**). Reaction of the ε-amino group of a protein lysyl residue (P-lys(ε)-NH_2) with **7** results in the formation of the tetrahedral intermediate (**8**). The tetrahedral intermediate (**8**) decomposes to thioacylated protein (**9**) plus HF. Interestingly, some of the 1,1,2,2-tetrafluoroethanethiolate (**2**) resulting from the β-elimination reaction with TFEC reacts directly with the ε-amino group of lysine residues generating a structure (**10**) that contains a $-CF_2CF_2H$ grouping attached at the N.

12.8. Mechanisms Contributing to the Nephrotoxicity of Haloalkene Cysteine S-Conjugates – Toxicant Channeling

Haloalkene cysteine S-conjugates are especially toxic to mitochondria (e.g., Groves et al. 1993; Chen et al. 2001). Thus, any mechanism that demonstrates nephrotoxicity of haloalkene cysteine S-conjugates must take into account the susceptibility of renal mitochondria and the bioactivation of these compounds via mitochondrial cysteine S-conjugate β-lyases.

Toxicity of DCVC to kidney cells has been associated with (1) covalent modification of macromolecules, (2) depletion of nonprotein thiols (presumably mostly GSH), and (3) lipid peroxidation (Beuter et al. 1989; Chen et al. 1990). These effects may be attributable to formation of metabolites derived from a β-lyase reaction since, as mentioned above, AOA can partially protect against DCVC toxicity in renal tissues and in renal cells in culture. Mechanisms by which metabolites of DCVC and other nephrotoxic haloalkene cysteine S-conjugates alter thiol status may involve direct inhibition of glutathione reductase (Lock and Schnellmann 1990) and generation of oxidative stress that leads indirectly to oxidation of thiol compounds (Chen et al. 1990). Oxidation of DCVC to DCVC sulfoxide followed by formation of a glutathione S-conjugate resulting from the reaction of DCVC sulfoxide with GSH may also lead to oxidative stress (Sausen and Elfarra 1991; Lash et al. 1994). Other studies lead us to suggest an additional possibility, namely that oxidative stress may result in part from Michael addition of thiols to aminoacrylate generated in the β-lyase reaction. In experiments in which LLC-PK_1 cells were exposed to DCVC, loss of nonprotein thiols was about 40%–60% (Chen et al. 1990). Interestingly, the authors suggested that depletion of nonprotein thiols to this extent was insufficient to kill the cells. As cited earlier, BTC is relatively nontoxic, despite the fact that it is metabolized in vivo via cysteine S-conjugate β-lyases (Elfarra and Hwang 1990). We are unaware of any studies on GSH status in renal cells/tissue resulting from exposure to BTC. Evidently, even if GSH is depleted in renal cells exposed to BTC, this insult may not be sufficient to induce overt toxicity. The implication of the work by Chen et al. (1990) is that in order for a cysteine S-conjugate to exhibit toxicity, it must generate reactive sulfur-containing fragments that covalently add to macromolecules. The toxicity may be enhanced, perhaps synergistically, by oxidative stress and by Michael adduction between aminoacrylate and susceptible nucleophiles such as GS^- and protein sulfhydryls and/or by modification of coenzyme in susceptible PLP enzymes.

Adduct formation with reactive fragments generated from a cysteine S-conjugate β-lyase reaction in vivo has been studied extensively using TFEC. For example, Bruschi et al. (1993) showed that six kidney mitochondrial proteins are thioacylated after rats are administered TFEC. No thioacylation of cytosolic proteins was detected. The six proteins were identified as HSP60, mitHSP70, mitAspAT, aconitase, the E_2k (dihydrolipoamide succinyl transferase) enzyme component of the α-ketoglutarate dehydrogenase complex (KGDHC), the E_3 (dihydrolipoamide dehydrogenase) enzyme component of KGDHC, and the E_3 enzyme component of the branched-chain keto acid dehydrogenase complex (BCDHC) (Bruschi et al. 1993; Bruschi, Crabb and Stevens 1994; Bruschi, Lindsay and Crabb 1998; James et al. 2002). Interestingly, Lock and Schnellmann (1990) had previously reported that metabolites of haloalkene cysteine S-conjugates (DCVC, TFEC, PCBC) inhibited dihydrolipoyl dehydrogenase (E_3). Our findings that mitAspAT catalyzes a β-lyase reaction with TFEC in vitro and is syncatalytically inactivated in the process (Cooper et al. 2002) is consistent with the in vivo finding that this enzyme in kidney is thioacylated after administration of TFEC to rats. We also showed that a high-M_r β-lyase present in kidney co-purifies with HSP70 (Cooper et al. 2001). As cited earlier, the high-M_r β-lyase in rat kidney mitochondria contains mitAspAT. This finding provides a mechanism for the thioacylation of kidney mitHSP70 in rats administered TFEC. Conceivably, mitochondrial HSP60 may also associate with a PLP-containing enzyme that catalyzes a β-lyase reaction with TFEC.

Although the E_2k and E_3 enzyme components of KGDHC (and the E_3 enzyme component of BCDHC) are thioacylated in kidney mitochondria of rats administered TFEC, the E_2p (dihydrolipoamide acetyl transferase) and E_3 enzyme components of pyruvate dehydrogenase complex (PDHC) are not (Bruschi, Lindsay and Crabb 1998; James et al. 2002). Moreover, the specific activity of KGDHC, but not that of PDHC, is diminished in the kidneys of TFEC-treated rats. We have found that KGDHC, but not PDHC, is directly inhibited in PC12 cells exposed to 1-mM TFEC (Park et al. 1999). These findings are remarkable because E_3 is a common component of KGDHC, PDHC, and BCDHC (and the glycine cleavage system). In the presence of TFEC and purified GTK (a source of thioacylating moieties), purified PDHC is more resistant to in vitro inactivation than is purified KGDHC (Park et al. 1999). Moreover, there is some evidence that E_3 enzyme components are bound to the complex via E_2 enzyme components in PDHC, whereas E_3 enzyme components are bound to the complex via E_1 enzyme components in KGDHC (McCartney et al. 1998). Thus, part of the resistance of PDHC to thioacylation/inactivation in kidney mitochondria of TFEC-treated rats may be due to differences in the arrangement of its constituent enzymes. In addition, PDHC is not associated with any aminotransferases/β-lyases, whereas KGDHC is closely associated with mitAspAT. Thus, the susceptibility of KGDHC to thioacylation by a fragment derived from TFEC may be due to the proximity of mitAspAT or to actual co-localization with subunit enzymes (James et al. 2002; Park et al. 1999).

Several tricarboxylic acid cycle (TCA) and associated enzymes are arranged in supramolecular complexes (metabolons) that facilitate channeling of substrate from one enzyme to another. For example, mitAspAT is part of a metabolon affiliated or localized with KGDHC (see references cited in Cooper, Bruschi and Anders 2002). Based on our findings (Cooper et al. 2002, 2003) and those of Bruschi and colleagues (Bruschi, Lindsay and Crabb 1998; James et al. 2002), we have proposed that not only are metabolites channeled through supramolecular complexes in the TCA

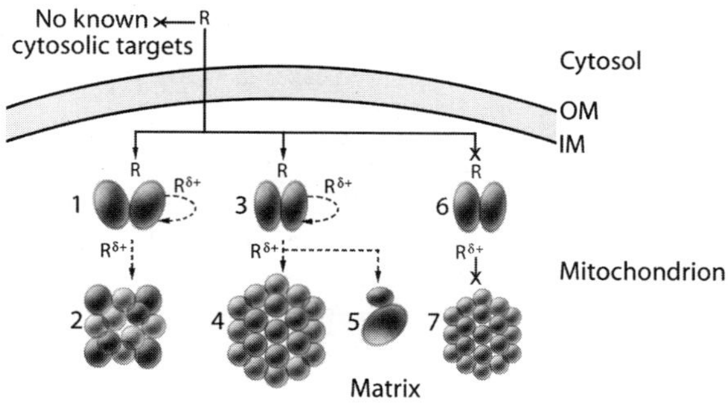

Figure 12.5 Model for toxicant channeling of β-lyase-derived TFEC products in mitochondria in vivo. TFEC (**R**) is transported into the mitochondrion where it is converted by cysteine S-conjugate β-lyases to toxicant(s) ($\mathbf{R}^{\delta+}$). The three mitochondrial α-keto acid dehydrogenase complexes (BCDHC, KGDHC, PDHC) are represented as multimeric units labeled **2**, **4**, and **6**, respectively. Mitochondrial cysteine S-conjugate β-lyases include the homodimeric $BCAT_m$ (**1**) and the homodimeric mitAspAT (**3**). The close juxtapositioning of $BCAT_m$ and mitAspAT to enzymes of energy metabolism results in channeling of toxicants to BCDHC (**2**) and KGDHC (**4**)/aconitase (**5**), respectively, resulting in their inactivation. PDHC (**6**) is not known to be associated with any aminotransferase/cysteine S-conjugate β-lyase and is not directly inactivated. The curved arrows represent syncatalytic inactivation of $BCAT_m$ and mitAspAT, respectively.
Abbreviations: IM, inner membrane; OM outer mitochondrial membrane. From Cooper and Pinto (2006).

cycle, but toxicants as well (Cooper, Bruschi and Anders 2002; Figure 12.5). This concept explains not only the susceptibility of KGDHC to TFEC-induced inactivation in rat kidney and cells in culture, but also the susceptibility of aconitase and BCDHC to thioacylation/inactivation. Aconitase is part of a metabolon that includes KGDHC and mitAspAT (Ovádi and Srere 2000). BCDHC is part of a metabolon that includes $BCAT_m$ (Van Horn et al. 2004).

Cysteine S-conjugate β-lyases are ubiquitous in the body. For example, mitAspAT, a major mitochondrial cysteine S-conjugate β-lyase, is present in every cell that contains mitochondria. How then can one explain the unusual susceptibility of kidney to halogenated cysteine S-conjugates? Many factors are presumably involved, including relative distribution of *N*-acetyltransferase, aminoacylases, cellular and mitochondrial uptake mechanisms, and concentrations of natural amino acid/α-keto acid substrates. However, a major contributing factor is likely to be the very large surface area of the renal proximal tubules coupled to the extraordinary high renal vascular perfusion. In humans, the kidneys receive 20% of the cardiac output; yet comprise $<1\%$ of the body weight (Pfaller and Gstraunthaler 1998).

Despite these factors, haloalkene cysteine S-conjugate-induced toxicity is not necessarily confined to renal tubules. As we have noted above, toxicity may also occur in the liver and occasionally in neural tissue, presumably as a consequence of the widespread occurrence of cysteine S-conjugate β-lyases.

12.9. Metabolism of Electrophiles Other than Haloalkenes via the Mercapturate/Cysteine S-Conjugate β-Lyase Pathways

The carbonic anhydrase inhibitor methazolamide is metabolized to both a glutathione S- and a cysteine S-conjugate. The latter is a substrate of cysteine S-conjugate β-lyase(s) in bovine kidney and liver homogenates (Kishida et al. 2001). Since cysteine S-conjugate β-lyases are also presumably present in eye tissues, the β-elimination reaction may account for the binding of a metabolite of methazolamide to macromolecules and for the specific ocular toxicity (Kishida et al. 2001).

Cisplatin is used to treat germ cell tumors, head and neck tumors, and cervical cancer even when the cancer has metastasized. Unfortunately, its effectiveness against other cancers is limited because at the doses required to exhibit anticancer properties it is toxic to renal proximal tubule cells and especially to the mitochondria in these cells (reviewed in Zhang and Hanigan 2003). DNA damage is the primary mechanism by which cisplatin kills tumor and other rapidly dividing cells. However, the renal proximal tubule cells are well-differentiated, nondividing cells that are not killed by other DNA-damaging agents. Evidence has been presented that damage to kidney cells is due to conversion of cisplatin to its glutathione S-conjugate and subsequently to its cysteine S-conjugate. The cysteine S-conjugate is then bioactivated by cysteine S-conjugate β-lyase(s) to generate a fragment containing a Pt-SH moiety (Eq. 5). This Pt-SH fragment is proposed to react with macromolecules at thiophilic centers (Zhang and Hanigan 2003).

$$(H_2N)_2Pt(Cl)SCH_2CH(NH_3^+)CO_2^- + H_2O \rightarrow CH_3C(O)CO_2^- + NH_4^+ + (H_2N)_2Pt(Cl)SH \quad (12.5)$$

After mice were treated with cisplatin, proteins in kidney mitochondria were more platinated than proteins in the cytosolic fraction (Zhang et al. 2006). Moreover, the platination was decreased in the mitochondrial fraction, but not in the cytosolic fraction, in mice pretreated with AOA. The specific activities of mitAspAT, aconitase, and especially KGDHC were decreased in LLC-PK_1 cells treated with cisplatin (Zhang et al. 2006). The specific activity of KGDHC was decreased even further in cisplatin-treated LLC-PK_1 cells overexpressing mitAspAT. The data are consistent with the hypothesis that the cisplatin cysteine S-conjugate is a β-lyase substrate of mitAspAT and that the released Pt-SH fragment reacts with proteins in kidney mitochondria especially KGDHC.

Another interesting example whereby cysteine S-conjugate β-lyases may contribute adversely to human health relates to exposure to breakdown products of inhalational anesthetic agents. Administration of various anesthetics can sometimes lead to damage to kidney, liver, and occasionally neural tissue (reviewed by Anders 2005). When an anesthetic gas is used in association with a desiccated carbon dioxide absorbent, severe heat buildup in the anesthetic circuit, particularly in the CO_2 absorber canister, can lead to conversion of trichloroethylene to dichloroacetylene, halothane to 2-bromo-2-chloro-1,1-difluoroethylene, sevoflurane to 2-(fluoromethoxy)-

1,1,3,3,3-pentafluoro-1-propylene (Compound A), and desflurane, isoflurane, and enflurane to CO. Dichloroacetylene, 2-bromo-2-chloro-1, 1-difluoroethylene, and Compound A form glutathione S-conjugates that undergo hydrolysis to cysteine S-conjugates, and subsequent bioactivation to toxic sulfur-containing fragments by cysteine S-conjugate β-lyases (Anders 2005). The cysteine S-conjugate derived from dichloroacetylene is DCVC. Glutathione S-conjugate formation with dichloroacetylene (Eq. 2) is much more rapid than is glutathione S-conjugate formation from trichloroethylene (Eq. 3) (Kanhai et al. 1991). Thus, assuming that the activities of γ-glutamyltransferase and aminopeptidase M/cysteinylglycinase are not limiting, toxic DCVC should form more readily from dichloroacetylene than from trichloroethylene in vivo (Kanhai et al. 1991). The above-mentioned findings have spurred the development of newer anesthetic gas ventilators that minimize the risk of conversion of anesthetic gases to toxic breakdown products (Anders 2005). Toxic effects of trichloroethylene exposure to base have been well documented particularly to the facial nerves in humans (reviewed by Anders 2004). However, whereas compound A has been found to be nephrotoxic to rats and toxic to isolated human kidney tubules, injury to human kidneys in vivo appears to be minimal (Anders 2004; Kharasch et al. 2005). Most likely the difference between rats and humans resides in the lower overall renal cysteine S-conjugate β-lyase activity in humans than in rats.

2,4′,5-Trichlorobiphenyl (a polychlorinated biphenyl or PCB) is metabolized through the mercapturate pathway (Bakke, Bergman and Larsen 1982). This PCB is thought to be converted to an epoxide by the action of P450 enzymes. The epoxide then reacts with GS^- to form the corresponding glutathione S-conjugate, which is eventually converted to the mercapturate and excreted in the bile. However, several other metabolites were also detected in the feces of rats administered 2,4′,5-trichloro[^{14}C]biphenyl, namely 2,4′,5-trichlorobiphenyls ring-substituted with -SCH_3, -$S(O)CH_3$, or -$S(O_2)CH_3$ (Bakke, Bergman and Larsen 1982). Evidently, the glutathione S-conjugate of trichlorobiphenyl is converted to the corresponding cysteine S-conjugate, which then undergoes a β-lyase reaction with subsequent formation of a trichlorobiphenyl metabolite containing an -SH substituent that is methylated and partially oxidized. It is not clear whether the -SH-substituted PCB is more toxic (i.e., bioactivated) relative to the parent PCB. Metabolism of PCBs through the mercapturate/cysteine S-conjugate β-lyase pathways deserves more study.

4-Amino-2,6-dichlorophenol is nephrotoxic in Fischer 344 rats. Both AOA and acivicin are protective (Hong et al. 1997; Song, Lang and Chen 1999), suggesting that nephrotoxicity involves conversion of a glutathione S-conjugate metabolite to a cysteine S-conjugate followed by a β-lyase reaction.

It is well known that high doses of acetaminophen are hepatotoxic especially to alcoholics and diabetics, but the exact mechanism is not known. The cytochrome P450 enzyme CYP2E1 appears to be a contributing factor in acetaminophen hepatotoxicity (e.g. Cheung et al. 2005). Acetaminophen is oxidized in vivo to a reactive quinoneimine by the action of CYP2E1. The quinoneimine can react with protein -SH groups and also with GSH to form a semistable *ipso* adduct or a relatively stable adduct at the C3 position (reviewed in Monks and Jones 2002). If these glutathione S-conjugates are converted to the cysteine S-conjugates in vivo then they might be substrates of cysteine S-conjugate β-lyases. This possibility appears to have been largely overlooked. However, it is interesting that when [^{14}C]paracetamol (acetaminophen) was administered to hamsters, a small amount of labeled methyl 2-hydroxy-5-acetamidophenylsulfone was detected in the urine (Wong et al. 1976). Formation of this sulfone may be rationalized by invoking a β-lyase reaction on the cysteine S-conjugate of acetaminophen followed by methylation and oxidation of the sulfur.

12.10. Conclusion

Conversion of an electrophile to the corresponding mercapturate and excretion represents detoxification. However, the mercapturate pathway may sometimes bioactivate (toxify) an electrophile. If the cysteine S-conjugate formed in the mercapturate pathway contains a good electron-withdrawing group attached to the sulfur, it may undergo a β-elimination reaction. This reaction is catalyzed by several PLP-containing enzymes (cysteine S-conjugate β-lyases) that are normally involved in amino acid metabolism. If the eliminated sulfur-containing fragment is reactive (e.g., by adding to macromolecules) the parent cysteine S-conjugate may be toxic especially to the kidneys. Electrophiles that are bioactivated by this mechanism include halogenated alkenes and drugs such as methazolamide and cisplatin. Some PCBs and aminophenols may also be metabolized in part by pathways involving cysteine S-conjugate β-lyases. However, the contribution of the β-lyase reaction to the toxicity of these compounds is not clear. Mitochondrial enzymes of energy metabolism are especially vulnerable to reactive fragments generated from toxic cysteine S-conjugates, by a process that we have termed toxicant channeling. Humans are exposed to a large number of exogenously and endogenously produced electrophiles. It is, therefore, possible that cysteine S-conjugate β-lyases contribute to mitochondrial dysfunction of aging and disease.

In view of (1) the large number of mammalian cysteine S-conjugate β-lyases identified to date, (2) their overlapping specificities, (3) their widespread occurrence in tissues, and (4) their presence in different subcellular compartments (e.g., cytosol, mitochondria, and peroxisomes), the potential of these enzymes for generating toxic products in different subcellular compartments, not only in the kidneys but also in other tissues, is highly significant. We suggest that bioactivation of some natural products, certain drugs, and endogenously produced electrophiles via pathways that include cysteine S-conjugate β-lyases may be more common than is generally appreciated.

Acknowledgements. Part of the work cited from the authors' laboratory was supported by NIH grant RO1 ES8421. We thank Dr. Antonio Artigues, the University of Kansas Medical Center for Mass spectral analysis of TFEC-inactivated mitAspAT.

References

Anders, M. W. 2004. Glutathione-dependent bioactivation of haloalkanes and haloalkenes. Drug Metab. Rev. 36:583–594.

Anders, M. W. 2005. Formation and toxicity of anesthetic degradation products. Annu. Rev. Pharmacol. Toxicol. 45:147–176.

Anders, M. W., and Dekant, W. 1994. aminoacylases Aov. Pharmacol. 27, 431–448.

Anders, M. W., and Dekant, W. 1998. Glutathione-dependent bioactivation of haloalkenes. Annu. Rev. Pharmacol. Toxicol. 38:501–537.

Anderson, P. M., and Schultze, M. O. 1965. Cleavage of *S*-(1,2-dichlorovinyl)-L-cysteine by an enzyme of bovine origin. Arch. Biochem. Biophys. 111:593–602.

Bakke, J. E., Bergman, Å. L., and Larsen, G. L. 1982. Metabolism of 2,4′, 5-trichlorophenyl by the mercapturate pathway. Science 217:645–647.

Beuter, W., Cojocel. C., Müller, W., Donaubauer, H. H., and Mayer, D. 1989. Peroxidative damage and nephrotoxicity of dichlorovinylcysteine. J. Appl. Toxicol. 9:181–186.

Bhattacharya, R. K., and Schultze, M. O. 1967. Enzymes from bovine and turkey kidneys which cleave *S*-(1,2-dichlorovinyl)-L-cysteine. Comp. Biochem. Physiol. 22:723–735.

Bhattacharya, R. K., and Schultze, M. O. 1972. Properties of DNA treated with *S*-(1,2-dichlorovinyl)-L-cysteine and a lyase. Arch. Biochem. Biophys. 153:105–115.

Blackmore, M., Whitwell, C., Morton, J. K., Gray, T. J., and Lock, E. A. 2002. The effects of haloalkene cysteine conjugates on cytosolic free calcium levels in LLC-PK_1 cells – studies using digital imaging fluorescence microscopy. Toxicology 175:143–152.

Brauch, H., Weirich, G., Klein, B., Rabstein, S., Bolt, H. M., and Bruning, T. 2004. VHL mutations in renal cell cancer: Does occupational exposure to trichloroethylene make a difference? Toxicol. Lett. 151:301–310.

Bruschi, S. A., West, K. A., Crabb, J. W., Gupta, R. S., and Stevens, J. L. 1993. Mitochondrial HSP60 (P1 protein) and HSP70-like protein (mortalin) are major targets for modification during *S*-(1,1,2,2-tetrafluoroethyl)-L-cysteine-induced toxicity. J. Biol. Chem. 268:23157–23161.

Bruschi, S. A., Crabb, J. W., and Stevens, J. L. 1994. The E3 subunit of 2-oxoglutarate, branched-chain α-keto acid, and malate dehydrogenase are adducted during nephrotoxic cysteine-conjugate injury. Toxicologist 14:428 (Abstract).

Bruschi S. A., Lindsay J. G., and Crabb J. W. 1998. Mitochondrial stress protein recognition of inactivated dehydrogenases during mammalian cell death. Proc. Natl. Acad. Sci. USA 95:13413–13418.

Bull, R. J., Orner, G. A., Cheng, R. S., Stillwell, L., Stauber, A. J., Sasser, L. B., Lingohr, M. K., and Thrall, B. D. 2002. Contribution of dichloroacetate and trichloroacetate to liver tumor induction in mice by trichloroethylene. Toxicol. Appl. Pharmacol. 182:55–65.

Cavallini, D., Federici, G., Bossa, F., and Granata, F. 1973. The protective effect of thiosulfate upon the inactivation of aspartate aminotransferase by aminoacrylic-acid-producing substrates. Eur. J. Biochem. 39:301–304.

Chasseaud, L. F. 1976. Conjugation with glutathione and mercapturic acid excretion. In Glutathione: Metabolism and Function, eds. I. M. Arias, and W. B. Jakoby, pp. 77–114, New York: Raven Press.

Chatfield, D. H., and Hunter, W. H. 1973. The metabolism of acetamidothiazoles in the rat. 2-Acetamido-4-chloromethylthiazole. Biochem. J. 134:879–884.

Chen, Q., Jones, T. W., Brown, P. C., and Stevens, J. L. 1990. The mechanism of cysteine conjugate cytotoxicity in renal epithelial cells. Covalent binding leads to thiol depletion and lipid peroxidation. J. Biol. Chem. 265:21603–21611.

Chen, Q., Jones, T. W., and Stevens, J. L. 1994. Early cellular events couple binding of reactive metabolites to cell killing by nephrotoxic cysteine conjugates. J. Cell Physiol. 161:293–302.

Chen, Y., Cai, J., Anders, M. W., Stevens, J. L., and Jones, D. P. 2001. Role of mitochondrial dysfunction in *S*-(1,2-dichlorovinyl)-L-cysteine-induced apoptosis. Toxicol. Appl. Pharmacol. 170:172–180.

Cheung, C., Yu, A.-M., Ward, J. M., Krausz, K. W., Akiyama, T. E., Feigenbaum, L., and Gonzalez, F. J. 2005. The *CYP2E1*-humanized transgenic mouse: role of CYP2E1 in acetaminophen hepatotoxicity. Drug Metab. Dispos. 33:449–457.

Colucci, D. F., and Buyske, D. A. 1965. The biotransformation of a sulfonamide to a mercaptan and to mercapturic acid and glucuronide conjugates. Biochem. Pharmacol. 14:457–466.

Cooper, A. J. L. 1998. Mechanisms of cysteine S-conjugate β-lyases. Adv. Enzymol. 72:199–238.

Cooper, A. J. L., and Tate, S. S. 1997. Enzymes involved in processing of glutathione conjugates. In Comprehensive Toxicology: Vol. 3. Biotransformations, Series eds. I. G. Sipes, C. A. McQueen, and A. J. Gandolfi, Volume ed. F. P. Guengerich, pp. 329–363, Oxford: Elsevier Press

Cooper, A. J. L., and Pinto, J. T. 2006. Cysteine S-conjugate β-lyases. Amino Acids 30:1–15.

Cooper, A. J. L., Wang, J., Gartner, C. A., and Bruschi, S. A. 2001. Co-purification of mitochondrial HSP70 and mature protein disulfide isomerase with a functional rat kidney high-M_r cysteine *S*-conjugate β-lyase. Biochem. Pharmacol. 62:1345–53.

Cooper, A. J. L., Bruschi, S. A., Iriarte, A., and Martinez-Carrion, M. 2002. Mitochondrial aspartate aminotransferase catalyses cysteine S-conjugate β-lyase reactions. Biochem. J. 368: 253–261.

Cooper, A. J. L., Bruschi, S. A., and Anders, M. W. 2002. Toxic, halogenated cysteine *S*-conjugates and targeting of mitochondrial enzymes of energy metabolism. Biochem. Pharmacol. 64: 553–564.

Cooper, A. J. L., Bruschi, S. A., Conway, M., and Hutson, S. M. 2003. Human mitochondrial and cytosolic branched-chain aminotransferases are cysteine *S*-conjugate β-lyases, but turnover leads to inactivation. Biochem. Pharmacol. 65:181–192.

Cummings, B. S., Parker, J. C., and Lash, L. H. 2000. Role of cytochrome P450 and glutathione S-transferase alpha in the metabolism and cytotoxicity of trichloroethylene in rat kidney. Biochem. Pharmacol. 95:531–543.

Cummings, B. S., and Lash, L. H. 2000. Metabolism of trichloroethylene and *S*-(1,2-dichlorovinyl)-L-cysteine in freshly isolated human proximal tubular cells. Toxicol. Sci. 53:458–466.

Davis, M. E. 1988. Effects of AT-125 on the nephrotoxicity of hexachloro-1,3-butadiene in rats. Toxicol. Appl. Pharmacol. 95:44–52.

Dekant, W. 2003. Biosynthesis of toxic glutathione conjugates from halogenated alkenes. Toxicol. Lett. 144:49–54.

Dekant, W., Vamvakas, S., and Anders, M. W. 1994. Formation and fate of nephrotoxic and cytotoxic glutathione *S*-conjugates: Cysteine conjugate β-lyase pathway. Adv. Pharmacol. 27:114–162.

Elfarra, A. A., and Hwang, I. Y. 1990. In vivo metabolites of *S*-(2-benzothiazolyl)-L-cysteine as markers of in vivo cysteine conjugate β-lyase and thiol glucuronosyl transferase activities. Drug Metab. Dispos. 18:917–922.

Elfarra, A. A., Jakobson, I., and Anders, M. W. 1986. Mechanism of *S*-(1,2-dichlorovinyl)glutathione-induced nephrotoxicity. Biochem. Pharmacol. 35:283–288.

Elfarra, A. A., Lash, L. H., and Anders, M. W. 1987. α-Ketoacids stimulate renal cysteine conjugate β-lyase activity and potentiate the cytotoxicity of *S*-(1,2-dichlorovinyl)-L-cysteine. Mol. Pharmacol. 31:208–212.

Eyre, R. J., Stevens, D. K., Parker, J. C., and Bull, R. J. 1995. Renal activation of trichloroethene and *S*-(1,2-dichlorovinyl)-L-cysteine and cell proliferative response in the kidneys of F344 rats and B6C3F1 mice. J. Toxicol. Environ. Health 46:465–481.

Fisher, M. B., Hayden, P. J., Bruschi, S. A., Dulik, D. M., Yang, Y., Ward, A. J., and Stevens, J. L. 1993. Formation, characterization, and immunoreactivity of lysine thioamide adducts from fluorinated nephrotoxic cysteine conjugates in vitro and in vivo. Chem. Res. Toxicol. 6:223–230.

Groves, C. E., Hayden, P. J., Lock, E. A., and Schnellmann, R. G. 1993. Differential cellular effects in the toxicity of haloalkenes and haloalkene cysteine conjugates to rabbit renal proximal tubules. J. Biochem. Toxicol. 8:49–56.

Hargus, S. J., Fitzsimmons, M. E., Aniya, Y., and Anders, M. W. 1991. Stereochemistry of the microsomal glutathione *S*-transferase catalyzed addition of glutathione to chlorotrifluoroethene. Biochemistry 30:717–721.

Harris, J. W., Dekant, W., and Anders, M. W. 1992. In vivo detection and characterization of protein adducts resulting from bioactivation of haloethene cysteine *S*-conjugates by ^{19}F NMR: chlorotrifluoroethene and tetrafluoroethene. Chem. Res. Toxicol. 5:34–41.

Hayden, P. J., and Stevens, J. L. 1990. Cysteine conjugate toxicity, metabolism and binding to macromolecules in isolated rat kidney mitochondria. Mol. Pharmacol. 37:468–476.

Hayden, P. J., Ichimura, T., McCann, D. J., Pohl, L. R., and Stevens, J. L. 1991. Detection of cysteine conjugate metabolite adduct formation with specific mitochondrial proteins using antibodies raised against halothane metabolite adducts. J. Biol. Chem. 266:18415–18418.

Hayden, P. J., Welsh, C. J., Yang, Y., Schaefer, W. H., Ward, A. J., and Stevens, J. L. 1992. Formation of mitochondrial phospholipid adducts by nephrotoxic cysteine conjugate metabolites. Chem. Res. Toxicol. 5:232–237.

Hayes, J. D., Flanagan, J. U., and Jowsey, I. T. 2005. Glutathione transferases. Annu. Rev. Pharmacol. Toxicol. 45:51–88.

Hong, S. K., Anestis, D. K., Ball, J. G., Valentovic, M. A., Brown, P. I., and Rankin, G. O. 1997. 4-Amino-2,6-dichlorophenol nephrotoxicity in the Fischer 344 rat: Protection by ascorbic acid, AT-125, and aminooxyacetic acid. Toxicol. Appl. Pharmacol. 147:115–125.

James, E. A., Gygi, S. P., Adams, M. L., Pierce, R. H., Fausto, N., Aebersold, R. H., Nelson, S. D., and Bruschi, S. A. 2002. Mitochondrial aconitase modification, functional inhibition, and evidence for a supramolecular complex of the TCA cycle by the renal toxicant *S*-(1,1,2,2-tetrafluoroethyl)-L-cysteine. Biochemistry 28:6789–6797.

Jolivette, L. J., and Anders, M. W. 2002. Structure–activity relationship for the biotransformation of haloalkenes by rat liver microsomal glutathione transferase 1. Chem. Res. Toxicol. 15:1036–1041.

Jolivette, L. J., and Anders, M. W. 2003. Computational and experimental studies on the distribution of addition and substitution products of the microsomal glutathione transferase 1-catalyzed conjugation of glutathione with fluoroalkenes. Chem. Res. Toxicol. 16:137–144.

Jones, T. W., Qin, C., Schaeffer, V. H., and Stevens, J. L. 1988. Immunohistochemical localization of glutamine transaminase K, a rat kidney cysteine conjugate β-lyase, and the relationship to the segment specificity of cysteine conjugate nephrotoxicity. Mol. Pharmacol. 34:621–627.

Kanhai, W., Koob, M., Dekant, W., and Henschler, D. 1991. Metabolism of ^{14}C-dichloroacetylene in rats. Xenobiotica 21:905–910.

Kharasch, E. D., Schroeder, J. L., Sheffels, P., and Liggitt, H. D. 2005. Influence of sevoflurane on the metabolism and renal effects of compound A in rats. Anesthesiology 103:1183–1188.

Kishida, K., Saida, N., Yamamura, N., Iwai, Y., and Sasabe, T. 2001. Cysteine conjugate of methazolamide is metabolized by β-lyase. J. Pharm. Sci. 90:224–233.

Koob, M., and Dekant, W. 1991. Bioactivation of xenobiotics by formation of toxic glutathione conjugates. Chem. Biol. Interact. 77:107–136.

Lash, L. H., and Anders, M. W. 1986. Cytotoxicity of *S*-(1,2-dichlorovinyl) glutathione and *S*-(1,2-dichlorovinyl)-L-cysteine in isolated rat kidney cells. J. Biol. Chem. 261:13076–13081.

Lash, L. H., and Anders, M. W. 1989. Uptake of nephrotoxic *S*-conjugates by isolated rat proximal tubules. J. Pharmacol. Exp. Ther. 248:531–537.

Lash, L. H., Elfarra, A. A., and Anders, M. W. 1986. Renal cysteine conjugate β-lyase: Bioactivation of nephrotoxic cysteine *S*-conjugates in mitochondrial outer membrane. J. Biol. Chem. 261:5930–5935.

Lash, L. H., Nelson, R. M., Van Dyke, R., and Anders, M. W. 1990. Purification and characterization of human kidney cytosolic conjugate β-lyase activity. Drug Metab. Dispos. 18:50–54.

Lash, L. H., Sausen, P. J., Duescher, R. J., Cooley, A. J., and Elfarra, A. A. 1994. Roles of cysteine conjugate β-lyase and *S*-oxidase in nephrotoxicity: Studies with *S*-(1,2-dichlorovinyl)-L-cysteine and *S*-(1,2-dichlorovinyl)-L-cysteine sulfoxide. J. Pharmacol. Exp. Ther. 269:374–383

Lash, L. H., Putt, D. A., Hueni, S. E., Krause, R. J., and Elfarra, A. A. 2003. Roles of necrosis, apoptosis, and mitochondrial dysfunction in *S*-(1,2-dichlorovinyl)-L-cysteine sulfoxide-induced cytotoxicity in primary cultures of human renal proximal tubular cells. J. Pharmacol. Exp. Ther. 305:1163–1172.

Lock, E. A., and Schnellmann, R. G. 1990. The effect of haloalkene cysteine conjugates on rat renal glutathione reductase and lipoyl dehydrogenase activities. Toxicol. Appl. Pharmacol. 104:180–190.

Lock, E. A., Sani, Y., Moore, R. B., Finkelstein, M. B., Anders, M. W., and Seawright, A. A. 1996. Bone marrow and renal injury associated with haloalkene cysteine conjugates in calves. Arch. Toxicol. 70:607–619.

Marjot, R., and McLeod, A. A. 1989. Chronic non-neurological toxicity from volatile substance abuse. Hum. Toxicol. 8:301–306.

McCartney, R. G., Rice, J. E., Sanderson, S. J., Bunik, V., Lindsay, H., and Lindsay, J. G. 1998. Subunit interactions in the mammalian α-ketoglutarate dehydrogenase components. J. Biol. Chem. 237:24159–24164.

McLellan, L. I., Wolf, C. R., and Hayes, J. D. 1989. Human microsomal glutathione S-transferase. Its involvement in the conjugation of hexachlorobuta-1,3-diene with glutathione. Biochem. J. 258:87–93.

Monks, T. J., and Jones, D. C. 2002. The metabolism and toxicity of quinones, quinonimines, quinone methides, and quinone-thioethers. Curr. Drug Metab. 3:425–438.

Morino, Y., and Okamoto, M. 1973. Labeling of the active site of cytoplasmic aspartate aminotransferase by β-chloro-L-alanine. Biochem. Biophys. Res. Commun. 50:1061–1067.

Müller, M., Birner, G., Sander, M., and Dekant, W. 1998. Reactivity of haloketenes with nucleobases: Reactions in vitro with DNA. Chem. Res. Toxicol. 11:464–470.

Odum, J., and Green, T. 1984. The metabolism and nephrotoxicity of tetrafluoroethylene in the rat. Toxicol. Appl. Pharmacol. 76:306–318.

Oesch, F., and Wolf, C. R. 1989. Properties of the microsomal and cytosolic glutathione transferases involved in hexachloro-1:3-butadiene conjugation. Biochem. Pharmacol. 38:353–359.

Ovádi, J., and Srere, P. A. 2000. Macromolecular compartmentation and channeling. Int. Rev. Cytol. 192:255–280.

Park, S. B., Osterloh, J. D., Vamvakas, S., Hashmi, M., Anders, M. W., and Cashman, J. R. 1992. Flavin-containing monooxygenase-dependent stereoselective *S*-oxygenation and cytotoxicity of cysteine *S*-conjugates and mercapturates. Chem. Res. Toxicol. 5:193–201.

Park, L. C. H., Gibson, G. E., Bunik, V., and Cooper, A. J. L. 1999. Inhibition of select mitochondrial enzymes in PC12 cells exposed to *S*-(1,1,2,2-tetrafluo- roethyl)-L-cysteine. Biochem. Pharmacol. 58:1557–1565.

Pfaller, W., and Gstraunthaler, G. 1998. Nephrotoxicity testing in vitro – what we know and what we need to know. Environ. Health Perspect. 106 (Suppl. 2): 559–569.

Sausen, P. J., and Elfarra, A. A. 1991. Reactivity of cysteine *S*-conjugate sulfoxides: Formation of *S*-[1-chloro-2-(*S*-glutathionyl)vinyl]-L-cysteine sulfoxide by the reaction of *S*-(1,2-dichlorovinyl)-L-cysteine sulfoxide with glutathione. Chem. Res. Toxicol. 4:655–660.

Schaeffer, V. H., and Stevens, J. L. 1987a. The transport of *S*-cysteine conjugates in LLC-PK1 cells and its role in toxicity. Mol. Pharmacol. 31:506–512.

Schaeffer, V. H., and Stevens, J. L. 1987b. Mechanism of transport for toxic cysteine conjugates in rat kidney cortex membrane vesicles. Mol. Pharmacol. 32:293–298.

Song, H., Lang, C. A., and Chen, T. S. 1999. The role of *p*-aminophenol-induced nephrotoxicity in the mouse. Drug Chem. Toxicol. 22:529–544.

Stevens, J. L. 1985. Isolation and characterization of a rat liver enzyme with both cysteine conjugate β-lyase and kynureninase activity. J. Biol. Chem. 260:7945–7950.

Stevens, J. L., and Jones, D. P. 1989. The mercapturic acid pathway: Biosynthesis, intermediary metabolism, and physiological disposition. In Glutathione. Chemical, Biochemical and Medicinal Aspects, Part B, eds. D. Dolphin, R. Poulson, and O. Avramović, pp 45–84. New York: Wiley.

Stevens, J. L., Robbins, J. D., and Byrd, R. A. 1986. A purified cysteine conjugate β-lyase from rat kidney cytosol. Requirement for an α-keto acid or an amino acid oxidase for activity and identity with soluble glutamine transaminase K. J. Biol. Chem. 261:15529–15537.

Tateishi, M., Suzuki, S., and Shimizu, H. 1978a. The metabolism of bromazepam in the rat – identification of mercapturic acid and its conversion in vitro to methylthio-bromazepam. Biochem. Pharmacol. 27:809–810.

Tateishi, M., Suzuki, S., and Shimizu, H. 1978b. Cysteine conjugate β-lyase in rat liver. A novel enzyme catalyzing formation of thiol-containing metabolites of drugs. J. Biol. Chem. 253:8854–8859.

Ueno, H., Likos, J. J., and Metzler, D. E. 1982. Chemistry of the inactivation of cytosolic aspartate aminotransferase by serine *O*-sulfate. Biochemistry 21:4387–4393.

Uttamsingh, V., Baggs, R. B., Krenitsky, D. M., and Anders, M. W. 2000. Immunohistochemical localization of the acylases that catalyze deacylation of *N*-acetyl-L-cysteine and haloalkene-derived mercapturates. Drug Metab. Dispos. 28:625–632.

Van Horn, C. G., Wallin, R., Fujii, H., and Hutson, S. M. 2004. Evidence for a direct protein–protein interaction between the leucine catabolic enzymes. FASEB J. 18:A848 (Abstract).

Vamvakas, S., and Köster, U. 1993. The nephrotoxin dichlorovinylcysteine induces expression of the protooncogenes *c-fos* and *c-myc* in LLC-PK1 cells – a comparative investigation with growth factors and 12-*O*-tetradecanoylphorbolacetate. Cell Biol. Toxicol. 9:1–13.

Villar, M. T., Niatsetskaya, Z. V., Artigues, A., Cooper, A. J. L. Inactivation of rat liver mitochondrial aspartate aminotransferase by a halogenated cysteine *S*-conjugate. Presented at the 8th International Symposium on Mass Spectrometry in the Health and Life Sciences: Molecular and Cellular Proteomics, San Francisco, August, 2007.

Wallin, A., Gerdes, R. G., Morgenstern, R., Jones, T. W., and Ormstad, K. 1988. Features of microsomal and cytosolic glutathione conjugation of hexachlorobutadiene in rat liver. Chem. Biol. Interact. 68:1–11.

Werner, M., Birner, G., and Dekant, W. 1996. Sulfoxidation of mercapturic acids derived from tri- and tetrachloroethene by cytochrome P450 3A: A bioactivation reaction in addition to deacetylation and cysteine conjugate β-lyase mediated cleavage. Chem. Res. Toxicol. 9:41–49.

Wolf, C. R., Berry, P. N., Nash, J. A., Green, T., and Lock, E. A. 1984. Role of microsomal and cytosolic glutathione *S*-transferases in the conjugation of hexachloro-1:3-butadiene and its possible relevance to toxicity. J. Pharmacol. Exp. Ther. 228:202–208.

Wong, L. T., Solomonraj, G., and Thomas, B. H. 1976. Metabolism of [^{14}C]paracetamol and its interaction with aspirin in hamsters. Xenobiotica 6:575–584.

Wright, S. H., Wunz, T. M., North, J., and Stevens, J. L. 1998. Na-dependent transport of *S*-(1,2-dichlorovinyl)-L-cysteine by renal brush border membrane vesicles. J. Pharmacol. Exp. Ther. 285:162–169.

Wu, C., and Schaum, J. 2000. Exposure assessment of trichloroethylene. Environ. Health Perspect. 108 (Suppl. 2):359–363.

Zhang, L., and Hanigan, M. H. 2003. Role of cysteine *S*-conjugate β-lyase in the metabolism of cisplatin. J. Pharmacol. Exp. Ther. 306:988–994.

Zhang, L., Cooper, A. J. L., Krasnikov, B. F., Xu, H., Bubber, P., Gibson, G. E., and Hanigan, M. H. 2006. Cisplatin-induced toxicity is associated with platinum deposition in mouse kidney mitochondria in vivo and with selective inactivation of α-ketoglutarate dehydrogenase complex in LLC-PK_1 cells. Biochemistry 45:8959–8977.

13

Bioactivation of Xenobiotics in Lung: Role of CYPs and FMOs

David E. Williams
Department of Environmental and Molecular Toxicology and The Linus Pauling Institute, Oregon State University, Corvallis, OR 97331, USA
e-mail: david.williams@oregonstate.edu

Keywords: Genetic Polymorphisms · Redox Cycling · Thioureas · Paraquat · 3-Methylindole

13.1. Introduction

The human lung exhibits a number of unique properties that makes it an excellent mode of drug/xenobiotic absorption, as well as a target for toxicity due to bioactivation to toxic metabolite(s). The lung has a very large surface area, a very thin endothelial layer for diffusion into blood, receives 100% of the cardiac output, and is a complex organ of more than 40 different cell types with multiple physiological functions in addition to gas exchange. There have been excellent reviews on this subject (e.g., Dahl and Lewis 1993) and this review is not intended to cover all lung toxicants and all diseases associated with xenobiotic exposure. Certainly there are omissions and examples that could have been included, and the author apologizes in advance for those shortcomings. The goal of this review is to provide the reader with some representative examples of toxicities induced in the lung by activation of xenobiotics. This review will not cover incidences of lung toxicities from exposure to toxic agents not requiring bioactivation, although it is recognized that these events are extremely important from the standpoint of human health; examples would be the Bhopal tragedy, the worst chemical (methylisocyanate) industrial event to date; the continuing cases of mesothelioma, resulting from asbestos exposure; a multitude of lung diseases, including asthma, associated with ozone inhalation or particulate matter; and cancer from inhalation of radon.

13.2. Tools for the Study of Xenobiotic Bioactivation and Lung Toxicity in Humans

13.2.1. Animal Models

Rodent models have been used extensively to study the metabolism and toxicity of xenobiotics in the lung. In addition to the usual caveats in

A.A. Elfarra (ed.), *Advances in Bioactivation Research*, DOI: 10.1007/978-0-387-77300-1_13,

extrapolation of animal data to man, differences in the structure/function of the human lung and most animal models have to be kept in mind; for example, the rat is an obligatory nose-breather. Advances in computer modeling and imaging are being used to bridge this gap (Marton et al. 2001; Minard et al. 2006). One of the greatest uses of animal models and xenobiotic-dependent human lung disease are mouse models of lung cancer (Malkinson 1992; Sargent et al. 2002; Witschi et al. 2002). One advantage is the potential for identification of important genes or loci (Manenti et al. 2003), as the complete mouse genome is available, as are transgenic mouse models for the further study of the role of a particular gene in the etiology of cancer (or other diseases) of the lung (Glasser and Nogee 2006). The A/J strain has proven especially useful for studies on inhibition and promotion of cancer, as it is very responsive to known or suspected human carcinogens and has a relatively short time to tumor appearance (Bogen and Witschi 2002; Castonguay, Pepin and Stoner 1991).

13.2.2. Human Lung Cell Lines

In most cases, transformed cell lines, such as A549 or BEAS-2B cells have been utilized to study mechanisms of xenobiotic toxicity (Andreescu, Sadik and McGee 2005; Biswal et al. 2002; Hukkanen et al. 2000; Lin et al. 2004; Marano et al. 2002; Tsuji and Walle 2006; Yang, Cardona and Barile 2002). Caution should be used in interpretation of data from such studies in light of the fact that, as with other transformed cell lines, the levels of xenobiotic-metabolizing enzymes differ markedly from the original tissue (Castell, Donato and Gomez-Lechon 2005) and some cell lines may actually be quite heterogeneous and differ markedly from batch to batch (Watanabe et al. 2002). One alternative would be the use of primary cells, but those are difficult to acquire and not many studies have appeared employing such cells (Crawford et al. 1998). One alternative approach is to produce stable transfected human lung cell lines that express the cytochrome P450s (CYPs), or other xenobiotic-metabolizing enzymes, at higher levels (Sheets, Yost and Carlson 2004; Van Vleet et al. 2002). Another approach involves the use of lung slices from organ donors (Fisher et al. 1994). The advantages of tissue slices are that they maintain cell–cell and cell–matrix communication, which may be important in the toxicity of certain xenobiotics. Tissue slices also maintain higher levels of CYP over time than primary cell cultures. Finally, with the availability of standardized microarrays, it will be possible to determine the impact of xenobiotics, which are bioactivated by lung cells, on expression of genes in pulmonary tissue (Cheng et al. 2003; Hellmann, Fields and Doolittle 2001; Schultz et al. 2004; Verheyen et al. 2004).

13.3. Xenobiotic-Metabolizing Enzymes in the Lung

Liver is the primary organ for xenobiotic metabolism in most mammals, including humans. Other organs, including lungs, are capable of xenobiotic metabolism and, in certain cases, the pulmonary contribution may match or exceed that of liver. The composition of phase 1 and phase 2 xenobiotic-metabolizing enzymes and transporters are distinct in the lung and this composition plays a major role in what determines whether or not a xenobiotic will be toxic in the lung.

13.3.1. Cytochrome P450s

As in liver, CYPs are the major enzymes responsible for xenobiotic metabolism. With respect to xenobiotic (and especially drug) metabolism, the lung has not been studied as extensively as other organs, such as liver and intestine for which one can construct a CYP pie chart (Paine et al. 2006) showing the relative amounts of the various enzymes. The composition of CYPs in the human lung and their contribution to xenobiotic metabolism has been summarized in excellent reviews by Hukkanen et al. (2002) and Ding and Kaminsky (2003). The information given in Table 13.1 draws heavily from those reviews and also incorporates some additional information. The listings of substrates, inducers, and inhibitors are only examples and not intended to be comprehensive.

Table 13.1 Composition of CYPS in the human lung.

CYP	Substrate	Inducer	Inhibitor	References
1A1	PAHs[a]	Smoking	ANF[b]	Kim et al. (2004) Choudhary et al. (2005) Mollerup et al. (1999) Anttila et al. (1992) Thum et al. (2006)
1A2[c]	Phenacetin			Antilla et al. (1992) Choudhary et al. (2005)
1B1	PAHs estrogen	Smoking, BaP[d] cancer	3,4-DMF[e]	Kim et al. (2004) Spivack et al. (2001) Choudhary et al. (2005) Jiang et al. (2006) Tsuji and Walle (2006)
2A6[f]	Coumarin	(liver only)	8-methoxy- psoralen	Crawford et al. (1998) Nakajima et al. (1996) Su and Ding (2004) Tiano et al. (1994) Tyndale and Sellers (2001)
2A13	Nicotine, NNK AFB_1[g]		8-methoxy- psoralen	Bao et al. (2005) He et al. (2004) Jalas, Ding and Murphy (2003) Smith et al. (2003) Su et al. (2000) Von Weymarn et al. (2005) Zhu et al. (2006)
2B6[h]	S-mephenytoin	CAR[i], PXR[j] ligands	Bupropion	Ekins et al. (1998) Wang and Negishi (2003) Kim et al. (2005)
2D6[k]	Bufuralol	None	Fluoxetine	Bernauer et al. (2006)
2E1	Dimethyl- nitrosamine butadiene	Ethanol	Disulfiram	Runge et al. (2001) Csanady, Guengerich and Bond (1992)

Table 13.1 (continued)

CYP	Substrate	Inducer	Inhibitor	References
2F1	3-methyl-indole naphthalene			Carr et al. (2003b) Lanza et al. (1999) Nichols et al. (2003) Wan et al. (2005)
2J2	Ebastine arachidonic acid		Terfenadine derivatives	Lafite et al. (2006) Wu et al. (1996) Zeldin et al. (1996)
2S1	?	TCDD		Rivera, Saarikoski and Hankinson (2002) Wang, He and Hong (2005)
3A4/5[l]	Steroids	Glucocorticoids		Anttila et al. (1997) Hukkanen et al. (2003)
4B1[m]	Fatty acids 4-ipomeanol 3-methylindole primary aryl amines			Zheng et al. (2003) Poch et al. (2005) Lo-Guidice et al. (2002) Henne et al. (2001) Baer and Rettie (2006) Baer, Rettie and Henne (2005)

[a] Polycyclic aromatic hydrocarbons.
[b] αNaphthoflavone.
[c] Indicates evidence of expression at the mRNA levels, but is not present at significant amounts.
[d] Benzo[*a*]pyrene.
[e] 3′,4′,-dimethoxyflavone.
[f] CYP2A6 is predominantly found in liver where it plays a role in metabolism of coumarin, nicotine, and the tobacco-specific nitrosamine, NNK. The major CYP2A in human lung is 2A13 (the earlier studies citing significant expression of 2A6 in the lung were probably the result of the inability of antibodies to distinguish the two forms and the difficulty in separation on standard SDS-PAGE gels). Recently a peptide-derived antibody, specific for CYP2A13 has been developed by Zhu et al. (2006).
[g] Aflatoxin B_1.
[h] CYP2B6 is expressed at much higher levels in liver, where it is inducible by CAR and PXR ligands. A splice variant, CYP2B7, is expressed in lung, but is inactive.
[i] Constitutive androstane receptor.
[j] Pregnane X receptor.
[k] Other studies (e.g., Kivistö et al., 1997) do not find significant levels of CYP2D6 in lung.
[l] Unlike liver, where CYP3A4 makes up half of the total CYP and CYP3A4>>3A5, the CYP3A subfamily is expressed at low levels in the lung, predominantly as 3A5.
[m] Human CYP4B1 is unusual in binding heme covalently and having a significant portion catalytically inactive. For this reason, and the difficulty in expressing human CYP4B1, its actual contribution to xenobiotic metabolism in lung is uncertain.

13.3.1.1. The CYPs that are Selectively Expressed in the Human Lung are CYPs 2A13, 2F1, 2S1, and 4B1

The finding that CYP1A2 is expressed at very low levels (if at all) in the lung in both human and fetal mice is interesting given that the phenotype of the *Cyp1A2* null mouse is neonatal lethality from respiratory distress (Pineau et al. 1995), suggesting an important role for this CYP in lung development. Other CYP RNAs detected in the human lung include CYP2R1, 2U1, and 2 W1 (Choudhary et al. 2005). Of course, in order for CYPs to catalyze xenobiotic (or endobiotic) metabolism, NADPH cytochrome P450 oxidoreductase (POR) must be present, and it is not surprising that immunohistochemical studies have demonstrated similar distribution for these components of the microsomal mixed-function oxidase system within the lung (Bernauer et al. 2006; Hall et al. 1989; Kivisto et al. 1995). The CYPs and PORs are located primarily in bronchial and bronchiolar epithelial cells, Clara cells (nonciliated cuboidal secretory cells), and type II alveolar cells. (Czerwinski et al. 1994; Hall et al. 1989).

13.3.2. Flavin-Containing Monooxygenases

The flavin-containing monooxygenases (FMOs) are a family of enzymes that, like the CYPs, utilize molecular oxygen and NADPH to metabolize xenobiotics and some endobiotics. Much of the work describing the properties of this enzyme was led by the late Dr. Daniel M. Ziegler at the University of Texas at Austin (reviewed in Ziegler 1988, 1993, 2002; Cashman et al. 1995; Krueger and Williams 2005). Five FMOs (1–5) are expressed in humans, all located in a cluster on the long arm of chromosome 1 (Hernandez et al. 2004). In most mammals, including primates, the major, if not sole, FMO in pulmonary microsomes is FMO2. In fact, the first evidence that FMO could exist in more than a single form was obtained independently at the same time in the laboratories of Dr. Ernst Hodgson at North Carolina State and Dr. Bettie Sue Masters at the Medical College of Wisconsin (Tynes et al. 1985; Williams et al. 1985). Subsequent studies by these laboratories and others demonstrated that, unlike nonhuman primates, where FMO2 protein is expressed in high amounts in the lung, most human lung samples were negative (Yueh, Krueger and Williams 1997; Dolphin et al. 1998; Krueger et al. 2001; Zhang and Cashman 2006). Further examination characterized an interesting genetic polymorphism in expression of FMO2. All Caucasians and Asians, genotyped to date, have two *FMO2*2* (g.23,238C>T) alleles, encoding for a truncated and enzymatically inactive protein (FMO2.2), whereas approximately 27% of individuals of African descent and 2–7% of Hispanics possess at least one *FMO2*1* allele, coding for the full-length and enzymatically active FMO2.1 protein (Dolphin et al. 1998; Whestine et al. 2000; Krueger et al. 2002a, 2002b, 2004, 2005; Furnes et al. 2003).

If active human FMO2 enzyme is expressed in the lung, this may render these individuals more susceptible to toxicity upon exposure to xenobiotics containing thiocarbamide and related structural moieties. These compounds represent one of the few examples of a chemical class for which FMO oxygenation produces a toxic metabolite (Henderson et al. 2004a; Smith and Crespi 2002; Krieter et al. 1984). The toxicity arises from an initial S-oxygenation to form the reactive sulfenic acid, which is capable of further oxygenation to sulfinic acid or redox cycling with glutathione. The generation of these reactive sulfur groups produces oxidative stress and ultimately, cell death. An example, which is discussed in more detail below, is α-naphthylthiourea (ANTU), a rodenticide known to be a selective pulmonary toxicant (Boyd and Neal 1976). On the contrary, for compounds such as phorate (Henderson et al. 2004b; Usmani et al. 2004), in which case FMO S-oxygenation produces a less-toxic metabolite than the parent compound or a CYP-dependent metabolite, the presence of active FMO2 in the lung would be predicted to be beneficial.

13.3.3. Other Phase I Xenobiotic-Metabolizing Enzymes

In addition to CYP and FMO monooxygenases and POR, the human lung contains other phase I enzymes capable of xenobiotic bioactivation (or inactivation). These enzymes include (but are not limited to) epoxide hydrolase (EH), carboxylesterase, prostaglandin synthase (COX1 and COX2) (Maciag, Sithanandam and Anderson 2004; Martey et al. 2004; Tong, Ding and Tai 2006; Wiese, Thompson and Kadlubar 2001), myeloperoxidase (Petruska et al. 1992; London, Lehman and Taylor 1997), lipoxygenase (Bedard et al. 2002), alcohol dehydrogenase (ADH), and amine oxidase (Dahl and Lewis 1993; Andres et al. 2001; Castell, Donato and Gomez-Lechon 2005; Smith, Curtis and Eling 1991; Smith and Harrison 1997; Yang, Cardona and Barile 2002; Zhang, Wang and Prakash 2006). In the examples that follow, we will not present an example specific to all of these enzymes. For the most part, the activities of these enzymes result in the production of a less-toxic compound, although there certainly are exceptions. Epoxide hydrolase can be thought of as a bioactivating enzyme for some of the polycyclic aromatic hydrocarbons (PAHs) carcinogenic to the lung as they catalyze the hydrolysis of the first epoxides formed by CYP1A1/2 or 1B1 (e.g., the *anti*- and *syn*-7,8-epoxides of BaP). Other researchers have noted that the role for xenobiotic co-oxidation by enzymes such as COX, myeloperoxidase, and lipoxygenase may be of greater significance in extrahepatic tissues, such as the lung, where their amount, relative to the CYPs, is greater. COX2 has been noted to increase in lung tumors and that may explain why COX and lipoxygenase inhibitors are effective chemopreventive agents in animal models (such as the A/J mouse) of lung cancer (Castonguay and Rioux 1997; Jalbert and Castonguay 1992; Rioux and Castonguay 1998a, 1998b; Yao et al. 2000) and perhaps in humans as well (Krysan et al. 2006; Mao et al. 2005, 2006).

13.3.4. Phase II Xenobiotic-Metabolizing Enzymes in Human Lung

A number of phase II conjugating enzymes have been described in the human lung. A number of studies have examined the effect of genetic polymorphisms in expression (often in conjunction with CYP1A1) of these enzymes and susceptibility to disease, mostly cancer (see section below on Genetic Polymorphisms). Among the glutathione-S-transferases (GSTs, reviewed in Hayes, Flanagan and Jowsey 2005) present in the human lung are mGST, GSTA1, GSTA2, GSTP1 (highest GST in lung), GSTM1, GSTM3, and GSTT1 (low expression in most samples). The conjugation of an electrophile by glutathione (GSH) through the activity of a GST usually (with a few notable exceptions, e.g., Sherratt et al. 1997) produces a nontoxic, easily excretable metabolite. The role of GSTs in inactivation of lung procarcinogens, such as epoxides of PAHs, may play an important protective role in the lung. The studies examining expression of GSTs of various classes and the individual allelic variants are discussed below in the section on genetic polymorphisms.

Two forms of *N*-acetyltransferase (NAT1 and NAT2) are present in the human lung (Boukouvala and Sim 2005; Chen et al. 2003; Hsia et al. 2002; Windmill et al. 2000) and some evidence exists for variations in their expression being important in cancer susceptibility, but these are probably the least understood of the phase II enzymes when it comes to the human lung (Hengstier et al. 1998; Mace et al. 1998; McCarver and Hines 2002). Given the ability of the lung to take up amines from the blood and the presence of carcinogenic amines such as 4-aminobiphenyl in tobacco smoke, a clearer understanding of the role of NAT1 and NAT2 in xenobiotic metabolism is needed.

Humans express 17 UDP-glucuronosyltransferases (UGTs). The UGTs are comprised of two families. The nine UGTs in the 1 family (1A1 and 1A3-10) are all derived from a single gene. Exons 2–5 are identical, but alternative splicing and different functional promoters determine the composition of exon 1. The UGTs in the 2A (2A1) and 2B (2B4, 2B7, 2B10, 2B11, 2B15, 2B17, and 2B28) subfamilies are the products of distinct genes (Wells et al. 2004). As with the CYP and FMO phase I xenobiotic-metabolizing enzymes, the UGTs exhibit broad substrate specificity, tissue- and development-specific expression and responsiveness to inducers (Dellinger et al. 2006; Fang et al. 2002; Gong et al. 2001; Iyer et al. 2003; Kuehl and Murphy 2003; Oguri et al. 2004; Ren et al. 2000; Strassburg et al. 1999; Turgeon et al. 2001, 2003; Uchaipichat et al. 2006; Yueh et al. 2001; Zheng, Fang and Lazarus 2002). UDP-glucuronosyltransferases may play an important role in lung cancer cells acquiring resistance to therapeutic drugs (Oguri et al. 2004) and in the detoxication of the lung procarcinogens BaP and 4-(methylnitrosamino)-1-(3-pyridyl)-1-butanone (NNK).

The final two phase II enzymes in the human lung mentioned here are the sulfotransferases (SULTs) and NAD(P)H quinone oxidoreductases (NQO1 and NQO2). SULTs conjugate numerous xenobiotics and steroids, producing a very polar derivative easily excreted in urine (Falany 1997). The regulation of the level of steroids by SULTs (estrogens, dehydroepiandrosterone), other hormones, and neurotransmitters may play an important role in the physiology of the lung, especially during development (He, Frost and Falany 2005; Her et al. 1998; McCarver and Hines 2002; Richard et al. 2001). SULTs can also bioactivate prodrugs, an example being minoxidil (Waldon et al. 1989). In the case of certain alkylated PAHs, for example, 7,12-dimethylbenz[*a*]anthracene (DMBA), CYP-dependent hydroxylation of the 7-methyl group followed by sulfation produces a reactive mutagenic and carcinogenic electrophile (Flesher, Horn and Lehner 1997). NQO1 and NQO2 serve to catalyze the two-electron reduction of quinones and related structures (Jaiswal 1994; Joseph et al. 1994; Long and Jaiswal 2000). Quinones can covalently bind to macromolecules or undergo redox cycling through one-electron reductions (Bolton et al. 2000). The lung is sensitive to quinones, given the high oxygen tension and presence of enzymes such as POR capable of catalyzing one-electron reductions. The high levels of oxygen help to drive formation of reactive-oxygen species (ROS) during redox cycling, ultimately leading to pulmonary toxicity. One example of this redox cycling in lung, paraquat, is given in more detail below. The expression of NQO may be related to susceptibility to lung diseases, such as cancer (Sunaga et al. 2002; Xu et al. 2001).

13.3.5. Xenobiotic Transporters (Phase III Enzymes)

Increasingly, the important role that drug transporters play in the toxicology of xenobiotics has been recognized. These transporters are now sometimes referred to as phase III enzymes. In addition to the ATP-binding cassette (ABC) transporters, such as p-glycoprotein, multidrug resistance proteins (MRP1, MRP2, MRP3), and breast cancer resistance protein (BCRP) (Leslie, Deeley and Cole 2001; Narasaki et al. 1996; Perez-Tomas 2006), the lung also expresses lung resistance protein (LRP) or Ral-interacting protein (RLIP76/RALBP1), not members of the ABC family (Drake et al. 2007; Leslie, Deeley and Cole 2005; Perez-Tomas 2006; Singhal et al. 2005; Stuckler et al. 2005). These transport proteins were first studied as their upregulation during neoplastic development conferred resistance to the lung tumor cells to a number of therapeutic agents, including cisplatin, doxorubicin, vinblastine, mitomycin-C, and others. These transporters now are appreciated to have a wider function, that is, they serve as the major conduit for the transport of xenobiotics and xenobiotic metabolites out of the cell. An example of great relevance to the human lung is the MRP1 export of NNAL, the major metabolite of the lung carcinogen and tobacco-specific nitrosamine NNK (Leslie et al. 2001).

13.4. Genetic Polymorphisms in Drug-Metabolizing Enzymes and Susceptibility to Disease

Almost without exception, human phase I and phase II xenobiotic-metabolizing enzymes exhibit genetic polymorphisms in expression, often in an ethnic-dependent fashion (Hirvonen 1999; Gonzalez 1995; Nebert, McKinnon and Puga 1996; Yang et al. 2002). There have been numerous studies examining the link between expression of certain variants and lung disease, with the majority of the studies focusing on lung cancer (or biomarkers of lung cancer risk) (Hengstier et al. 1998). One aim of such studies is to identify subpopulations that have the highest risk from exposure. It has been known for many years that certain ethnic groups have a higher risk for development of lung diseases. Genetic polymorphisms in expression of enzymes involved in metabolism of the xenobiotics associated with the etiology of the disease, such as lung cancer, have been the driver for these studies.

Given the role of CYP1A1 and CYP1B1 in bioactivation of PAH lung carcinogens and inactivation by GSTM1, many studies have focused on expression of CYP1A1 and/or CYP1B1 (examples are found in Anttila et al. 2001; Georgiadis et al. 2005; Kim et al. 2004; London et al. 1995; Song et al. 2001; Taioli et al. 1998; Wenzlaff et al. 2005), GSTs (mostly GSTM1) (examples found in Baur et al. 2006; Benhamou et al. 2002; Coles et al. 2000; Cote et al. 2005; Crawford et al. 2000; Ford et al. 2000; Houlston 1999; Matsuzoe et al. 2001; Perera et al. 2002; Risch et al. 2001; Sorenson et al. 2004; Stucker et al. 1999, 2002; Sweeney et al. 2003), or combinations of CYP1A1 and GSTM1 (Alexandrov et al. 2002; Anttila et al. 1994; Bartsch et al. 2000; Hung et al. 2003; Le Marchand et al. 1998; Peluso et al. 2004; Schoket et al. 1998; Shields et al. 1993; Smith et al. 2001). The hypothesis under test, supported by a number of studies, is that individuals with both high levels of CYP1A1 or 1B1 (greater bioactivation) and null variants of GSTM1 (greater inactivation) would exhibit the greatest risk to diseases, such as cancer, associated with PAH exposure to lung. The examination of polymorphisms in other CYPs, that is, 2C9 (London et al. 1996b), 2D1 (Caporaso et al. 1992), and 2E1 (London et al. 1996a; Wu et al. 1997) and association with lung cancer, has revealed a weaker relationship than the CYP1A1/1B1 and GSTM1 studies.

Another CYP polymorphism examined is in the CYP2A subfamily (2A6 and 2A13), as these are the CYPs with the highest activity toward nicotine and NNK (Ariyoshi et al. 2002; Brown von Weymarn and Murphy 2005; Fujieda et al. 2004; He et al. 2004; London et al. 1999; Loriot et al. 2001; Miyamoto et al. 1999; Tan et al. 2001; Su et al. 2000; Wang et al. 2003, 2006), lung toxicants and/or carcinogens (see review by Jalas, Hecht and Murphy 2005). As discussed in the first section, the major CYP responsible for NNK bioactivation in the human lung is 2A13. CYP2A13 is highly expressed in the lung and 2A6 is not; 2A13 also has a catalytic efficacy for bioactivation of NNK that is 30-fold greater than 2A6 (Su et al. 2000). To date, there are at least nine allelic variants of CYP2A13 and evidence has been presented with expressed enzymes demonstrating reduction in nicotine and NNK metabolism by some variants (e.g., CYP2A13 R257C) which has also been associated with reduction in lung cancer risk in a human population (Wang et al. 2003).

Epoxide hydrolase genetic polymorphisms have also been associated with lung cancer risk (Wu et al. 2001) and with emphysema (Smith and Harrison 1997). A possible correlation between NQO1, smoking, and lung cancer has also been described (Rosvold et al. 1995).

13.5. Examples of Xenobiotic Bioactivation in Lung by POR (Paraquat), CYP (3-Methyindole), and FMO (α-Naphthylthiourea)

Paraquat is a quaternary ammonium bipyridyl herbicide that is responsible for numerous accidental poisonings and suicides. As a diamine, paraquat is rapidly and efficiently taken up from the general circulation and accumulates in alveolar epithelial cells (type I and type II) and Clara cells (Bus and Gibson 1984; Han et al. 2006; Smith, 1985, 1987; Smith, Rose and Wyatt 1978). One-electron reduction of paraquat produces the radical shown below in Figure 13.1, which in turn is rapidly oxidized back to

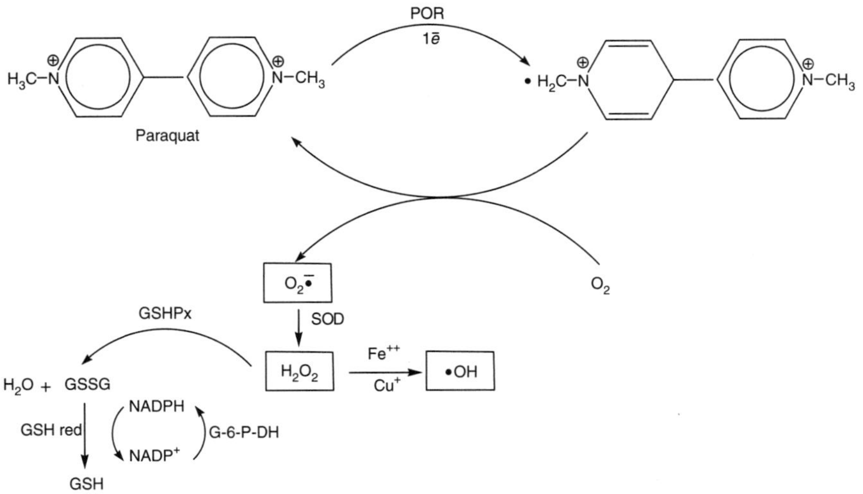

Figure 13.1 POR bioactivation of paraquat.

paraquat by molecular oxygen with generation of superoxide anion radical. In the presence of superoxide dismutase, superoxide anion radical is converted to hydrogen peroxide. In the presence of transition metals, such as Fe^{+2} or Cu^{+1}, the extremely reactive hydroxyl radical is produced through the Fenton reaction. In addition to the formation of these ROS, H_2O_2 can also result in depletion of reducing equivalents, due to the requirement of glutathione peroxidase (needed to regenerate GSH) for NADPH (catalyzed by glucose-6-phosphate dehydrogenase). The high concentration of oxygen in the lung serves to drive this toxic cycle faster, with death ensuing from respiratory failure from anoxia followed by a severe fibrosis. Treatment with hyperbaric oxygen is counter-indicated, as this only serves to drive the cycle faster. It is not surprising that, unless treated early with agents that alter absorption and accumulation in lung, little can be done for the patient short of a lung transplant.

3-Methylindole (3-MI), produced by ruminal bacteria reductive metabolism of tryptophan and indole-3-carbinol from plants, is a species-specific pulmonary toxin (Carlson and Breeze 1984). The species specificity in toxicity appears to be due to the presence in cattle and goats of a CYP (CYPF) with high selectivity toward production of the 3-methyleneindoleine metabolite, which is thought to be responsible for the binding of 3-MI to macromolecules and toxicity in lung cells expressing CYP2F (Huijzer et al. 1989; Kaster and Yost, 1997; Lanza and Yost 2001; Lanza et al. 1999; Loneragan et al. 2001; Ramakanth et al. 1994; Regal et al. 2001). Much of the work describing the metabolism of 3-MI and the role of various CYPs has been performed in the laboratory of Dr. Garold Yost of the University of Utah. Other CYPs also metabolize 3-MI, but do not exhibit the selectivity toward dehydrogenation (Figure 13.2). Members of the CYP4B subfamily are also active in carrying out the dehydrogenation of 3-MI (Carr et al. 2003a), but for reasons given above related to expression of active CYP4B1 in the human lung, are not likely to play a major role in bioactivation of 3-MI in the general population. Humans express CYP2F1 selectively in lung (Carr et al. 2003b) and CYP2F1, as other members of this subfamily, is very efficient at

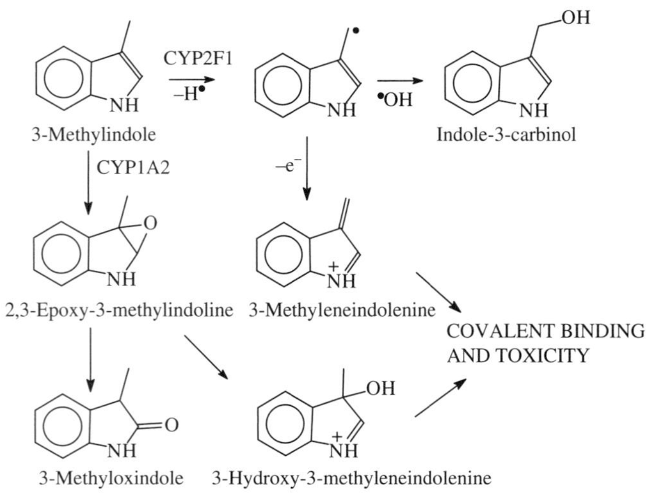

Figure 13.2 CYP2F1 bioactivation of 3-methylindole.

bioactivation of 3-MI to 3-methyleneindoleine (Nichols et al. 2003). Based on these findings, 3-MI and related structures should be pneumotoxic in humans as well.

Flavin-containing monooxygenases oxygenate the sulfur moiety of thiocarbamides to produce the reactive sulfenic acid (Hardwick et al. 1991; Henderson et al. 2004a; Krieter et al. 1984; Nagata, Williams and Ziegler 1990; Onderwater et al. 1998; Poulsen, Hyslop and Ziegler 1979; Smith and Crespi 2002; Ziegler 1982). In some cases, a second oxygenation to the sulfinic acid is carried out (Figure 13.3). The pulmonary form, FMO2, produces the sulfenic acid from a number of thioureas, including ANTU, known to be a pneumotoxin in a number of species (Henderson et al. 2004a). Human FMO produces a single major metabolite from ANTU, which we have demonstrated by liquid chromatography-mass spectrometry (LC-MS) and MS-MS to be the sulfenic acid (Henderson et al. 2004a). If the reactions are carried out in the presence of glutathione, the sulfenic acid metabolite is no longer detectable (0.2 m M GSH eliminates 70% of the sulfenic acid and no metabolite is detected at 1 m M GSH and above) and the ratio of GSSG/GSH is markedly increased (Henderson et al. 2004a). These results are consistent with a redox cycle, proposed by us and others. If the sulfenic acid is sufficiently reactive with GSH, the parent compound will be regenerated resulting in the depletion of GSH and ultimately NADPH (Figure 13.3).

The laboratory of Dr. Paul Ortiz de Montellano has recently described an FMO (EtaA) in the bacteria responsible for tuberculosis (*Mycobacterium tuberculosis*) that S-oxygenates the prodrugs ethionamide (ETA) and thiacetzaone (TAZ) (second-line drugs for treatment of tuberculosis) to the sulfenic acid derivatives and ETA carboxamidopyridine and TAZ carbodiimide, thought to be responsible for the effectiveness against *M. tuberculosis* (Qian and de Montellano 2006; Vannelli et al. 2002) and probably the adverse and serious side effects, including hepatotoxicity (Newton 1975). Human FMO1 and FMO3 (Qian and de Montellano

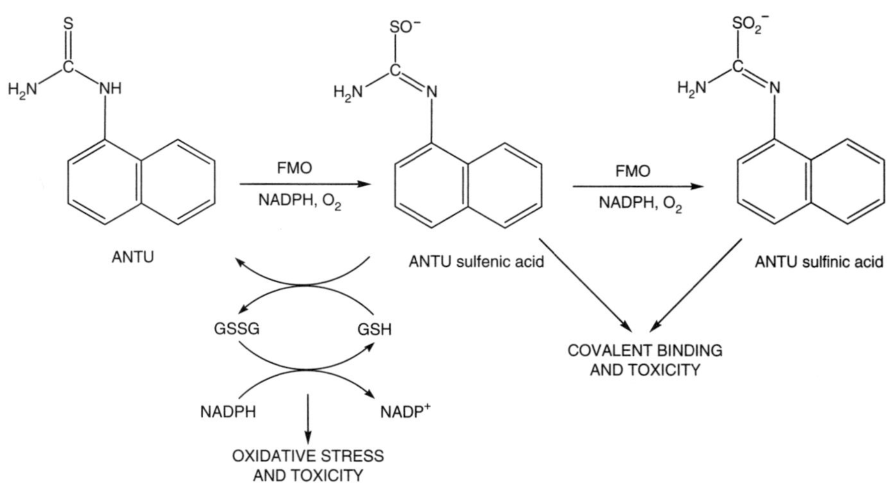

Figure 13.3 FMO2 bioactivation of alpha-naphthylthiourea.

2006) as well as FMO2 (our laboratory, unpublished) are also effective in oxygenation of ETA and TZU, forming the same products. An interesting question arises with respect to the FMO2 genetic polymorphism in lung. Would the 27% of African-Americans and 2–7% of Hispanics who possess active FMO2 require a higher dose (if FMO2 metabolized the prodrug before reaching its target) or are the active metabolites of FMO2 available to kill the bacteria, perhaps requiring a smaller and less toxic dose?

13.6. Future Directions

As can be seen from the three examples given here, paraquat, 3-MI, and α-naphthylthiourea, bioactivated by POR, CYP, and FMO, respectively, formation of reactive intermediates capable of directly or indirectly producing ROS and causing oxidative stress is a common theme for xenobiotic-dependent pulmonary toxicity. Although outside the scope of this review, the same can be said for other agents toxic to lung that generate acute or chronic inflammation (asbestos, atmospheric particulate matter, etc.). The high oxygen tension in the lung is one of the contributing factors to this phenomenon. It is not surprising that GSH and the enzymes required to maintain high levels of GSH are so important in the lung (Rahman et al., 1999). Strategies for maintenance and enhancement of antioxidant power in the lung should be a priority of individuals at risk of exposure. In addition to what we already know about the importance of oxidative stress in xenobiotic-dependent lung toxicity, there is a need to understand how nanomaterials, which are rapidly revolutionalizing our everyday life, impact lung health. There is already evidence that the lung is a primary target organ for nano-xenobiotic-dependent toxicity (Borm 2002; Donaldson et al. 2002, 2006; Muller et al. 2005) and the emerging field of nanotoxicology should be supported by investigators concerned with the health of the human pulmonary system.

Acknowledgments. The author wishes to thank Dr. Garold Yost of the University of Utah for supplying the figure on the metabolism of 3-methyindole and Ms. Sandy Segna of Oregon State University for editing this text. The work described in this review article, conducted in the author's laboratory, has been supported by NIH grants HL038650 and ES00210.

References

Alexandrov, K., Cascorbi, I., Rojas, M., Bouvier, G., Kriek, E., and Bartsch, H. 2002. *CYP1A1* and *GSTM1* genotypes affect benzo[*a*]pyrene DNA adducts in smokers' lung: Comparison with aromatic/hydrophobic adduct formation. Carcinogenesis 23:1969–1977.

Andreescu, S., Sadik, O. A., and McGee, D. W. 2005. Effect of natural and synthetic estrogens on A549 lung cancer cells: correlation of chemical structures with cytotoxic effects. Chem. Res. Toxicol. 18:466–474.

Andres, N., Lizcano, J. M., Rodriguez, M. J., Romera, M., Unzeta, M., and Mahy, N. 2001. Tissue activity and cellular localization of human semicarbazide-sensitive amino oxidase. J. Histochem. Cytochem. 49:209–217.

Anttila, S., Hirvonen, A., Husgafvel-Pursiainen, K., Karjalainen, A., Nurminen, T., and Vainio, H. 1994. Combined effect of CYP1A1 inducibility and *GSTM1* polymorphism on histological type of lung cancer. Carcinogenesis 15:1133–1135.

Anttila, S., Hukkanen, J., Hakkola, J., Stjernvall, T., Beaune, P., Edwards, R. J., Boobis, A. R., Pelkonen, O., and Raunio, H. 1997. Expressions and localization of CYP3A4 and CYP3A5 in human lung. Am. J. Respir. Cell Mol. Biol. 16:242–249.

Anttila, S., Tuominen, P., Hirvonen, A., Nurminen, M., Karjalainen, A., Hankinson, O., and Elovaara, E. 2001. CYP1A1 levels in lung tissue of tobacco smokers and polymorphisms of *CYP1A1* and aromatic hydrocarbon receptor. Pharmacogenetics 11:501–509.

Anttila, S., Vainio, H., Hietanen, E., Camus, A.-M., Malaveille, C., Brun, G., Husgafvel-Pursiainen, K., Heikkilä, L., Karjalainen, A., and Bartsch, H. 1992. Immunohistochemical detection of pulmonary cytochrome P4501A and metabolic activities associated with P4501A1 and P4501A2 isozymes in lung cancer patients. Environ. Hlth. Perspect. 98:179–182.

Ariyoshi, N., Miyamoto, M., Umetsu, Y., Kunitoh, H., Dosaka-Akita, H., Sawamura, Y.-I., Yokota, J., Nemoto, N., Sato, K., and Kamataki, T. 2002. Genetic polymorphism of *CYP2A6* gene and tobacco-induced lung cancer risk in male smokers. Cancer Epidemiol. Biomarkers Prev. 11:890–894.

Baer, B. R., and Rettie, A. E. 2006. CYP4B1: An enigmatic P450 at the interface between xenobiotic and endobiotic metabolism. Drug Metab. Rev. 38:451–476.

Baer, B. R., Rettie, A. E., and Henne, K. R. 2005. Bioactivation of 4-ipomeanol by CYP4B1: Adduct characterization and evidence for an enedial intermediate. Chem. Res. Toxicol. 18:855–864.

Bao, Z., He, X.-Y., Ding, X., Prabhu, S., and Hong, J.-Y. 2005. Metabolism of nicotine and cotinine by human cytochrome P450 2A13. Drug Metab. Dispos. 33:258–261.

Bartsch, H., Nair, U., Risch, A., Rojas, M., Wikman, H., and Alexandrov, K. 2000. Genetic polymorphism of *CYP* genes, alone or in combination, as a risk modifier of tobacco-related cancers. Cancer Epidemiol. Biomarkers Prev. 9:3–28.

Baur, M., Herbarth, O., Aust, G., Hengstier, J. G., Dotzauer, A., Graebsch, C., and Schmuecking, E. 2006. Expression patterns and novel splicing variants of glutathione-S-transferase isoenzymes of human lung and hepatocytes cell lines. Cell Tissue Res. 324:423–432.

Bedard, L. L., Smith, G. B. J., Reid, K. R., Petsikas, D., and Massey, T. E. 2002. Investigation of the role of lipoxygenase in bioactivation of 4-(methylnitrosamino)-1-(3-pyridyl-1-butanone (NNK) in human lung. Chem. Res. Toxicol. 15:1267–1273.

Benhamou, S., Lee, W. J., Alexandrie, A.-K., Boffetta, P., Couchardy, C., Dutkiewicz, D., Brockmöller, J., Clapper, M. L., Daly, A., Dolzan, V., Ford, J., Gaspari, L., Haugen, A., Hirvonen, A., Husgafvel-Pursiainen, K., Ingelman-Sundberg, M., Kalina, I., Kihara, M., Kremers, P., Le Marchand, L., London, S. J., Nazar-Stewart, V., Onon-Kihara, M., Rannug, A., Romkes, M., Ryberg, D., Seidegard, J., Shields, P., Strange, R. C., Stucker, I., To-Figueras, J., Brennan, P., and Taioli, E. 2002. Meta- and pooled analysis of the effects of glutathione S-transferase M1 polymorphisms and smoking on lung cancer risk. Carcinogenesis 23:1343–1350.

Bernauer, U., Hirsch-Heinrich, B., Tonnies, M., Peter-Matthias, W. and Gundert-Remy, U. 2006. Characterization of the xenobiotic-metabolizing cytochrome P450 expression pattern in human lung tissue by immunochemical and activity determination. Toxicol. Lett. 164:278–288.

Biswal, S., Acquaah-Mensah, G., Datta, K., Wu, X., and Kehrer, J. P. 2002. Inhibition of cell proliferation and AP-1 activity by acrolein in human A549 lung adenocarcinoma cells due to thiol imbalance and covalent modifications. Chem. Res. Toxicol. 15:180–186.

Bogen, K. T., and Witschi, H. 2002. Lung tumors in A/J mice exposed to environmental tobacco smoke: estimated potency and implied human risk. Carcinogenesis 23:511–519.

Bolton, J. L., Trush, M. A., Penning, T. M., Dryhurst, G., and Monks, T. J. 2000. Role of quinones in toxicology. Chem. Res. Toxicol. 13:135–160.

Borm, P. J. 2002. Particle toxicology: From coal mining to nanotechnology. Inhal. Toxicol. 14:311–324.

Boukouvala, S., and Sim, E. 2005. Structural analysis of the genes for human arylamine *N*-acetyltransferases and characterization of alternative transcripts. Basic Clin. Pharmacol. Toxicol. 96:343–351.

Boyd, M. R., and Neal, R. A. 1976. Studies on the mechanism of toxicity and of development of tolerance to the pulmonary toxin, alpha-naphthythiourea (ANTU). Drug Metab. Dispos. 4:314–322.

Brown, K. M., von Weymarn, L. B., and Murphy, S. E. 2005. Identification of *N*-(hydroxymethyl) norcotinine as a major product of cytochrome P450 2A6, but not cytochrome P450 2A13-catalyzed cotinine metabolism. Chem. Res. Toxicol. 18:1792–1798.

Bus, J. S., and Gibson, J. E. 1984. Paraquat: Model for oxidant-initiated toxicity. Environ. Hlth. Perspect. 55:37–46.

Caporaso, N. E., Shields, P. G., Landi, M. T., Shaw, G. L., Tucker, M. A., Hoover, R., Sugimura, H., Weston, A., and Harris, C. C. 1992. The debrisoquine metabolic phenotype and DNA-based assays: Implications of misclassification for the association of lung cancer and the debrisoquine metabolic phenotype. Environ. Hlth. Perspect. 98:101–105.

Carlson, J. R., and Breeze, R. G. 1984. Ruminal metabolism of plant toxins with emphasis on indolic compounds. J. Animal Sci. 58:1040–1049.

Carr, B. A., Ramakanth, S., Dannan, G. A., and Yost, G. S. 2003a. Characterization of pulmonary CYP4B2, a specific catalyst of methyl oxidation of 3-methylindole. Mol. Pharmacol. 63:1137–1147.

Carr, B. A., Wan, J., Hines, R. N., and Yost, G. S. 2003b. Characterization of the human lung *CYP2F1* gene and identification of a novel lung-specific binding motif. J. Biol. Chem. 278:15473–15483.

Cashman, J. R., Park, S. B., Berkman, C. E., and Cashman, L. E. 1995. Role of hepatic flavin-containing monooxygenase in drug and chemical metabolism in adult humans. Chem. Biol. Interact. 96:33–46.

Castell, J. V., Donato, M. T., and Gomez-Lechon, M. J. 2005. Metabolism and bioactivation of toxicants in the lung. The in vitro cellular approach. Exp. Toxicol. Pathol. 57 Suppl 1:189–204.

Castonguay, A., Pepin, P., and Stoner, G. D. 1991. Lung tumorigenicity of NNK given orally to A/J mice: its application to chemopreventive efficacy studies. Exp. Lung Res. 17:485–499.

Castonguay, A., and Rioux, N. 1997. Inhibition of lung tumourigenesis by sulindac: Comparison of two experimental models. Carcinogenesis 18:491–496.

Chen, Y. S., Ho, C. C., Cheng, K. C., Tyan, Y. S., Hung, C. F., Tan, T. W., and Chung, J. G. 2003. Curcumin inhibited the arylamines *N*-acetyltransferase activity, gene expression and DNA adduct formation in human lung cancer cells (A549). Toxicol. In Vitro 17:323–333.

Cheng, R. Y., Zhao, A., Alvord, W. G., Powell, D. A., Bare, R. M., Masuda, A., Takahashi, T., Anderson, L. M., and Kasprzak, K. S. 2003. Gene expression dose–response changes in microarrays after exposure of human peripheral lung epithelial cells to nickel (II). Toxicol. Appl. Pharmacol. 191:22–39.

Choudhary, D., Jansson, I., Stoilov, I., Sarfarazi, M., and Schenkman, J. B. 2005. Expression patterns of mouse and human CYP orthologs (families 1–4) during development and in different adult tissues. Arch. Biochem. Biophys. 436:50–61.

Coles, B., Yang, M., Lang, N. P., and Kadlubar, F. F. 2000. Expression of hGSTP1 alleles in human lung and catalytic activity of the native protein variants towards 1-chloro-2,4-dinitrobenzene, 4-vinylpyridine and (+)-anti-benzo[a]pyrene-7,8-diol-9,10-oxide. Cancer Lett. 156:167–175.

Cote, M. L., Kardia, S. L. R., Wenzlaff, A. S., Land, S. J., and Schwartz, A. G. 2005. Combinations of glutathione S-transferase genotypes and risk of early-onset lung cancer in Caucasians and African Americans: A population-based study. Carcinogenesis 26:811–819.

Crawford, E. L., Khuder, S. A., Durham, S. J., Frampton, M., Utell, M., Thilly, W. G., Weaver, D. A., Ferencak, W. J., Jennings, C. A., Hammersley, J. R., Olson, D. A. and Willey, J. C. (2000). Normal bronchial epithelial cell expression of glutathione transferase P1, glutathione transferase M3, and glutathione peroxidase is low in subjects with bronchogenic carcinoma. Cancer Res. 60:1609–1618.

Crawford, E. L., Weaver, D. A., DeMuth, J. P., Jackson, C. M., Khuder, S. A., Frampton, M. W., Utell, M. J., Thilly, W. G., and Willey, J. C. 1998. Measurement of cytochrome P450 2A6 and 2E1 gene expression in primary human bronchial epithelial cells. Carcinogenesis 19:1867–1871.

Csanady, G. A., Guengerich, F. P., and Bond, J. A. 1992. Comparison of the biotransformation of 1,3-butadiene and its metabolite, butadiene monoepoxide, by hepatic and pulmonary tissues from humans, rats and mice. Carcinogenesis 13:1143–1153.

Czerwinski, M., McLemore, T. L., Gelboin, H. V., and Gonzalez, F. J. 1994. Quantification of CYP2B7, CYP4B1, and CYPOR messenger RNAs in normal human lung and lung tumors. Cancer Res. 54:1085–1091.

Dahl, A. R., and Lewis, J. L. 1993. Respiratory tract uptake of inhalants and metabolism of xenobiotics. Annu. Rev. Pharmacol. Toxicol. 32:383–407.

Dellinger, R. W., Fang, J. L., Chen, G., Weinberg, R., and Lazarus, P. 2006. Importance of UDP-glucuronosyltransferase 1A10 *UGT1A10) in the detoxification of polycyclic aromatic hydrocarbons: decreased glucuronidative activity of the UGT1A10 139lys isoform. Drug Metab. Dispos. 34:943–949.

Ding, X., and Kaminsky, L. S. 2003. Human extrahepatic cytochromes P450: Function in xenobiotic metabolism and tissue-selective chemical toxicity in the respiratory and gastrointestinal tracts. Annu. Rev. Pharmacol. Toxicol. 43:149–173.

Dolphin, C. T., Beckett, D. J., Janmohamed, A., Cullingford, T. E., Smith, R. L., Shephard, E. A., and Phillips, I. R. 1998. The flavin-containing monooxygenase 2 gene (FMO2) of humans, but not of other primates, encodes a truncated, nonfunctional protein. J. Biol. Chem. 273:30599–30607.

Donaldson, K., Aitken, R., Tran, L., Stone, V., Duffin, R., Forrest, G., and Alexander, A. 2006. Carbon nanotubes: A review of their properties in relation to pulmonary toxicology and workplace safety. Toxicol. Sci. 92:5–22.

Donaldson, K., Brown, D., Clouter, A., Duffin, R., MacNee, W., Renwick, L., Tran, L., and Stone, V. 2002. The pulmonary toxicology of ultrafine particles. J. Aerosol. Med. 15:213–220.

Drake, K. J., Singhai, J., Yadav, S., Nadkar, A., Pungaliya, C., Singhal, S. S., and Awasthi, S. 2007. RALBP1/RLIP76 mediates multidrug resistance. Int. J. Oncol. 30:139–144.

Ekins, S., Vandenbranden, M., Ring, B. J., Gillespie, J. S., Yang, T. J., Gelboin, H. V., and Wrighton, S. A. 1998. Further characterization of the expression in liver and catalytic activity of CYP2B6. J. Pharmacol. Exp. Therap. 286:1253–1259.

Falany, C. N. 1997. Enzymology of human cytosolic sulfotransferases. FASEB J. 11:206–216.

Fang, J. L., Beland, F. A., Doerge, D. R. Wiener, D., Guillemette, C., Marques, M. M., and Lazarus, P. 2002. Characterization of benzo(a)pyrene-trans-7,8-dihydrodiol glucuronidation by human tissue microsomes and overexpressed UDP-glucuronosyltransferase enzymes. Cancer Res. 62:1978–1986.

Fisher, R. L., Smith, M. S., Hasal, S. J., Hasal, K. S., Gandolfi, A. J., and Brendel, K. 1994. The use of human lung slices in toxicology. Human Exp. Toxicol. 13:466–471.

Flesher, J. W., Horn, J., and Lehner, A. F. 1997. 7-Sulfooxymethyl-12-methylbenz[a]anthracene is an exceptionally reactive electrophilic mutagen and ultimate carcinogen. Biochem. Biophys. Res. Commun. 231:144–148.

Ford, J. G., Li, Y., O'Sullivan, M. M., Demopoulos, R., Garte, S., Taioli, E., and Brandt-Rauf, P. W. 2000. Glutathione S-transferase M1 polymorphism and lung cancer risk in African-Americans. Carcinogenesis 21:1971–1975.

Fujieda, M., Yamazaki, H., Saito, T., Kiyotani, K., Gyamfi, A., Sakurai, M., Dosaka-Akita, H., Sawamura, Y., Yokota, J., Kunitoh, H.,and Kamataki, T. 2004. Evalution of *CYP2A6* genetic polymorphisms as determinants of smoking behavior and tobacco-related lung cancer risk in male Japanese smokers. Carcinogenesis 25:2451–2458.

Furnes, B., Feng, J., Sommer, S. S., and Schlenk, D. 2003. Identification of novel variants of the flavin-containing monooxygenase gene family in African Americans. Drug Metab. Dispos. 31:187–193.

Georgiadis, P., Topinka, J., Vlachodimitropoulos, D., Stoikidou, M., Gioka, M., Stephanou, G., Autrup, H., Demopoulos, N. A., Katsouyanni, K., Sram, R., and Kyrtopoulos, S. A. 2005. Interactions between CYP1A1 polymorphisms and exposure to environmental tobacco smoke in the modulation of lymphocyte bulky DNA adducts and chromosomal aberrations. Carcinogenesis 26:93–101.

Glasser, S. W., and Nogee, L. M. 2006. Genetically engineered mice in understanding the basis of neonatal lung disease. Semin. Perinatol. 30:341–349.

Gong, Q.-H., Cho, J. W., Huang, T., Potter, C., Gholami, N., Basu, N. K., Kubota, S., Carvalho, S., Pennington, M. W., Owens, I. S., and Popescu, N. C. 2001. Thirteen UDPglucuronosyltransferase genes are encoded at the human *UGT1* gene complex locus. Pharmacogenetics 11:357–368.

Gonzalez, F. J. 1995. Genetic polymorphism and cancer susceptibility: Fourteenth Sapporo Cancer Seminar. Cancer Res. 55:710–715.

Hall, P. M., Stupans, I., Burgess, W., Birkett, D. J., and McManus, M. E. 1989. Immunochemical localization of NADPH-cytochrome P450 reductase in human tissues. Carcinogenesis 10:521–530.

Han, J. F., Wang, S. L., He, X. Y., Lium C. Y., and Hong, J. Y. 2006. Effect of genetic variation on human cytochrome P450 reductase-mediated paraquat cytotoxicity. Toxicol. Sci. 91:42–48.

Hardwick, S. J., Skamarauskas, J. T., Smith, L. L., Upshall, D. G., and Cohen, G. M. 1991. Protection of rats against the effects of alpha-naphthylthiourea (ANTU) by elevation of nonprotein sulphydryl levels. Biochem. Pharmacol. 42:1203–1208.

Hayes, J. D., Flanagan, J. U., and Jowsey, I. R. 2005. Glutathione transferases. Annu. Rev. Pharmacol. Toxicol. 45:51–88.

He, D., Frost, A. R., and Falany, C. N. 2005. Identification and immunohistochemical localization of sulfotransferase 2B1b (SULT2B1b) in human lung. Biochim. Biophys. Acta 1724:119–126.

He, X.-Y., Shen, J., Ding, X., Lu, A. Y. H., and Hong, J.-Y. 2004. Identification of critical amino acid residues of human CYP2A13 for the metabolic activation of 4-(methylnitrosamino)-1-(3-pyridyl)-1-butanone, a tobacco-specific carcinogen. Drug Metab. Dispos. 32:1516–1521.

Hellmann, G. M., Fields, W. R., and Doolittle, D. J. 2001. Gene expression profiling of cultured human bronchial epithelial and lung carcinoma cells. Toxicol. Sci. 61:154–163.
Henderson, M. C., Krueger, S. K., Stevens, J. F., and Williams, D. E. 2004a. Human flavin-containing monooxygenase form 2 S-oxygenation: Sulfenic acid formation from thioureas and oxidation of glutathione. Chem. Res. Toxicol. 17:633–640.
Henderson, M. C., Krueger, S. K., Siddens, L. K., Stevens, J. F. and Williams, D. E. 2004b. S-Oxygenation of the thioether organophosphate insecticides phorate and disulfoton by human lung flavin-containing monooxygenase 2. Biochem. Pharmacol. 68:959–967.
Hengstier, J. G., Arand, M., Herrero, M. E., and Oesch, F. 1998. Polymorphisms of *N*-acetyltransferases, glutathione S-transferases, microsomal epoxide hydrolase and sulfotransferases: Influence on cancer susceptibility. Recent Results Cancer Res. 154:47–85.
Henne, K. R., Kunze, K. L., Zheng, Y. M., Christmas, P., Soberman, R. J., and Rettie, A. E. 2001. Covalent linkage of prosthetic heme to CYP4 family P450 enzymes. Biochemistry 40:12925–12931.
Her, C., Wood, T. C., Eichier, E. E., Mohrenweiser, H. W., Ramagli, L. S., Siciliano, M. J., and Weinshilboum, R. M. 1998. Human hydroxysteroid sulfotransferase SULT2B1: Two enzymes encoded by a single chromosome 19 gene. Genomics 53:284–295.
Hernandez, D., Janmohamed, A., Chandan, P., Phillips, I. R., and Shephard, E. A. 2004. Organization and evolution of the flavin-containing monooxygenase genes of human and mouse: Identification of novel gene and pseudogene clusters. Pharmacogenetics 14:117–130.
Hirvonen, A. 1999. Polymorphisms of xenobiotic-metabolizing enzymes and susceptibility to cancer. Environ. Hlth. Perspect. 107:37–47.
Houlston, R. S. 1999. Glutathione S-transferase M1 status and lung cancer risk: A meta-analysis. Cancer Epidemiol. Biomarkers Prev. 8:675–682.
Hsia, T. C., Chung, J. G., Lu, H. F., Ho, H. C., Yang, C. C., Lu, K. H. and Hung, C. F. 2002. The effect of paclitaxel on 2-aminofluorene-DNA adducts formation and arylamine *N*-acetyltransferase activity and gene expression in human lung tumor cells (A549). Fd. Chem. Toxicol. 40:697–703.
Huijzer, J. C., Adams, J. D. Jr., Jaw, J.-Y., and Yost, G. S. 1989. Inhibition of 3-methylindole bioactivation by the cytochrome P-450 suicide substrates 1-aminobenzotriazole and α-methylbenzylaminobenzotriazole. Drug Metab. Dispos. 17:37–42.
Hukkanen, J., Lassila, A., Päivärinta, Valanne, S., Sarpo, S., Hakkola, J., Pelkonen, O., and Raunio, H. 2000. Induction and regulation of xenobiotic-metabolizing cytochrome P450s in the human A549 lung adenocarcinoma cell line. Am. J. Respir. Cell Mol. Biol. 22:360–366.
Hukkanen, J., Pelkonen, O., Hakkola, J., and Raunio, H. 2002. Expression and regulation of xenobiotic-metabolizing enzymes in human lung. Crit. Rev. Toxicol. 32:391–411.
Hukkanen, J., Vaisanen, T., Lassila, A., Piipari, R., Anttila, S., Pelkonen, O., Raunio, H., and Hakkola, J. 2003. Regulation of CYP3A5 by glucocorticoids and cigarette smoke in human lung-derived cells. J. Pharmacol. Exp. Therap. 304:745–752.
Hung, R., Boffetta, P., Brockmöller, J., Butkiewicz, D., Cascorbi, I., Clapper, M. L., Garte, S., Haugen, A., Hirvonen, A., Anttila, S., Kalina, I., Le Marchand, L., London, S. J., Rannug, A., Romkes, M., Salagovic, J., Schoket, B., Gaspari, L., and Taioli, E. 2003. CYP1A1 and GSTM1 genetic polymorphisms and lung cancer risk in Caucasian non-smokers: a pooled analysis. Carcinogenesis 24:875–882.
Iyer, L. V., Ho, M. N., Shinn, W. M., Bradford, W. W., Tanga, M. J., Nath, S. S., and Green, C. E. 2003. Glucuronidation of 1′-hydroxyestragole (1-HE) by human UDP-glucuronosyltransferases UGT2B7 and UGT1A9. Toxicol. Sci. 73:36–43.
Jaiswal, A. K. 1994. Human NAD(P)H:quinone oxidoreductase 2. Gene structure, activity, and tissue-specific expression. J. Biol. Chem. 269:14502–14508.

Jalas, J. R., Ding, X. and Murphy, S. E. 2003. Comparative metabolism of the tobacco-specific nitrosamines 4-(methylnitrosamino)-1-(3-pyridyl)-1-butanone and 4-(methylnitrosamino)-1-(3-pyridyl)-1-butanol by rat cytochrome P4502A3 and human cytochrome P450 2A13. Drug Metab. Dispos. 31:1199–1202.

Jalas, J. R., Hecht, S. S., and Murphy, S. E. 2005. Cytochrome P450 enzymes as catalysts of metabolism of 4-(methylnitrosamino)-1-(3-pyridyl)-1-butanone, a tobacco specific carcinogen. Chem. Res. Toxicol. 18:95–110.

Jalbert, G., and Castonguay, A. 1992. Effects of NSAIDs on NNK-induced pulmonary and gastric tumorigenesis in A/J mice. Cancer Lett. 66:21–28.

Jiang, H., Vudathala, D. K., Blair, I. A., and Penning, T. M. 2006. Competing roles of aldo-keto reductase 1A1 and cytochrome P4501B1 in benzo[*a*]pyrene-7,8-diol activation in human bronchoalveolar H358 cells: Role of AKRs in P4501B1 induction. Chem. Res. Toxicol. 19:68–78.

Joseph, P., Xie, T., Xu, Y., and Jaiswal, A. K. 1994. NAD(P)H :Quinone oxidoreductase 1 (DT-diaphorase): Expression, regulation and role in cancer. Oncology Res. 6:525–532.

Kaster, J. K., and Yost, G. S. 1997. Production and characterization of specific antibodies: Utilization to predict organ- and species-selective pneumotoxicity of 3-methylindole. Toxicol. Appl. Pharmacol. 143:324–337.

Kim, J. H., Sherman, M. E., Curriero, F. C., Guengerich, F. P., Strickland, P. T., and Sutter, T. R. 2004. Expression of cytochromes P450 1A1 and 1B1 in human lung from smokers, non-smokers, and ex-smokers. Toxicol. Appl. Pharmacol. 199:210–219.

Kim, M. J., Kim, H., Cha, I. J., Park, J. S., Shon, J. H., Liu, K. H., and Shin, J. G. 2005. High-throughput screening of inhibitory potential of nine cytochrome P450 enzymes in vitro using liquid chromatography/tandem mass spectrometry. Rapid Commun. Mass Spectrom. 19:2651–2658.

Kivisto, K. T., Fritz, P., Linder, A., Friedel, G., Beaune, P., and Kroemer, H. K. 1995. Immunohistochemical localization of cytochrome P450 3A in human pulmonary carcinomas and normal bronchial tissues. Histochem. Cell Biol. 103:25–29.

Kivistö, K. T., Griese, E.-U., Stüven, T., Fritz, P., Friedel, G., Kroemer,, H. K., and Zanger, U. M. 1997. Analysis of CYP2D6 expression in human lung: Implications for the association between CYP2D6 activity and susceptibility to lung cancer. Pharmacogenetics 7:295–302.

Krieter, P. A., Ziegler, D. M., Hill, K. E., and Burk, R. F. 1984. Increased biliary GSSG efflux from rat livers perfused with thiocarbamide substrates for the flavin-containing monooxygenase. Mol. Pharmacol. 26:122–127.

Krueger, S. K., and Williams, D. E. 2005. Mammalian flavin-containing monooxygenases: structure/function, genetic polymorphisms and role in drug metabolism. Pharmacol. Therap. 106:357–387.

Krueger, S. K., Martin, S. R., Yueh, M.-F., Pereira, C. B., and Williams, D. E. 2002a. Identification of active flavin-containing monooxygenase isoform 2 in human lung and characterization of expressed protein. Drug Metab. Dispos. 30:34–41.

Krueger, S. K., Siddens, L. K., Henderson, M. C., Andreasen, E. A., Tanguay, R. L., Pereira, C. B., Cabacungan, E. T., Hines, R. N., Ardlie, K. G., and Williams, D. E. 2005. Haplotype and functional analysis of four flavin-containing monooxygenase isoform 2 (FMO2) polymorphisms in Hispanics. Pharmacogenetics Genomics 15:245–256.

Krueger, S. K., Siddens, L. K., Martin, S. R., Yu, Z., Pereira, C. B., Cabacungan, E. T., Hines, R. N., Ardlie, K. G., Raucy, J. L., and Williams, D. E. 2004. Differences in FMO2*1 allelic frequency between Hispanics of Puerto Rican and Mexican descent. Drug Metab. Dispos. 32:1337–1340.

Krueger, S. K., Williams, D. E., Yueh, M. F., Martin, S. R., Hines, R. N., Raucy, J. L., Dolphin, C. T., Shephard, E. A., and Phillips, I. R. 2002b. Genetic polymorphisms of flavin-containing monooxygenase (FMO). Drug Metab. Rev. 34:523–532.

Krueger, S. K., Yueh, M.-F., Martin, S. R., Pereira, C. B., and Williams, D. E. 2001. Characterization of expressed full-length and truncated FMO2 from rhesus monkey. Drug Metab. Dispos. 29:693–700.

Krysan, K., Reckamp, K. L., Sharma, S., and Dubinett, S. M. 2006. The potential and rationale for COX-2 inhibitors in lung cancer. Anticancer Agents Med. Chem. 6:209–220.

Kuehl, G. E., and Murphy, S. E. 2003. N-Glucuronidation of nicotine and cotinine by human liver microsomes and heterologously expressed UDP-glucuronosyltransferases. Drug Metab. Dispos. 31:1361–1368.

Lafite, P., Dijols, S., Buisson, D., Machery, A. C., Zeldin, D. C., Dansette, P. M., and Mansuy, D. 2006. Design and synthesis of selective, high-affinity inhibitors of human cytochrome P450 2 J2. Med. Chem. Lett. 16:2777–2780.

Lanza, D. L., and Yost, G. S. 2001. Selective dehydrogenation/oxygenation of 3-methylindole by cytochrome P450 enzymes. Drug Metab. Dispos. 29:950–953.

Lanza, D. L., Code, E., Crespi, C. L., Gonzalez, F. J., and Yost, G. S. 1999. Specific dehydrogenation of 3-methylindole and epoxidation of naphthalene by recombinant human CYP2F1 expressed in lymphoblastoid cells. Drug Metab. Dispos. 27:798–803.

Le Marchand, L., Sivaraman, L., Pierce, L., Seifried, A., Lum, A., Wilkens, L. R. and Lau, A. F. 1998. Associations of *CYP1A1*, *GSTM1*, and *CYP2E1* polymorphisms with lung cancer suggest cell type specificities to tobacco carcinogens. Cancer Res. 58:4858–4863.

Leslie, E. M., Ito, K., Upadhyaya, P., Hecht, S. S., Deeley, R. G., and Cole, S. P. 2001. Transport of the beta-*O*-glucuronide conjugate of the tobacco-specific carcinogen 4-(methylnitrosamino)-1-(3-pyridyl)-1-butanol (NNAL) by the multidrug resistance protein 1 (MRP1). Requirement for glutathione or a non-sulfur-containing analog. J. Biol. Chem. 276:27846–27854.

Leslie, E. M., Deeley, R. G., and Cole, S. P. 2001. Toxicological relevance of the multidrug resistance protein 1, MRP1 (ABCC1) and related transporters. Toxicology 167:3–23.

Leslie, E. M., Deeley, R. G., and Cole, S. P. 2005. Multidrug resistance proteins: role of P-glycoprotein, MRP1, MRP2, and BCRP (ABCG2) in tissue defense. Toxicol. Appl. Pharmacol. 204:216–237.

Lin, P., Chang, Y.-C., Chen, C.-H., Yang, W.-J., Cheng, Y.-H., and Chang, L. W. 2004. A comparative study on the effect of 2,3,7,8-tetrachlorodibenzo-*p*-dioxin, polychlorinated biphenyl 126 and estrogen in human bronchial epithelial cells. Toxicol. Appl. Pharmacol. 195:83–91.

Lo-Guidice, J.-M., Allorge, D., Cauffiez, C., Chevalier, D., Lafitte, J.-J., Lhermitte, M., and Broly, F. 2002. Genetic polymorphism of the human cytochrome P450 CYP4B1: Evidence for a non-functional allelic variant. Pharmacogenetics 12:367–374.

London, S. J., Daly, A. K., Cooper, J., Carpenter, C. L., Navidi, W. C., Ding, L., and Idle, J. R. 1996a. Lung cancer risk in relation to the *CYP2Ea Rsa I* genetic polymorphism among African-Americans and Caucasians in Los Angeles County. Pharmacogenetics 6:151–158.

London, S. J., Daly, A. K., Leathart, J. B. S., Navidi, W. C., and Idle, J. R. 1996b. Lung cancer risk in relation to the *CYP2C9*1/CYP2C9*2* genetic polymorphism among African-Americans and Caucasians in Los Angeles County, California. Pharmacogenetics 6:527–533.

London, S. J., Daly, A. K., Fairbrother, K. S., Holmes, C., Carpenter, C. L., Navidi, W. C., and Idle, J. R. 1995. Lung cancer risk in African-Americans in relation to a race-specific *CYP1A1* polymorphism. Cancer Res. 55:6035–6037.

London, S. J., Idle, J. R., Daly, A. K., and Coetzee, G. A. 1999. Genetic variation of CYP2A6, smoking, and risk of cancer. Lancet 353:898–899.

London, S. J., Lehman, T. A., and Taylor, J. A. 1997. Myeloperoxidase genetic polymorphism and lung cancer risk. Cancer Res. 57:5001–5003.

Loneragan, G. H., Gould, D. H., Mason, G. L., Garry, F. B., Yost, G. S., Lanza, D. L., Miles, D. G., Hoffman, B. W., and Mills, L. J. 2001. Association of 3-methyleneindolenine, a toxic metabolite of 3-methylindole, with acute interstitial pneumonia in feedlot cattle. Amer. J. Vet. Res. 62:1525–1530.

Long, D. J., 2nd, and Jaiswal, J. K. 2000. NRH:Quinone oxidoreductase2 (NQO2). Chem.-Biol. Interact. 129:99–112.

Loriot, M.-A., Rebuissou, S., Oscarson, M., Cenee, S., Miyamoto, M., Ariyoshi, N., Kamataki, T., Hemon, D., Beaune, P., and Stucker, J. 2001. Genetic polymorphisms of cytochrome P450 2A6 in a case–control study on lung cancer in a French population. Pharmacogenetics 11:39–44.

Mace, K., Bowman, E. D., Vautravers, P., Shields, P. G., Harris, C. C., and Pfeifer, A. M. 1998. Characterization of xenobiotic-metabolising enzyme expression in human bronchial mucosa and peripheral lung tissues. Eur. J. Cancer 34:914–920.

Maciag, A., Sithanandam, G., and Anderson, L. M. 2004. Mutant K-*ras*^{V12} increases COX-2, peroxides and DNA damage in lung cells. Carcinogenesis 25:2231–2237.

Malkinson, A. M. 1992. Primary lung tumors in mice: an experimentally manipulable model of human adenocarcinoma. Cancer Res. 52:2670S–2776S.

Manenti, G., Galbiati, F., Noci, S., and Dragani, T. A. 2003. Outbred CD-1 mice carry the susceptibility at the pulmonary adenoma susceptibility 1 (*Pas1*) locus. Carcinogenesis 24:1143–1148.

Mao, J. T., Cui, X., Reckamp, K., Liu, M., Krysan, K., Dalwadi, H., Sharma, S., Hazra, S., Strieter, R., Gardner, B., and Dubinett, S. M. 2005. Chemoprevention strategies with cyclooxygenase-2 inhibitors for lung cancer. Clin. Lung Cancer 7:30–39.

Mao, J. T., Fishbein, M. C., Adams, B., Roth, M. D., Goodglick, L., Hong, L., Burdick, M., Strieter, E. R., Holmes, C., Tashkin, D. P., and Dubinett, S. M. 2006. Celecoxib decreases Ki-67 proliferative index in active smokers. Clin. Cancer Res. 12:314–320.

Marano, F., Boland, S., Bonvallot, V., Baulig, A., and Baeza-Squiban, A. 2002. Human airway epithelial cells in culture for studying the molecular mechanisms of the inflammatory response triggered by diesel exhaust particles. Cell Biol. Toxicol. 18:315–320.

Martey, C. A., Pollock, S. J., Turner, C. K., O'Reilly, K. M., Baglole, C. J., Phipps, R. P., and Sime, P. J. 2004. Cigarette smoke induces cyclooxygenase-2 and microsomal prostaglandin E2 synthase in human lung fibroblasts: Implications for lung inflammation and cancer. Am. J. Physiol. Lung Cell. Mol. Physiol. 287:L981-L991.

Marton, T. B., Zhang, Z., Yu, G., and Musante, C. J. 2001. Three-dimensional computer modeling of the human upper respiratory tract. Cell Biochem. Biophys. 35:255–261.

Matsuzoe, D., Hideshima, T., Iwasaki, A., Yoneda, S., Kawahara, K., Shirakusa, T., and Kimura, A. 2001. Glutathione S-transferase μ1 null genotype is associated with K-*ras* gene mutation in lung adenocarcinoma among smokers. Carcinogenesis 22:1327–1330.

McCarver, D. G., and Hines, R. N. 2002. The ontogeny of human drug-metabolizing enzymes: Phase II conjugation enzymes and regulatory mechanisms. J. Pharmacol. Exp. Therap. 300:361–366.

Minard, K. R., Einstein, D. R., Jacob, R. E., Kabilan, S., Kuprat, A. P., Timchalk, C., Trease, L. L., and Corley, R. A. 2006. Application of magnetic resonance (MR) inaging for the development and validation of computational fluid dynamic (CFD) models of the rat respiratory system. Inhalation Toxicol. 18:787–794.

Miyamoto, M., Umetsu, Y., Dosaka-Akita, H., Sawamura, Y., Yokota, J., Kunitoh, H., Nemoto, N., Sato, K., Ariyoshi, N., and Kamataki, T. 1999.

CYP2A6 gene deletion reduces susceptibility to lung cancer. Biochem. Biophys. Res. Commun. 261:658–660.

Mollerup, S., Ryberg, D., Hewer, A., Phillips, D. H., and Haugen, A. 1999. Sex differences in lung CYP1A1 expression and DNA adduct levels among lung cancer patients. Cancer Res. 59:3317–3320.

Muller, J., Huaux, F., Moreau, N., Misson, P., Heilier, J.-F., Delos, M., Arras, M., Fonseca, A., Nagy, J. B., and Lison, D. 2005. Respiratory toxicity of multi-wall carbon nanotubes. Toxicol. Appl. Pharmacol. 207:221–231.

Nagata, T., Williams, D. E., and Ziegler, D. M. 1990. Substrate specificities of rabbit lung and porcine liver flavin-containing monooxygenases: Differences due to substrate size. Chem. Res. Toxicol. 3:372–376.

Nakajima, M., Yamamoto, T., Nunoya, K.-I., Yokoi, T., Nagashima, K., Inoue, K., Funae, Y., Shimada, N., Kamataki, T., and Kuroiwa, Y. 1996. Role of human cytochrome P4502A6 in C-oxidation of nicotine. Drug Metabol. Dispos. 24:1212–1217.

Narasaki, F., Matsuo, I., Ikuno, N., Fukuda, M., Soda, H., and Oka, M. 1996. Multidrug resistance-associated protein (MRP) gene expression in human lung cancer. Anticancer Res. 16:2079–2082.

Nebert, D. W., McKinnon, R. A., and Puga, A. 1996. Human drug-metabolizing enzyme polymorphisms: Effects on toxicity and cancer. DNA Cell. Biol. 15:273–280.

Newton, R. W. 1975. Side effects of drugs used to treat tuberculosis. Scott. Med. J. 20:47–49.

Nichols, W. K., Mehta, R., Skordos, K., Mace, K., Pfeifer, A. M., Carr, B. A., Minko, T., Burchiel, S. W., and Yost, G. S. 2003. 3-Methylindole-induced toxicity to human bronchial epithelial cell lines. Toxicol. Sci. 71:229–236.

Oguri, T., Takahashi, T., Miyazaki, M., Isobe, T., Kohno, N., Mackenzie, P. I., and Fujiwara, Y. 2004. UGT1A10 is responsible for SN-38 glucuronidation and its expression in human lung cancers. Anticancer Res. 24:2893–2896.

Onderwater, R. C., Commandeur, J. N., Groot, E. J., Sitters, A., Menge, W. M., and Vermeulen, N. P. 1998. Cytotoxicity of a series of mono- and di-substituted thioureas in freshly isolated rat hepatocytes: A preliminary structure–toxicity relationship study. Toxicology 125:117–129.

Paine, M. F., Hart, H. L., Ludington, S. S., Haining, R. L., Rettie, A. E., and Zeldin, D. C. 2006. The human intestinal cytochrome P450 "pie". Drug Metab. Dispos. 34:880–886.

Peluso, M., Neri, M., Margarino, G., Mereu, C., Munnia, A., Ceppi, M., Buratti, M., Felletti, R., Stea, F., Quaglia, R., Puntoni, R., Taioli, E., Garte, S., and Bonassi, S. 2004. Comparison of DNA adduct levels in nasal mucosa, lymphocytes and bronchial mucosa of cigarette smokers and interaction with metabolic gene polymorphisms. Carcinogenesis 25:2459–2465.

Perera, F. P., Mooney, L. A., Stampfer, M., Phillips, D. H., Bell, D. A., Rundle, A., Cho, S., Tsai, W.-Y., Ma, J., Blackwood, A., and Tang, D. 2002. Associations between carcinogen-DNA damage, glutathione S-transferase genotypes, and risk of lung cancer in the prospective Physicians' Health Cohort Study. Carcinogenesis 23:1641–1646.

Perez-Tomas, R. 2006. Multidrug resistance: retrospect and prospects in anticancer drug treatment. Curr. Med. Chem. 13:1859–1876.

Petruska, J. M., Mosebrook, D. R., Jakab, G. J., and Trush, M. A. 1992. Myeloperoxidase-enhanced formation of (±)-trans-7,8-dihydroxy-7,8-dihydrobenzo[*a*]pyrene-DNA adducts in lung tissue in vitro: A role of pulmonary inflammation in the bioactivation of a procarcinogen. Carcinogenesis 13:1075–1081.

Pineau, T., Fernandez-Salguero, P., Lee, S .S. T., McPhail, T., Ward, J. M., and Gonzalez, F. J. 1995. Neonatal lethality associated with respiratory distress in mice lacking cytochrome P4501A2. Natl. Acad. Sci. USA 92:5134–5138.

Poch, M. T., Cutler, N. S., Yost, G. S., and Hines, R. N. 2005. Molecular mechanisms regulating human *CYP4B1* lung-selective expression. Drug Metab. Dispos. 33:1174–1184.

Poulsen, L. L., Hyslop, R. M., and Ziegler, D. M. 1979. S-Oxygenation of N-substituted thioureas catalyzed by the pig liver microsomal FAD-containing monooxygenase. Arch. Biochem. Biophys. 198:78–88.

Qian, L., and de Montellano, P. R. 2006. Oxidative activation of thiaacetazone by the *Mycobacterium tuberculosis* flavin monooxygenase EtaA and human FMO1 and FMO3. Chem. Res. Toxicol. 19:443–449.

Rahman, Q., Abidi, P., Afaq, F., Schiffmann, D., Mossman, B. T., Kamp, D. W., and Athar, M. 1999. Glutathione redox system in oxidative lung injury. Crit. Rev. Toxicol. 29:543–568.

Ramakanth, S., Thornton-Manning, J. R., Wang, H., Maxwell, H., and Yost, G. S. 1994. Correlation between pulmonary cytochrome P450 transcripts and the organ-selective pneumotoxicity of 3-methylindole. Toxicol. Lett. 71:77–85.

Regal, K. A., Laws, G. M., Yuan, C., Yost, G. S., and Skiles, G. L. 2001. Detection and characterization of DNA adducts of 3-methylindole. Chem. Res. Toxicol. 14:1014–1024.

Ren, Q., Murphy, S. E., Zheng, Z., and Lazarus, P. 2000. O-Glucuronidation of the lung carcinogen 4-(methylnitrosamino)-1-(3-pyridyl)-1-butanol (NNAL) by human UDP-glucuronosyltransferases 2B7 and 1A9. Drug Metab. Dispos. 28:1352–1360.

Richard, K., Hume, R., Kaptein, E., Stanley, E. L., Visser, T. J., and Coughtrie, M. W. 2001. Sulfation of thyroid hormone and dopamine during human development: Ontogeny of phenol sulfotransferases and arylsulfatase in liver, lung, and brain. J. Clin. Endocrinol. Metab. 86:2734–2742.

Rioux, N., and Castonguay, A. 1998a. Inhibitors of lipoxygenase: A new class of cancer chemopreventive agents. Carcinogenesis 19:1393–1400.

Rioux, N., and Castonguay, A. 1998b. Prevention of NNK-induced lung tumorigenesis in A/J mice by acetylsalicylic acid and NS-398. Res. 58:5354–5360.

Risch, A., Wikman, H., Thiel, S., Schmezer, P., Edler, L., Drings, P., Dienemann, H., Kayser, K., Schulz, V., Spiegelhalder, B. and Bartsch, H. 2001. Glutathione-S-transferase M1, M3, T1 and P1 polymorphisms and susceptibility to non-small-cell lung cancer subtypes and hamartomas. Pharmacogenetics 11:757–764.

Rivera, S. P., Saarikoski, S. T., and Hankinson, O. 2002. Identification of a novel dioxin-inducible cytochrome P-450. Mol Pharmacol. 61:255–259.

Rosvold, E. A., McGlynn, K. A., Lustbader, E. D., and Buetow, K. H. 1995. Identification of an NAD(P)H:quinone oxidoreductase polymorphism and its association with lung cancer and smoking. Pharmacogenetics 5:199–206.

Runge, D. M., Stock, T. W., Lehmann, T., Taege, C., Bernauer, U., Stolz, D. B., Hofmann, S., and Foth, H. 2001. Expression of cytochrome P450 2E1 in normal human bronchial epithelia cells and activation by ethanol in culture. Arch. Toxicol. 75:335–345.

Sargent, L. M., Senft, J. R., Lowry, D. T., Jefferson, A. M., Tyson, F. L., Malkinson, A. M., Coleman, A. E., and Reynolds, S. H. 2002. Specific chromosomal aberrations in mouse lung adenocarcinoma cell lines detected by spectral karyotyping: a comparison with human lung adenocarcinoma. Cancer Res. 62:1152–1157.

Schoket, B., Phillips, D. H., Kostic, S., and Vincze, I. 1998. Smoking-associated bulky DNA adducts in bronchial tissue related to *CYP1A1 MspI* and *GSTM1* genotypes in lung patients. Carcinogenesis 19:841–846.

Schultz, M. A., Zhang, L., Gu, Y. Z., Baker, G. L., Fannuchi, M. V., Padua, A. M., Gurske, W. A., Morin, D., Penn, S. G., Jovanovich, S. B., Plopper, C. G., and Buckpitt, A. R. 2004. Gene expression analysis in response to lung toxicants: I. Sequencing and microarray development. Am. J. Respir. Cell Mol. Biol. 30:296–310.

Sheets, P. L., Yost, G. S., and Carlson, G. P. 2004. Benzene metabolism in human lung cell lines BEAS-2B and A549 and cells overexpressing CYP2F 1. J. Bio-Chem. Mol. Toxicol. 18:92–99.

Sherratt, P. J., Pulford, D. J., Harrison, D. J., Green, T., and Hayes, J. D. 1997. Evidence that human class Theta glutathione S-transferase T1-1 can catalyse the activation of dichloromethane, a liver and lung carcinogen in the mouse. Comparison of the tissue distribution of GSTT1-1 with that of classes Alpha, Mu and Pi GST in human. Biochem. J. 326(Pt. 3):837–846.

Shields, P. P., Bowman, E. D., Harrington, A. M., Doan, V. T., and Weston, A. 1993. Polycyclic aromatic hydrocarbon–DNA adducts in human lung and cancer susceptibility genes. Cancer Res. 53:3486–3492.

Singhal, S. S., Yadav, S., Singhal, J., Zajac, E., Awasthi, Y. C., and Awasthi, S. 2005. Depletion of FLIP76 sensitizes lung cancer cells to doxorubicin. Biochem. Pharmacol. 70:481–488.

Smith, B. J., Curtis, J. F., and Eling, T. E. 1991. Bioactivation of xenobiotics by prostaglandin H synthase. Chem. Biol. Interact. 79:245–264.

Smith, B. B. J., Harper, P. A., Wong, J. M. Y., Lam, M. S. M., Reid, K. R., Petsikas, D., and Massey, T. E. 2001. Human lung microsomal cytochrome P4501A1 (CYP1A1) activities: Impact of smoking status and CYP1A1, aryl hydrocarbon receptor, and glutathione S-transferase M1 genetic polymorphisms. Cancer Epidemiol. Biomarkers Prev. 10:839–853.

Smith, C. A., and Harrison, D .J. 1997. Association between polymorphism in genes for microsomal epoxide hydrolase and susceptibility to emphysema. Lancet 350:630–633.

Smith, G. B., Bend, J. R., Bedard, L. L., Reid, K. R., Petsikas, D., and Massey, T. E. 2003. Biotransformation of 4-(methylnitrosamino)-1-(3-pyridyl)-1-butanone (NNK) in peripheral human lung microsomes. Drug Metab. Dispos. 31:1134–1141.

Smith, L. L. 1985. Paraquat toxicity. Philos. Trans. R. Soc. Lond. B Biol. Sci. 311:647–657.

Smith, L. L. 1987. Mechanism of paraquat toxicity in lung and its relevance to treatment. Human Toxicol. 6:31–36.

Smith, L. L., Rose, M. S., and Wyatt, I. 1978. The pathology and biochemistry of paraquat. Ciba Found. Symp. 65:321–341.

Smith, P. B., and Crespi, C. 2002. Thiourea toxicity in mouse C3H/10T1/2 cells expressing human flavin-dependent monooxygenase 3. Biochem. Pharmacol. 63:1941–1948.

Song, N., Tan, W., Xing, D. and Lin, D. 2001. CYP1A1 polymorphism and risk of lung cancer in relation to tobacco smoking: A case-control study in China. Carcinogenesis 22:11–16.

Sorenson, M., Autrup, H., Tjonneland, A., Overvad, K., and Raaschou-Nielsen, O. 2004. Glutathione S-transferase T1 null-genotype is associated with an increased risk of lung cancer. Int. J. Cancer 110:219–224.

Spivack, S. D., Hurteau, G. J., Reilly, A. A., Aldous, K. M., Ding, X., and Kaminsky, L. S. 2001. CYP1B1 expression in human lung. Drug Metab. Dispos. 29:916–922.

Strassburg, C. P., Strassburg, A., Nguyen, N., Li, Q., Manns, M. P., and Tukey, R. H. 1999. Regulation and function of family 1 and family 2 UDP-glucuronosyltransferase genes (UGT1A, UGT2B) in human oesophagus. Biochem. J. 338(Pt. 2):489–498.

Stucker, I., de Waziers, I., Cenee, S., Bignon, J., Depierre, A., Millerson, B., Beaune, P., and Hemon, D. 1999. GSTM1, smoking and lung cancer: A case–control study. Int. J. Epidemiol. 28:829–835.

Stucker, I., Hirvonen, A., de Waziers, I., Cabelguenne, A., Mitrunen, K., Cénée, S., Koum-Besson, E., Hémon, D., Beaune, P., and Lorlot, M.-A. 2002. Genetic polymorphisms of glutathione S-transferases as modulators of lung cancer susceptibility. Carcinogenesis 23:1475–1481.

Stuckler, D., Singhal, J., Singhal, S. S., Yadav, S., Awasthi, Y. C., and Awasthi, S. 2005. RLIP76 transports vinorelbine and mediates drug resistance in non-small cell lung cancer. Cancer Res. 65:991–998.

Su, T., and Ding, X. 2004. Regulation of the cytochrome P450 2A genes. Toxicol. Appl. Pharmacol. 199:285–294.

Su, T., Bao, Z., Zhang, Q.-Y., Smith, T. J., Hong, J.-Y., and Ding, X. 2000. Human cytochrome P450 CYP2A13: Predominant expression in the respiratory tract and its high efficiency in metabolic activation of a tobacco-specific carcinogen, 4-(methylnitrosamino)-1-(3-pyridyl)-1-butanone. Cancer Res. 60:5074–5079.

Sunaga, N., Kohno, T., Yanagitani, N., Sugimura, H., Kunitoh, H., Tamura, T., Takei, T., Tsuchiya, S., Saito, R., and Yokota, J. 2002. Contribution of the NQO1 and GSTT1 polymorphisms to lung adenocarcinoma susceptibility. Cancer Epidemiol. Biomarkers Prev. 11:730–738.

Sweeney, C., Nazar-Stewart, V., Stapleton, P. L., Eaton, D. L., and Vaughan, T. L. 2003. Glutathione S-transferase M1, T1, and P1 polymorphisms and survival among lung cancer patients. Cancer Epidemiol. Biomarkers Prev. 12:527–533.

Taioli, E., Ford, J., Trachman, J., Li, Y., Demopoulos, R., and Garte, S. 1998. Lung cancer risk and CYP1A1 genotype in African Americans. Carcinogenesis 19:813–817.

Tan, W., Chen, G. F., Xing, D. Y., Song, C. Y., Kadlubar, F. F., and Lin, D. X. 2001. Frequency of CYP2A6 gene deletion and its relation to risk of lung and esophageal cancer in the Chinese population. Int. J. Cancer 95:96–101.

Thum, T., Erpenbeck, V. J., Moeller, J., Hohlfeld, J. M., Krug, N., and Borlak, J. 2006. Expression of xenobiotic metabolizing enzymes in different lung compartments of smokers and nonsmokers. Environ. Hlth. Perspect. 114:1655–1661.

Tiano, H. F., Wang, R.-L., Hosokawa, M., Crespi, C., Tindall, K. R., and Langenbach, R. 1994. Human CYP2A6 activation of 4-(methylnitrosamino)-1-(3-pyridyl)-1-butanone (NNK): Mutational specificity in the *gpt* gene of AS52 cells. Carcinogenesis 15:2859–2866.

Tong, M., Ding, Y., and Tai, H.-H. 2006. Reciprocal regulation of cyclooxygenase-2 and 15-hydroxyprostaglandin dehydrogenase expression in A549 human lung adenocarcinoma cells. Carcinogenesis 27:2170–2179.

Tsuji, P. A., and Walle, T. 2006. Inhibition of benzo[*a*]pyrene-activating enzymes and DNA binding in human bronchial epithelial BEAS-2B cells by methoxylated flavonoids. Carcinogenesis 27:1579–1585.

Turgeon, D., Carrier, J. S., Chouinard, S., and Belanger, A. 2003. Glucuronidation activity of the UGT2B17 enzymes toward xenobiotics. Drug Metab. Dispos. 31:670–676.

Turgeon, D., Carrier, J. S., Levesque, E., Hum, D. W., and Belanger, A. 2001. Relative enzymatic activity, protein stability, and tissue distribution of human steroid-metabolizing UGT2B subfamily members. Endocrinology 142:778–787.

Tyndale, R. F., and Sellers, E. M. 2001. Variable CYP2A6-mediated nicotine metabolism alters smoking behavior and risk. Drug Metab. Dispos. 29:548–552.

Tynes, R. E., Sabourin, P. J., and Hodgson, E. 1985. Identification of distinct hepatic and pulmonary forms of microsomal flavin-containing monooxygenase in the mouse and rabbit. Biochem. Biophys. Res. Commun. 126:1069–1075.

Uchaipichat, V., Mackenzie, P. I., Elliot, D., and Miners, J. O. 2006. Selectivity of substrate (trifluoperazine) and inhibitor (amitriptyline, androsterone, canrenoic acid, hecogenin, phenylbutazone, quinidine, quinine, and sulfinpyrazone) "probes" for human UDP-glucuronosyltransferases. Drug Metab. Dispos. 34:449–456.

Usmani, K. A., Karoly, E. D., Hodgson, E., and Rose, R. L. 2004. In vitro sulfoxidation of thioether compounds by human cytochrome P450 and flavin-containing monooxygenase isoforms with particular reference to the CYP2C subfamily. Drug Metab. Dispos. 32:333–339.

Vannelli, T. A., Dykam, A., and de Montellano, P. R. 2002. The antituberculosis drug ethionamide is activated by a flavoprotein monooxygenase. J. Biol. Chem. 277:12824–12829.

Van Vleet, T. R., Macé, K., and Coulombe, R. A. Jr. 2002. Comparative aflatoxin B1 activation and cytotoxicity in human bronchial cells expressing cytochromes P450 1A2 and 3A4. Cancer Res. 62:105–112.

Verheyen, G. R., Nuijten, J. M., Van Hummelen, P., and Schoeters, G. R. 2004. Microarray analysis of the effect of diesel exhaust particles on in vitro cultured macrophages. Toxicol. In Vitro 18:377–391.

Von Weymarn, L. B., Zhang, Q.-Y., Ding, X., and Hollenberg, P. F. 2005. Effects of 8-methoxypsoralen on cytochrome P450 2A13. Carcinogenesis 26:621–629.

Waldon, D. J., Buhl, A. E., Baker, C. A., and Johnson, G. A. 1989. Is minoxidil sulfate the active metabolite for hair growth? J. Invest. Dermatol. 92:538–545.

Wan, J., Carr, B. A., Cutler, S., Lanza, D. L., Hines, R. N., and Yost, G. S. 2005. SP1 and SP3 regulate basal transcription of the human CYP2F1 gene. Drug Metab. Dispos. 33:1244–1253.

Wang, H., and Negishi, M. 2003. Transcriptional regulation of cytochrome P450 2B genes by nuclear receptors. Curr. Drug Metab. 4:515–525.

Wang, H., Tan, W., Hao, B., Miao, X., Zhou, G., He, F., and Lin, D. 2003. Substantial reduction in risk of lung adenocarcinoma associated with genetic polymorphism in CYP2A13, the most active cytochrome P450 for the metabolic activation of tobacco-specific carcinogen NNK. Cancer Res. 63:8057–8061.

Wang, S.-L., He, X.-Y., and Hong, J.-Y. 2005. Human cytochrome P450 2S1: Lack of activity in the metabolic activation of several cigarette smoke carcinogens and in the metabolism of nicotine. Drug Metab. Dispos. 33:336–340.

Wang, S.-L., He, X.-Y., Shen, J., Wang, J.-S., and Hong, J.-Y. 2006. The missense genetic polymorphisms of human CYP2A13: Functional significance in carcinogen activation and identification of a null allelic variant. Toxicol. Sci. 94:38–45.

Watanabe, N., Dickinson, D. A., Krzywanski, D. M., Iles, K. E., Zhang, H., Venglarik, C. J., and Forman, H. J. 2002. A549 subclones demonstrate heterogeneity in toxicological sensitivity and antioxidant profile. Am. J. Physiol. Lung Cell Mol. Physiol. 283:L726-L736.

Wells, P. G., Mackenzi, P. I., Chowdhury, J. R., Buillemette, C., Gregory, P. A., Ishii, Y., Hansen, A. J., Kessler, F. K., Kim, P. M., Chowdhury, N. R., and Ritter, J. K. 2004. Glucuronidation and UDP-glucuronosyltransferases in health and disease. Drug Metab. Dispos. 32:281–290.

Wenzlaff, A. S., Cote, M. L., Bock, C. H., Land, S. J., Santer, S. K., Schwartz, D. R., and Schwartz, A. G. 2005. *CYP1A1* and *CYP1B1* polymorphisms and risk of lung cancer among never smokers: A population-based study. Carcinogenesis 26:2207–2212.

Whestine, J. R., Yueh, M.-F., Hopp, K. A., McCarver, D. G., Williams, D. E., Park, C.-S., Kang, J. H., Cha, Y.-N., Dolphin, C. T., Shephard, E. A., Phillips, I. R., and Hines, R. N. 2000. Ethnic differences in human flavin-containing monooxygenase 2 (FMO2) polymorphisms: Detection of expressed protein in African Americans. Toxicol. Appl. Pharmacol. 168:216–224.

Wiese, F. W., Thompson, P. A., and Kadlubar, F. F. 2001. Carcinogen substrate specificity of human COX-1 and COX- 2. Carcinogenesis 21:5–10.

Williams, D. E., Hale, S. E., Muerhoff, A. S., and Masters, B. S. S. 1985. Rabbit lung flavin-containing monooxygenase. Purification and induction during pregnancy. Mol. Pharmacol. 28:381–390.

Windmill, K. F., Gaedigk, A., Hall, P. M., Samaratunga, T., Grant, D. M., and McManus, M. E. 2000. Localization of *N*-acetyltransferases NAT1 and NAT2 in human tissues. Toxicol. Sci. 54:19–29.

Witschi, H., Espiritu, I., Dance, S. T., and Miller, M. S. 2002. A mouse lung tumor model of tobacco smoke carcinogenesis. Toxicol. Sci. 68:322–330.

Wu, S., Moomaw, C. R., Tomer, K. B., Falck, J. R., and Zeldin, D. C. 1996. Molecular cloning and expression of CYP2J2, a human cytochrome P450 arachidonic acid epoxygenase highly expressed in heart. J. Biol. Chem. 271:3460–3468.

Wu, X., Gwyn, K., Amos, C. I., Makan, N., Hong, W. K., and Spitz, M. R. 2001. The association of microsomal epoxide hydrolase polymorphisms and lung cancer risk in African-Americans and Mexican-Americans. Carcinogenesis 22:923–928.

Wu, X., Shi, H., Jiang, H., Kemp, B., Hong, W. K., Declos, G. L., and Spitz, M R. 1997. Associations between cytochrome *P4502E1* genotype, mutagen sensitivity, cigarette smoking and susceptibility to lung cancer. Carcinogenesis 18:967–973.

Xu, L. L., Wain, J. C., Miller, D. P., Thurston, S. W., Su, L., Lynch, T. J., and Christiani, D. C. 2001. The NAD(P)H:Quinone oxidoreductase 1 gene polymorphism and lung cancer: differential susceptibility based on smoking behavior. Cancer Epidemiol. Biomarkers Prev. 10:303–309.

Yang, A., Cardona, D. L., and Barile, F. A. 2002. In vitro cytotoxicity testing with fluorescence-based assays in cultured human lung and dermal cells. Cell Biol. Toxicol. 18:97–108.

Yang, M., Coles, B. F., Delongchamp, R., Lang, N. P., and Kadlubar, F. F. 2002. Effects of the ADH3, CYP2E1, and GSTP1 genetic polymorphisms on their expressions in Caucasian lung tissue. Lung Cancer 38:15–21.

Yao, R., Rioux, N., Castonguay, A., and You, M. 2000. Inhibition of COX-2 and induction of apoptosis: Two determinants of nonsteroidal anti-inflammatory drugs' chemoprevention efficacies in mouse lung tumorigenesis. Exp. Lung Res. 26:731–742.

Yueh, M.-F., Krueger, S. K., and Williams, D. E. 1997. Pulmonary flavin-containing monooxygenase (FMO) in rhesus macaque: Expression of FMO2 protein, mRNA and analysis of the cDNA. Biochim. Biophys. Acta 1350:267–271.

Yueh, M.-F., Nguyen, N., Famourzadeh, M., Strassburg, C. P., Oda, Y., Guengerich, F. P., and Tukey, R. H. 2001. The contribution of UDP-glucuronosyltransferase 1A9 on CYP1A2-mediated genotoxicity by aromatic and heterocyclic amines. Carcinogenesis 22:943–950.

Zeldin, D. C., Foley, J., Ma, J., Boyle, J. E., Pascual, J. M. S., Moomax, C. R., Tomer, K. B., Steenbergen, C., and Wu, S. 1996. CYP2 J subfamily P450s in the lung: Expression, localization, and potential functional significance. Mol. Pharmacol. 50:1111–1117.

Zhang, J., and Cashman, J. R. 2006. Quantitative analysis of *FMO* gene mRNA levels in human tissues. Drug Metab. Dispos. 34:19–26.

Zhang, J. Y., Wang, Y., and Prakash, C. 2006. Xenobiotic-metabolizing enzymes in human lung. Curr. Drug Metab. 7:939–948.

Zheng, Y. M., Henne, K. R., Charmley, P., Kim, R. B., McCarver, D. G., Cabacungan, E. T., Hines, R. N., and Rettie, A. E. 2003. Genotyping and site-directed mutagenesis of a cytochrome P450 meander Pro-X-Arg motif critical to CYP4B1 catalysis. Toxicol. Appl. Pharmacol. 186:119–126.

Zheng, Z., Fang, J.-L., and Lazarus, P. 2002. Glucuronidation: An important mechanism for detoxification of benzo[*a*]pyrene metabolites in aerodigestive tract tissues. Drug Metab. Dispos. 30:397–403.

Zhu L.-R., Thomas, P. E., Lu, G., Reuhl, K. R., Yang, G.-Y., Wang, L.-D., Wang, S.-L., Yang, C. S., He, X.-Y., and Hong, J.-Y. 2006. CYP2A13 in human respiratory tissues and lung cancers: an immunohistochemical study with a new peptide-specific antibody. Drug Metab. Dispos. 34:1672–1676.

Ziegler, D. M. 1982. Functional groups bearing sulfur. In Metabolism of Functional Groups, eds. W. B. Jakoby, J. R. Bend, and J. Caldwell, pp. 171–184. New York: Academic Press
Ziegler, D. M. 1988. Flavin-containing monooxygenases: Catalytic mechanism and substrate specificities. Drug Metab. Rev. 19:1–32.
Ziegler, D. M. 1993. Recent studies on the structure and function of multisubstrate flavin-containing monooxygenases. Annu. Rev. Pharmacol. Toxicol. 33:179–199.
Ziegler, D. M. 2002. An overview of the mechanism, substrate specificities and structure of FMOs. Drug Metab. Rev. 34:503–511.

14

Generation of Reactive Metabolites and Associated DNA Adducts from Benzene, Butadiene, and PAH in Bone Marrow. Their Effects on Hematopoiesis and Impact on Human Health

Colin Jefcoate and Michele Larsen
Department of Pharmacology and Center for Molecular and Environmental Toxicology, University of Wisconsin Madison, Madison, WI 53706, USA
e-mail: jefcoate@wisc.edu

Keywords: DMBA · BP · Benzene and Butadiene

14.1. Introduction

The bone marrow (BM) is the site of hematopoietic developmental processes, which originate from hematopoietic stem cell (HSC) progenitors. Their differentiation generates myeloid, erythroid, and lymphoid lineages that populate the blood, lymphatic system, and spleen. These cells migrate from the BM to sites of injury throughout the body (Alison et al. 2006; Greten et al. 2004). The BM plays a critical role in controlling hematopoiesis, angiogenesis, immune responses, and stromal responses to tissue injury. Thus, chemical affects in the BM manifest broad toxic and carcinogenic systemic consequences. The BM also provides a key site for tumor initiation by reactive chemicals, resulting in a variety of lymphomas and leukemias (Forrest et al. 2005; Boffetta, Jourenkova and Gustavsson 1997; Mastrangelo, Fadda and Marzia 1996; Recio, Saranko and Steen 2000). Benzene, butadiene, and polycyclic hydrocarbons (PAHs) disrupt each BM processes in this way.

Each of these chemicals produces multiple reactive metabolites (Figure 14.1 a–c), which will target not only DNA, but many proteins that contribute to the complex processes of hematopoiesis and cancer. It is unlikely that a single reactive metabolite is responsible. Indeed, we suspect that synergy may occur between chemicals that are toxic to cells in different ways, such as via oxidative stress or through reactive electrophiles. These mechanisms are cooperative since oxidative stress depletes cell glutathione (GSH), which, in turn, diminishes the protection against

A.A. Elfarra (ed.), *Advances in Bioactivation Research*, DOI: 10.1007/978-0-387-77300-1_14,

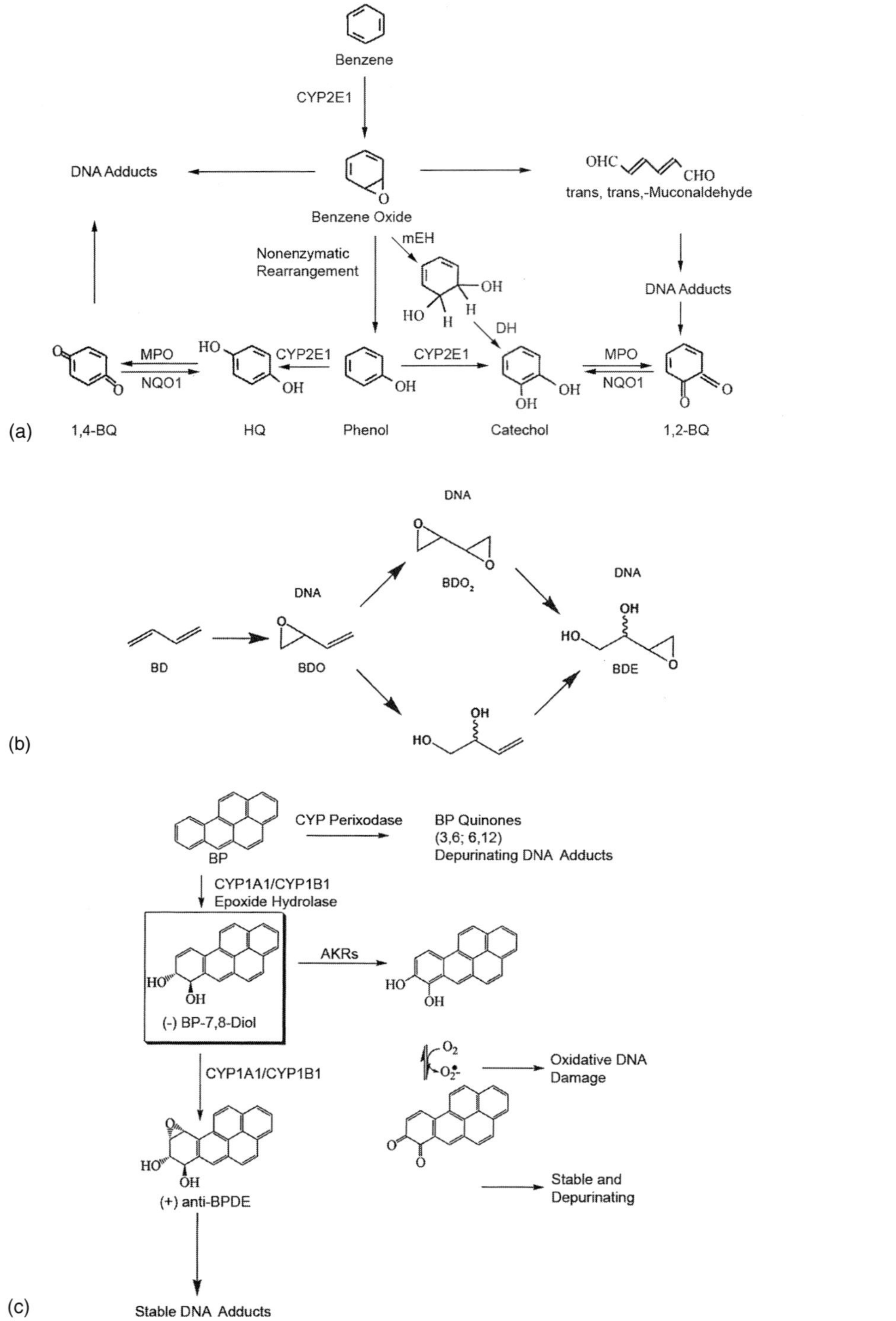

Figure 14.1 Benzene, butadiene, and benzo[a]pyrene are each metabolized to epoxides, dihydrodiols, and dihydrodiol epoxides, but also form other products. (**a**) Pathways for metabolism of Benzene. (**b**) Pathways for 1,3 Butadiene. (**c**) Pathways for Benzo[a] pyrene.

reactive electrophiles. This cooperation between reactive metabolites requires more recognition in the real world of pollutant mixtures.

DNA adducts typically form from reactions of reactive electrophilic metabolites with deoxyguanine (dG) or deoxyadenine (dA). These adducts have been detected in BM by DNA post-labeling (Moorthy et al. 2003) and, more recently, by mass spectrometry (MS) (Turteltaub and Mani 2003). They provide the means to trap and identify reactive metabolites, while also producing an important source of toxicity and mutations. Post-labeling does not detect all DNA reactions with reactive metabolites since depurination may subsequently result in the formation of DNA strand breaks. The excreted purine–metabolite adducts is however no longer linked to the site of in vivo damage. DNA modification, indicated by sites of mutation in key target genes (e.g., p53), provides complementary information, but also reflects modifications that survive DNA repair processes and positive growth selection (Bauer et al.1995).

These mechanisms of toxicity extend well beyond DNA damage. For example, we have found that the effects of PAHs in BM are largely attenuated by deleting the tumor necrosis factor α (TNFα receptor in mice. Tumor necrosis factor α, and other suppressors of hematopoietic steps, may be elevated by metabolites or cooperate with metabolite-initiated responses (Galvan et al. 2006). Deletion of protein kinase R, possibly a mediator of TNFα, also attenuates PAH effects downstream of metabolism. P53–/– mice are resistant to many of the effects of PAHs and benzene on hematopoiesis. p53 mediates apoptosis in pre-B cells following PAH treatment of co-cultured stromal cells (Page et al. 2002, 2003, 2004).

Benzene, butadiene, and PAHs are each metabolized by CYPs in the liver and in peripheral sites, like the BM (Figure 14.1). Metabolism in the liver and extrahepatic sites may deliver reactive metabolites to the BM or, conversely, limit the delivery of the chemical to the BM for local activation. These general issues have been extensively studied for benzene (Bernauer et al. 2000; Bauer et al. 2003), for PAHs (Galvan et al. 2005 Uno et al. 2004), and, to a lesser extent, for butadiene (Irons et al. 2000; Bond and Medinsky 2001). These considerations add to the importance of understanding the pharmacokinetics in relation to the BM. The duration of this exposure is critical since the toxicity involves extended effects on BM cells as they progress through an extensive sequence of differentiation. The BM toxicity produced by repeated cycles of reactive metabolite-mediated DNA or protein damage and repair needs to be considered. The route of chemical administration (oral, inhalation, or intraperitoneal (i.p.)) is also critical (Uno et al. 2004). Oral administration removes much of the chemical through first-pass metabolism, typically leading to protocols where repeated administrations are used. Intraperitoneal administration produces single-dose toxicity, which aids in mechanistic dissection, but is obviously further from environmental exposures.

The metabolic activations of benzene, butadiene, and PAHs share several features, including considerable overlap in the participation of various enzymes (Figure 14.1; Waidyanatha et al. 2005; Recio et al. 2000; Palackal et al. 2002). Each is metabolized to epoxides by one or more forms of cytochrome 450 (CYPs), which can then undergo further metabolism by microsomal epoxide hydrolase (mEH) to form a *trans*-dihydrodiol (DH). Each can potentially undergo secondary CYP metabolism to form a dihydrodiol epoxide (DHE). While this sequence occurs for generation of bay-region PAH epoxides, alternative rearrangement to phenols is favored at other PAH positions and for benzene. The more stable butadiene epoxide readily undergoes a second CYP reaction to the diepoxide. The formation of DHEs also depends on the competing dehydrogenation to catechols. This is favored for the less-stable benzene DH compared to PAH DH. Specific deletion of CYPs and other genes involved in these pathways in mice has provided key insight into the important steps in these toxicity processes and has also linked these reactive metabolites to DNA adduct formation. Human deficiency polymorphisms have been similarly helpful, while also providing a link to the mechanisms of adverse health effects (Zhang et al. 2004). Some of these approaches will be outlined for each chemical.

The selectivity of the reactions of the reactive metabolites with DNA depends on the particular metabolite. In addition, some metabolites, notably quinones, undergo redox cycling to produce oxidative stress. This is indicated by 8-hydroxy dG modifications in DNA. Myeloperoxidase (MPO; Zhang et al. 2002), which is present at high levels in BM, effectively generates quinones from phenols, hydroquinols, and catechols. Myeloperoxidase can also directly convert PAHs to quinones and butadiene to the epoxide (Elfarra et al. 1996). Generation of phenols (from benzene or PAHs) may lead to detoxification through glucuronidation by UDP glucuronosyl transferases (UDPGTs) or sulfation by sulfotransferases (STs) (Auyeung, Kessler and Ritter 2003), but may also activate MPO by acting as a co-substrate. Quinones are removed by a combination of NADPH quinone reduction (NQO1) and conjugation by UDPGT or ST (Grove et al. 2000). Induction of quinone reductase and other phase 2 enzymes via dithiolethiones confers protection against quinone toxicity (Twerdok, Rembish and Trush 1992; Twerdok, Mosebrook and Trush 1992; Kwak et al. 2001). Orthoquinones differ from other quinones in that they form from DHs by dehydrogenation at aldo/keto reductase enzymes (AKR), followed by rapid oxidation by oxygen (Palackal et al. 2001, 2002). These quinones are typically poor substrates for NQO1 and react readily as electophiles at protein and DNA through a Michael addition reaction. This reactivity is the prime source of their toxicity, but also limits their presence.

Glutathione, GSH transferases (GSTs), and deficiencies in the human GST enzymes (mu-1 and theta-1 forms GSTM1 and GSTT1) play a key role in removing the reactive metabolites of benzene, butadiene, and PAHs (Sundberg et al. 2002). The common deficiencies provide a powerful means to link reactive metabolites from occupational exposures to disease outcomes. However, GSH/GST reactions with quinones can also enhance toxicity by forming GS-adducts. These products provide an even better source of oxygen radicals than the parent quinone (Bolton et al. 2000).

There is extensive overlap in the cellular processes initiated by reactive metabolites from each of these compounds (benzene, butadiene, and PAHs). Thus, much may be learnt from comparison of the BM response to each chemical. Importantly, these compounds are present in mixtures in diesel exhaust and tobacco smoke and, therefore, may combine their effects.

14.2. BM and Hematopoiesis

The BM is highly susceptible to toxicity from reactive metabolites, in part because of the extensive numbers of highly proliferative cells that participate in hematopoiesis (Figure 14.2). The various BM cell populations can be identified by means of interactions of specific cell surface markers with fluorescence-labeled antibodies. This labeling, in turn, allows physical separation by fluorescence-activated cell sorting (FACS). Antibody-conjugated magnetic beads are also effective for large-scale affinity separations of cell populations. Mixed BM cells or sorted cells are also further characterized by their differentiation in culture. Various supporting media have been developed, which selectively promote clonal expansion of progenitors for the specific lineages (Weissman 2000; Hardy and Hayakawa 2001). The colonies formed in this way provide a means to quantify the numbers of particular progenitor cells.

Different proportions of the cells arising from the BM distribute to the blood, thymus, lymphatic system, spleen, and other tissues. Effects of chemicals in the BM will, therefore, impact cell populations at these other sites. Several of these cell types contribute to innate immunity and, along with products of the mesenchymal lineage (endothelia, fibroblasts), migrate to the sites of chemical or physical injury to provide the first line of repair. Reactive metabolites also target the mesenchymal population, which provide support factors that direct the hematopoietic processes.

In response to appropriate stimuli, HSCs differentiate via long term (LT)- and short term (ST)-intermediate stem cells into precursors for three lineages: killer cells (NK), lymphoid cells, or myeloid cells. Lymphoid precursors further differentiate to cytotoxic T lymphocytes cells, which are programmed to move to the thymus, or B-lymphocytes, which carry

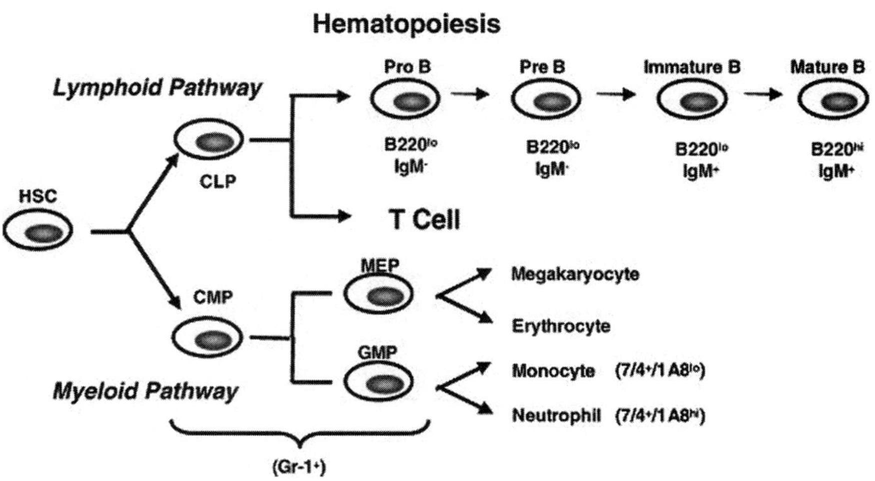

Figure 14.2 Scheme for bone marrow hematopoiesis showing lymphoid and myeloid differentiation. Scheme includes surface markers used to identify B-lymphocytes, myeloid, monocyte, and neutrophil populations. *Abbreviations*: CLPs, common lymphoid progenitors; CMPs, common myeloid progenitors; GMPs, granulocyte/monocyte progenitors; HSCs, hematopoietic stem cells; MEPs, megakaryocyte/erythrocyte progenitors.

out the antigen-initiated production of immunoglobulins. Myeloid precursors divide into two lineages that lead to, respectively, erythrocytes and megakaryotypes (produce platelets) or granulocytes, which are comprised of neutrophils and monocytes (Carsetti 2000; Weissman 2000). Monocytes terminally differentiate into macrophage, the major phagocytic cell type. Natural killer cells and macrophage provide a first line of defense against foreign cells and viruses (Innate immunity). Antigen-initiated antibody immune responses are mediated by recruitment of cytotoxic T cells and NK cells along with macrophage.

These differentiation processes in BM are regulated by chemokines, cytokines, and other protein factors that are released from specific stromal cells, which originate from mesenchymal stem cells. Lymphocytes develop through a discrete series of intermediate immature B-lymphocytes. These progenitor B cells, also known as pre-B cells, express immunoglobulin M (IgM) on their surface, but mature further in response to antigen stimulation. This maturation is facilitated by interleukin 7 (IL7) and stromal cell derived factor (SDF) from BM stromal cells (Grawunder, Melchers and Rolink 1993; Iguchi et al. 1997), but is also diminished by other factors, including interferon gamma (IFN-γ and TNFα which can arise from macrophage (Rusten et al. 1994, 1995; Mundle et al. 1999; Rebel et al. 1999; Kouro et al. 2001; Bryder et al. 2001). SDF1 and IL7 promote these steps through specific receptors (e.g., CXCR4 for SDF1) on the target progenitor cells (Tokoyoda et al. 2004).

The stromal cells are, for the most part, fibroblastic and include progenitors for bone-forming osteoblasts and various related specialized cells that support different stages of hematopoiesis. Adipocytes, which arise from an alternative differentiation of the stromal progenitors (Liu et al. 2007), release factors that may disrupt hematopoiesis, including leptin and adiponectin. These processes are critically affected by the local vasculature through transport of regulatory molecules, oxygen availability, and by factors released from the endothelia.

14.3. Chemical Disruption of Hematopoiesis

Reactive metabolites can disrupt these processes in many ways, particularly via decreased proliferation, enhanced apoptosis, or altered commitment to differentiation. In the case of stem cells or other multipotential cells, chemicals may also redirect subsequent lineage commitments. The supporting stroma may also exhibit a change in the release of paracrine factors, including growth factors, chemokines, cytokines, proteases and protease inhibitors, and matrix proteins. The complexity of these problems is enhanced by the diversity of cell types. There is of particular interest in low doses of chemicals, which are more environmentally relevant. Low doses also produce more subtle effects on differentiation, which can predominate over apoptosis. DNA is a key site for such interactions, not only because of the possibility for mutations, but also because of the signaling that arises when DNA adducts or strand breaks are recognized. This leads to activation of the ATM and ATR kinase pathways, which link to p53, NFκB, and Chk signaling processes (Heince et al. 2007). These signaling pathways, in turn, regulate cell proliferation and apoptosis (Guo, Faller and Vaziri 2002; Yoo et al. 2007; Wu et al. 2006).

Cancers (leukemias and lymphomas) probably arise from changes in proliferative control produced as a consequence of DNA damage or chromosomal rearrangement in HSC or proliferative cells (Reya and Clevers 2005). These effects arise from reactions of reactive metabolites with DNA or from other chemical effects that are directed to chromosomal stability and mitotic processes. Realignment of chromosomes can promote growth by placing a proliferative gene under control of a more frequently active promoter. Chemical effects on BM cell populations are often seen with only minimal detection of DNA adducts, thus suggesting the importance of these other targets (Whysner et al. 2004).

The toxic metabolites affect hematopoiesis, in part, through effects on the release of these stromal/endothelial factors, which control the hematopoietic niches of the BM. It is notable that benzene-exposed workers show decreased blood levels of CXCL4 and two other platelet-derived CXC chemokines (Vermeulen et al. 2005). The origins of this deficit, health implications, and information regarding whether this set of responses occurs for the other similarly acting chemicals remains to be determined.

Recent work indicates that the stem cell population is sustained during these chemical stresses, although with significant changes in gene expression (Faiola et al. 2004). The chemical stresses result in decreases in myeloid and lymphoid progenitor cells, either through effects on the fate of stem cells and other early progenitors or from apoptosis in the affected populations. The targeting of stem cells raises important questions about the chemical metabolism in these cells. Stem cells are characterized by high activity of ATP-dependent transporters, which results in low accumulation of Hoechst dyes relative to other cells (Reys and Clevers 2005). The responses of separated HSC populations have been characterized for PAHs and quinone metabolites (Zhu, Li and Trush 1995; Van Grevenynghe et al. 2005) and cytochrome P450 forms have been identified in human CD34+ stem cell populations (Soucek et al. 2005).

14.4. In Vitro and Ex Vivo Model System for BM Toxicity

The complexity of these in vivo controls over hematopoiesis has necessitated the generation of simpler model systems. For example, BM stromal cell lines (typically BMS2 cells) have been cultured with various hematopoietic progenitor cell lines, particularly pre-B cells (Yamaguchi et al. 1997a,b; Mann et al. 1999; Near et al. 1999). BMS2 is a fibroblastic, multipotential line derived from mouse BM stroma (Heidel et al. 1999). Polycyclic hydrocarbon metabolism can be provided by the BMS2 cells, while responses such as apoptosis and cell cycle changes have been characterized in the hematopoietic line. This approach is helpful in addressing detailed mechanism – for example, signaling mechanisms produced by reactive metabolites in pre-B cells and transfer of reactive metabolites between BMS2 cells and the pre-B cells. This model has been used to demonstrate paracrine-induced apoptosis in pre-B cells. Evidence has been provided for secretion of a large mediating protein (>50 kDa) from the BMS2 cells triggered by PAH reactive metabolites (Allen et al. 2003). Other, more complex systems utilize mixed BM cultures or co-cultures of separated stroma and hematopoietic cell (Wyman et al. 2002). Equivalent apoptotic pre-B cells are very difficult to detect in vivo after these chemical treatments due to the rapid removal of dying cells by macrophage (Dogusan, Montecino-Rodriguez and Dorshkind 2004).

Effects of reactive metabolites on progenitor cells in vivo can be measured by characterization of their subsequent ex vivo differentiation in culture. The effects can also be generated through in vitro incubations of BM cells with the test chemicals. Their commitment to the separate lineages is resolved by colony-formation assays for lymphoid or myeloid cells or FACS analysis of changes in the respective cell populations. These methods allow dissection of in vivo effects of the chemicals on the separate cell populations in the more controlled ex vivo environment.

The difficulty of reconstituting the physiology of the BM compartment in cell culture remains a major problem, particularly the control of the stem cell niche and the local role of vasculature (Reya and Clevers 2005). A further issue is that each of the many cell types has a distinct profile of enzymes involved in chemical metabolism. The extent of transfer of reactive metabolites between different cell types and different BM compartments also remains uncertain.

14.5. Benzene Disruption of Hematopoiesis and Initiation of Cancer

Benzene produces acute myeloid leukemia, as well as a variety of other leukemias (Snyder 2002). Detailed examination of DNA adducts generated from carcinogenic benzene treatment suggests that adduct formation correlates poorly with cancer development (Whysner et al. 2004). Chromosomal aberrations suggest clastogenic activity. Additionally, adducts from quinones readily undergo depurination resulting in strand breaks. Hemotoxicity is detectable in workers exposed to low doses of benzene (Lan et al. 2004). Kinetic considerations for benzene exposure and distribution to the BM have been determined for workers and for mouse models (Kim et al. 2006; Chen et al. 2007). All of the products generated from the pathway shown in Figure 14.1 have been detected in these in vivo studies. In the mouse, benzene is absorbed more slowly after intradermal exposure than after intragastric gavage. This retention results in more quinone conjugation.

Short-term responses include effects on hematopoiesis, which are particularly directed to progenitor cells (Morgan and Alvares 2005). Suppression of erythromyelopoiesis results in decreased leukocyte and erythrocyte levels in peripheral blood (Ross et al. 1996; Moran, Siegel and Ross 1999). By contrast, myeloid-derived granulocytes and neutrophils increase (Faiola et al. 2004). In BM, there is a nonspecific 40% loss of nucleated cells, but no change in stem cells (Yoon et al. 2003).

Microarray studies of mRNA from total BM cells, following extended high-level benzene exposure, show that some changes maximize within 5 days, while other changes occur more slowly (Yoon et al. 2003). A modest increase in gene expression is associated with cell cycle arrest at G1/S (p21), but larger increases are associated with G2/M arrest (cyclin G1, wee kinase) and apoptosis (caspase 11). These responses are consistent with activation of p53 resulting from DNA damage. Other notable changes include substantial increases in CYP2E1 and MPO, which are involved in benzene metabolism (see below), and metallothionein 1, which responds to and protects against oxidative stress. The role of p53 has been further defined by treatment of p53 knock out (KO) mice. Benzene responses divide into those that are removed by p53 deficiency (cell cycle, apoptosis, metallothionein) and those that are retained (CYP2E1, MPO). For example, chronic benzene exposure causes an S-phase arrest in myeloid precursors, which is dependent on p53 (Yoon et al. 2001, 2003). Other hematopoietic responses are only seen after p53 deletion, probably resulting from the protective role of p53. Thus, p53 mediates some toxicity, but provides protection against other changes.

Separation of HSCs, which represent about only $1/10^4$ cells after exposure to benzene (Faiola et al. 2004), shows some selective changes. For example, the increase in p21 is only seen in the total population, while increases in cyclin G and SDF1 or decreases in Pax 6 are unique to the HSC. These expression changes suggest that the fate of the HSC may, indeed, be affected by the treatment.

Since hematopoiesis depends on factors released from the adjacent stroma, these cells provide an important site of toxicity (Funk, Kincade and Witte 1994; Iguchi et al. 1997; Hahn et al. 2000). Ex vivo hematopoiesis of BM cells isolated after in vivo benzene treatment is substantially arrested and this suppression is largely dependent on changes in the supporting activity of the adherent stromal cells (Iguchi et al. 1997; Abraham 1996).

For exposed workers, BM effects of benzene can be recognized not only by changes in peripheral blood mononuclear cell populations, but also through gene expression changes in these cells, which are identified through microarray gene expression profiles (Forrest et al. 2005). In a study of workers exposed to benzene in Chinese chemical plants, a set of 19 cytokines or cytokine response genes were upregulated, while other markers were substantially downregulated (cJun and HSP70) (Forrest et al. 2005).

14.6. Benzene Metabolism and Formation of Reactive Metabolites in BM

The major products from in vivo benzene metabolism are phenol, *p*-hydroquinone/*p*-benzoquinone, and catechol/*o*-quinone (Figure 14.1). The formation of benzene epoxide and the ensuing conversion by mEH to benzene *trans*-dihydrodiol (BDH) have been established from reactions with liver microsomes (Glatt et al. 1989). Benzene epoxide also rearranges to phenol, undergoes rearrangement to oxepine, and CYP-mediated ring-opening to mucondialdehyde (Snyder 2002). Benzene *trans*-dihydrodiol is converted to *o*-quinone by peroxidases and to catechol by AKRs (Palackal et al. 2001). Benzene dihydrodiol epoxide (BDE) is formed from BDH

(Snyder et al. 1993; Waidyanatha, Sangaiah and Rappaport 2005). Benzene 1,2,4-triphenol, which is identified among benzene metabolites, may arise from BDE. Phenols are further metabolized via sulfation and glucuronidation. Orthoquinones and *p*-quinones are removed by reduction at NQO1 coupled to UDPGT to form quinone glucuronides (Lind 1985; Schrenk et al. 1996). Benzene epoxide reacts with glutathione catalyzed by GSTs to form phenyl GSH conjugates (Snyder 2002).

The activation of benzene depends on the presence of CYPs, particularly CYP2E1, mEH, AKR, and peroxidases, including MPO. CYP2E1 is appreciably expressed in BM stroma and, therefore, metabolism can be initiated close to the sites of toxicity (Bernauer et al. 2000). Each of the other enzymes is also present in BM. The contribution of liver metabolites depends on their effective transfer to BM. Phenol, *p*-hydroquinol, catechol, and possibly BDH are likely to transfer from liver to BM through circulating blood. The presence of these reactive metabolites has been detected through albumin adducts in the blood of Chinese workers exposed to 1–>10 ppm benzene (Lin et al. 2006). The dose–response increases were ordered: benzene epoxide>1,4 quinone>>1,2 quinone. These adducts suggest that metabolism in the liver can deliver reactive metabolites to the BM in exposed humans, although this depends on the speed of this albumin-trapping reaction in blood. They also form glutathione conjugates. These adducts and conjugates provide markers of benzene activation in humans (Snyder 2002; Kim et al. 2006; Waidyanatha, Sangaiah and Rappaport 2005). Benzene toxicity and the impact of gene deletions and polymorphisms can reasonably be explained by transfer of *p*-hydroquinol and catechol to the BM with subsequent activation to reactive quinones by MPO. The transfer of BDH and activation to BDE by CYP2E1 in BM provides another possibility.

Direct administrations of phenol, catechol, or *p*-hydroquinol each fail to reproduce the benzene BM toxicity. Mixtures of catechol and *p*-hydroquinol, however, reproduce many of the features of benzene toxicity in BM (Yoon et al. 2003). Benzene toxicity in BM is substantially removed in mice deficient in, respectively, CYP2E1 (Valentine et al. 1996) and mEH (Bauer et al. 2003).

CYP2E1 is appreciably expressed in BM and the activity correlates well with benzene toxicity, suggesting that local metabolism is a key factor (Bernauer et al. 2000). A mouse deficiency of NQO1 enhances toxicity (Long et al. 2002). NQO1 is poorly expressed in BM cells, but increases with benzene exposure, presumably through induction by quinone metabolites (Ross 2005). Low-activity human polymorphisms in NQO1 have been linked to enhanced risk of benzene-induced leukemia, further confirming their key roles (Moran, Siegel and Ross 1999; Ross 2005). Thus, one polymorphism of NQO1 (2/2 variant) is much more readily degraded through ubiquitination leading to a near-complete deficiency. Collectively, this suggests participation of a combination of metabolites: BDH from the role of mEH and *p*-benzoquinone from the protective role of NQO1. Combination of NQO1 deficiency and GST deficiencies increases the toxicity of benzene by 20-fold in exposed workers (Chen et al., 2007; Manini et al. 2006).

Benzene toxicity from occupational exposure is substantially enhanced by smoking. The combinatorial effect of benzene and smoking is greatly enhanced by polymorphisms in CYP2E1 (threefold) and, particularly, by the NQO1 low-activity allele (up to 20-fold) (Wan et al. 2002). CYP2E1 polymorphisms alone have little effect. The basis for this strong interaction remains to be determined, since components of cigarette smoke are also metabolized by these enzymes (nitrosamines, CYP2E1; PAH quinones, NQO1). Nevertheless, this dramatic effect clearly emphasizes the importance of synergy between components of environmental mixtures.

In contrast to *p*-quinones, *o*-quinones are poor substrates for NQO1, suggesting that the protective role of this enzyme in benzene toxicity derives from the *p*-benzoquinone. *o*-Quinones are more reactive electrophiles that readily react with cell nucleophiles, notably glutathione and protein cysteines. This reactivity, however, probably decreases availability to DNA or other specific targets. The mutagenesis of BDH, when activated by liver S9, appears to involve BDE as the prime contributor, while the alternative conversion to *o*-quinone by AKR diminishes mutagenesis (Glatt et al. 1989; Snyder et al. 1993).

DNA adducts, measured by accelerated mass spectrometry (AMS) to the lowest detectable level ($5\,ng\,kg^{-1}$), have been compared in liver and BM after administration of 14C-benzene to mice in vivo (Turteltaub and Mani 2003). DNA adducts in liver were maximum after 30 min, whereas peak BM adduct levels were reached in 6 h and were sustained longer. The order of BM adduct formation between mouse strains and rats (B6C3F1>DBA2>C57B6>rats) paralleled toxicity, suggesting that these reactive metabolites are also critical determinants of toxicity.

Reactions of both *o*- and *p*-quinones with DNA produce unstable adduct that result in depurination and strand breaks (Chakravarti et al. 2006). *p*-Benzoquinone, however, also forms more stable DNA adducts that can be detected by post-labeling. These quinone reactions with DNA have been directly linked to mutations (Gaskell et al. 2004; Xie et al. 2005).

Additionally, the greater stability of *p*-benzoquinone results in redox cycling with generation of oxygen radicals and hydrogen peroxide. 8-Hydroxy dG adducts are a likely additional outcome of these radical reactions (Bolton et al. 2000; Watanabe and Forman 2003). 8-Hydroxy dG adducts are commonly used as markers of oxidative stress through their detection in blood and urine (excretion after depurination) (Pilger and Raudiger 2006). Measurement of benzene exposure-mediated 8-hydroxy dG adduct levels has been equivocal, but these adducts can readily be measured for smokers (PAH quinones). These adducts cause mutations through G/T transversions and strand breaks.

Despite the detection of adducts in total BM populations, several studies show that effects on other targets, such as mitotic mechanisms, are perhaps more important. In addition, benzene and other chemical stressors enhance epigenetic changes that do not involve adducts, through effects on DNA methylation or DNA repair processes (Morgan and Alvares 2005). Benzene metabolites also target key enzyme activities. For example, *p*-quinone inhibits activation of precursor forms of cytokines by sulfhydryl-dependent proteases (Kalf, Renz and Niculescu 1996). We will discuss the important role of cytokines in BM effects of PAHs on hematopoiesis.

More important, is the target BM cell population. In a study that provides insights for other chemical stressors (Givers et al. 2001), effects of benzene on BM HSC and progenitor populations increased with time after exposure starting at 9 weeks and extending to 11 months. At this time, 15% of the cells showed aneuploidy and some specific chromosomal abnormalities. These experiments provide compelling evidence for the importance of metabolism of benzene and other chemicals within HSC niches.

14.7. 1,3-Butadiene and BM Toxicity

1,3-Butadiene (BD) is a gas, which is present in many of the sources that provide environmental benzene, including cigarette smoke and diesel emissions. BD is also extensively used in the plastics and rubber industries, often in association with styrene, which shares similar epoxide-mediated toxicities. BD induces chromosomal damage, clastogenic changes, and extensive DNA adducts at high doses, but also increases DNA repair activity (Vodicka et al. 2006).

BD differs from benzene in that electrophilic, but not oxidant stress metabolites are generated. BD is primarily metabolized to the monoepoxide (BMO) and diepoxide (DEB) and the respective DH derivatives, resulting from reaction at EH (Figure 14.1) (Elfarra, Krause and Selzer 1996; Scholdberg et al. 2005). These reactions are catalyzed by CYP2E1 and CYP2A6, while CYP3A4, additionally, converts BMO to DEB (Vodicka et al. 2006). Myeloperoxidases rather than CYPs have been implicated in the conversion of BD to BMO in BM cell lysates from humans and mice. Metabolism is enhanced by hydrogen peroxide, which is needed for MPO, but not by NADPH, which drives CYP metabolism (Maniglier-Poulet et al. 1995). Myeloperoxidase forms BMD, but not DEB (Elfarra, Krause and Selzer 1996). BD, therefore, differs from benzene through the greater stability of the epoxides and a decrease in oxidative stress metabolites. BMO and DEB are each generated at much higher levels in mice than in rats (4–8 and 25–100 times, respectively), consistent with the much greater toxicity in mice (Bond and Medinsky 2001).

Mice and humans exposed to BD each form BMO adducts with dG (7-alkyl) and dA (1-alkyl) in multiple tissues (Scholdberg et al. 2005). 1,2,3-Trihydroxybutyl adducts derived from DEB are also detectable in vivo (Vodicka et al. 2006).

Formation of valine–hemoglobin adducts provides evidence for circulating epoxides, which should also reach the BM (Swendberg et al. 2007). Mice are much more susceptible than rats, consistent with higher blood levels of the epoxides. Deletion of epoxide hydrolase enhances toxicity, suggesting that these epoxides contribute much more to toxicity than the DHE (Wickliffe et al. 2007). Serum analysis of workers in the Texan rubber industry found mean BD exposure levels of up to 2 ppm. Individuals in a high-exposure group exhibited lymphocyte mutations, which were increased by BD (Abdel-Rahman, Ammenheuser and Ward 2001). The frequency of mutations was also increased threefold by low-activity His/Tyr mutations of EH. A similar, more extensive study of Czech workers exposed to BD identified metabolites due to GSH conjugation as well as BMO- and BDE-derived hemoglobin adduct formation.

Metabolite-selective effects of GST genotype were observed. There was, however, no correlation between metabolite markers and lymphocyte HPRT mutations or chromosome aberrations despite reported exposures that were similar to those in the Texas study (Albertini et al. 2007). A second study of Chinese workers with similar exposures also failed to find a correlation between HPRT mutations or chromosome aberrations and either GST or EH polymorphisms, although metabolites were not characterized in this study (Zhang et al. 2004). Differences between the responsive Texan workers and the apparently unresponsive Czech and Chinese groups may reflect higher-than-estimated exposures in the Texas analyses and also possibly other active components in the exposures. In light of benzene effects on mitotic processes, mutations in lymphocytes are not necessarily an indicator of critical BM effects, notably on HSC populations.

The mutagenic activities of BMO and DEB have been compared in lymphoblastoid cell lines. While DEB and BMO each produce AT-to-TA transversions, DEB is much more potent and produces large deletions, which may arise from bifunctional crosslinking (Recio, Saranko and Steen 2000). The responses to BD, however, suggest that both mechanisms cooperate in providing the toxicity. In vivo treatment with BD and either BMO or BDO each cause specific mutations in mouse lung, but not in the BM of the same mice (Saranko et al. 2001). In vitro treatment of BM cells with the epoxides produces similar mutations to those seen in lung cells. This suggests that the mutations are produced in the mouse BM, but at a low frequency. When human BM progenitor cell populations were treated separately with BMO, DEB, and the DHE (Irons et al. 2000), only DEB inhibited lymphoid and erythroid colony formation. These activities were comparable to those of benzoquinone. The greater effectiveness of DEB-induced DNA changes adds weight to the need to focus on such changes in human samples.

14.8. PAH Activation and BM Toxicity

Polycyclic hydrocarbonss produce many of the same effects as benzene on BM cells, including immunosuppression and cancer (Thurmond et al. 1987; Boffetta, Jourenkova and Gustavsson 1997). In mice, doses of 25 mg kg^{-1} of 7,12-dimethylbenz[a]anthracene (DMBA), administered intraperitoneally, produce maximum effects on BM (Heidel et al. 1999). There is 50–70% suppression of both myeloid and lymphoid lineages between 24 and 48 h of exposure. In contrast, benzo(a)pyrene (BP) causes scarcely any depletion of BM cells. Intraperitoneal administration produces a broad distribution of PAH with blood levels that remain relatively constant between 6 and 24 h, with proportionate levels in the BM (Galvan et al. 2005). The lipophilic PAHs primarily distribute into fat and reach the liver through the blood. This systemic distribution after i.p. administration is represented schematically in Figure 14.3. Slow transfer to the liver decreases the effectiveness of liver metabolism.

After i.p. administration, BP-mediated activation of the AhR produces a much larger induction of CYP1A1 than the weaker AhR activator,

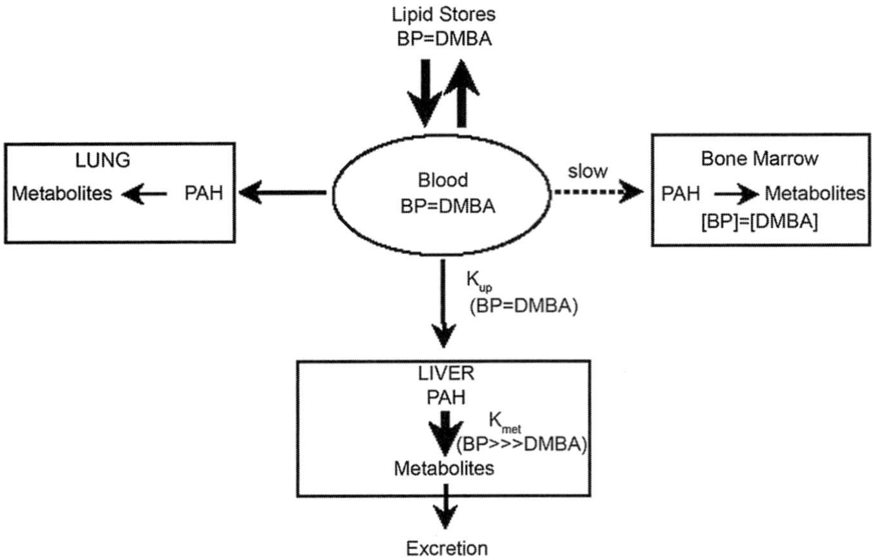

Figure 14.3 Scheme showing systemic equilibration of PAHs after intraperitoneal injection. Most of the lipophilic PAHs distribute into body fat from where there is distribution into blood and then to liver (high metabolism), lung (typical of tissues with moderate metabolism), and bone marrow (the toxicity target). In liver, uptake is slower than metabolism with the consequence that increased metabolism through induction of CYP1A1 depletes liver PAHs (BP<<DMBA), but has little immediate effect on blood levels. Bone marrow levels of PAH are proportional to blood levels and, therefore, not much affected by high liver metabolism. This contrasts with orally administered PAHs, which enter the liver first and where the enhanced metabolism rapidly lowers blood and bone marrow PAH levels.

DMBA. Since BP is a much better substrate for CYP1A1-mediated metabolism than DMBA, the resultant increase in CYP1A1 expression level leads to decreased intrahepatic BP levels relative to equivalent DMBA administration (Galvan et al. 2005). This does extend to differential effects on blood and BM PAH levels in the key 12–24-h period of BM toxicity. In AhRd mice, the receptor binds PAH weakly and there is no induction of CYP1A1. The diminished hepatic activity similarly does not initially affect blood or BM levels of the PAHs. Remarkably, however, this loss of AhR induction restores BP-initiated BM toxicity to levels seen with DMBA. Slow transfer of PAHs into the liver from lipid storage appears to limit the systemic effects of increased liver metabolism. The similar levels of BP and DMBA reaching the BM in normal and AhRd mice contrast with the large differences in toxicity. The restoration of BP toxicity in AhRd mice points to an AhRd-mediated protection against reactive metabolites. This difference between BP and DMBA is not specific to BM toxicity. These observations provided the first clue that BM metabolism was central to these toxicity effects.

By contrast, intragastric PAHs enter the liver through portal circulation and are substantially removed in a first pass by CYP-mediated metabolism. For BP, blood levels peak within 2–3 h and decline to near zero in 5 h (Uno et al. 2004). Even within this short period, the much greater AUC in CYP1A1–/– mice demonstrates that CYP1A1 is a key contributor. AhR induction of liver CYP1A1 enhances clearance and diminishes transfer of PAHs to BM. However, because of this effective clearance, PAH toxicity with orally administered PAH typically requires multiple administrations of PAH. Thus, the protective role of liver metabolism against PAH toxicity is substantially dependent on the route of administration.

14.9. Reactive PAH Metabolites and Formation of DNA Adducts

Most investigations have used either DMBA or BP (Thurmond et al. 1987; Wyman et al. 2002) as model PAHs, with potent carcinogenic and immunosuppressive activities. In vivo, PAHs are found as complex mixtures formed through partial combustion processes. Such mixtures have been examined with respect to metabolism, DNA adduct formation, and carcinogenesis in a mouse epidermis model, but not as yet for BM effects (Marston et al. 2001; Kleiner et al. 2004). The activation process involves two CYP-dependent steps (Palackal et al. 2001; Shimada and Guengerich 2006; Conney et al. 1994), the first of which converts the PAH to a non-K-region *trans*-dihydrodiol (PAHDH), and the second of which results in formation of syn- and anti-dihydrodiol epoxides (PAHDE) (Figure 14.1). PAHDE have been linked to the initiation of carcinogenesis through covalent binding to purines of DNA, which result in mutations through error-prone replication (Loechler 1995). The DHEs form on benzene rings in the so-called bay and fjord locations. In these structures, the metabolized ring is puckered by trans-bay steric interactions from either the methyl groups or benzene rings. The out-of-plane structure increases reactivity of the epoxide ring. For DMBA, the active bay-region configuration is provided by the 3,4 dihydrodiol 1,2 epoxide isomers. For BP, equivalent activity is provided by the 7,8 dihydrodiol 9,10 epoxide isomers. There are four isomers of each PAHDE (syn- and anti-epoxides, each with optical isomers), which differ in their reactivity with the stereo-selective DNA.

While most PAH toxicity studies focus on PAHDE, their various quinone derivatives are extensively formed and also contribute substantially to toxicity. PAHDH are converted by a second competing pathway to *o*-quinones, through dehydrogenation by members of the AKR family and auto-oxidation (Palackal et al. 2002). These PAH *o*-quinone metabolites, like the benzene *o*-quinone, are reactive electrophiles, which attack proteins and DNA. Their reaction with DNA predominantly forms depurinating DNA adducts and strand breaks. The PAH *o*-quinones also exhibit distinct toxic effects, including inhibition of microsomal Ca-ATPases, PKCs, and protein phosphatases. Other PAH quinones arise from the parent PAHs through an initial electron abstraction by peroxidases or P450 cytochromes or from further metabolism of PAH phenol metabolites. These quinones are typically less electrophilic than *o*-quinones and *p*-benzoquinone, but are more subject to 1e-redox cycling due to the stability of the intermediate semiquinones. BP forms these quinones much more readily than DMBA, where the preferred peroxidative 1e-reaction leads to H-abstraction from the methyl groups. This results in the predominant formation of hydroxymethyl products. This redox cycling of quinones with oxygen generates oxyradicals that produce DNA damage, principally through initial formation of 8 hydroxy dG.

Two-electron reduction by NQO1 prevents this cycling (Kerzee and Ramos 2000; Long et al. 2000, 2001, 2002; Moorthy et al. 2003). Quinones also readily react with glutathione to form GS-derivatives, which become more active in redox cycling due to the electron-donor property of the S-substituent (Bolton et al. 2000).

While we have focused on PAH metabolites as a source of toxicity, it is important to recognize that activation of the AhR alone disrupts hematopoiesis (Murante and Gasiewicz 2000). Sufficient PAHs reach the BM to increase CYP1B1 levels (Figure 14.5). Several features of the BM response to PAHs suggest that the AhR involvement is limited to induction of PAH-metabolizing enzymes: (1) the effects on progenitor populations are different from those of 2,3,7,8-tetrachlorodibenzo dioxin TCDD, a potent AhR ligand, which is metabolized extremely slowly; (2) AhRd mice, which are scarcely induced by BP, respond more extensively; (3) DMBA, a weak inducer, is much more toxic.

14.10. Enzymes Involved in Activation and Detoxification

The conversions of PAHs to PAHDH and then to PAHDE, respectively, by CYP1A1 and CYP1B1 is selective to the individual PAH. The epoxidation of PAHDH by either CYP1A1 or CYP1B1 competes with the conversion to *o*-quinones by AKR. There are multiple forms of AKR1C that are effective in the metabolism of PAHDH, which are distributed across many tissues (Burczynski and Penning 2000). Mercaptoethanol and *N*-acetyl cysteine have been used to trap PAH *o*-quinone generated through metabolism of PAHDH by recombinant AKR forms (Jin and Penning 2007). Mass spectrometry has been used to identify the *o*-quinone-thiol conjugates. Although peroxidation of PAHs by 1e abstraction is catalyzed by CYPs, this reaction is much more likely to be mediated by the high levels of MPO in BM. Thus, BP is converted to a mixture of quinones (1,6-; 3,6-; 6,12-) when incubated with BM cell lysates (Legraverend et al. 1983). Recent work has linked MPO to adverse effects of BP on polymorphonuclear leukocytes (Kumar et al. 2006).

AhR-mediated PAH induction responses also differ between tissues and, notably, between liver and BM. As noted above, the activation of the AhR is highly PAH-dependent (BP>>DMBA) (Schmidt and Bradfield 1996). CYP1A1 is significantly expressed in mouse liver only after activation of AhR. CYP1B1 is not expressed at detectable protein levels in mouse liver hepatocytes, even after AhR activation, but is expressed extensively in extrahepatic tissues (Savas et al. 1994; Sutter et al. 1994; Bhattacharyya et al. 1995).

The loss of DMBA toxicity in the BM of CYP1B1-null mice has established a key role for CYP1B1 in the activation process. The decline in BM toxicity is matched by a loss of PAHDE adducts (Galvan et al. 2003; Heidel, Czuprynski and Jefcoate 1998; Heidel et al. 2000; Figure 14.4). CYP1B1 is constitutively expressed in many extrahepatic tissues to higher levels than CYP1A1. BM is only one of many tissues expressing CYP1B1. These tissues are targets for PAH toxicity and carcinogenicity (Savas et al.

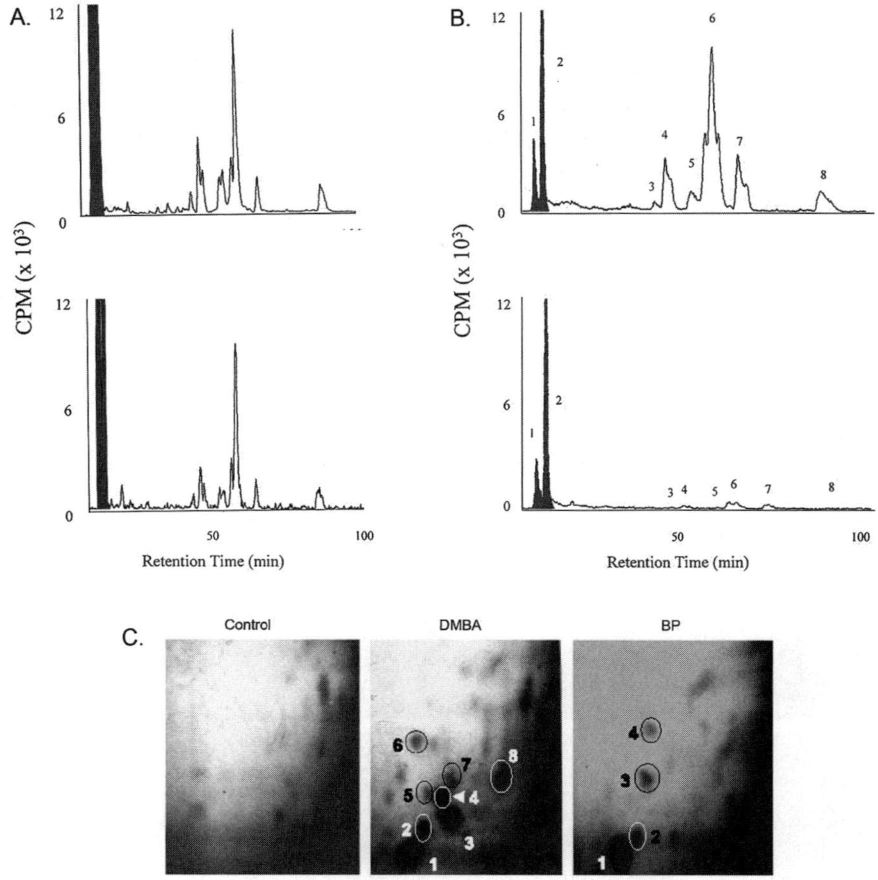

Figure 14.4 DMBA and BP adducts on bone marrow DNA measured by post-labeling using either 33-P (HPLC) or 32-P (2D-electrophoresis). (**a**) DMBA 3,4 dihydrodiol 1,2 epoxide adducts from co-culture of DMBA with BMS2 and pre-B mouse cell lines. 33-P labeled dG and dA adducts are similar in BMS2 cells (upper) where activation occurs and in pre-B cells (lower), which is the site of toxicity and largely devoid of metabolism. (**b**) DMBA adducts similarly analyzed in bone marrow DNA from wild-type mice (upper) and CYP1B1–/– mice (lower). The distribution of adducts is very similar in the in vitro and in vivo models reflecting similar proportions of DMBE isomers. 1–8 represent the (+) and (–) syn- and anti-DE adducts with dG and dA. DMBA and BP adducts on bone marrow DNA are compared by 32-P post-labeling. The numbering represents positions of adduct identified with standards. 3 and 4 correspond to dihydrodiol epoxide adducts, 1 and 2 are likely to be quinone adducts, and 5–8 are unknown.

1994; Bhattacharyya et al. 1995). In humans, the expression is much higher in tumors than in surrounding normal tissues (McFadyen and Murray 2005). Stromal fibroblasts, including those in BM, express constitutive levels of CYP1B1 that are inducible after AhR activation. The BMS2 mouse BM stromal line expresses CYP 1B1 at modest levels, but effectively generates DMBA–DE adducts that closely match those generated from exposure of BM cells to DMBA (Figure 14.4a). Co-cultured pre-B cells, which have no metabolic activity, generate a similar set of adducts, indicating effective transfer of DMBA–DE from BMS2 cells (Figure 14.4b). These BM stromal cells, like other fibroblasts, express negligible levels of CYP1A1. Mouse endothelial cells, which line the vasculature of the BM, also typically express CYP1B1 (Tang, Jefcoate and Sheibani unpublished). In situ hybridization has demonstrated the presence of CYP1B1 mRNA in BM, which is increased appreciably following various PAH exposure (Galvan et al. 2005). Expression is detectable under basal conditions and is enhanced more by BP than DMBA, in accord with AhR activation (Figure 14.5).

DNA post-labeling shows that DMBA more readily forms PAHDE–DNA adducts in BM than BP (Galvan et al. 2005), even in AhRd mice, where BP is as toxic as DMBA (Figure 14.4C) (Moorthy, unpublished). This increase in adducts for DMBA compared to BP occurs despite similar CYP1B1-mediated metabolism to PAHDH in microsomal preparations. The DMBA adducts are absent in CYP1B1–/– mice, indicating similar critical roles for CYP1B1 in PAHDE production as in toxicity

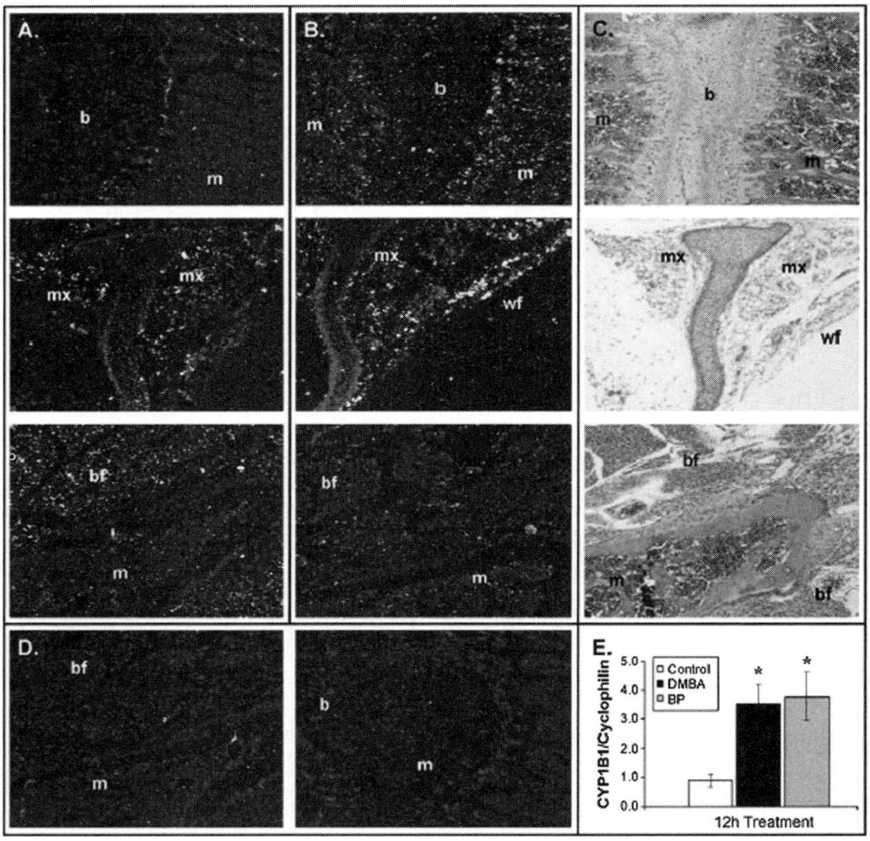

Figure 14.5 Levels and distribution of cytochrome P450 1B1 in bone marrow determined by qRT-PCR and in situ hybridization after treatment with BP. Mice were exposed to BP (50 mg kg^{-1}, i.p.) for 24 h prior to sacrifice and removal of the sternum for sectioning. In situ hybridization and H/E staining are shown for serial sections taken from three separate sections of the sternum comprising bone, matrix, and fat. CYP levels are much lower in absence of BP. (**a**) CYP1A1 antisense probe. (**b**) CYP1B1 antisense probe. (**c**) H and E staining. (**d**) Sense control. (**e**) QRT-PCR of mRNA 12 h after comparable 12-h treatments.
CYP1A1 was only detected in brown fat (bf) attached to the outside of sternum. CYP1B1 is seen in white fat (wf), in the matrix (m), and in mixed fat/matrix populations (mx).

(Galvin et al. 2003; Figure 14.4B). The BM levels of CYP1B1, which are higher after BP treatment, also do not correlate with either toxicity or adduct formation (Galvan et al. 2005; Figure 14.5). This is consistent with the hypothesis that BP metabolism is diverted to products that generate toxcity without producing adducts, and which can be protected by the greater AhR induction provided by BP. The effective toxicity of benzene quinones and their preferential formation by BP than by DMBA supports this view.

The absence of CYP1B1 in liver establishes an extrahepatic role for CYP1B1 participation in BM toxicity. Reverse transcriptase-polymerase chain reaction (RT–PCR) shows that CYP1B1 mRNA increases appreciably in BM cells 12 h after treatment with either PAH. Basal CYP1B1 levels and DMBA metabolism are each relatively high in cultured BM stroma and are partially retained in AhR–/– cells. Since there is only a modest increase after addition of TCDD (Heidel et al. 2000), it appears that other regulatory mechanisms contribute to this expression.

Experiments in AhRd, CYP1B1–/–, and CYP1B1–/–AhRd mice indicate two features of the PAH toxicity process: (1) CYP1B1 is essential for activation of PAHs in BM, but is not a limiting factor in toxicity in normal or AhRd mice; (2) AhR activates a limiting protective process, which may, therefore, involve conjugation processes.

Three families of conjugation enzymes react with the principle PAH metabolites (phenols, PAHDH, PAHDE, and quinones). One or more of these enzymes may, therefore, provide this AhR-induced removal of reactive BP metabolites in BM. These reactions are, of course, also involved in the metabolism of benzene. The UDPGTs, STs, and GSTs each exist in multiple forms, demonstrating different specificity for PAH metabolites and different regulation by AhR. The forms participating in reactions with PAH metabolites are likely to be different from those participating in benzene metabolism. UDPGT1A forms are involved in further conjugation of PAH phenols and hydroquinones and, to a lesser extent, PAHDH. NQO1 provides protection by converting quinones to hydroquinones that can then be glucuronidated. Several forms of the enzymes (UDPGTs, GSTs, and NQO1) are induced by PAHs through AhR activation (Long et al. 2000, 2001) and these forms are typically involved in conjugation of the primary PAH metabolites. NQOI also has endogenous functions in BM cells (Long et al. 2002)

Nrf2 provides another important activation pathway. This protein is anchored in the cytoplasm through complex formation with KEAP1, but is released to the nucleus when the latter is activated by oxidative or electrophilic stress. Nrf2 forms heterodimers with maf family proteins that recognize a sequence that has been identified as the antioxidant response element (ARE) (Ma et al. 2004). Recent functional promoter analyses of NQO1 and UDPGT1A7 show that AhR and Nrf2 function synergistically through complexes with ARE and XRE in the respective promoters (Auyeung, Kessler and Ritter 2001, 2003; Jemnitz, Veres and Vereczkey 2002; Grove et al. 2000). Polycyclic hydrocarbon quinones and benzene quinones effectively activate Nrf2. This leads to induction of NQO1, which initiates the excretion of these quinones. The induction of NQO1 and UDPGT1A forms in BM by BP or BP metabolites may account for the AhR-dependent attenuation of BP toxicity.

14.11. Liver Metabolism of PAHs versus BM Metabolism

As with the other BM toxicants, it is critical to determine whether bioactivation occurs in the liver or in the BM. This is a particular issue in PAH toxicity for three reasons: (1) CYP1A1 is highly induced in liver; (2) basal CYP1B1 is not expressed in hepatocytes; (3) basal CYP1B1 is appreciable in BM (Galvan et al. 2005). The effectiveness of CYP1B1 deletion in preventing DMBA-induced tumors argues that peripheral activation is critical for tumorigenesis (Buters et al. 1999, 2003). The essential role of CYP1B1 in BM toxicity and DNA adduct formation leads to a similar conclusion (Heidel et al. 2000). The poor correlation between CYP1B1 expression levels (BP AhRd~DMBA WT>BP WT) indicate that CYP1B1 is essential, but not a limiting factor. In other words, very little BM CYP1B1 metabolism is sufficient to initiate toxicity.

We have recently found that CYP1B1 deletion does not affect the levels of either PAHs or PAHDH in blood, which determine the transfer from liver to BM (Larsen and Jefcoate, unpublished). This resistance to CYP1B1 deletion establishes that the activation does not depend on transfer of PAH or PAHDH to BM. Activation of PAH or PAHDH is, therefore, mediated by CYP1B1 in BM.

As noted earlier, liver metabolism plays a larger role for PAHs administered intragastrically because intestinal uptake directly transfers the PAH to liver (Galvan et al. 2005; Uno et al. 2004). The generation of a conditional liver deletion of P450 oxidoreductase (OxR) provides the means to completely prevent all NADPH-driven, hepatic P450-mediated metabolism (Gu et al. 2003). Preliminary experiments suggest, however, that diminished liver metabolism of i.p.-administered PAHs leads to a compensatory enhanced metabolism in extrahepatic tissues.

14.12. Disruption of Hematopoietic Maturation by PAHs

A single i.p. administration of DMBA to C57Bl/6 mice produces over 70% loss of BM hematopoietic cells 24–48 h after treatment, but does not affect adherent stromal cells. This cell loss is observed in H/E-stained BM sections (Figure 14.6) and, more quantitatively, when cells eluted from the femurs of treated animals are analyzed by FACS. DMBA treatment substantially reduced the number of BM cells of both the lymphoid (Figure 14.6) and myeloid lineages (Figure 14.7; Heidel et al.1999, 2000; Mann et al. 1999; Yamaguchi et al. 1997a, 1997b; Galvan et al. 2006).

Fluorescence-activated cell sorting analyses showed that DMBA decreases precursor lymphocytes, but not mature lymphocytes. There was a loss of granulocytes, but an increase in BM HSC (Galvan et al. 2006). These data suggest that PAHs act early in hematopoiesis and affect both myeloid and lymphoid lineages. More detailed analysis of the BM cell populations shows that although BP does not change the total number of cells, there are effects on myeloid populations that selectivity differ from those of DMBA (Figure 14.7). This could reflect a difference in the type of reactive metabolites generated (e.g., quinones rather than PAHDE). Although DMBA decreases BM progenitor cells, stem cell populations

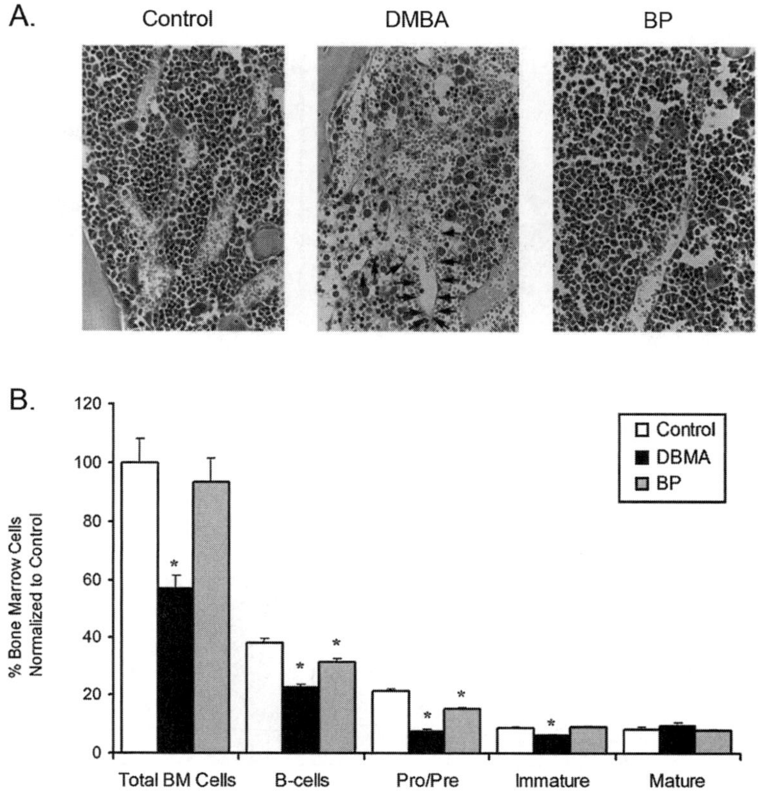

Figure 14.6 Effects of DMBA on BM cells are much greater than the effects of an equivalent dose of BP. Mice were treated with oil controls and either BP or DMBA (50 mg kg^{-1} i.p.) for 48 h. (**a**) H and E staining of sternum sections shows depletion of cells by DMBA is much greater than by BP. (**b**) FACS analysis of bone marrow cells eluted from femurs. Total BM cells are compared with the total B cell population and pro/pre progenitor B cells. Immature B cells and mature B cells are each determined by selective cell surface markers.

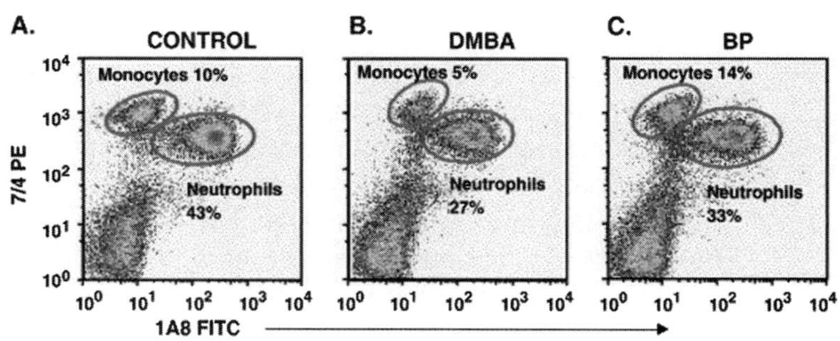

Figure 14.7 FACS analysis of myeloid cells after the treatments shown in Figure 6 shows distinct effects of DMBA and BP on monocyte and neutrophil populations.

increase (Figure 14.8). This is consistent with the slow proliferation of these cells. The increase may arise from a decrease in differentiation to the progenitors. The formation of granulocytes and lymphoid progenitors from HSCs are similarly decreased, consistent with equal effects on each pathway (Galvan et al. 2006).

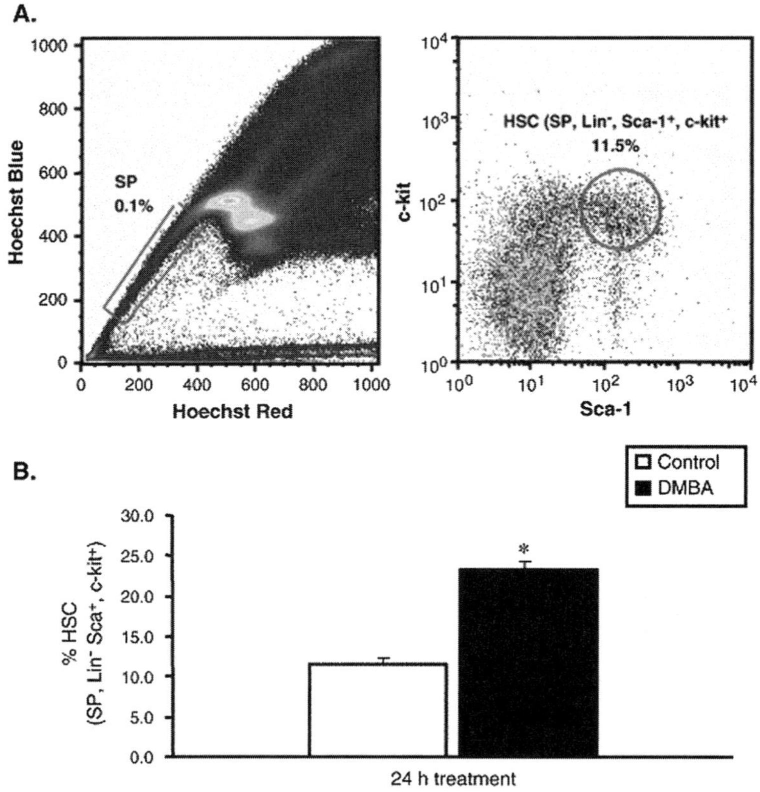

Figure 14.8 DMBA enhances the proportion of hematopoietic stem cells (HSC), while decreasing total bone marrow cells. (**a**) FACS Separation of HSC. *Left*: Isolation of side fraction, SP (0.1% of total cells) based on effective depletion of Hoechst dyes; *Right*: Separation of HSC (Lin$^-$, Sca$^+$, kit$^+$) from side fraction (11.5% of SP). (**b**) Percent of HSC recovered from side fraction after control and DMBA treatments. Total cells and side fraction declined by 30% after DMBA treatment, reflecting a small, but significant net increase in HSC cells.

Co-culture of pre-B cells with BM fibroblasts in the presence of low concentrations of DMBA (<0.3 μM) produces apoptosis (Yamaguchi et al. 1997b). Importantly, this response, which required CYP1B1 expression in fibroblast cells, was removed when pre-B cells were derived from p53–/– mice (Page et al. 2003). The effects of conditioned media from DMBA-treated BMS2 cells on pre-B cells support this hypothesis (Allen et al. 2003). Analysis of the active conditioned media implicates a high–molecular-weight protein (greater than 50 kDa).

Polycyclic hydrocarbons induce apoptosis in a pre-B cell line, but only when BM stromal cells are present at the time of PAH exposure (Wyman et al. 2002; Mann et al. 1999; Near et al. 1999; Yamaguchi et al. 1997; Heidel et al. 1999). We did not detect apoptotic cells after DMBA exposures in vivo, possibly because of rapid removal of apoptotic cells by macrophage. We have used p53–/– mice to show that p53 plays an essential role in both the toxicity and in the in vitro apoptotic responses. p53 is activated by DNA damage and, therefore, the reactive metabolites derived from PAHs may generate toxic effects through signaling derived from DNA damage. ATM kinase mediates such responses through p53. PolyADP ribosylation by PARP enzymes plays a key role in the phosphorylation of p53 by ATM (Heince et al. 2007). Presumably, the role of p53 in PAHs, benzene, and possibly BD toxicity involve similar processes. Thus, p53–/– pre-B cells do not respond in vitro to reactive DMBA metabolites generated by CYP1B1 in BM stromal cells. These p53-linked responses are mediated by activation of caspases 8 and 9 (Page et al. 2002, 2003), much as for benzene (Yoon et al. 2003).

Exposure to the potent AhR agonist, TCDD, which is not metabolized by P450 cytochromes, causes pre-B cell apoptosis in vitro and comparable toxicity in vivo (Thurmond and Gasiewicz 2000). TCDD exposure in vivo impaired the responsiveness of HSCs (lin- CD34- c-kit+ Sca-1+ cells) when challenged in vitro (Sakai et al. 2003). AhR activation by PAH alone may affect HSC, but is not sufficient for these effects, thus implicating reactive metabolites.

14.13. Cooperation of PAH Metabolites and TNFα in BM Toxicity

TNFα is essential for this PAH-mediated damage in the BM. TNFα participation in the response to benzene and BD is also likely, but has not been tested. This requirement for TNFα in PAH responses has been inferred from the effects of deleting the TNF receptor 1 (TNFR1), which is very specific for TNFα effects on cells. TNFRI-null mice are completely resistant to DMBA-initiated BM toxicity (Page et al. 2004). TNFα is produced by stromal cells in response to a variety of stress stimuli (Galvan et al. 2003). Tumor necrosis factor α binds to TNFRI (p55), which mediates the majority of the biological effects of TNFα and to TNFRII (p75), which plays a modulatory role (Declercq et al. 1998; Guoqing and Goeddel 2002; Miscia et al. 2002; Rusten and Jacobsen 1995; Rusten et al. 1994). Tumor necrosis factor binds to TNFR1 and TNFRII to initiate either apoptotic cell death or inflammation through NF-κB (Guoqing and Goeddel 2002; Mundle et al. 1999) and AP-1 completes (Arnott et al. 2002). TNF-Tumor necrosis factor α exerts multiple cell-type-selective effects that alter the progress of hematopoiesis in the BM (Bryder et al. 2001; Rebel et al. 1999).

A similar dissociation of PAHs and TNFα has been seen in the skin. Polycyclic hydrocarbonss stimulate epidermal expression of TNFα and other inflammatory cytokines (Casale et al. 2000). TNFα-null mice are resistant to PAH-induced skin tumor formation (Moore et al. 1999; Suganuma 1999). Similarly, TNFα may enhance the effects of PAH metabolites in the BM.

TNFα stimulates double-stranded RNA-activated protein kinase R (PKR), which inhibits translation (Gil and Esteban 2000; Williams 1999). We have shown that DMBA effects on BM cells are lost in PKR–/– mice (Page et al. 2004). DMBA treatment causes activation of PKR in wild type, but not in TNFR–/– mice. This suggests that PKR activation mediates effects of TNFα in the BM. Recent work shows that PKR plays an essential role in the cell response to bulky DNA adducts, similar to those formed by PAHDE (Bergeron et al. 2000). Protein kinase R may, therefore, coordinate independent effects of PAHDE on

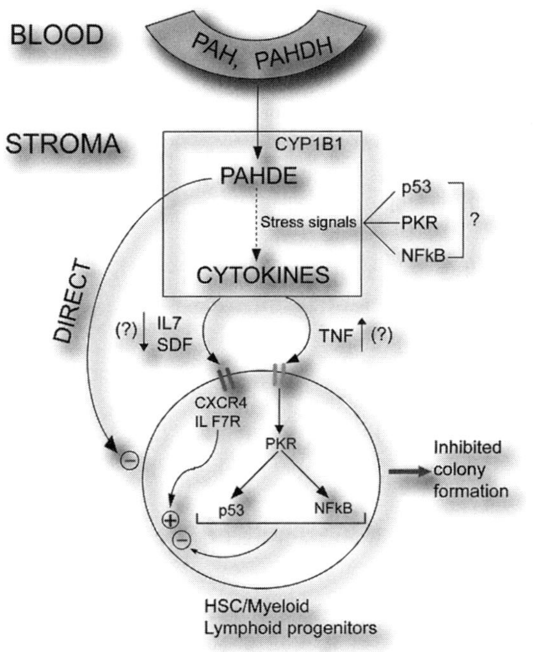

Figure 14.9 Scheme of PAH effects on hematopoietic cells in bone marrow involving activation by CYP1B1 in stromal cells. PAH or PAHDH reaching BM from blood are metabolized by CYP1B1 in stroma (fibroblasts, endothelia, macrophage) to dihydrodiol epoxides or quinones. These reactive chemicals activate p53 and other stress responses in the stroma to increase or decrease cytokines and other proteins that regulate hematopoiesis. For example, IL7, SDF1 exert selective stimulatory effects on progenitor differentiation through their cognate receptors (ILF7-R, CXLR4), while TNFα exerts suppression effects through TNFR. Reactive metabolites from stroma also transfer to hematopoietic cells and cause apoptosis in combination with signaling effects of TNFα. Synergy between p53 pathways activated by reactive metabolites, effects on DNA, and TNFα/PKR signaling may converge on apoptotic pathways.

hematopoietic cells and a more general stress activation of TNFα. Protein kinase R can also activate p53. This cooperation between PAH metabolites, TNFα, p53, and PKR is currently under investigation in our group of investigators.

In vivo BP and DMBA treatment increases TNFα mRNA in BM cells immediately after elution from the femur (Galvan et al. 2006), consistent with the finding that TNFα signaling is required for DMBA-stimulated BM toxicity. This less than twofold effect probably reflects large increases in immunoreactive TNFα in a subset of cells.

Figure 14.9 provides a simple overview of how we envision TNFα and PAH-derived reactive metabolites as well as reactive metabolites from benzene and BD might adversely affect susceptible populations of BM cells. Reactive metabolites from stromal metabolism may either act directly on progenitor cells or indirectly through altered cytokine release. Reactive metabolites affect release of TNFα from stroma in response to DNA damage, p53, and NF-κB activations. TNFα, either directly or through enhancing chemical stress effects, suppresses hematopoietic progenitor cells. The effects of other cytokines (IL7 or SDF1) may be decreased through similar stress pathways.

14.14. Conclusions

There is considerable mechanistic overlap in the toxicity of these chemicals. Many of the same questions arise concerning the extent to which the reactive metabolites are generated exclusively in the BM or derive from hepatic precursors. More extensive knowledge of participating enzymes in the BM is advancing this understanding. DNA-adduct and protein-adduct analyses provide a measure of reactive metabolites, and have been used extensively in occupational health studies, particularly in comparison to lymphocyte mutations and chromosomal abnormalities. However, the relationship between BM changes and observed responses in blood cells requires more study.

Direct DNA damage does not provide the only route to such responses. Epigenetic effects on DNA methylation, chromatin structure effects on DNA repair processes, and chromosomal damage from effects on mitotic regulation, each provide new directions for assessing toxicity. For PAHs, and probably for the other chemicals, inflammatory cytokines, notably TNFα, critically mediate the effects of reactive metabolites on hematopoietic progenitor cells, which are primarily targeted. Effects of the chemicals on the stromal support processes have been implicated in the BM effects of benzene and PAHs and are likely to extend to butadiene.

While extrapolation from rodent models is useful, differences between rats and mice warrant caution in interpreting human data. More recent work has used microarray mRNA expression studies based on blood samples to identify novel responses and risk markers. The chemical-mediated changes observed in HSCs provide an important direction to understanding the long-term effects of these chemicals, including cancer.

References

Abdel-Rahman, S. Z., Ammenheuser, M. M., and Ward, J. B. 2001. Human sensitivity to 1,3-butadiene: role of human microsomal epoxide hydrolase polymorphisms. Carcinogenesis 22:415–422.

Abraham, N. G. 1996. Hematopoietic effects of benzene inhalation assessed by long-term bone marrow culture. Environ. Health Perspect. 104 Suppl. 6:1277–1282.

Albertini, R. J., Shram, R. J., Vacek, P. M., Lynch, J., Rossner, P., Niclas, J. A., McDonald, J. D., Boysen, G., Georgieva, N., and Swendberg, J. A. 2007. Molecular epidemiology studies in 1,3-butadiene exposed Czech workers. Chem. Biol. Interact. 166:63–77.

Alison, M. R., Lovell, M. J., Direkze, N. C., Wright, N. A., and Poulsom, R. 2006. Stem cell plasticity and tumor formation. Eur. J. Cancer 42:1247–1256.

Allen, L. L., Mann, K. K., Matulka, R. A., Ryn, H. Y., Schlezinger, J. J., and Sherr, D. H. 2003. Bone marrow stromal B cell interactions in polycyclic aromatic hydrocarbon-induced pro/pre-B cell apoptosis. Toxicol. Sci. 76:357–365.

Arnott, C. H., Scott, K. A., Moore, R. J., Hewer, A., Phillips, D. H., Parker, P., Balkwill, F. R., and Owens, D. M. 2002. Tumour necrosis factor-alpha mediates tumour promotion via a PKC alpha- and AP-1-dependent pathway. Oncogene 21:4728–4738.

Auyeung, D. J., Kessler, F. K., and Ritter, J. K. 2001. An alternative promoter contributes to tissue- and inducer-specific expression of the rat UDP-glucuronosyltransferase 1A6 gene. Toxicol. Appl. Pharmacol. 174:60–68.

Auyeung, D. J., Kessler, F. K., and Ritter, J. K. 2003. Mechanism of rat UDP-glucuronosyltransferase 1A6 induction by oltipraz: evidence for a contribution of the aryl hydrocarbon receptor pathway. Mol. Pharmacol. 63:119–127.

Bauer, A. K., Faiola, B., Abernethy, D. J., Marchan, R., Pluta, L. J., Wong, V. A., and Loechler, E. L. 1995. How are potent bulky carcinogens able to induce such a diverse array of mutations? Mol. Carcinog. 13:213–219.

Bauer, A. K., Faiola, B., Abernethy, D. J., Marchan, R., Pluta, L. J., Wong, V. A., Gonzalez, F. J., Butterworth, B. E. Borghoff, S. J., Everitt, J. I., and Recio, L. 2003. Male mice deficient in microsomal epoxide hydrolase are not susceptible to benzene-induced toxicity. Toxicol. Sci. 72:201–209.

Bergeron, J., Benlimame, N., Zeng-Rong, N., Ziao, D., Scrivens, P. J., Koromilas, A. E., and Alaoui-Jamali, M. A. 2000. Identification of the interferon-inducible double-stranded RNA-dependent protein kinase as a regulator of cellular response to bulky adducts. Cancer Res. 60:6800–6804.

Bernauer, U., Vieth, B., Ellrich, R., Heinrich-Hirsch, B., Janig, G. R., and Gundert-Remy, U. 2000. CYP2E1 expression in bone marrow and its intra and inter species variability; approaches for a more reliable extrapolation from one species to another in the risk assessment of chemicals. Arch. Toxicol. 73:618–624.

Bhattacharyya, K. K., Brake, P. B., Eltom, S. E., Otto, S. A., and Jefcoate, C. R. 1995. Identification of a rat adrenal cytochrome P450 active in polycyclic hydrocarbon metabolism as rat CYP1B1. J. Biol. Chem. 270:11595–11602.

Boffetta, P., Jourenkova, N., and Gustavsson, P. 1997. Cancer risk from occupational and environmental exposure to polycyclic aromatic hydrocarbons. Cancer Causes Control 8:444–472.

Bolton, J. L., Trush, M. A., Penning, G. A., Dryhurst, G., and Monks, T. J. 2000. Role of quinones in toxicology. Chem. Res. Toxicol. 13:135–160.

Bond, J. A., and Medinsky, M. A. 2001. Insights into the toxicokinetics and toxicodynamics of 1,3-butadiene. Chem. Biol. Interact. 135–136:599–614.

Bryder, D., Ramsfjell, V., Dybedal, I. Theilgaard-Monch, K., Hogerkorp, C.M., Adolfsson, J., Borge, O.J., and Jacobson, S.E. 2001. Self-renewal of multipotent long-term repopulating hematopoietic stem cells is negatively regulated by Fas and tumor necrosis factor receptor activation. J. Exp. Med. 194:941–952.

Burczynski, M. E., and Penning, T. M. 2000. Genotoxic polycyclic aromatic hydrocarbon ortho-quinones generated by aldo–keto reductases induce CYP1A1 via nuclear translocation of the aryl hydrocarbon receptor. Cancer Res. 60:908–915.

Buters, J. T., Sakai, S., Richter, T., Pineau, T., Alexander, D. L., Savas, U., Doehmer, J., Ward, J. R., Jefcoate, C. R., and Gonzalez, F. J. 1999. Cytochrome P4501B1 determines susceptibility to 7,12-dimethylbenz[a]anthracene-induced lymphomas. Proc. Natl. Acad. Sci. U.S.A. 96:1977–1982.

Carsetti, R. 2000. The development of B cells in the bone marrow is controlled by the balance between cell-autonomous mechanisms and signals from the microenvironment. J. Exp. Med. 191:5–8.

Casale, G. P., Cheng, Z., Liu, J., Cavalieri, E. L., and Singhal, M. 2000. Profiles of cytokine mRNAs in the skin and lymph nodes of SENCAR mice treated epicutaneously with dibenzo[a,l]pyrene or dimethylbenz[a]anthracene reveal a direct correlation between carcinogen-induced contact hypersensitivity and epidermal hyperplasia. Mol. Carcinog. 27:125–140.

Chakravarti, D., Zahid, M., Backora, M., Myers, E. M., Gaikwad, N., Weisenburger, D. D., Cavalieri, E. L., Rogan, E. G., and Joshi, S. S. 2006. Orthoquinones of benzene and estrogens induce hyperproliferation of human peripheral blood mononuclear cells. Leuk. Lymphoma 47:2635–2644.

Chen, Y., Li, G., Yin, S., Xu, J., Ji, Z., Xiu, X., Liu, L., and Ma, D. 2007. Genetic polymorphisms involved in toxicant-metabolizing enzymes and the risk of chronic benzene poisoning in Chinese occupationally exposed populations. Xenobiotica 37:103–112.

Conney, A. H., Chang, R. L., Jerina, D. M., and Wei, S. J. 1994. Studies on the metabolism of benzo[a]pyrene and dose-dependent differences in the mutagenic profile of its ultimate carcinogenic metabolite. Drug Metab. Rev. 26:125–163.

Declercq, W., Denecker, G., Fiers, W., and Vandenabeele, P. 1998. Cooperation of both TNF receptors in inducing apoptosis: involvement of the TNF-receptor-associated factor binding domain of the TNF receptor 75. J. Immunol. 161:390–399.

Dogusan, Z., Montecino-Rodriguez, E., and Dorshkind, K. 2004. Macrophages and stromal cells phagocytose apoptotic bone marrow-derived B lineage cells. J. Immunol. 172:4717–4723.

Elfarra, A. A., Krause, R. J., and Selzer, R. R. 1996. Biochemistry of 1,3-butadiene metabolism and its relevance to 1,3-butadiene-induced carcinogenicity. Toxicology 113:23–30.

Faiola, B., Fuller, E. S., Wong, V. A., and Recio, L. 2004. Gene expression profile in bone marrow and hematopoietic stem cells in mice exposed to inhaled benzene. Mutat. Res. 549:195–212.

Forrest, M. S., Lan, Q., Hubbard, A. E., Zhang, L., Vermeulen, R., Zhao, X., Li, G., Wu, Y-Y., Shen, M., Yin, S., Chanock, S. J., Rothman, N., and Smith, M. T. 2005. Discovery of novel biomarkers by microarray analysis of peripheral blood mononuclear cell gene expression in benzene-exposed workers. Environ. Health Perspect. 113:801–807.

Funk, P. E., Kincade, P. W., and Witte, P. L. 1994. Native associations of early hematopoietic stem cells and stromal cells isolated in bone marrow cell aggregates. Blood 83:361–369.

Galvan, N., Jaskul-Sztul, R., MacWilliams, P. S., Czuprynski, C. J., and Jefcoate, C. R. 2003. Bone marrow cytotoxicity of benzo[a]pyrene is dependent on CYP1B1, but is diminished by Ah receptor-mediated induction of CYP1A1 in liver. Toxicol. Appl. Pharmacol. 193:84–96.

Galvan, N., Teske, D. E., Zhou, G., Moorthy, B., MacWilliams, P. S., Czuprynski, C. J., and Jefcoate, C. R. 2005. Induction of CYP1A1 and CYP1B1 in liver and lung by benzo(a)pyrene and 7,12-dimethylbenz(a)anthracene do not affect distribution of polycyclic hydrocarbons to target tissue: role of AhR and CYP1B1 in bone marrow cytotoxicity. Toxicol. Appl. Pharmacol. 202:244–257.

Galvan, N., Page, T. J., Czuprynski, C. J, Jefcoate, C. R. 2006. Benzo(a)pyrene and 7,12 dimethylbenzantanthracene differentially affect bone marrow cells of lymphoid and myeloid lineages. Toxicol. Appl. Pharmacol. 213:105–116.

Gaskell, M., McLuckie, K. I. E., and Farmer, P. B. 2004. Comparison of the repair of DNA damage induced by the benzene metabolites hydroquinone and *p*-benzoquinone: a role for hydroquinone in benzene genotoxicity. Carcinogenesis 26:673–680.

Gil, J., and Esteban, M. 2000. Induction of apoptosis by the dsRNA-dependent protein kinase (PKR): mechanism of action. Apoptosis 5:107–114.

Givers, C. R., Wong, R., Moore, D. H., and Pallavicini, M. G. 2001. Persistence of aneuploid immature/primitive hematopoietic sub-populations in mice 8 months after benzene exposure. Mutat. Res. 491:127–136.

Glatt, H., Padykula, R., Berchtold, G. A., Ludewig, G., Platt, K. L., Klein, J., and Oesch, F. 1989. Multiple activation pathways of benzene leading to products with varying genotoxic characteristics. Environ. Health Perspect. 82:81–89.

Grawunder, U., Melchers, F., and Rolink, A. 1993. Interferon-gamma arrests proliferation and causes apoptosis in stromal cell/interleukin-7-dependent normal murine pre-B cell lines and clones in vitro, but does not induce differentiation to surface immunoglobulin-positive B cells. Eur. J. Immunol. 23:544–551.

Greten, F. R., Eckmann, L., Greten, T. F., Park, J. M., Li, Z. W., Egan, L. J., Kagnoff, M. F., and Karin, M. 2004. IKKβ links inflammation and tumorigenesis in a mouse model of colitis-associated cancer. Cell 118:285–296.

Grove, A. D., Llewellyn, G. C., Kessler, F. K., White, K. L. Jr., Crespi, C. L., and Ritter, J. K. 2000. Differential protection by rat UDP-glucuronosyltransferase

1A7 against benzo[a]pyrene-3,6-quinone- versus benzo[a]pyrene-induced cytotoxic effects in human lymphoblastoid cells. Toxicol. Appl. Pharmacol. 162:34–43.

Gu, J., Weng, Y., Zhang, Q. Y., Cui, H., Behr, M., Wu, L., Yang, W., Zhang, L., and Ding, X. 2003. Liver-specific deletion of the NADPH-cytochrome P450 reductase gene. J. Biol. Chem. 278:25895–25901.

Guo, N., Faller, D. V., and Vaziri, C. 2002. Carcinogen-induced S-phase arrest is Chk1 mediated and caffeine sensitive. Cell Growth Differentiation 13:77–86.

Guoqing, C., and Goeddel, D. V. 2002. TNF-R1 signaling: a beautiful pathway. Science 296:1634–1635.

Hahn, B. K., Piktel, D., Gibson, L. F., and Landreth, K. S. 2000. Hematopoiesis: the role of stromal integrin interactions in pro-B cell proliferation. Hematology 5:153–160.

Hardy, R. R., and Hayakawa, K. 2001. B cell development pathways. Annu. Rev. Immunol. 19:595–621.

Heidel, S. M., Czuprynski, C. J., and Jefcoate, C. R. 1998. Bone marrow stromal cells constitutively express high levels of cytochrome P4501B1 that metabolizes 7,12-dimethylbenz[a]anthracene. Mol. Pharmacol. 54:1000–1006.

Heidel, S. M., Holston, K., Buters, J. M. T., Gonzalez, F. J., Jefcoate, C. R., and Czuprynski, C. J. 1999. Bone marrow stromal cell cytochrome P4501B1 is required for preB cell apoptosis induced by 7,12-dimethylbenz[a]anthracene. Mol. Pharmacol. 56:1317–1323.

Heidel, S. M., MacWilliams, P. S., Baird, W. M., Dashwood, W. D., Buters, J. T. M., Gonzalez, F. J., Larsen, M. C., Czuprynski, C. J., and Jefcoate, C. R. 2000. Cytochrome P4501B1 mediates induction of bone marrow cytotoxicity and preleukemia cells in mice treated with 7,12-dimethylbenz[a]anthracene. Cancer Res. 60:3454–3460.

Heince, J.-F., Koslov, S., Dawson, V. L., Dawson, T. M., Hendzel, M. J., Lavin, M. F., and Poirier, G. G. 2007. ATM signaling network is modulated by a novel PAR-dependent in the early response to DNA damaging agents. J. Biol. Chem. 282:16441–16453.

Iguchi, A., Okuyama, R., Koguma, M., Obinata, M., and Yanai, N. 1997. Selective stimulation of granulopoiesis in vitro by established bone marrow stromal cells. Cell Struct. Funct. 22:357–364.

Irons, R. D., Pyatt, D. W., Stillman, W. S., Som, D. B., Claffey, D. J., and Ruth, J. A. 2000. Comparative toxicity of known and putative metabolites of 1,3-butadiene in human CD34(+) bone marrow cells. Toxicology 150:99–106.

Jemnitz, K., Veres, Z., and Vereczkey, L. 2002. Coordinate regulation of UDP-glucuronosyltransferase UGT1A6 induction by 3-methylcholanthrene and multidrug resistance protein MRP2 expression by dexamethasone in primary rat hepatocytes. Biochem. Pharmacol. 63:2137–2144.

Jin, Y., and Penning, T. M. 2007. Aldo–keto reductases and bioactivation/detoxication. Ann. Rev. Pharm. Toxicol. 47:263–92.

Kalf, G. F., Renz, J. F., and Niculescu, R. 1996. *p*-Benzoquinone, a reactive metabolite of benzene, prevents the processing of pre-interleukins-1 alpha and -1 beta to activate cytokines by inhibition of the processing enzymes, calpain, and interleukin-1 beta converting enzyme. Environ. Health Perspect. 104 Suppl. 6:1251–1256.

Kerzee, J. K., and Ramos, K. S. 2000. Activation of c-Ha-ras by benzo(a)pyrene in vascular smooth muscle cells involves redox stress and aryl hydrocarbon receptor. Mol. Pharmacol. 58:152–158.

Kim, S., Vermeulen, R., Waidjanatha, S., and Rappaport, S. M. 2006. Modeling human metabolism of benzene following occupational and environmental exposure. Cancer Epidemiol. Biomarkers Prev. 15:2246–2252.

Kleiner, H. E., Vulimiri, S. V., Hatten, W. B., Reed, M. J., Nebert, D. W., Jefcoate, C. R., DiGiovanni, J. 2004. Role of cytochrome P4501 family members in the metabolic activation of polycyclic aromatic hydrocarbons in mouse epidermis. Chem. Res. Toxicol. 17:1667–1674.

Kouro, T., Medina, K. L., Oritani, K., and Kincade, P.W. 2001. Characteristics of early murine B-lymphocyte precursors and their direct sensitivity to negative regulators. Blood 97:2708–2715.

Kumar, A., Patel, S., Gupta, Y. K., and Singh, M. P. 2006. Involvement of endogenous nitric oxide in myleoperoxidase mediated benzo(a)pyrene induced polymorphonuclear leukocytes injury. Mol. Cell. Biochem. 286:43–51.

Kwak, M. K., Egner, P. A., Dolan, P. M., Ramos-Gomez, M., Groopman, J. D., Itoh, K., Yamamoto, M., and Kensler, T. W. 2001. Role of Phase 2 enzyme induction in chemoprotection by dithiolethiones. Mutat. Res. 480:305–315.

Lan, Q., Zhang, L., Li, G., Vermeulen, R., Weinberg, R. S., Dosemeci, M., Rappaport, S. M., Shen, M., Alter, B. P., Wu, Y., Kopp, W., Waidyanatha, S., Rabkin, C., Guo, W., Chanock, S., Hayes, R. B., Linet, M., Kim, S., Yin, S., Rothman, N., and Smith, M. T. 2004. Hematotoxicity in workers exposed to low levels of benzene. Science 306:1774–1776.

Legraverend, C., Harrison, D. E., Ruscetti, F. W., and Nebert, D. W. 1983. Bone marrow toxicity induced by oral benzo[a]pyrene: protection resides at the level of the intestine and liver. Toxicol. Appl. Pharmacol. 70:390–401.

Lin, Y.S., McKelvey, Waidyanatha, S., and Rappaport, S.M. 2006. Variability of albumin adducts of 1,4-benzoquinone, a toxic metabolite of benzene, in human volunteers. Biomarkers 11:14–27.

Lind, C. 1985. Formation of benzo[a]pyrene-3,6-quinol mono- and diglucuronides in rat liver microsomes. Arch. Biochem. Biophys. 240:226–235.

Liu, T. M., Martina, M., Hutmacher, D. W., Lee, E. H., and Lim, B. 2007. Identification of common pathways mediating differentiation of bone marrow- and adipose tissue-derived human mesenchymal stem cells into three mesenchymal lineages. Stem Cells 25:750–760.

Loechler, E. L. 1995. How are potent bulky carcinogens able to induce such a diverse array of mutations? Mol. Carcinogenesis 13:213–219.

Long, D. J. 2 nd, Waikel, R. L., Wang, X. J., Perlaky, L., Roop, D. R., and Jaiswal, A. K. 2000. NAD(P)H:quinone oxidoreductase 1 deficiency increases susceptibility to benzo(a)pyrene-induced mouse skin carcinogenesis. Cancer Res. 60:5913–5915.

Long, D. J. 2 nd, Waikel, R. L., Wang, X. J., Roop, D. R., and Jaiswal, A. K. 2001. NAD(P)H:quinone oxidoreductase 1 deficiency and increased susceptibility to 7,12-dimethylbenz[a]-anthracene-induced carcinogenesis in mouse skin. J. Natl. Cancer Inst. 93:1166–1170.

Long, D. J. 2 nd, Gaikwad, A., Multani, A., Pathak, S., Montgomery, C. A., Gonzalez, F. J., and Jaiswal, A. K. 2002. Disruption of the NAD(P)H:quinone oxidoreductase 1 (NQO1) gene in mice causes myelogenous hyperplasia. Cancer Res. 62:3030–3036.

Ma, Q., Kinneer, K., Bi, Y., Chan, J. Y., and Kan, Y. W. 2004. Induction of murine NAD(P)H:quinone oxidoreductase by 2,3,7,8-tetrachlorodibenzo-*p*-dioxin requires the CNC (cap 'n' collar) basis leucine zipper transcription factor Nrf2 (nuclear factor erythroid 2-related factor 2): cross-interaction between AhR (aryl hydrocarbon receptor) and Nrf2 signal transduction. Biochem. J. 377:205–213.

Maniglier-Poulet, C., Cheng, X., Ruth, J. A., and Ross, D. 1995. Metabolism of 1,3-butadiene to butadiene monoxide in mouse and human bone marrow cells. Chem. Biol. Interact. 97:119–129.

Manini, P., De Palma, G., Andreoli, R., Poli, D., Mozzoni, P., Folesani, G., Mutti, A., and Apostoli, P. 2006. Environmental and biological monitoring of benzene exposure in a cohort of Italian taxi drivers. Toxicol. Lett. 167:142–151.

Mann, K. K., Matulka, R. A., Hahn, M. E., Trombino, A. F., Lawrence, B. P., Kerkvliet, N. I., and Sherr, D. H. 1999. The role of polycyclic aromatic hydrocarbon metabolism in dimethylbenz[a]anthracene-induced pre-B lymphocyte apoptosis. Toxicol. Appl. Pharmacol. 161:10–22.

Marston, C. P., Periera, C., Ferguson, J., Fischer, K., Hedstrom, O., Dashwood, W. M., and Baird, W. M. 2001. Effect of a complex environmental mixture from coal tar containing polycyclic aromatic hydrocarbons (PAH) on the tumor initiation, PAH-DNA binding and metabolic activation of carcinogenic PAH in mouse epidermis. Carcinogenesis 22:1077–1086.

Mastrangelo, G., Fadda, E., and Marzia, V. 1996. Polycyclic aromatic hydrocarbons and cancer in man. Environ. Health Perspect. 104:1166–1170.

McFadyen, M. C., and Murray, G. T. 2005. Cytochrome P4501B1, a novel anticancer therapeutic target. Future Oncol. 1:252–259.

Miscia, S., Marchisio, M., Grilli, A., Di Valerio, V., Centurione, L., Sabatino, G., Garaci, F., Zauli, G., Bonvini, E., and Di Baldassarre, A. 2002. Tumor necrosis factor alpha (TNF-alpha) activates Jak1/Stat3-Stat5B signaling through TNFR-1 in human B cells. Cell Growth Differ. 13:13–18.

Moore, R. J., Owens, D. M., Stamp, G., Arnott, C., Burke, F., East, N., Holdsworth, H., Turner, L., Rollins, B., Pasparakis, M., Kollias, G., and Balkwill, F. 1999. Mice deficient in tumor necrosis factor-alpha are resistant to skin carcinogenesis. Nat. Med. 5:828–831.

Moorthy, B., Miller, K. P., Jiang, W., Williams, E. S., Kondraganti, S. R., and Ramos, K. S. 2003. Role of cytochrome P4501B1 in benzo[a]pyrene activation to DNA-binding metabolites in mouse vascular smooth muscle cells: evidence from ^{32}P-postlabeling for formation of 3-hydroxybenzo[a]pyrene and benzo[a]pyrene-3,6-quinone as major proximate genotoxic intermediates. J. Pharmacol. Exp. Ther. 305:394–401.

Morgan, G. J., and Alvares, C. L. 2005. Benzene and the hematopoietic cell. Chem. Biol. Interact. 153/154:217–222.

Moran, J. L., Siegel, D., and Ross, D. 1999. A potential mechanism underlying the increased susceptibility of individuals with a polymorphism in NADPH quinone reductase 1 (NQO1) to benzene toxicity. Proc. Natl. Acad. Sci. U.S.A. 96:8150–8155.

Mundle, S.D., Reza, S., Ali, A., Mativi, Y., Shetty, V., Venugopal, P., Gregory, S.A., and Raza, A. 1999. Correlation of tumor necrosis factor alpha (TNF alpha) with high caspase 3-like activity in myelodysplastic syndromes. Cancer Lett. 140:201–207.

Murante, F. G., and Gasiewicz, T. A. 2000. Hematopoietic progenitor cells are sensitive targets of 2,3,7,8-tetrachlorodibenzo-*p*-dioxin in C57Bl/6 J mice. Toxicol. Sci. 54:374–383.

Near, R. I., Matulka, R. A., Mann, K. K., Gogate, S. U., Trombino, A. F., and Sherr, D. H. 1999. Regulation of preB cell apoptosis by aryl hydrocarbon receptor/transcription factor-expressing stromal/adherent cells. Proc. Soc. Exp. Biol. Med. 221:242–252.

Page, T. J., O'Brien, S., Jefcoate, C. R., and Czuprynski, C. J. 2002. 7,12-Dimethylbenz[a]anthracene-induces apoptosis in murine pre-B cells through a caspase 8 dependent pathway. Mol. Pharmacol. 62:313–319.

Page, T. J., O'Brien, S., Holston, K., Macwilliams, P., Jefcoate, C. R., and Czuprynski, C. J. 2003. 7,12-Dimethylbenz[a]anthracene-induced bone marrow toxicity is p53 dependent. Toxicol. Sci. 74:85–92.

Page, T. J., Macwilliams, P., Suresh, M., Jefcoate, C. R., and Czuprynski, C. J. 2004. 7,12-Dimethylbenz[a]anthracene-induced bone marrow hypocellularity is dependent on signaling through both the TNFR and PKR. Toxicol. Appl. Pharmacol. 198:21–28.

Palackal, N. T., Burczynski, M. E., Harvey, R. G., and Penning, T. M. 2001. The ubiquitous aldehyde reductase (AKR1A1) oxidizes proximate carcinogen trans-dihydrodiols to *o*-quinones: potential role in polycyclic aromatic hydrocarbon activation. Biochemistry 40:10901–10910.

Palackal, N. T., Lee, S. H., Harvey, R. G., Blair, I. A., and Penning, T. M. 2002. Activation of polycyclic aromatic hydrocarbon trans-dihydrodiol proximate carcinogens by human aldo–keto reductase (AKR1C) enzymes and their functional overexpression in human lung carcinoma (A549) cells. J. Biol. Chem. 277:24799–24808.

Pilger, A., and Rudiger, H.W. 2006. 8-Hydroxy-2'-deoxyguanosine as a marker of oxidative DNA damage related to occupational and environmental exposures. Int. Arch. Occup. Environ. Health 80:1–15.

Rebel, V.I., Hartnett, S., Hill, G.R., Lazo-Kallanian, S.B., Ferrara, J.L., and Sieff, C.A. 1999. Essential role for the p55 tumor necrosis factor receptor in regulating hematopoiesis at a stem cell level. J. Exp. Med. 190:1493–1504.

Recio, L., Saranko, C. J., and Steen, A. M. 2000. 1,3-Butadiene: cancer, mutations, and adducts. Part II: roles of two metabolites of 1,3-butadiene in mediating its in vivo genotoxicity. Res. Rep. Health Eff. Inst. 92:49–87.

Reya, T., and Clevers, H. 2005. Wnt signaling in stem cells and cancer. Nature 434:843–849.

Ross, D., Siegel, D., Schattenberg, D. G., Sun, X. M., and Moran, J. L. 1996. Cell-specific activation and detoxification of benzene metabolites in mouse and human bone marrow: identification of target cells and a potential role for modulation of apoptosis in benzene toxicity. Environ Health Perspect. 104 Suppl 6:1177–1182.

Ross, D. 2005. Functions and distribution of NQO1 in human bone marrow: potential clues to benzene toxicity. Chem. Biol. Interact. 153-154:137–146.

Rusten, L.S., and Jacobsen, S.E. 1995. Tumor necrosis factor (TNF)-alpha directly inhibits human erythropoiesis in vitro: role of p55 and p75 TNF receptors. Blood 85:989–996.

Rusten, L.S., Jacobsen, F.W., Lesslauer, W., Loetscher, H., Smeland, E.B., and Jacobsen, S.E. 1994. Bifunctional effects of tumor necrosis factor alpha (TNF alpha) on the growth of mature and primitive human hematopoietic progenitor cells: involvement of p55 and p75 TNF receptors. Blood. 83:3152–3159.

Sakai, R., Kajiume, T., Inoue, H., Kanno, R., Miyazaki, M., Ninomiya, Y., and Kanno, M. 2003. TCDD treatment eliminates the long-term reconstitution activity of hematopoietic stem cells. Toxicol. Sci. 72:84–91.

Saranko, C. J., Meyer, K. G., Pluta, L. J., Henderson, R. F., Recio, L. 2001. Lung specific mutagenicity and mutational spectrum in B6C3F1 laci transgenic mice following inhalation exposure to 1,2-epoxybutene. Mutat. Res. 473:37–49.

Savas, U., Bhattacharyya, K.K., Christou, M., Alexander, D.L. and Jefcoate, C.R. 1994. Mouse cytochrome P-450EF, representative of a new 1B subfamily of cytochrome P-450s. Cloning, sequence determination, and tissue expression. J. Biol. Chem. 269:14905–14911.

Schmidt, J. V., and Bradfield, C. A. 1996. Ah receptor signaling pathways. Ann. Rev. Cell. Dev. Biol. 12:55–89.

Scholdberg, T. A., Merritt, W. K., Dean, S. M., Kowalcyzk, A., Harris, C. M., Harris, T. M., Rizzo, C. J., Lloyd, R. S., and Stone, M. P. 2005. Structure of an oligodeoxynucleotide containing a butadiene oxide-derived N1 beta-

hydroxyalkyl deoxyinosine adduct in the human N-ras codon 61 sequence. Biochemistry 44:3327–3337.
Schrenk, D., Orzechowski, A., Schwarz, L. R., Snyder, R., Burchell, B., Ingelman-Sundman, M., and Bock, K. W. 1996. Phase II metabolism of benzene. Environ. Health Perspect. 104:1183–1188.
Shimada, T., and Guengerich, F.P. 2006. Inhibition of human cytochrome P450 1A1-, 1A2-, and 1B1-mediated activation of procarcinogens to genotoxic metabolites by polycyclic aromatic hydrocarbons. Chem. Res. Toxicol. 19:288–294.
Snyder, R. 2002. Benzene and leukemia. Crit. Rev. Toxicol. 32:155–202.
Snyder, R., Chepiga, T., Yang, C. S., Thomas, H., Platt, K., and Oesch, F. 1993. Benzene meabolism by reconstituted cytochromes P450 2B1 and 2E1 and its modulation by cytochrome b5, microsomal epoxide hydrolase, and glutathione transferases: evidence for an important role of microsomal epoxide hydrolase in the formation of hydroquinone. Toxicol. Appl. Pharmacol. 122:172–181.
Soucek, P., Anzenbacher, P., Skoumalova, I., and Dvorak, M. 2005. Expression of cytochrome P450 genes in Cd34+ hematopoietic stem and progenitor cells. Stem Cells 23:1417–1422.
Suganuma, M., Okabe, S., Marino, M. W., Sakai, A., Sueoka, E., and Fujiki, H. 1999. Essential role of tumor necrosis factor alpha (TNF-alpha) in tumor promotion as revealed by TNF-alpha-deficient mice. Cancer Res. 59:4516–4518.
Sundberg, K., Dreij, K., Seidel, A., and Jernstrom, B. 2002. Glutathione conjugation and DNA adduct formation of dibenzo[a,l]pyrene and benzo[a]pyrene diol epoxides in V79 cells stably expressing different human glutathione transferases. Chem. Res. Toxicol. 15:170–179.
Sutter, T.R., Y.M. Tang, C.L. Hayes, Y.Y.P. Wo, E.W. Jabs, X. Li, H. Yink, C.W. Cody, and Greenlee, W.F. 1994. Complete cDNA sequence of a human dioxin-inducible mRNA identifies a new gene subfamily of cytochrome p450 that maps to chromosome 2. J. Biol. Chem. 269:13092–13099.
Swendberg, J. A., Boysen, G., Georgieva, G., Bird, M. G., Lewis, R. J. 2007. Future directions in butadiene risk assessment. Chem. Biol. Interact. 116:78–83.
Thurmond, L.M., Lauer, L.D., House, R.V., Cook, J.C., and Dean, J.H. 1987. Immunosuppression following exposure to 7,12- dimethylbenz[a]anthracene (DMBA) in Ah-responsive and Ah-nonresponsive mice. Toxicol. Appl. Pharmacol. 91:450–460.
Thurmond, T. S., and Gasiewicz, T. A. 2000. A single dose of 2,3,7,8-tetrachlorodibenzo-*p*-dioxin produces a time- and dose-dependent alteration in the murine bone marrow B-lymphocyte maturation profile. Toxicol. Sci. 58:88–95.
Tokoyoda, K., Egawa, T., Sugiyama, T., Choi, B., and Nagasawa, T. 2004. Cellular niches controlling B lymphocyte behavior within bone marrow during development. Immunity 20:707–718.
Turteltaub, K. W., and Mani, C. 2003. Benzene metabolism in rodents at doses relevant to human exposure from urban air. Res. Rep. Health Eff. Inst. 113:1–26.
Twerdok, L. E., Mosebrook, D. R., and Trush, M. A. 1992. Comparison of oxidant-generation and BP-diol activation by bone marrow cells from C57Bl/6 and DBA/2 mice: implications for risk of bone marrow toxicity induced by polycyclic hydrocarbons. Toxicol. Appl. Pharmacol. 112:266–272.
Twerdok, L. E., Rembish, S. J., and Trush, M. A. 1992. Induction of quinone reductase and glutathione in bone marrow cells by 1,2-dithiole-3-thione: effects on hydroquinone-induced toxicity. Toxicol. Appl. Pharmacol. 112:273–281.
Uno, S., Dalton, T. P., Derkenne, S., Curran, C. P., Miller, M. L., Shertzer, H. G., and Nebert, D. W. 2004. Oral exposure to benzo[a]pyrene in the mouse: detoxication by inducible cytochrome P450 is more important than metabolic activation. Mol. Pharmacol. 65:1225–1237.

Valentine, J.L., Lee, S.S., Seaton, M.J., Asgharian, B., Farris, G., Corton, J.C., Gonzalez, F.J., and Medinsky, M.A. 1996. Reduction of benzene metabolism and toxicity in mice that lack CYP2E1 expression. Toxicol. Appl. Pharmacol. 141:205–213.

Van Grevenynghe, J., Bernard, M., Lanouet, S., Le Berre, C., Fest, T., and Fardel, O. 2005. Human CD34-positive hematopoietic cells constitute targets for carcinogenic polycyclic aromatic hydrocarbons. J. Pharm. Exp. Therap. 314:693–702.

Vermeulen, R., Lan, Q., Zhang, L., Gunn, L., McCarthy, D., Woodbury, R. L., McGuire, M., Poduct, V. N., Li, G., Chattergee, N., Mu, R., Yin, S., Rothman, N., and Smith, M. T. 2005. Decreased levels of CXC-chemokines in serum of benzene-exposed workers identified by array-based proteomics. Proc. Natl. Acad. Sci. U.S.A. 102:17041–17046.

Vodicka, P., Stetina, R., Smerak, P., Vodickova, L., Naccarati, A., Barta, I., and Hemminki, K. 2006. Micronuclei, DNA single strand breaks, and DNA repair activity in mice exposed to 1,3-butadiene by inhalation. Mutat. Res. 608:49–57.

Waidyanatha, S., Sangaiah, R., and Rappaport, S. M. 2005. Characterization and quantification of cysteine adducts of benzene diol epoxide. Chem. Res. Toxicol. 18:1178–1185.

Wan, J., Shi, J., Hui, L., Wu, D., and Hu, D. 2002. Association of genetic polymorphisms in CYP2E1, MPO, NQO1, GSTM1, and GSTT1 with benzene poisoning. Environ. Hlth Perspect. 110:1213–1218.

Watanabe, N., and Forman, H. J. 2003. Autoxidation of extracellular hydroquinones is a causative event for the cytoxicity of menadione and DMNQ in A549-S cells. Arch. Biochem. Biophys. 411:145–157.

Weissman, I. L. 2000. Stem cells: units of development, units of regeneration, and units in evolution. Cell 100:157–168.

Whysner, J., Reddy, M. V., Ross, P. M., Mohan, M., and Lax, E. A. 2004. Genotoxicity of benzene and its metabolites. Mutat. Res. 566:99–130.

Wickliffe, J. K., Herring, S. M., Hallberg, L. M., Galbert, L. A., Masters, O. E. 3rd., Ammenheuser, M. M., Xie, J., Friedberg, E. C., Lloyd, R. S., Abdel-Rahman, S. Z., and Ward, J. B., Jr. 2007. Detoxification of olefinic epoxides and nucleotide excision repair of epoxide-mediated DNA damage: insights from animal models examining human sensitivity to 1,3-butadiene. Chem. Biol. Interact. 166:226–231.

Williams, B. R. G. 1999. PKR: a sentinel kinase for cellular stress. Oncogene 18:6112–6120.

Wu, Z. H., Shi, Y., Tibbetts, R. S., Miyamoto, S. 2006. Molecular linkage between the kinase ATM and NFκB signaling in response to genotoxic signaling. Science 311:1141–1146.

Wyman, A., Lavin, A. L., Wilding, G. E., and Gasiewicz, T. A. 2002. 2,3,7,8-Tetrachlorodibenzo-*p*-dioxin does not directly alter the phenotype of maturing B cells in a murine coculture system. Toxicol. Appl. Pharmacol. 180:164–177.

Xie, Z., Zhang, Y., Guliaev, A. B., Shen, H., Hang, B., Singer, B., and Wang, Z. 2005. The *p*-benzoquinone DNA adducts derived from benzene are highly mutagenic. DNA Repair 4:1399–1409.

Yamaguchi, K., Matulka, R. A., Shneider, A. M., Tosselli, P., Trombino, A. F., Yang, S., Hafer, L. J., Mann, K. K., Tao, X., Tilly, J. L., Near, R. I., and Sherr, D. H. 1997a. Induction of preB cell apoptosis by 7,12-dimethylbenz[a]anthracene in long-term primary murine bone marrow cultures. Toxicol. Appl. Pharmacol. 147:190–203.

Yamaguchi, K., Near, R. I., Matulka, R. A., Schneider, A., Tosselli, P., Trombino, A. F., and Sherr, D. H. 1997b. Activation of the aryl hydrocarbon receptor/

transcription factor and bone marrow stromal cell-dependent preB cell apoptosis. J. Immunol. 158:2165–2173.

Yoo, H. Y., Kumagai, A., Shevchenko, A., and Dunphy, W. G. 2007. ATM-dependent activation of ATR occurs through phosphorylation of TOPBPI by ATM. J. Biol. Chem. 282:17501–17506.

Yoon, B. I., Hirabayashi, Y., Kawasaki, Y., Kodama, Y., Kaneko, T., Kim, D. Y., and Inoue, T. 2001. Mechanism of action of benzene toxicity: cell cycle suppression I hematopoietic progenitor cells (CFU-GM). Exp. Hematol. 29:278–285.

Yoon, B. I., Kitada, K., Kawasaki, Y., KatsuhideI, I., Kodama, Y., Inoue, T., and Hirobayashi, Y. 2003. Mechanisms of benzene induced hematoxicity and leukemogenicity: cDNA microarray analyses using mouse bone marrow tissue. Environ. Health Perspect. 111:1411–1420.

Zhang, R., Brennan, M. L., Shen, Z., MacPherson, J. C., Schmitt, D., Molenda, C. E., and Hazen, S. L. 2002. Myeloperoxidase functions as a major enzymatic catalyst for initiation of lipid peroxidation at sites of inflammation. J. Biol. Chem. 277:46116–46122.

Zhang, L., Hayes, R. B., Guong, W., McHale, C. M., Yin, S., Wiencke, J. K., O'Neill, J. P., Rothman, N., Li, G. L., and Smith, M. T. 2004. Lack of increased genetic damage in 1,3-butadiene exposed Chinese workers studied in relation to EPHX1 and GST phenotypes. Mutat. Res. 558:63–74.

Zhu, H., Li, Y., and Trush, M. A. 1995. Characterization of benzo[a]pyrene quinone-induced toxicity to primary cultured bone marrow stromal cells from DBA/2 mice: potential role of mitochondrial dysfunction. Toxicol. Appl. Pharmacol. 130:108–120.

15

Butadiene-Mediated Mutagenesis and Carcinogenesis

Jonathan B. Ward[1], Jeffrey K. Wickliffe[1], Michael P. Stone[2], Thomas M. Harris[2], Priscilla H. Fernandes[3,4] and R. Stephen Lloyd[3]
[1]*Department of Preventive Medicine and Community Health, The University of Texas Medical Branch, TX 77555-1110, USA*
[2]*Department of Chemistry, Center for Molecular Toxicology, Vanderbilt University, Nashville, TN 37235, USA*
[3]*Center for Research on Occupational and Environmental Toxicology, Department of Molecular and Medical Genetics, Oregon Health and Science University, Portland, OR 97239, USA*
[4]*Department of Molecular and Human Genetics, Baylor College of Medicine, Houston, TX 77021, USA*
e-mail: lloydst@ohsu.edu

Keywords: Base Substitution Mutations · Frameshift Mutations · Deletion Mutations · DNA Crosslinks · DNA Repair · Transgenic Mice · *Hprt* Mutations · TK6 Human Lymphoblastoid Cells · *Salmonella typhimurium*

15.1. Exposure to Butadiene

1,3-Butadiene (BD) ($CH_2=CH–CH=CH_2$) is a four-carbon, doubly unsaturated chemical that exists as a volatile gas at ambient temperatures and has a mild gasoline-like odor. It ranks 36th in chemicals produced in the US (http://www.osha.gov/SLTC/butadiene/index.html) with a global annual production of > 12 billion pounds, with > 4 billion pounds being produced in the US alone. It is produced through the processing of petroleum and is mainly used in the production of synthetic rubber, plastics, and resins. Exposure to BD mainly occurs in the workplace, including the following industries: synthetic elastomer (rubber and latex) production, petroleum refining, secondary lead smelting, water treatment, agricultural fungicides, production of nylon, and the use of fossil fuels. Exposure to the general population occurs predominantly by inhalation of cigarette smoke, automobile exhaust, or polluted air found in close proximity to chemical, plastic, or rubber production facilities. Additional

A.A. Elfarra (ed.), *Advances in Bioactivation Research*, DOI: 10.1007/978-0-387-77300-1_15,

exposure can result from ingestion of foods that are contaminated from storage in BD-containing plastic containers.

15.2. Human Epidemiology and Carcinogenesis

Epidemiological studies have been reported for workers exposed to BD, both in the manufacture of the monomer and in the styrene-butadiene rubber (SBR) industry. The largest study of monomer production workers involved 2795 individuals employed for at least 6 months between 1952 and 1994 (Divine and Hartman 1996; Divine and Hartman 2001; Divine, Wendt and Hartman 1993). In addition, there were three smaller studies of monomer production workers (Cowles et al. 1994; Downs, Crane and Kim 1987; Ward et al. 1996). Hematological malignancies, mainly lymphomas, were observed in one of the small studies and in the earlier update of the large cohort study. However, these findings were not consistent. Overall, the evidence for cancer induction in monomer production workers has been weak and without dose-related responses. Positive correlations between exposure to BD in monomer production workers and malignancies were only seen in workers employed prior to 1950. These findings were different for the SBR workers, in which there was an increased risk of leukemia associated with exposure to BD in the largest SBR industry study consisting of 17 924 men from eight North American SBR plants (Delzell et al. 1996; Graff et al. 2005; Matanoski et al. 1993; Meinhardt et al. 1982; Santos-Burgoa et al. 1992; Sathiakumar et al. 2005). No increases in other lymphohematopoietic malignancies were observed. Only job categories with relatively high BD exposures showed excess leukemia deaths. In June, 2007, an IARC review committee reclassified butadiene as a Group 1 carcinogen based on the conclusion that there was “sufficient evidence” of a carcinogenic effect in humans (Grosse et al. 2007).

15.3. Rodent Carcinogenesis

Given the limited evidence for an association between BD exposure and leukemia in epidemiological findings, investigators have examined the effect of BD and select metabolites on rodents using carcinogenesis as an endpoint. In mice, BD was found to be a carcinogen, inducing tumors at multiple sites in both sexes but to a much lesser extent in rats (Melnick et al. 1990; Owen and Glaister 1990; Owen et al. 1987). Mice developed tumors from exposure to BD concentrations that were as much as three orders of magnitude lower than those that caused cancer in rats (Melnick et al. 1990; Owen et al. 1987). A two-year study of chronic inhalation exposure of female and male mice to BD concentrations as low as 20 and 62.5 ppm, respectively, increased the incidence of lymphomas as well as adenomas and carcinomas of the lung and liver. In both sexes, excess tumors of the heart, forestomach, Harderian gland, and mammary glands were seen with exposures to 200 ppm (Melnick et al. 1990). At the same dose or higher, an increase in lymphocytic lymphomas in B6C3F1 mice was observed (Huff et al. 1985). More recently, brain tumors were induced in B6C3F1 mice on exposure to BD (Kim et al. 2005). Mice have proven

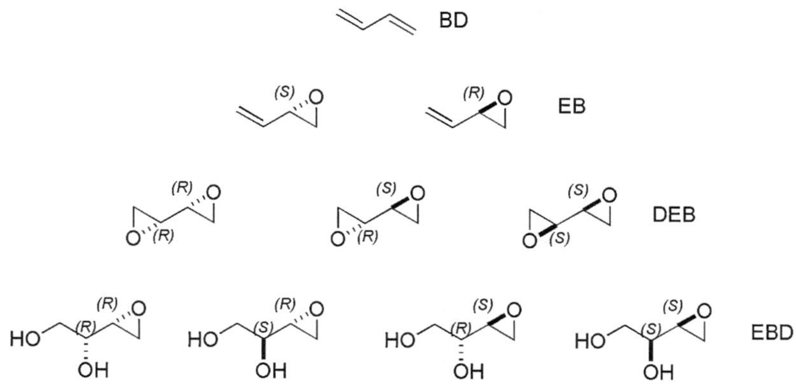

Figure 15.1. Structure of BD and key reactive metabolic intermediates: EB, DEB, and EBD

particularly sensitive to the mutagenic effects of inhaled BD, as well as the epoxide metabolites (Cochrane and Skopek 1994a; Meng et al. 1998a, 1998b, 1999a, 1999b, 2000, 2004).

15.4. Metabolic Activation

Given the interspecies variability in cancer susceptibility associated with BD, significant attention has been focused on the metabolic fates of BD following inhalation. Although the pathways for the metabolic activation and detoxification have been extensively reviewed (Elfarra, Krause and Kemper 2001; Elfarra et al., 2001), we will briefly highlight key intermediates here (Figure 15.1).

BD is oxidized by cytochrome P-450 2E1 and 2A6 to 3,4-epoxy-1-butene (EB) (Csanady, Guengerich and Bond 1992; Duescher and Elfarra 1994); both enantiomers are observed. EB may be further oxidized by either cytochrome P-450 2E1 or 3A4 to form 1,2:3,4-diepoxybutane (DEB). All three stereoisomers arise, that is, the *R,R*, *S,S*, and *R,S* (meso) forms. EB can be hydrolyzed by epoxide hydrolase (EH) to form 3-butene-1,2-diol (Cheng and Ruth 1993; Malvoisin and Roberfroid 1982; Nauhaus et al. 1996) that is subsequently metabolized by cytochrome P-450 to form hydroxymethylvinyl ketone (HMVK) (Kemper, Elfarra and Myers 1998). 3-Butene-1,2-diol and DEB can undergo cytochrome-mediated oxidation and hydrolysis, respectively, to form 3,4-epoxy-1,2-butanediol (EBD) (Boogaard and Bond 1996; Cheng and Ruth 1993; Malvoisin and Roberfroid 1982). These electrophilic species (EB, DEB, EBD, and HMVK) react with nucleophilic sites in DNA and will be reviewed below.

15.5. DNA Adducts

15.5.1. Reactions of EB

EB reacts with nucleophiles at both C_α and C_β with pure nucleophilic reactions favoring attack at C_α and acid-catalyzed reactions favoring C_β.

The reactions of EB with DNA and its constituent nucleosides have been studied extensively (Citti et al. 1984; Koc et al. 1999; Koivisto et al. 1995, 1996, 1997, 1998; Kumar et al. 1996; Leuratti et al. 1993b; Neagu et al. 1994; Selzer and Elfarra, 1996a, 1996b, 1997a, 1999; Tretyakova et al., 1996, 1997a, 1998). Reaction of EB with single-stranded (ss) and double-stranded (ds) DNA has been found to give mainly the N7-(2-hydroxy-3-buten-1-yl) and (1-hydroxy-3-buten-2-yl) adducts of 2′-deoxyguanosine (dGuo), formed in comparable amounts (Blair et al. 2000; Citti et al. 1984; Kumar et al. 1996; Neagu et al. 1994; Selzer and Elfarra 1999; Tretyakova et al. 1997a). Reaction occurs to a lesser extent with dAdo and dCyd. Adducts of dAdo at N1 convert to N^6 adducts via a Dimroth rearrangement which occurs during isolation of the nucleosides by enzymatic degradation of the DNA. The N1 dAdo adducts alternatively undergo hydrolysis of the 6-amino group to give the analogous dIno derivatives. The N3 adducts of dAdo are less stable than N7 adducts of dGuo and readily deglycosylate. Adducts are formed at the N3 position of dCyd which rapidly deaminate to give the analogous dUri derivatives. The rate of reactions at the N7 position of dGuo are not significantly altered by formation of ds DNA but the reactions at other nucleophilic sites in DNA are significantly suppressed by Watson–Crick base pairing.

A limitation on these studies has been that the complex mixtures of products that result from the butadiene monoepoxide (EB) reactions with DNA preclude complete separation and identification of all of the minor products, which although minor in quantity may make major contributions to the genotoxicity of EB. The EB studies have been carried out using racemic EB which adds to the complexity of reaction mixtures by producing diastereomeric mixtures of adducted nucleosides. Consequently, reactions of EB with the individual nucleosides have also been carried out to simplify the separations and to provide an opportunity for more thorough characterization of the individual adducts and thus a more complete description of the reaction potential of DNA.

A study of the reaction of guanine with EB has been carried out (Citti et al. 1984; Kumar et al. 1996; Neagu et al. 1994; Selzer and Elfarra 1996b). Guo was used rather than dGuo. The N7-substituted ribonucleosides deglycosylate more slowly than their 2′-deoxy analogs facilitating direct observation of the N7-substituted nucleosides rather than only the bases derived from them. Reaction occurred mainly at N7; diastereomeric forms of both the C_α and C_β regioisomers were observed. In addition, the diastereoisomeric pair of adducts arising by attack of N^2 on C_β were observed along with even smaller amounts of N1 adducts arising also by attack on C_β. The N^2 and N1 adducts, but not the N7, were thermally stable.

A similar study of the reaction of EB with Ado gave five diastereoisomeric pairs of adducts (Selzer and Elfarra 1996a). The N1 adducts resulting from attack on both the C_α and C_β positions of EB were characterized along with the analogous N^6 adducts arising by Dimroth rearrangement. In addition, a diastereomeric pair of 1-substituted inosines, resulting from attack at the C_β position of EB, were observed. It is known that adducts of epoxides at the N1 position of dAdo are prone to deamination particularly when the hydroxyl group is primary; the deamination process involves intramolecular attack on C6 of adenine by the hydroxyl group (Barlow et al. 1997; Fujii, Saito and Terahara 1986; Kim et al. 2000; Qian and Dipple 1995; Selzer and Elfarra 1996a). The reaction of EB with dCyd gave four diastereomeric pairs of adducts (Selzer and Elfarra 1997b). They were identified as the diastereomeric pairs of adducts arising from attack of N3 on the C_α position of EB, the dUri resulting from both the C_α and C_β adducts of dCyt, and O^6 adducts arising from attack on C_β of dCyt. The dCyt adduct arising by attack on C_β of EB was not observed, but it can be inferred that this adduct had been formed but deaminated too rapidly to be detected. The C_α dCyt adduct was thermally unstable and readily deaminated to form the analogous dUri. The dUri adducts were found to be thermally stable at physiological pH.

Although thymine adducts had not been observed in the reactions of EB with DNA, the reaction of EB with thymidine gave the two pairs of diastereomeric adducts arising from attack of O^4 on the C_α and C_β positions of EB (Selzer and Elfarra 1997a). The rate of formation was significantly slower than the rates for formation of adducts with the other nucleosides, which accounts for the fact that thymine adducts had not been observed in the reactions of EB with DNA (Selzer and Elfarra 1999). These adducts were thermally stable at physiological pH.

15.5.2. Reactions of EBD and DEB

The reactions of DEB and EBD with DNA and its constituent nucleosides have been studied extensively by several research groups (Blair et al. 2000; Koc et al. 1999; Koivisto et al. 1999; Leuratti et al. 1993a, 1993b, 1994; Loeber et al. 2006; Mabon et al. 1996; Millard et al. 2006; Millard and White 1993; Millard and Wilkes 2001; Oe et al. 1999; Park et al. 2004, 2005; Park and Tretyakova 2004; Tretyakova et al. 1996, 1997b, 1997c, 1998; Yunes et al. 1996; Zhang and Elfarra 2003, 2005; Zhao, Koskinen and Hemminki 1998; Zhao et al. 2000). Both EBD and DEB react with DNA primarily at the N7 position of guanine and secondarily with adenine (Koivisto et al. 1999). Both react with high regioselectivity with the terminal C_α of the epoxide. The main products resulting from the reactions of EBD and DEB with DNA are the N7-(2,3,4-trihydroxybutyl) and N7-(2-hydroxy-3, 4-epoxybut-1-yl) adducts, respectively. Both of these adducts are thermally unstable and undergo deglycosylation. The epoxide moiety of the 2-hydroxy-3,4-epoxybut-1-yl derived from DEB is relatively stable to hydrolysis, although it does undergo hydrolysis on storage. In mouse inhalation experiments with BD, the N7-(2,3,4-trihydroxybutyl) adducts were also observed (Koivisto et al. 1999). On the basis of control experiments, they were able to conclude that 98% of these adducts arose from EBD adduction of DEB rather than from DEB and the reaction showed high selectivity for the 2*R*-diol-3*S*-epoxide.

The reactions of DEB with dGuo have been studied by Zhang and Elfarra (2003, 2004, 2005, 2006). The presence of the second epoxide leads to a number of possibilities for secondary reactions of initially formed 2-hydroxy-3,4-epoxybuty-1-yl adducts. In the context of DNA, this reactivity leads to the potential for crosslinking reactions, which have been modeled by Zhang and Elfarra (2006) in nucleosides.

DEB and EBD react with the N1 position of dAdo. The N1 adducts readily undergo rearrangement to the isomeric N^6 adducts by a base-catalyzed Dimroth rearrangement (Barlow et al. 1997; Leuratti et al. 1993a, 1993b, 1994; Qian and Dipple 1995; Selzer and Elfarra 1996a; Tretyakova et al. 1996, 1997b; Zhao, Koskinen and Hemminki 1998; Zhao et al. 2000). The N1 adducts are also prone to demination giving the analogous inosine N1 adducts (Selzer and Elfarra 1996a). In ds DNA the N1 position is protected by Watson–Crick base pairing and the N3 position becomes the preferential site of attack (Tretyakova et al. 1996, 1997b, 1998; Zhao et al. 2000). The N3 adducts readily depurinate leaving an abasic site in the DNA.

15.5.3. Crosslink Formation by DEB

DEB is a *bis*-electrophile and consequently is capable of forming intrastrand and interstrand DNA crosslinks and DNA–protein conjugates (Loeber et al. 2006). All three stereoisomers of DEB are produced metabolically, with the *S,S* stereoisomer being the most cytotoxic and genotoxic. A fused seven-member ring system at the N1 and N2 positions of dG, 7,8-dihydroxy-3-(2-deoxy-b-D-erythro-pentofuranosyl)-3,5,6,7,8,9-hexahydro-1,3-diazepino[1,2-a]purin-11(11H)one, was also characterized (Zhang and Elfarra 2004). Incubation of the N1 adducts with dG led to formation of a pair of N7-dG–N1-dG crosslinked adducts, diastereomers of 20-deoxy-1-[4-(2-amino-1,7-dihydro-6H-purin-6-on-7-yl)-2,3-dihydroxybutyl]-dG (Zhang and Elfarra 2006). The dominant crosslink formed by DEB arises from the N7 adduct of dGuo reacting with a second dGuo at the N7 position (Park et al. 2005; Park and Tretyakova 2004; Zhang and Elfarra 2006). Interstrand crosslinks arise in ds DNA with strong preference for a 5′-GNC-3′ sequence context (Millard et al. 2006; Millard and White 1993; Millard and Wilkes 2001; Park et al. 2005). The efficiency of cross-linking varies, with *S,S*- > *R,R*- > *R,S*-DEB (Millard et al. 2006). In a study of DNA duplexes containing a 5′-GGC-3′/3′-CCG-5′ sequence by Tretyakova's group, the *S,S* stereoform of DEB gives mainly 1,3 inter-chain crosslinks, although a small fraction of 1,2 interstrand and intras-trand crosslinks were also observed (Park et al. 2005; Park and Tretyakova 2004). The *R,R* form of the diepoxide gave mainly the 1,3 interchain crosslink, whereas the meso form, that is, the *R,S* form, gave comparable amounts of 1,2 and 1,3 intrastrand crosslinks, but little of the interstrand crosslink. Different crosslinking specificities of DEB stereo-isomers provide a likely basis for their distinct biological activities.

To a lesser extent, guanine–adenine interstrand crosslinks are also formed in ds DNA treated with racemic DEB (Park et al. 2004). Crosslinks were observed between the N7 position of dGuo and mainly the N1 position of dAdo with lesser quantities of crosslinks to the N3, N^6, and N7 of dAdo also being formed. The N1 interstrand crosslink arises primarily in a 1,3 sequence context. Although the dAdo–dGuo crosslinks are an order of magnitude less abundant than the dGuo–dGuo crosslinks, the dGuo cross-links to the N1 and N^6 positions of dAdo are more hydrolytically stable than the dGuo–dGuo crosslinks and, if formed in vivo, may accumulate to a larger extent in target tissues. The formation of guanine–adenine adducts may contribute to base pair substitution and deletion mutations at A:T base pairs following exposures to BD (Park et al. 2004).

DNA containing N7-(2-hydroxy-3,4-epoxybut-1′-yl)-guanine adducts has been found to form conjugates with the DNA repair protein O^6-alkylguanine DNA alkyltransferase (AGT) (Loeber et al. 2006). The crosslinking sites were found to be the alkyl acceptor site, Cys145, and a neighboring active site residue, Cys150. The chemical structure of the crosslink was established as 1-(*S*-cysteinyl)-4-(guan-7-yl)-2,3-butanediol (Loeber et al. 2006). Significantly, a correlation between cellular expression of AGT and the cytotoxic and mutagenic activity of DEB has been noted (Valadez et al. 2004).

15.5.4. Reactions of HMVK

The HMVK metabolite of BD yielded cyclic 1,N^2-dG adducts with dGuo (Powley et al. 2003).

15.6. Mutagenic Effects of BD

15.6.1. Introduction

This section will review the evidence that BD is a mutagen in rodents and in humans. Our analyses will address (1) data on the relationship between dose and mutagenic response, (2) treatment duration and response, (3) organ specificity, (4) age effects and response, (5) the mutagenic effects of specific metabolites of BD, (6) the spectrum of mutations induced by BD and its metabolites, and (7) the effect of biotransformation of BD on its mutagenicity. The evidence for mutagenic effects of BD in exposed human populations and the possible importance of polymorphisms in a BD-metabolizing enzyme will be reviewed and discussed. The objective of this discussion is both to discern whether its mutagenic characteristics support an argument that BD poses a cancer risk to exposed populations and to provide a context for the studies of the possible mutagenic effects of specific BD DNA adducts.

15.6.2. Evidence that BD and its Epoxide Metabolites are Mutagens

Since BD is not a biologically reactive compound, in order to assess its mutagenic capacity in bacterial test systems, BD was incubated in the presence of a preinduced rat liver microsomal preparation (S9) and was demonstrated to be mutagenic in *S. typhimurium* TA 1530 (de Meester et al. 1980). Adler et al. (1997) found that the three epoxide metabolites of BD were mutagenic in *S. typhimurium* with or without metabolic activation. In cultured mammalian cells BD has failed to demonstrate a mutagenic effect, most likely due to inadequate metabolic activation (McGregor et al. 1991). Thus, in most mammalian cell culture studies, the mutagenicity of the epoxide metabolites of BD was investigated. Cochrane and Skopek (1994a) evaluated the mutagenic effects of EB, EBD, and DEB in TK6 human lymphoblastoid cells. They measured mutation at two loci, the X-linked *Hprt* locus and the autosomal *tk* locus (in heterozygous cells). All three metabolites were mutagenic at both loci. Dose–response curves demonstrated that the order of potency was DEB>>EBD>EB, with DEB being about 100-fold more potent than EB. Human TK6 lymphoblasts treated with 400-μM EB or 4-μM DEB showed increased *Hprt* mutant frequencies (MFs) with both epoxides, with DEB >> EB (Steen, Meyer and Reico 1997a, 1997b).

The most definitive demonstrations of the mutagenic effects of BD come from numerous studies in mice and rats. In an inhalation exposure study by Cochrane and Skopek (1994b), the mutagenic effects of BD were assessed at the *Hprt* locus in spleen lymphocytes in male B6C3F1 mice. Exposure to 625 ppm BD, 6 h per day, 5 days per week for 2 weeks, resulted in an average *Hprt* MF of 6.2×10^{-6} as compared to 1.2×10^{-6} in air controls. Both EB and DEB administered by intraperitoneal (i.p.) injection generated positive dose responses, with DEB being more potent than EB. When exposure times were limited to 5 days, an increase in *Hprt* MF in male mice was statistically significant at 1300-ppm BD but not at lower doses (Tates et al. 1994).

Additionally, a series of studies of BD led by Recio were conducted in transgenic mice that had inserts of lambda phage containing the *Esche- richia coli lac* repressor gene (*lacI*) or the structural gene for β-galactosidase *(lacZ)*. Concentrations of BD ranged from 62.5 to 1250 ppm. At these concentrations, BD produced a dose-related increase in MF in the lung (Recio et al. 1993), bone marrow (Recio and Goldsworthy 1995), and spleen (Recio, Pluta and Meyer 1998).

An even more detailed understanding of the relative mutagenic potency of BD and its metabolites, as well as the role of gender and species (mouse versus rat), were provided by a group led by Walker. The *Hprt* assay was conducted using lymphocytes from the spleen or thymus. There were several key findings from these studies. First, they confirmed that BD, EB, and DEB were all mutagenic in mice and rats (Meng et al. 1998a, 1999a, 1999b). Second, they determined that 4–5-week-old mice were more sensitive to BD than mice 8–9 weeks of age, mice were more sensitive than rats, and females were more sensitive to BD than males (Meng et al. 2007b). A valuable aspect of their assay protocol was that they usually necropsied mice at weekly intervals following the termination of exposure, which allowed them to determine the time of peak manifestation of mutations. In addition, they were able to calculate the area under the manifestation curve to determine the mutagenic potency of a treatment (Meng et al. 1998a). This was a more useful parameter for comparing different treatment characteristics than comparing peak MF manifestation. They calculated that the mutagenic potency of BD is about five-fold greater in mice than in rats (Meng et al. 1998a). The low mutagenic potency of BD in the rat has been suggested to be a function of the extent of formation of DEB, rather the ability of DEB to induce mutations (Meng et al. 1999b). The shape of the dose–response curve in mice is supralinear, with the rate of increase in MF being most rapid at the lowest doses, but leveling off as exposure rises to concentrations that saturate biotransformation enzymes. In mice, the lowest exposure at which a significant increase in *Hprt* MF was demonstrated was 3 ppm for 6 hours per day, 5 days per week for 2 weeks (Meng et al. 2001). This exposure level is within the range of human occupational exposure.

In several of the animal mutagenesis studies, the spectra of mutations induced by BD and its metabolites were investigated (Cochrane and Skopek 1994b; Meng et al., 2000, 2007a; Recio et al. 1993; Recio and Meyer 1995; Sisk et al. 1994). Although the details of these investigations differ, the overall conclusions are that (1) BD and its epoxides induce mutations at both GC and AT base pairs with similar susceptibility, (2) a variety of base substitution and frameshift mutations can be generated, and (3) deletion mutations are also generated, probably as a response to interstrand DNA crosslinks created by DEB.

15.6.3. Mutagenic Effects of BD in Human Studies

Three groups of investigators have studied the mutagenic effects of BD in the lymphocytes of workers from either BD monomer production plants or SBR plants in the USA, China, and the Czech Republic. Early investigations of workers in a Texas monomer plant showed a strong correlation between *Hprt* VF (variant frequency is the term used for this autoradiographic assay) and butenediol urine metabolite levels, and that workers in the highest exposure areas had higher VFs (Ward et al. 1994). A follow-up study in the same plant produced a similar result and two studies in a neighboring SBR plant also produced consistent results, associating *Hprt* VF with exposure to BD (Ammenheuser et al. 2001; Ward et al. 1996, 2001). Using the cloning assay, it was further demonstrated that BD-exposed workers had a higher MF than nonexposed workers, and they had a higher proportion of exon deletion mutations (Ma et al. 2000). This finding is consistent with evidence for induction of deletions by BD and DEB in mice and in cultured cells.

These results, however, were not consistent with the studies done in China (Hayes et al. 1996, 2000), or the study performed in the Czech Republic (Albertini et al. 2003), in which there were no significant differences between exposed and nonexposed groups. In the Czech study, the highest frequencies of *Hprt* mutant cells were seen in the control group, mostly because several control subjects had very high values. Mean VFs in the monomer and polymer sections of the plant were similar to the values seen in the Texas plants at similar exposure levels.

The reasons for the inconsistencies in the detection of mutations associated with BD in exposed humans are not known but may involve exposure to other environmental mutagens, both in the work and home environment. In the Texas studies, it was discovered that workers who carried polymorphic variants that reduced the activity of microsomal epoxide hydrolase (mEH) were sensitive to the mutagenic effects associated with BD. Workers with the high-activity forms of the gene were less sensitive (Abdel-Rahman et al. 2003, 2005; Abdel-Rahman, Ammenheuser and Ward 2001). In mutagenicity studies conducted in mice lacking mEH activity, there was a parallel increase in sensitivity to BD (Wickliffe et al. 2003). These findings are also discussed in the section on the effects of modulation of BD metabolism. Humans are clearly less sensitive to the carcinogenic effects of BD than mice, based on the cancer rates observed in workers (Delzell et al. 1996) compared to rats in mouse bioassays (Melnick et al. 1990). However, the demonstrated mutagenicity of BD and its metabolites in mice and rats suggests that there is no fundamental reason to believe that BD is not mutagenic in humans. The question is primarily one of exposure level and duration and possibly genetic susceptibility of individuals. Although an increase in the frequency of mutations has been observed in only some groups of humans occupationally exposed to BD, it is likely that the observed increase in leukemia in workers (Delzell et al. 1996) does result from mutagenic events associated with BD exposure.

15.6.4. Modulation of Mutagenicity

Since rodents and humans share similar pathways for the biotransformation of BD (review in Jackson et al. 2000) and repair of adducted DNA, human polymorphisms in the genes encoding both the toxifying (CYP2E1) and detoxifying enzymes (mEH, GSTs) could cause certain individuals to be more susceptible to the possible carcinogenic effects of BD (Abdel-Rahman et al. 2003, 2005; Abdel-Rahman, Ammenheuser and Ward 2001). Due to the relative ease with which the mouse genome can be manipulated, studies have been conducted using mice that are deficient in mEH to examine sensitivity associated with a reduced capacity for hydrolytic detoxification. In addition, mice deficient in DNA repair have also been examined to determine which DNA repair pathways are important in maintaining genomic integrity potentially compromised by the reactive metabolites of BD. These studies are summarized below.

15.6.4.1. Disruption of mEH

Microsomal epoxide hydrolase is one of the principal enzymes responsible for detoxifying the reactive epoxide intermediates of BD. Mice have been exposed to BD by inhalation, and EB and DEB by i.p. injection. As measured by the *Hprt* mutation assay, mice without a functional mEH are significantly more sensitive to the mutagenic effects of BD and the epoxide metabolites in comparison to mEH-proficient mice. mEH-deficient mice exhibit a fivefold increase in the frequency of *Hprt* mutations following exposure to 20-ppm BD by inhalation (Wickliffe et al. 2003). mEH-deficient mice also exhibit a 16-fold and twofold increase in the frequency of *Hprt* mutations following exposure to 240 mg kg^{-1} EB and 30 mg kg^{-1} DEB, respectively (Wickliffe et al. 2003, 2007). The results with DEB are misleading since the toxicity of this compound was apparent compared to both BD and EB, thus leading to a "muted" response with respect to mutagenicity. Taken together, these results indicate that mEH is critically important in the detoxification of the genotoxic metabolites of BD.

15.6.4.2. Disruption of DNA Repair

Based on the variety of adducts that have been detected in biological samples and the remaining potential adducts that have been synthesized, several DNA repair mechanisms are likely involved in recognizing and repairing DNA damage caused by the reactive metabolite BD. Studies have initially focused on repair pathways primarily responsible for DNA crosslink adducts because of the substantial mutagenicity that these lesions pose. Mice deficient in the global genome repair subpathway of nucleotide excision repair (NER) were exposed to BD by inhalation and EB by i.p.

injection (Wickliffe et al. 2006, 2007). These mice, lacking a functional *Xpc* gene, are significantly more sensitive to the effects of BD (20 ppm as described previously; two-fold increase in *Hprt* mutations) and EB (300 mg kg^{-1} i.p.; 2.8-fold increase in *Hprt* mutations). This indicates that NER is one of the pathways involved in the recognition and repair of BD-induced DNA adducts. A pilot experiment has also been conducted, based on the number of relatively simple nucleotide modifications (i.e., alkylpurines) suggested by previous research, that examined the role that methylpurine glycosylase (Mpg) may play in excising damaged purines. This experiment (exposure to 62.5-ppm BD for 2 weeks), though limited by a small sample size, suggests that Mpg is not involved in repairing modified purines and that either an alternate repair process is involved, or downstream repair processes are involved, or these lesions are simply bypassed in an error-free manner such that genomic integrity is maintained. One limitation of the preceding studies in mice is the lack of information regarding adduct formation. These studies indicate that NER is involved in repairing DNA modified by BD-epoxides. It is also likely that other repair mechanisms are crucial to the maintenance of genomic integrity (i.e., nonhomologous end-joining), but these remain to be elucidated.

15.7. Structure–Function Analyses of Mutagenicity

15.7.1. Overall Experimental Strategy

As described above, a large number of DNA adducts have been identified and mutation spectra characterized using several assays. In order to correlate specific adducts with a mutagenic signature, we have taken a reductionist approach by synthesizing oligodeoxynucleotides (ODNs) containing site- and stereo-specific BD adducts, establishing the mutagenic spectra of each in either prokaryotic or eukaryotic mutation assays and solving the nuclear magnetic resonance (NMR) solution structures of these DNAs. Although for a few mutagens, one can design syntheses to yield a stereochemically defined lesion at a single site in an ODN, this approach fails for the BD-derived epoxides because of reactions with numerous nucleophilic sites. Two alternative synthetic approaches are available for preparation of ODNs containing adducts of the epoxides of BD and of other electrophiles. The first of these is assembly of the adducted ODN using an adducted phosphoramidite (Figure 15.2, top scheme). This method has wide versatility, but the requirement for orthogonal protection of the hydroxyl groups on the butadienyl moiety is a complication to this approach.

An alternative approach for preparation of adducted ODNs is post-oligomerization (Figure 15.2, bottom scheme). The method is limited to cases in which adducts are linked to exocyclic amino groups. This synthetic approach reverses the nucleophile–electrophile relationship between the nucleoside and mutagen. A halopurine or similar entity replaces the Gua or Ade. For example, 6-halopurine is used as a replacement for Ade and 2-halohypoxanthine as a replacement for Gua. The nucleophilic partner in these condensation reactions will be an amine equivalent of the

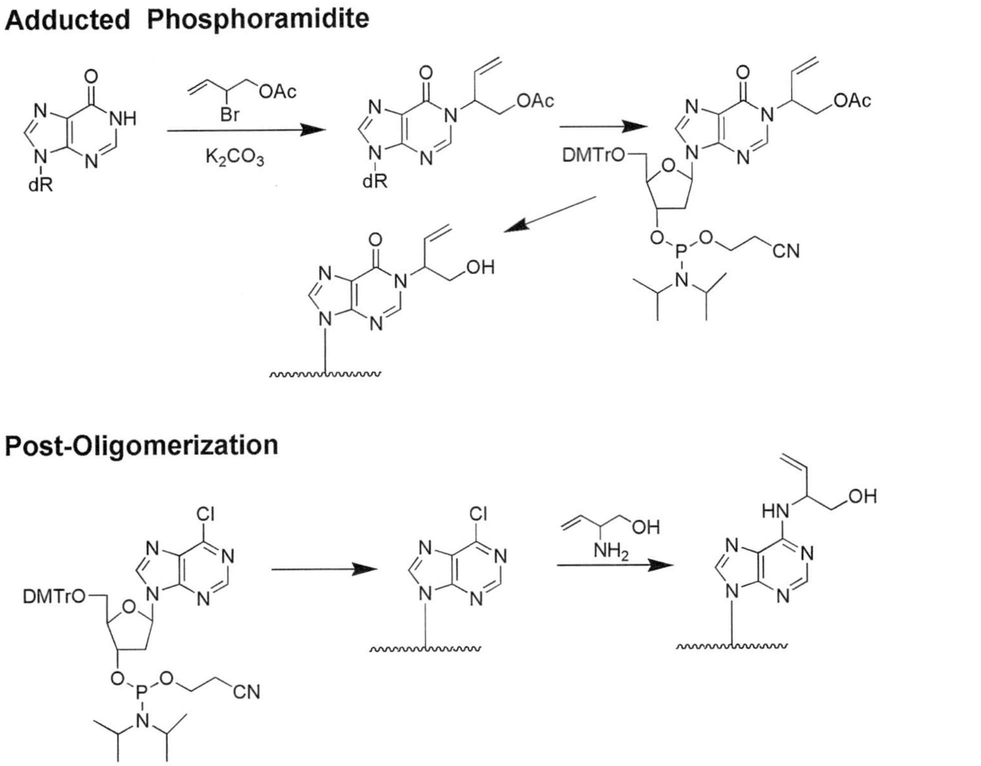

Figure 15.2. Synthetic approaches for the preparation of ODNs containing site-specific DNA lesions. The top scheme shows the use of a previously adducted phosphoramidite in the ODN construction. The bottom scheme illustrates the post-oligomerization strategy.

electrophile. For example, with epoxides the nucleophilic species will be the corresponding amino alcohol. This strategy avoids entirely the need for orthogonal protection of hydroxyl groups. A further benefit of the method is that the stereochemistry and regiochemistry of the adducts of epoxides are controlled by the choice of amino alcohols.

Irrespective of how the adducted ODNs are prepared, utmost care must be taken to assure the constitution and purity of the materials before they are committed to further studies. For NMR studies, a modest level of such impurities can be tolerated; up to ~5% of incorrect oligomeric entities will usually escape detection in two-dimensional nuclear Overhauser effect spectroscopy (NOESY) and other two dimensional NMR spectroscopy. For mutation studies, the purity is of utmost importance to be able to have confidence in small effects that may be observed. As a minimum standard of the purity of an adducted ODN, the sample should be homogeneous as determined by capillary gel electrophoresis, and the molecular weight determined by mass spectrometry (MS). An enzymatic digestion with phosphodiesterases to give the constituent nucleosides should be carried out so that high-performance liquid chromatography (HPLC) analyses can be used to establish that the nucleosides, including the adducted nucleoside(s), are present in the correct stoichiometric proportions and that the adducted nucleoside exists as a single diastereomer.

15.7.2. Chemistry by which DNAs have been Prepared Containing Structurally Defined, Site-Specific BD Lesions

15.7.2.1. N^6-dAdo, 1-Hydroxy-3-buten-2-yl Adducts

EB reacts with nucleophiles to give a mixture of products arising by attack at C1 and C2. The N^6 1-hydroxy-3-buten-2-yl lesion arises in DNA mainly or entirely by attack of Ade N1 rather than N^6 on EB (Kim et al. 2000). Oxirane ring-opening occurs with inversion of configuration at C_β. Rearrangement of the N1 adduct to the N^6 occurs via the Dimroth rearrangement. The N^6 adduct retains the configuration of the EB moiety at C_β. Consequently, the *R* and *S* epoxides yield the *S* and *R* lesions, respectively.

For the synthesis of EB-adducted ODNs, the phosphoramidite reagent prepared from 6-chloropurine 2′-deoxyriboside was inserted into ODNs (Carmical et al. 2000b; Kim et al. 1998; Nechev et al. 2001). The exocyclic amino groups of the other nucleosides were protected with 4-*tert*-butylphenoxyacetyl groups to facilitate deprotection of the resulting chloropurine-containing ODNs without displacement of the halo-substituent. It is advantageous to remove the halopurine-containing ODN from the solid matrix, remove the protective groups, and purify the ODN prior to carrying out the condensation. Condensations with the enantiomerically pure, configurationally defined amino alcohols (Ohfune and Kurokawa 1984) were carried out in dimethylsulfoxide (DMSO) containing diisopropylethylamine with a large excess (~100-fold) of the 2*R* and 2*S* amino alcohols, yielding the (2*R*)- and (2*S*)-1-hydroxy-3-buten-2-yl adducts of dAdo; Figure 15.3a).

15.7.2.2. N^6-dAdo, 2,3,4-Trihydroxybutyl-1-yl Adducts

Reactions of (2*R*,3*R*)- and (2*S*,3*S*)-DEB with nucleophiles occur at the terminal position to give adducts having 2*R*,3*R* and 2*S*,3*S* configurations, respectively. With the meso diepoxide, that is, (2*R*,3*S*)-DEB, the terminal positions are not equivalent and two diastereomeric products, the (2*R*,3*S*)- and (2*S*,3*R*)-2,3,4-trihydroxybutyl-1-yl adducts, would be formed.

To date, ODNs bearing N^6-dAdo adducts have only been prepared for the 2*R*,3*R* and 2*S*,3*S* stereoisomers (Carmical et al. 2000b; Nechev et al. 2001). The post-oligomerization synthetic strategy has been employed using (2*R*,3*R*)- and (2*S*,3*S*)-1-amino-2,3,4-butanetriol. The 2*R*,3*R* stereoisomer was prepared by reaction of dimethyl 2,3-*O*-benzylidine-D-tartrate with one equivalent of ammonia to give the monoamide followed by reduction with $LiAlH_4$ and deprotection. However, lack of availability of L-tartaric acid or its derivatives necessitated the use of 3,4-*O*-isopropylidene-L-threonate for preparation of the 2*S*,3*S* stereoisomer. The threonate was converted to the amide by treatment with ammonia. Reaction with $LiAlH_4$ reduction and deprotection gave the (2*S*,3*S*)-aminotriol. The N^6-dAdo adducts were prepared by treatment of 6-chloropurine 2′-deoxyriboside with the amines as described above. ODNs containing N^6-trihydroxybutyl adducts (Figure 15.3b) were prepared in good yields by the procedure that had been used for the 2-hydroxy-3-buten-1-yl adducts of EB.

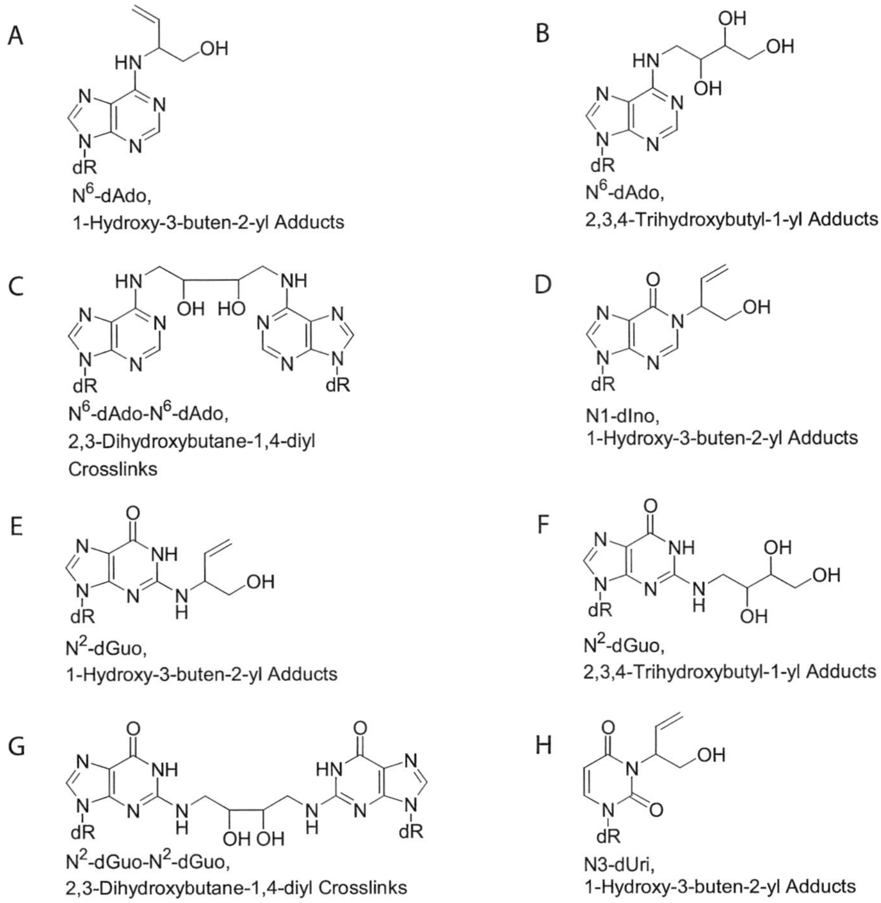

Figure 15.3. Structures of key BD-derived DNA adducts.

15.7.2.3. N^6-dAdo-N^6-dAdo, 2,3-Dihydroxybutane-1,4-diyl Intrastrand Crosslinks of DEB

Intrastrand DEB-derived crosslinks have been constructed between N^6 positions of adjacent adenines (Figure 15.3c) in an 11-mer ODN using a modification of the post-oligomerization procedure (Kanuri et al. 2002; Kowalczyk et al. 2002). The enantiomeric 2*R*,3*R* and 2*S*,3*S* diamines were prepared from dimethyl 2,3-*O*-benzylidenetartrate (Carmical et al. 2000a). The *bis*(amide) was formed by ammonolysis of the *bis*(ester). Reduction with $LiAlH_4$, followed by deprotection of the hydroxyl groups gave the diamine in good yield. The diastereomeric *bis*-nucleosides were prepared by reaction of the diamines with 6-chloropurine 2′-deoxyriboside.

An 11-mer ODN was prepared having 6-chloropurine residues at adjacent positions near the middle of the chain. For synthesis of ODN containing intrachain crosslinks, condensations with the diamines were carried out using a 25% excess of the ODNs in order to avoid 2:1 adducts of diamine with the ODNs. Basic conditions were needed to avoid formation of the amine salt during the course of the reaction. The diastereomeric crosslinked ODNs were obtained in purified yields of 25–30%.

15.7.2.4. N1-dIno, 1-Hydroxy-3-buten-2-yl Adducts

The N1 position of dAdo is a major site of reaction with electrophilic reagents. However, the N1 adduct is unstable and readily undergoes Dimroth rearrangement to the N^6 adduct or hydrolysis of the amino group to yield the analogous N1-substituted inosine (Selzer and Elfarra 1996a). The latter reaction is of importance with adducts of epoxides where the hydroxyl group participates in the hydrolysis of the amino group (Fujii, Saito and Terahara 1986). This reaction becomes prominent when the hydroxyl group is primary. As a consequence, the N1-(1-hydroxy-3-buten-1-ol) adduct derived from EB is prone to deamination to form the analogous dIno derivative (Figure 15.3d).

ODNs containing N1 adducts of dIno cannot be prepared by the post-oligomerization approach; neither is it feasible to prepare them by direct adduction. As a consequence the ODNs had to be prepared from adducted phosphoramidites (Kowalczyk, Harris and Harris 2001). Syntheses were carried out using racemic 2-bromo-3-buten-1-ol with the hydroxyl group protected as the acetate to block epoxide formation and the dIno protected as the 1,1,3,3-tetraisopropyl-1,3-disiloxanediyl derivative. Although a mixture of isomeric products was obtained, the correct isomer was isolated (as a diastereomeric mixture) and after removal of the silyl protection, converted to the phosphoramidite derivative. Assembly of the ODN proceeded normally with the diastereomers of the resulting ODN being readily resolved by HPLC. The absolute configuration at C_β of the butenyl fragments was established by enzymatic digestion. An authentic sample of the 2*S* adduct was prepared by the reaction of (2*R*)-EB with inosine; the reaction proceeds with inversion of configuration at C_β leading to the 2*S* adduct.

15.7.2.5. N^2-dGuo, 1-Hydroxy-3-buten-2-yl, and N^2-dGuo, 2,3, 4-Trihydroxybut-1-yl Adducts

The N7 position is the most nucleophilic site in guanine. Consequently, the synthesis of N^2-adducted dGuos and ODNs containing adducted dGuos must rely on indirect methods. Syntheses of BD adducts have been achieved using 2-fluoro-dIno in which the O^6 position has been protected with the trimethylsilylethyl group (Harris and Harris 2000; Nechev et al. 2001). The trimethylsilylethyl group offers advantage over other alkyl groups commonly used to protect the O^6 position in that it is readily removed with tetrabutylammonium fluoride. dGuos bearing (2*R*)- and (2*S*)-(1-hydroxy-3-buten-2-yl) adducts (Figure 15.3e) were prepared in good yields by the reaction of the protected 2-fluoro-dIno with the individual enantiomers of 2-amino-3-buten-1-ol (Nechev et al. 2001). The trimethylsilylethyl group was then removed by treatment with dilute acetic acid to give the adducted nucleosides in excellent yields.

For the synthesis of ODNs, a 12-mer ODN was assembled with silyl-protected 2-fluoro-dIno inserted at the desired position in the DNA sequence (Carmical et al. 2000c; Nechev et al. 2001). The ODN was deprotected with the trimethylsilylethyl group fully retained, and after HPLC purification, the ODN was treated with the individual enantiomers of 2-amino-3-buten-1-ol. The remaining trimethylsilyl protection was removed by treatment with weak acid.

The N^2 2,3,4-trihydroxybut-1-yl adducts of dGuo (Figure 15.3f) are prepared by reaction of the aminotriol with silyl-protected 2-fluoro-dIno by the procedures used above for the EB adducts (Carmical et al. 2000c; Harris and Harris 2000; Nechev et al. 2001).

15.7.2.6. N^2-dGuo-N^2-dGuo, (2R,2R)- and (2S,3S)-2, 3-Dihydroxybutane-1,4-diyl Intrastrand Crosslinks

ODNs have been prepared containing 2*R*,2*R* and 2*S*,3*S* DEB intrastrand crosslinks between adjacent dGuo residues (Figure 15.3 g) (Carmical et al. 2000a). Reaction of the enantiomeric 2*R*,3*R* and 2*S*,3*S* diamines with silyl-protected 2-fluoro-dIno gave the diastereomeric *bis*(nucleosides) having the BD-derived tether between N^2 positions. The crosslinked ODNs were prepared by reaction of the enantiomeric diamines with an ODN containing silyl-protected 2-fluoro-dIdo at adjacent positions. In theory, the diamine should be the limiting reagent to maximize the yield of crosslinked material as opposed to having two diamine molecules react with each molecule of the ODN. However, on account of the sluggishness of reactions of the 2-fluoro-dIno, it was found to be more effective to use 1.5–2.5 equivalents of the diamine to promote the reaction. Even with this stoichiometry, relatively good yields of the crosslinked species were obtained which suggests that the second condensation, that is, the ring-closure reaction, proceeds faster than the first condensation. After removal of the silyl protection by treatment with aqueous acetic acid, the crosslinked ODNs were purified by HPLC and then characterized by matrix-assisted laser desorption ionization time-of-flight mass spectrometry (MALDI-TOF MS), capillary gel electrophoresis (CGE), and enzymatic digestion to the constituent nucleosides. It is noteworthy that the presence of the crosslink did not appear to retard significantly the enzymatic digestion.

15.7.2.7. N3-dUri, 1-hydroxy-3-buten-2-yl adducts

The N3 adduct of dCyt is hydrolytically unstable and readily deaminates to give the analogous adducted dUri (Figure 15.3 h). The synthesis of an ODN containing this lesion was carried out using racemic 3-butene-1,2-diol, which was converted to the 1-*O*-tosyl-2-*O*-(dimethyl-*t*-butylsilyl) derivative (Fernandes et al., 2006). The condensation of the tosylate with the 5′-*O*-(dimethoxytrityl)-3′-*O*-(4-toluoyl) derivative of dUri was carried out and, after the removal of the 3′-*O*-toluoyl group, the phosphoramidite reagent was prepared. A 12-mer ODN was prepared by automated synthesis using this phosphoramidite reagent. The *tert*-butyldimethylsilyl protecting group was removed from the hydroxyl group of the butenyl side chain by treatment with tetrabutylammonium fluoride and tributylammonium hydrofluoride. The diastereomeric ODNs were not resolved by HPLC or CGE, but after enzymatic digestion to nucleosides, HPLC analysis showed baseline separation of the diastereomeric nucleosides. This procedure could readily be adapted for the preparation of ODNs containing individual diastereomers of the dUri adducts of EB by using (2*R*)- and (2*S*)-3-butene-1,2-diol.

15.7.3. Mutagenesis Conferred by Replication of DNAs Containing Specific BD Adducts

15.7.3.1. Vector Design and Mutagenesis Assay

In order to ascertain the mutagenic potential of specific BD lesions, we have utilized two well-established ss vectors that were designed for prokaryotic and eukaryotic replication, M13mp7L2 and pMS2, respectively. These ss vectors possess regions of self-complementarity that form stable ds stem-loop structures at ambient temperatures. Within this stem structure, a unique restriction enzyme site is created that can be efficiently cleaved by addition of *Eco*RI to M13mp7L2 or *Eco*RV to pMS2. Thus, the resulting DNA molecules are cleaved at precise locations such that knowledge of the sequences at the 5′ and 3′ ends of the ss DNA allows for further manipulation and engineering of defined ODNs into these linear molecules and converting them into adduct-containing ss circular DNAs using scaffolding ODNs. The design of the scaffold perfectly positions the modified DNA to be ligated at a fixed position in the ss vector. These closed circular DNAs are then transformed into and replicated in either *E. coli* or COS-7 cells. In the case of the M13mp7L2 vector, phage plaques were formed in soft agarose overlays and these plaques sequentially transferred to nitrocellulose filters and subsequently hybridized with radioactive probes that could detect single-base substitutions. For transformation of pMS2-modified vectors, these DNAs are replicated in COS-7 cells for 48 h and the autonomously replicated DNAs harvested and transformed into *E. coli* and selected for antibiotic resistance. Bacterial colonies are transferred to filters and then probed with defined ODNs for detection of point mutations and deletions.

15.7.3.2. Mutagenicity and Structural Analyses of N^6-dAdo BD Adducts

M13 replication of DNAs containing the (2*R*)- and (2*S*)-1-hydroxy-3-buten-2-yl adducts of dAdo BD resulted in no detectable mutagenesis (< 0.025% mutation frequency) (Carmical et al. 2000b). In contrast, replication of DNAs containing the (2*R*,3*R*)- and (2*S*,3*S*)–2,3,4-trihydroxybut-1-yl N^6-dAdo adducts yielded 0.14% and 0.25% mutation frequency per replication event, respectively. Although these lesions were very weakly miscoding, the mutagenic spectra were very distinct with the *R,R* isomer giving exclusively A-to-G transition mutations, while the *S,S* isomer yielded only A-to-C transversion mutations. Analyses of in vitro replication bypass studies using purified *E. coli* DNA polymerases I, II, III revealed that none of these lesions caused any significant block to replication bypass (Carmical et al. 2000b).

The solution structures of both the (2*R*,3*R*)-(2,3,4-trihydroxybutyl)-N^6-dAdo and (2*S*,3*S*)-(2,3,4-trihydroxybutyl)-N^6-dAdo adducts (Figure 15.4) were determined in the following complementary oligodeoxynucleotides: d(CGGA<u>CXA</u>GAAG)·d(CTTCTTGTCCG), where the numbering of the nucleotides is given as superscripted 1–11 and 12–22 for each ODN, respectively (Merritt et al. 2004; Scholdberg et al. 2004). These ODNs contain codon 61 (underlined) of the human *N-ras* proto-oncogene. In both instances, NMR spectroscopy revealed that the BD triol moiety was oriented in the major groove of the DNA with modest structural perturbations localized to the site of adduction at $X^6 \cdot T^{17}$, and its nearest-neighbor base pairs $C^5 \cdot G^{18}$ and $A^7 \cdot T^{16}$. All sequential NOE connectivities arising from DNA protons were observed. Torsion angle analysis from correlation spectroscopy (COSY) data suggested the deoxyribose sugar at X^6 remained in the C2′-endo conformation. However, structural refinement of the two adducts suggested stereospecific differences in hydrogen bonding between the hydroxyl groups located at the β- and γ-carbons of the BD moiety, and T^{17} O^4 of the modified base pair $X^6 \cdot T^{17}$. For the *R,R* stereoisomer, a hydrogen bond was predicted between the γ-OH and T^{17} O^4, whereas for the *S,S* stereoisomer, a hydrogen bond was predicted between the β-OH and T^{17} O^4 (Figure 15.4b). This difference positioned the two adducts differently in the major groove. The minimal structural perturbations induced by these major groove adducts correlated with their facile bypass by three *E. coli* DNA polymerases in vitro and their weak mutagenicities as described above (Carmical et al. 2000b).

In order to model the structure of the mispaired intermediate of the *S,S* stereoisomer, an NMR-derived solution structure was determined for this lesion mismatched with dG, the intermediate that generated A-to-G mutations (Scholdberg et al. 2005a). In the major conformation, base pair $X^6 \cdot G^{17}$ oriented "face-to-face". Both nucleotide X^6 and G^{17} were intrahelical and in the *anti* conformation about the glycosyl bond. Hydrogen bonding was suggested between X^6 N1 and G^{17} N1H, and between X^6 N^6H and G^{17} O^6. The BDT moiety allowed formation of a stable A • G mismatch.

Collectively, these data reveal that the major groove adducts are unlikely to contribute significantly to the in vivo mutagenesis at adenine residues. These data are very consistent with the lack of mutagenesis conferred by other site-specific N^6-adenine lesions, including *R*- and *S*-β-styrene oxide (Kanuri et al. 2001) and six different stereoisomers of benzo[*a*]pyrene-7,8-dihydrodiol 9,10-epoxide adducts (Chary et al. 1995).

15.7.3.3. Mutagenecity and Structural Analyses of N^6-dAdo-N^6-dAdo, 2,3-Dihydroxybutane-1,4-diyl Intrastrand Crosslinks

An additional set of lesions that can be derived from an initial reaction of DEB with DNA containing adjacent adenine residues is of an N1,N1 crosslink that can rearrange to the N^6,N^6-DEB crosslink. ODNs containing both the *R,R* or *S,S* stereoisomers were synthesized as described above, engineered into prokaryotic and eukaryotic ss vectors and replicated (Kanuri et al. 2002). The mutation frequencies of both lesions were nearly 10-fold higher in COS-7 cells than in *E. coli*. Replication of the intrastrand crosslink was highly mutagenic (54% per event), with all the mutations being point mutations at the 3′ adenine and yielding 40% A-to-G, 9% A-to-C, and 5% A-to-T. In contrast, the *S,S* crosslink was significantly less mutagenic (20%) with the spectra being 13% A-to-G, 6% A-to-T and 1% A-to-C.

Replication of these same lesions in *E. coli* produced more modest levels of mutagenesis (*R,R* 8% and *S,S* 2.8%) with nearly all the mutations being A-to-G transitions (Kanuri et al. 2002). The DNA polymerase responsible for inducing these mutations was investigated by conducting mutagenesis studies in isogenic *E. coli* strains that were either wild-type or only differed by inactivation of DNA polymerase II, IV, or V (Kanuri et al. 2005).

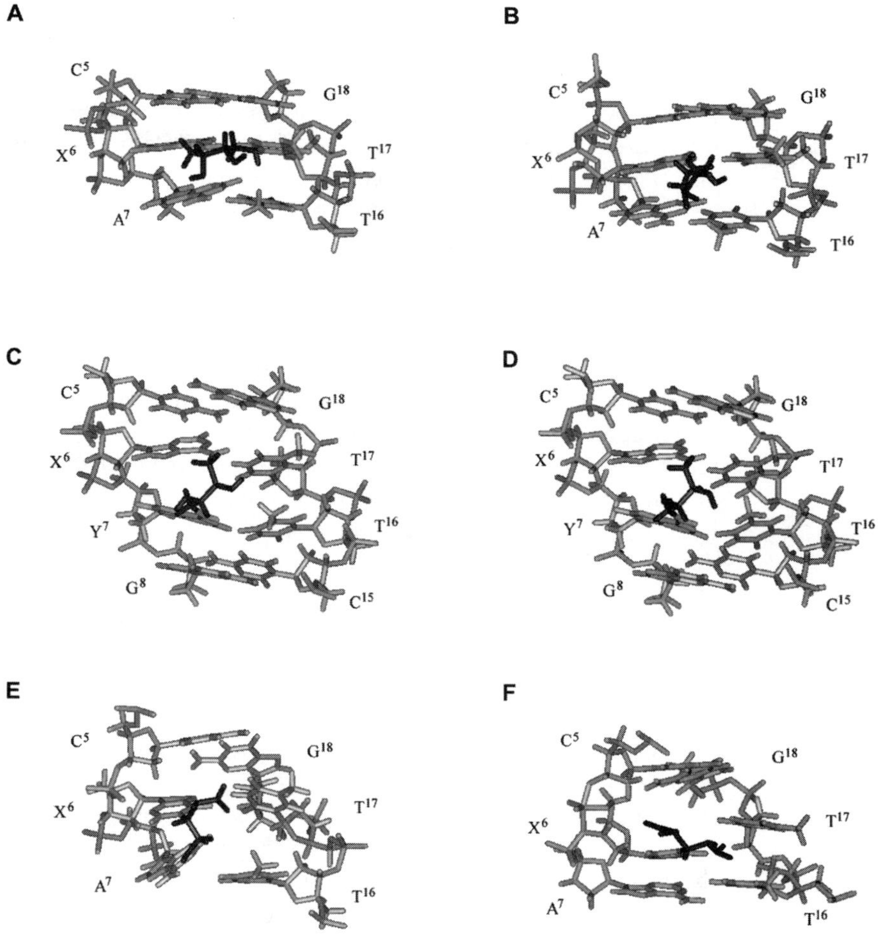

Figure 15.4. NMR-derived solution structures of DNAs containing various BD-derived DNA Adducts. (**a**) (2*R*,3*R*)-N^6-(2,3,4-trihydroxybut-1-yl)-deoxyadenosine; (**b**) (2*S*,3*S*)-N^6-(2,3,4-trihydroxybut-1-yl)-deoxyadenosine; (**c**) (2*S*,3*S*)-N6-(2,3-dihydroxybutyl)-deoxyadenosyl crosslink conformation I; (**d**) (2*S*,3*S*)-N^6-(2,3-dihydroxybutyl)-deoxyadenosyl crosslink conformation II; (**e**) N1-(1-hydroxy-3-buten-2*R*-yl)-2′-deoxyinosine; (**f**) (2S)-N1-(1-hydroxy-3-buten-2-yl)-deoxyinosine.

Mutation frequencies and spectra were indistinguishable among the wild type, pol IV and pol V strains. However, no mutations were ever detected in the pol II$^-$ strain, thus strongly implicating this polymerase in the mutagenic replication bypass of these crosslinks.

Solution structural studies of both the *(R,R)*- and *(S,S)*-N^6-dAdo-N^6-dAdo, 2,3-dihydroxybutane-1,4-diyl intrastrand crosslinks of DEB were determined in the ODN 5′-d(CGGACXYGAAG)•d(CTTCTCGTCCG)-3′, where XY are the crosslink sites (Merritt et al. 2005a; Xu et al. 2007). Both the *R,R* and *S,S* intrastrand crosslinks were accommodated in the major groove of duplex DNA. For the *R,R* crosslink, at the 5′-side of the crosslink there was a break in Watson–Crick base pairing at base pair $X^6 \cdot T^{17}$, whereas at the 3′-side of the crosslink at base pair $Y^7 \cdot T^{16}$ base pairing was intact. An increase in base pair opening was observed at base pair $X^6 \cdot T^{17}$, accompanied by a shift in the phosphodiester backbone torsion angle β P5′-O5′-C5′-C4′ at nucleotide X^6. The DNA helix was not bent by the presence of the four-carbon crosslink, as determined from gel mobility assays of multimers containing nonhydroxylated four-carbon N^6,N^6-dA crosslinks. The potential presence of a hydrogen bond between the hydroxyl group located on the β-carbon of the four-carbon crosslink and T^{17} O^4, perhaps stabilized the base pair opening at $X^6 \cdot T^{17}$, and protected the T^{17} imino proton from solvent exchange. The opening of base pair $X^6 \cdot T^{17}$ altered base stacking patterns at the crosslink site and induced slight unwinding of the DNA duplex.

For the *S,S* intrastrand DNA crosslink, Watson–Crick base pairing was perturbed at base pair $X^6 \cdot T^{17}$, whereas base pairing was intact at base pair $Y^7 \cdot T^{16}$. The crosslink appeared to exist in two conformations in rapid exchange on the NMR time scale. In the first conformation (Figure 15.4c), a hydrogen bond formed between the β-OH and T^{16} O^4, whereas in the second (Figure 15.4d) a hydrogen bond formed between the β-OH and T^{17} O^4. In contrast to the *R,R* crosslink, the *anti* conformation of the two hydroxyl groups at C_β and C_γ with respect to the C_β–C_γ bond resulted in a decreased twist between base pairs $X^6 \cdot T^{17}$ and $Y^7 \cdot T^{16}$, and an approximate 10° bending of the duplex. These conformational differences may account, in part, for the differential mutagenicity of the (*S,S*)- and (*R,R*)-BD-(61-2,3) crosslinks, and suggest that stereochemistry plays a role in modulating biological responses to these crosslinks.

15.7.3.4. Mutagenicity and Structural Analyses of N1-dIno, 1-Hydroxy-3-buten-2-yl Adducts

As described above, BD adduction at N1 of adenine and subsequent Dimroth rearrangement, can lead to the formation of N^6 adducts, but these N1 lesions can also undergo spontaneous deamination to yield the (R and S)-N1-(1-hydroxy-3-buten-2-yl)-dIno adducts. Using the M13 vector, replication gave exceptionally high mutagenic yields, with the *S* isomer producing point mutations of 67% I-to-G, 12% I-to-C, and 11% I-to-T, while the *R* isomer gave 54% I-to-G, 34% I-to-C, and 3% I-to-T (Rodriguez et al., 2001). Since the original base pair was an A:T, the overall mutagenic frequencies are $\geq 90\%$ per replication event. When the same lesions were incorporated into the eukaryotic pMS2 vector and replicated through COS-7 cells, although both stereoisomers were strongly mutagenic, the *S* isomer was more mutagenic yielding a 95% mutation frequency versus 59% for the *R* isomer (Kanuri et al. 2002). The *S* isomer yielded 79% I-to-G, 10% I-to-C, and 6% I-to-T, while the *R* isomer produced 48% I-to-G, 7% I-to-C, and 4% I-to-T. These data suggest that during replication, the dIno adduct was recognized as a dGuo adduct. However, since N1-dIno adducts should be unable to participate in Watson–Crick base pairing with dCyt, it was proposed that incorporation of dCTP opposite the N1-dIno adducts occurred by rotation of the glycosyl bond. This would position the modified base into the *syn* conformation, enabling formation of a protonated dIno • dCyt Hoogsteen-type pair during translesion synthesis.

The solution structures of both the (2R and 2S)-N1-(1-hydroxy-3-buten-2-yl)-dIno (Figure 15.4e, and f, respectively) adducts were determined in the sequence described above (Merritt et al. 2005b; Scholdberg et al. 2005b). The stereoisomeric N1-dIno butenyl adducts were both oriented in the major groove. For both dIno adducts, ^{1}H NMR revealed a weak C^5 H1′-to-X^6 H8 NOE, followed by an intense X^6 H8-to-X^6 H1′ NOE. Simultaneously the X^6 H8-to-X^6 H3′ NOE was weak. The resonance arising from the T^{17} imino proton was not observed. The modified dIs were both in the *syn* conformation about the glycosyl bond with a glycosyl bond angle of 83°; T^{17}, the complementary nucleotide, was stacked into the helix, but not hydrogen bonded with the adducted inosine.

These structures provide a plausible hypothesis as to why these N1-dIno adducts strongly code for the incorporation of dCTP during translesion DNA replication, irrespective of stereochemistry. Rotation of the N1-dIno adduct into the *syn* conformation may facilitate incorporation of dCTP via Hoogsteen-type templating with dIno, generating A-to-G mutations. However, conformational differences between adducts with *R* and *S* stereochemistry suggest that adduct stereochemistry plays a secondary role in modulating the biological response.

15.7.3.5. Mutagenicities of DNAs Containing N^2 Guanine Adducts of R *and* S *EB and* R,R *and* S,S *DEB*

As described in previous sections, ODNs containing site-specific *R* and *S* EB and *R,R* and *S,S* DEB lesions were synthesized for replication studies in a prokaryotic vector (Carmical et al. 2000c) and used in an in vitro eukaryotic polymerase assay (Minko et al. 2001). Replication of M13 vectors carrying each of these four defined lesions was greatly reduced (between 200- and 2000-fold, depending on the lesion); however, those DNAs that were replicated were copied in a nearly error-free manner, such that mutation frequencies were generally $< 0.05\%$ (Carmical et al. 2000c). Consistent with the severe blockage of these lesions in the in vivo replication bypass, in vitro syntheses using purified *E. coli* polymerases I, II, and III, all revealed a near-complete blockage one nucleotide prior to the lesions.

To date, the only replication bypass study conducted using a eukaryotic polymerase revealed that yeast polymerase eta (η) would modestly replicate past these lesions, albeit with a 200–300 fold reduction in overall catalytic efficiency relative to control guanine (Minko et al. 2001). Incorporation opposite the *S* stereoisomers was nearly 10-fold more efficient than the corresponding *R* adducts. It would be of considerable interest to test whether polymerase kappa (κ) could bypass these lesions in light of its ability to bypass other bulky N^2 guanine lesions (Avkin et al. 2004; Choi, Angel and Guengerich 2006; Ogi et al. 2002; Zhang et al. 2002).

15.7.3.6. Mutagenicity of N^2-dGuo-N^2-dGuo, 2,3-Dihydroxybutane-1, 4-diyl Intrastrand Crosslinks

Given our understanding of the replication and mutagenicity of the EBD adducts on N^2 of guanine and the paucity of data concerning replication of aliphatic intrastrand crosslinks ODNs containing N^2-dGuo-N^2-dGuo, (2*R*,2*R*)-, and (2*S*,3*S*)-2,3-dihydroxybutane-1,4-diyl intrastrand crosslinks were synthesized as described above. These 8-mer DNAs were engineered into the M13mp7L2 vector and introduced into *E. coli* (Carmical et al. 2000a). Both stereoisomeric species were severe blocks to replication bypass, reducing plaque formation by $> 10^4$. Analyses of the mutagenic spectra of the limited progeny phage revealed that the *S,S* stereoisomer was approximately 10-fold more mutagenic than its *R,R* counterpart, with a mixture of every possible point mutation. Additionally, an approximate equal frequency of deletions was also detected, suggesting that the severe block to replication could be overcome by transient slippage of the blocked primer. Also consistent with these lesions being severe blocks to in vivo replication bypass, analyses of in vitro reaction of *E. coli* polymerase I, II and III revealed total blockage of synthesis one nucleotide prior to the lesions (Carmical et al. 2000a).

Since these lesions were such strong blocks to replication bypass, it was postulated that they may be sufficiently distorting to the structure of the duplex DNA that they would be readily recognized and removed by the NER system. However, neither of the duplex DNAs was efficiently incised by UvrABC or was bound by UvrA protein. These data suggest that these lesions could persist in cells and pose major challenges to genomic replication and integrity.

15.7.3.7. Mutagenicity of N3-dUri, 1-Hydroxy-3-buten-2-yl Adducts

Although most of the research has focused on purine adducts, N3 cytosine adducts are formed upon reaction with EB, but these lesions rapidly deaminate to the corresponding uracil adduct. Oligodeoxynucleotides containing a mixture of *R* and *S* stereoisomers of the N3-dUri adducts were engineered into the pMS2 vector and replicated in COS-7 cells. These lesions were extraordinarily mutagenic with the overall mutation frequency being 97%. Only point mutations were detected with 53% C(U)-to-T, 32.5% C(U)-to-A, and 11% C(U)-to-G (Fernandes et al. 2006). Even though the in vivo replication of these adducted DNAs did not appear to be compromised based on the yield of progeny vectors, in vitro replication of DNAs containing these lesions showed that both polymerases δ and ε were blocked one nucleotide prior to the lesions. However, polymerase η could incorporate every nucleotide opposite the adduct, and polymerase zeta (ζ) and polymerase η could extend all primer mismatches opposite the lesions (Fernandes and Lloyd 2007). Collectively, these data suggest that deaminated cytosine adducts may play a role in the overall mutagenic spectra following BD exposure.

Overall, these data demonstrate that many BD-modified base adducts, including N^2 guanine (minor groove) and N^6 adenine (major groove) are only weakly mutagenic in either eukaryotic or prokaryotic assay systems, while deaminated adenine and cytosine BD adducts are extremely mutagenic. We also speculate that the deaminated poducts of butadiene-modified N1-dA and N3-dC would also be mutagenic if formed in cells, but to date, these lesions have not been detected in animal exposure models. Further, perturbation of metabolic pathways favoring increases in the concentration and half-life of the diepoxide intermediate or interference with the NER pathway promote mutagenesis.

Acknowledgements. We thank Drs. Amanda K. McCullough, Marinel Ammenheuser, and Wen Xu for their insightful comments and recommendations.

References

Abdel-Rahman, S. Z., Ammenheuser, M. M., and Ward, J. B., Jr. 2001. Human sensitivity to 1,3-butadiene: role of microsomal epoxide hydrolase polymorphisms. Carcinogenesis 22:415–423.

Abdel-Rahman, S. Z., Ammenheuser, M. M., Omiecinski, C. J., Wickliffe, J. K., Rosenblatt, J. I., and Ward, J. B., Jr. 2005. Variability in human sensitivity to 1,3-butadiene: influence of polymorphisms in the 5′-flanking region of the microsomal epoxide hydrolase gene (EPHX1). Toxicol. Sci. 85:624–631.

Abdel-Rahman, S. Z., El-Zein, R. A., Ammenheuser, M. M., Yang, Z., Stock, T. H., Morandi, M., and Ward, J. B., Jr. 2003. Variability in human sensitivity to 1,3-butadiene: influence of the allelic variants of the microsomal epoxide hydrolase gene. Environ. Mol. Mutagen. 41:140–146.

Adler, I. D., Kliesch, U., Nylund, L., and Peltonen, K. 1997. In vitro and in vivo mutagenicity of the butadiene metabolites butadiene diolepoxide, butadiene monoepoxide and diepoxybutane. Mutagenesis 12:339–345.

Albertini, R. J., Sram, R. J., Vacek, P. M., Lynch, J., Nicklas, J. A., van Sittert, N. J., Boogaard, P. J., Henderson, R. F., Swenberg, J. A., Tates, A. D., et al. 2003. Biomarkers in Czech workers exposed to 1,3-butadiene: a transitional epidemiologic study. Res. Rep. Health Eff. Inst. 1–141; discussion 143–162.

Ammenheuser, M. M., Bechtold, W. E., Abdel-Rahman, S. Z., Rosenblatt, J. I., Hastings-Smith, D. A., and Ward, J. B., Jr. 2001. Assessment of 1,3-butadiene exposure in polymer production workers using HPRT mutations in lymphocytes as a biomarker. Environ. Health Perspect. 109:1249–1255.

Avkin, S., Goldsmith, M., Velasco-Miguel, S., Geacintov, N., Friedberg, E. C., and Livneh, Z. 2004. Quantitative analysis of translesion DNA synthesis across a benzo[a]pyrene-guanine adduct in mammalian cells: the role of DNA polymerase kappa. J. Biol. Chem. 279:53298–53305.

Barlow, T., Ding, J., Vouros, P., and Dipple, A. 1997. Investigation of hydrolytic deamination of 1-(2-hydroxy-1-phenylethyl)adenosine. Chem. Res. Toxicol. 10:1247–1249.

Blair, I. A., Oe, T., Kambouris, S., and Chaudhary, A. K. 2000. 1,3-Butadiene: cancer, mutations, and adducts. Part IV: Molecular dosimetry of 1,3-butadiene. Res. Rep. Health. Eff. Inst. 151–190; discussion 211–259.

Boogaard, P. J., and Bond, J. A. 1996. The role of hydrolysis in the detoxification of 1,2:3,4-diepoxybutane by human, rat, and mouse liver and lung in vitro. Toxicol. Appl. Pharmacol. 141:617–627.

Carmical, J. R., Kowalczyk, A., Zou, Y., Van Houten, B., Nechev, L. V., Harris, C. M., Harris, T. M., and Lloyd, R. S. 2000a. Butadiene-induced intrastrand DNA cross-links: a possible role in deletion mutagenesis. J. Biol. Chem. 275:19482–19489.

Carmical, J. R., Nechev, L. V., Harris, C. M., Harris, T. M., and Lloyd, R. S. 2000b. Mutagenic potential of adenine N^6 adducts of monoepoxide and diolepoxide derivatives of butadiene. Environ. Mol. Mutagen. 35:48–56.

Carmical, J. R., Zhang, M., Nechev, L., Harris, C. M., Harris, T. M., and Lloyd, R. S. 2000c. Mutagenic potential of guanine N^2 adducts of butadiene mono- and diolepoxide. Chem. Res. Toxicol. 13:18–25.

Chary, P., Latham, G. J., Robberson, D. L., Kim, S. J., Han, S., Harris, C. M., Harris, T. M., and Lloyd, R. S. 1995. In vivo and in vitro replication consequences of stereoisomeric benzo[a]pyrene-7,8-dihydrodiol 9,10-epoxide adducts on adenine N^6 at the second position of N-ras codon 61. J. Biol. Chem. 270:4990–5000.

Cheng, X., and Ruth, J. A. 1993. A simplified methodology for quantitation of butadiene metabolites. Application to the study of 1,3-butadiene metabolism by rat liver microsomes. Drug Metab. Dispos. 21:121–124.

Choi, J. Y., Angel, K. C., and Guengerich, F. P. 2006. Translesion synthesis across bulky N^2-alkyl guanine DNA adducts by human DNA polymerase kappa. J. Biol.Chem. 281:21062–21072.

Citti, L., Gervasi, P. G., Turchi, G., Bellucci, G., and Bianchini, R. 1984. The reaction of 3,4-epoxy-1-butene with deoxyguanosine and DNA in vitro: synthesis and characterization of the main adducts. Carcinogenesis 5:47–52.

Cochrane, J. E., and Skopek, T. R. 1994a. Mutagenicity of butadiene and its epoxide metabolites: I. Mutagenic potential of 1,2-epoxybutene, 1,2,3,4-diepoxybutane and 3,4-epoxy-1,2-butanediol in cultured human lymphoblasts. Carcinogenesis 15:713–717.

Cochrane, J. E., and Skopek, T. R. 1994b. Mutagenicity of butadiene and its epoxide metabolites: II. Mutational spectra of butadiene, 1,2-epoxybutene and diepoxybutane at the hprt locus in splenic T cells from exposed B6C3F1 mice. Carcinogenesis 15:719–723.

Cowles, S. R., Tsai, S. P., Snyder, P. J., and Ross, C. E. 1994. Mortality, morbidity, and haematological results from a cohort of long-term workers involved in 1,3-butadiene monomer production. Occup. Environ. Med. 51:323–329.

Csanady, G. A., Guengerich, F. P., and Bond, J. A. 1992. Comparison of the biotransformation of 1,3-butadiene and its metabolite, butadiene monoepoxide, by hepatic and pulmonary tissues from humans, rats and mice. Carcinogenesis 13:1143–1153.

de Meester, C., Poncelet, F., Roberfroid, M., and Mercier, M. 1980. The mutagenicity of butadiene towards *Salmonella typhimurium*. Toxicol. Lett. 6:125–130.

Delzell, E., Sathiakumar, N., Hovinga, M., Macaluso, M., Julian, J., Larson, R., Cole, P., and Muir, D. C. 1996. A follow-up study of synthetic rubber workers. Toxicology 113:182–189.

Divine, B. J., and Hartman, C. M. 1996. Mortality update of butadiene production workers. Toxicology 113:169–181.

Divine, B. J., and Hartman, C. M. 2001. A cohort mortality study among workers at a 1,3 butadiene facility. Chem. Biol. Interact. 135–136:535–553.

Divine, B. J., Wendt, J. K., and Hartman, C. M. 1993. Cancer mortality among workers at a butadiene production facility. IARC Sci. Publ. 127:345–362.

Downs, T. D., Crane, M. M., and Kim, K. W. 1987. Mortality among workers at a butadiene facility. Am. J. Ind. Med. 12:311–329.

Duescher, R. J., and Elfarra, A. A. 1994. Human liver microsomes are efficient catalysts of 1,3-butadiene oxidation: evidence for major roles by cytochromes P450 2A6 and 2E1. Arch. Biochem. Biophys. 311:342–349.

Elfarra, A. A., Krause, R. J., and Kemper, R. A. 2001. Cellular and molecular basis for species, sex and tissue differences in 1,3-butadiene metabolism. Chem. Biol. Interact. 135–136:239–248.

Elfarra, A. A., Moll, T. S., Krause, R. J., Kemper, R. A., and Selzer, R. R. 2001. Reactive metabolites of 1,3-butadiene: DNA and hemoglobiin adduct formation and potential roles in carcinogenicity. In Biological Reactive Intermediates VI. Dansette, P. M., et al., eds. pp. 93–103. New York: Kluwer Academic/Plenum Publishers.

Fernandes, P. H., Hackfeld, L. C., Kozekov, I. D., Hodge, R. P., and Lloyd, R. S. 2006. Synthesis and mutagenesis of the butadiene-derived N3 2′-deoxyuridine adducts. Chem. Res. Toxicol. 19:968–976.

Fernandes, P. H., and Lloyd, R. S. 2007. Mutagenic bypoass of the butadience-derived 2′-deoxyuridine adducts by polymerases eta and zeta. Mut. Res. 625:40–49.

Fujii, R., Saito, R., and Terahara, N. 1986. Purines. XXVII. Hydrolytic deamination versus Dimroth rearrangement in the 9-substituted purine ring. Effect of an omega-hydroxyalkyl group at the 1-position. Chem. Pharm. Bull. 34:1094–1107.

Graff, J. J., Sathiakumar, N., Macaluso, M., Maldonado, G., Matthews, R., and Delzell, E. 2005. Chemical exposures in the synthetic rubber industry and lymphohematopoietic cancer mortality. J. Occup. Environ. Med. 47:916–932.

Grosse, Y., Baan, R., Straif, K., Secretan, B., El Ghissassi, F., Bouvard, V., Altieri, A., and Cogliano, V. 2007. Carcinogenicity of 1,3-butadiene, ethylene oxide, vinyl chloride, vinyl fluride, and vinyl bromide. Lancet Oncology 8:679–680.

Harris, T. M., and Harris, C. M. 2000. Synthesis of N^2 substituted deoxyguanosine nucleosides from 2-fluoro-O^6-(trimethylsilylethyl)-2′-deoxyinosine. In Current Protocols in Nucleic Acid Chemistry, ed. A. L. Boyle, pp. 1.3.1–1.3.15. Hoboken: J. Wiley & Sons.

Hayes, R. B., Xi, L., Bechtold, W. E., Rothman, N., Yao, M., Henderson, R., Zhang, L., Smith, M. T., Zhang, D., Wiemels, J., et al. 1996. Hprt mutation frequency among workers exposed to 1,3-butadiene in China. Toxicology 113:100–105.

Hayes, R. B., Zhang, L., Yin, S., Swenberg, J. A., Xi, L., Wiencke, J., Bechtold, W. E., Yao, M., Rothman, N., Haas, R., et al. 2000. Genotoxic markers among butadiene polymer workers in China. Carcinogenesis 21:55–62.

http://www.osha.gov/SLTC/butadiene/index.html.

Huff, J. E., Melnick, R. L., Solleveld, H. A., Haseman, J. K., Powers, M., and Miller, R. A. 1985. Multiple organ carcinogenicity of 1,3-butadiene in B6C3F1 mice after 60 weeks of inhalation exposure. Science 227:548–549.

Jackson, M. A., Stack, H. F., Rice, J. M., and Waters, M. D. 2000. A review of the genetic and related effects of 1,3-butadiene in rodents and humans. Mutat. Res. 463:181–213.

Kanuri, M., Finneman, J., Harris, C. M., Harris, T. M., and Lloyd, R. S. 2001. Efficient nonmutagenic replication bypass of DNAs containing beta-adducts of styrene oxide at adenine N(6). Environ. Mol. Mutagen. 38:357–360.

Kanuri, M., Nechev, L. V., Kiehna, S. E., Tamura, P. J., Harris, C. M., Harris, T. M., and Lloyd, R. S. 2005. Evidence for *Escherichia coli* polymerase II mutagenic bypass of intrastrand DNA crosslinks. DNA Repair (Amst) 4:1374–1380.

Kanuri, M., Nechev, L. V., Tamura, P. J., Harris, C. M., Harris, T. M., and Lloyd, R. S. 2002. Mutagenic spectrum of butadiene-derived N1-deoxyinosine adducts and N^6,N^6-deoxyadenosine intrastrand cross-links in mammalian cells. Chem. Res. Toxicol. 15:1572–1580.

Kemper, R. A., Elfarra, A. A., and Myers, S. R. 1998. Metabolism of 3-butene-1,2-diol in B6C3F1 mice. Evidence for involvement of alcohol dehydrogenase and cytochrome P450. Drug Metab. Dispos. 26:914–920.

Kim, H. Y., Finneman, J. I., Harris, C. M., and Harris, T. M. 2000. Studies of the mechanisms of adduction of 2′-deoxyadenosine with styrene oxide and polycyclic aromatic hydrocarbon dihydrodiol epoxides. Chem. Res. Toxicol. 13:625–637.

Kim, H.-Y., Finneman, J. I., Harris, C. M., and Harris, T. M. 1998. Synthesis and adduction of fully deprotected oligodeoxynucleosides containing 6-chloropurine. Tetrahedron Lett. 39:6803–6806.

Kim, Y., Hong, H. H., Lachat, Y., Clayton, N. P., Devereux, T. R., Melnick, R. L., Hegi, M. E., and Sills, R. C. 2005. Genetic alterations in brain tumors following 1,3-butadiene exposure in B6C3F1 mice. Toxicol. Pathol. 33:307–312.

Koc, H., Tretyakova, N. Y., Walker, V. E., Henderson, R. F., and Swenberg, J. A. 1999. Molecular dosimetry of N-7 guanine adduct formation in mice and rats exposed to 1,3-butadiene. Chem. Res. Toxicol. 12:566–574.

Koivisto, P., Adler, I. D., Pacchierotti, F., and Peltonen, K. 1998. DNA adducts in mouse testis and lung after inhalation exposure to 1,3-butadiene. Mutat. Res. 397:3–10.

Koivisto, P., Adler, I. D., Sorsa, M., and Peltonen, K. 1996. Inhalation exposure of rats and mice to 1,3-butadiene induces N^6-adenine adducts of epoxybutene detected by ^{32}P-postlabeling and HPLC. Environ. Health Perspect. 104 Suppl 3:655–657.

Koivisto, P., Kilpelainen, I., Rasanen, I., Adler, I. D., Pacchierotti, F., and Peltonen, K. 1999. Butadiene diolepoxide- and diepoxybutane-derived DNA adducts at N7-guanine: a high occurrence of diolepoxide-derived adducts in mouse lung after 1,3-butadiene exposure. Carcinogenesis 20:1253–1259.

Koivisto, P., Kostiainen, R., Kilpelainen, I., Steinby, K., and Peltonen, K. 1995. Preparation, characterization and ^{32}P-postlabeling of butadiene monoepoxide N6-adenine adducts. Carcinogenesis 16:2999–3007.

Koivisto, P., Sorsa, M., Pacchierotti, F., and Peltonen, K. 1997. ^{32}P-postlabelling/HPLC assay reveals an enantioselective adduct formation in N7 guanine residues in vivo after 1,3-butadiene inhalation exposure. Carcinogenesis 18:439–443.

Kowalczyk, A., Carmical, J. R., Zou, Y., Van Houten, B., Lloyd, R. S., Harris, C. M., and Harris, T. M. 2002. Intrastrand DNA cross-links as tools for studying DNA replication and repair: two-, three-, and four-carbon tethers between the N^2 positions of adjacent guanines. Biochemistry 41:3109–3118.

Kowalczyk, A., Harris, C. M., and Harris, T. M. 2001. Synthesis and characterization of oligodeoxynucleotides containing an N1 beta-hydroxyalkyl adduct of 2′-deoxyinosine. Chem. Res. Toxicol. 14:746–753.

Kumar, R., Vodicka, P., Koivisto, P., Peltonen, K., and Hemminki, K. 1996. ^{32}P-postlabelling of diastereomeric 7-alkylguanine adducts of butadiene monoepoxide. Carcinogenesis 17:1297–1303.

Leuratti, C., Jones, N. J., Marafante, E., Kostiainen, R., Peltonen, K., and Waters, R. 1994. DNA damage induced by the environmental carcinogen butadiene: identification of a diepoxybutane-adenine adduct and its detection by ^{32}P-postlabelling. Carcinogenesis 15:1903–1910.

Leuratti, C., Jones, N. J., Marafante, E., Peltonen, K., Kostiainen, R., and Waters, R. 1993a. Biomonitoring of exposure to 1,3-butadiene: detection by high-performance liquid chromatography and ^{32}P-postlabelling of an adenine adduct formed by diepoxybutane. IARC Sci. Publ. 124:143–150.

Leuratti, C., Marafante, E., Jones, N. J., and Waters, R. 1993b. Detection by HPLC-^{32}P-postlabelling of DNA adducts formed after exposure to epoxybutene and diepoxybutane. IARC Sci. Publ. 124:277–282.

Loeber, R., Rajesh, M., Fang, Q., Pegg, A. E., and Tretyakova, N. 2006. Cross-linking of the human DNA repair protein O^6-alkylguanine DNA alkyltransferase to DNA in the presence of 1,2,3,4-diepoxybutane. Chem. Res. Toxicol. 19:645–654.

Ma, H., Wood, T. G., Ammenheuser, M. M., Rosenblatt, J. I., and Ward, J. B., Jr. 2000. Molecular analysis of hprt mutant lymphocytes from 1,3-butadiene-exposed workers. Environ. Mol. Mutagen 36:59–71.

Mabon, N., Moorthy, B., Randerath, E., and Randerath, K. 1996. Monophosphate ^{32}P-postlabeling assay of DNA adducts from 1,2:3,4-diepoxybutane, the most genotoxic metabolite of 1,3-butadiene: in vitro methodological studies and in vivo dosimetry. Mutat. Res. 371:87–104.

Malvoisin, E., and Roberfroid, M. 1982. Hepatic microsomal metabolism of 1,3-butadiene. Xenobiotica 12:137–144.

Matanoski, G., Francis, M., Correa-Villasenor, A., Elliott, E., Santos-Burgoa, C., and Schwartz, L. 1993. Cancer epidemiology among styrene-butadiene rubber workers. IARC Sci. Publ. 124:363–374.

McGregor, D., Brown, A. G., Cattanach, P., Edwards, I., McBride, D., Riach, C., Shepherd, W., and Caspary, W. J. 1991. Responses of the L5178Y mouse lymphoma forward mutation assay: V. Gases and vapors. Environ Mol Mutagen 17:122–129.

Meinhardt, T. J., Lemen, R. A., Crandall, M. S., and Young, R. J. 1982. Environmental epidemiologic investigation of the styrene-butadiene rubber industry. Mortality patterns with discussion of the hematopoietic and lymphatic malignancies. Scand. J. Work Environ. Health 8:250–259.

Melnick, R. L., Huff, J., Chou, B. J., and Miller, R. A. 1990. Carcinogenicity of 1,3-butadiene in C57BL/6 x C3H F1 mice at low exposure concentrations. Cancer Res. 50:6592–6599.

Meng, Q., Henderson, R. F., Chen, T., Heflich, R. H., Walker, D. M., Bauer, M. J., Reilly, A. A., and Walker, V. E. 1999a. Mutagenicity of 1,3-butadiene at the Hprt locus of T-lymphocytes following inhalation exposures of female mice and rats. Mutat. Res. 429:107–125.

Meng, Q., Henderson, R. F., Long, L., Blair, L., Walker, D. M., Upton, P. B., Swenberg, J. A., and Walker, V. E. 2001. Mutagenicity at the Hprt locus in T cells of female mice following inhalation exposures to low levels of 1,3-butadiene. Chem. Biol. Interact. 135–136:343–361.

Meng, Q., Henderson, R. F., Walker, D. M., Bauer, M. J., Reilly, A. A., and Walker, V. E. 1999b. Mutagenicity of the racemic mixtures of butadiene monoepoxide and butadiene diepoxide at the Hprt locus of T-lymphocytes following inhalation exposures of female mice and rats. Mutat. Res. 429:127–140.

Meng, Q., Recio, L., Reilly, A. A., Wong, B. A., Bauer, M., and Walker, V. E. 1998a. Comparison of the mutagenic potency of 1,3-butadiene at the hprt locus of T-lymphocytes following inhalation exposure of female B6C3F1 mice and F344 rats. Carcinogenesis 19:1019–1027.

Meng, Q., Redetzke, D. L., Hackfeld, L. C., Hodge, R. P., Walker, D. M., and Walker, V. E. 2007a. Mutagenicity of stereochemical configurations of 1,2-epoxybutene and 1,2:3,4-diepoxybutane in human lymphblastoid cells. Chem. Biol. Interact. 166:207–218.

Meng, Q., Singh, N., Heflich, R. H., Bauer, M. J., and Walker, V. E. 2000. Comparison of the mutations at Hprt exon 3 of T-lymphocytes from B6C3F1 mice and F344 rats exposed by inhalation to 1,3-butadiene or the racemic mixture of 1,2:3,4-diepoxybutane. Mutat. Res. 464:169–184.

Meng, Q., Skopek, T. R., Walker, D. M., Hurley-Leslie, S., Chen, T., Zimmer, D. M., and Walker, V. E. 1998b. Culture and propagation of Hprt mutant T-lymphocytes isolated from mouse spleen. Environ. Mol. Mutagen. 32:236–243.

Meng, Q., Walker, D. M., McDonald, J. D., Henderson, R. F., Carter, M. M., Cook, D. L., Jr, McCash, C. L., Torres, S. M., Bauer, M. J., et al. 2007b. Age-, gender-, and species-dependent mutagenicity in T cells of mice and rats exposed by inhalation to 1,3-butadiene. Chem Biol Interact. 166:121–131.

Meng, Q., Walker, D. M., Scott, B. R., Seilkop, S. K., Aden, J. K., and Walker, V. E. 2004. Characterization of Hprt mutations in cDNA and genomic DNA of T-cell mutants from control and 1,3-butadiene-exposed male B6C3F1 mice and F344 rats. Environ. Mol. Mutagen. 43:75–92.

Merritt, W. K., Nechev, L. V., Harris, T. M., Harris, C. M., Llyod, R. S., and Stone, M. P. 2005a. Structure of the 1,4-bis(2′-deoxyadensin-N^6-yl)-2S,3R-butanediol cross-link arising from alkylation of the human N-ras codon 61 by butadiene diepoxide. Biochemistry 44:10081–10092.

Merritt, W. K., Kowalczyk, A., Scholdberg, T. A., Dean, S. M., Harris, T. M., Harris, C. M., Lloyd, R. S., and Stone, M. P. 2005b. Dual roles of glycosyl torsion angle conformation and stereochemical configuration in butadiene oxide-derived N1 beta-hydroxyalkyl deoxyinosine adducts: A structural perspective. Chem. Res. Toxicol. 18:1098–1107.

Merritt, W. K., Scholdberg, T.A., Nechev, L. V., Harris, T. M., Harris, C. M., Llyod, R. S., and Stone, M. P. 2004. Stereospecific structural perturbations arising from adenine N^6 butadiene triol adducts in duplex DNA. Chem. Res. Toxicol. 17:1007–1019.

Millard, J. T., and White, M. M. 1993. Diepoxybutane cross-links DNA at 5′-GNC sequences. Biochemistry 32:2120–2124.

Millard, J. T., and Wilkes, E. E. 2001. Diepoxybutane and diepoxyoctane interstrand cross-linking of the 5S DNA nucleosomal core particle. Biochemistry 40:10677–10685.

Millard, J. T., Hanly, T. C., Murphy, K., and Tretyakova, N. 2006. The 5′-GNC site for DNA interstrand cross-linking is conserved for diepoxybutane stereoisomers. Chem. Res. Toxicol. 19:16–19.

Minko, I. G., Washington, M. T., Prakash, L., Prakash, S., and Lloyd, R. S. 2001. Translesion DNA synthesis by yeast DNA polymerase eta on templates containing N^2-guanine adducts of 1,3-butadiene metabolites. J. Biol. Chem. 276:2517–2522.

Nauhaus, S. K., Fennell, T. R., Asgharian, B., Bond, J. A., and Sumner, S. C. 1996. Characterization of urinary metabolites from Sprague–Dawley rats and B6C3F1 mice exposed to [1,2,3,4-^{13}C]butadiene. Chem. Res. Toxicol. 9:764–773.

Neagu, I., Koivisto, P., Neagu, C., Kaltia, S., Kostiainen, R., and Peltonen, K. 1994. Alkylation of purine bases with 3,4-epoxy-1-butene, a reactive metabolite of 1,3-butadiene. IARC Sci. Publ. 125:419–422.

Nechev, L. V., Zhang, M., Tsarouhtsis, D., Tamura, P. J., Wilkinson, A. S., Harris, C. M., and Harris, T. M. 2001. Synthesis and characterization of nucleosides and oligonucleotides bearing adducts of butadiene epoxides on adenine N^6 and guanine N^2. Chem. Res. Toxicol. 14:379–388.

Oe, T., Kambouris, S. J., Walker, V. E., Meng, Q., Recio, L., Wherli, S., Chaudhary, A. K., and Blair, I. A. 1999. Persistence of N7-(2,3,4-trihydroxybutyl)guanine adducts in the livers of mice and rats exposed to 1,3-butadiene. Chem. Res. Toxicol. 12:247–257.

Ogi, T., Shinkai, Y., Tanaka, K., and Ohmori, H. 2002. Pol kappa protects mammalian cells against the lethal and mutagenic effects of benzo[a]pyrene. Proc. Natl. Acad. Sci. U S A 99:15548–15553.

Ohfune, Y., and Kurokawa, N. 1984. Synthesis of the serine equivalent, (2R)-and (2S)-3-butenol derivatives. Synthetic approaches to the metal chelating polyamino acid, "aspergillomarasmine A". Tetrahedron Lett. 25:1071–1074.

Owen, P. E., and Glaister, J. R. 1990. Inhalation toxicity and carcinogenicity of 1,3-butadiene in Sprague–Dawley rats. Environ. Health Perspect. 86:19–25.

Owen, P. E., Glaister, J. R., Gaunt, I. F., and Pullinger, D. H. 1987. Inhalation toxicity studies with 1,3-butadiene. 3. Two year toxicity/carcinogenicity study in rats. Am. Ind. Hyg. Assoc. J. 48:407–413.

Park, S., and Tretyakova, N. 2004. Structural characterization of the major DNA-DNA cross-link of 1,2,3,4-diepoxybutane. Chem. Res. Toxicol. 17:129–136.

Park, S., Anderson, C., Loeber, R., Seetharaman, M., Jones, R., and Tretyakova, N. 2005. Interstrand and intrastrand DNA-DNA cross-linking by 1,2,3,4-diepoxybutane: role of stereochemistry. J. Am. Chem. Soc. 127:14355–14365.

Park, S., Hodge, J., Anderson, C., and Tretyakova, N. 2004. Guanine-adenine DNA cross-linking by 1,2,3,4-diepoxybutane: potential basis for biological activity. Chem. Res. Toxicol. 17:1638–1651.

Powley, M. W., Jayaraj, K., Gold, A., Ball, L. M., and Swenberg, J. A. 2003. 1,N^2-propanodeoxyguanosine adducts of the 1,3-butadiene metabolite, hydroxymethylvinyl ketone. Chem. Res. Toxicol. 16:1448–1454.

Qian, C., and Dipple, A. 1995. Different mechanisms of aralkylation of adenosine at the 1- and N^6-positions. Chem. Res. Toxicol. 8:389–395.

Recio, L., and Goldsworthy, T. L. 1995. The use of transgenic mice for studying mutagenicity induced by 1,3-butadiene. Toxicol. Lett. 82–83:607–612.

Recio, L., and Meyer, K. G. 1995. Increased frequency of mutations at A:T base pairs in the bone marrow of B6C3F1 lacI transgenic mice exposed to 1,3-butadiene. Environ. Mol. Mutagen. 26:1–8.

Recio, L., Bond, J. A., Pluta, L. J., and Sisk, S. C. 1993. Use of transgenic mice for assessing the mutagenicity of 1,3-butadiene in vivo. IARC Sci. Publ. 124:235–243.

Recio, L., Pluta, L. J., and Meyer, K. G. 1998. The in vivo mutagenicity and mutational spectrum at the lacI transgene recovered from the spleens of B6C3F1 lacI transgenic mice following a 4-week inhalation exposure to 1,3-butadiene. Mutat. Res. 401:99–110.

Rodriguez, D. A., Kowalczyk, A., Ward, J. B., Jr., Harris, C. M., Harris, T. M., and Lloyd, R. S. 2001. Point mutations induced by 1,2-epoxy-3-butene N1 deoxyinosine adducts. Environ. Mol. Mutagen. 38:292–296.

Santos-Burgoa, C., Matanoski, G. M., Zeger, S., and Schwartz, L. 1992. Lymphohematopoietic cancer in styrene-butadiene polymerization workers. Am. J. Epidemiol. 136:843–854.

Sathiakumar, N., Graff, J., Macaluso, M., Maldonado, G., Matthews, R., and Delzell, E. 2005. An updated study of mortality among North American synthetic rubber industry workers. Occup. Environ. Med. 62:822–829.

Scholdberg, T. A., Merritt, W. K., Dean, S. M., Kowalcyzk, A., Harris, C. M., Harris, T. M., Rizzo, C. J., Lloyd, R. S., and Stone, M. P. 2005b. Structure of an oligodeoxynucleotide containing a butadiene oxide-derived N1 beta-hydroxyalkyl deoxyinosine adduct in the human N-ras codon 61 sequence. Biochemistry 44:3327–3337.

Scholdberg, T.A., Nechev, L. V., Merritt, W. K., Harris, T. M., Harris, C. M., Llyod, R. S., and Stone, M. P. 2004. Structure of a site specific major groove (2S,3S)-N^6-(2,3,4-trihydroxybutyl)-2′-deoxyadenosyl DNA adduct of butadiene diol epoxide. Chem. Res. Toxicol. 17:717–730.

Scholdberg, T.A., Nechev, L. V., Merritt, W. K., Harris, T. M., Harris, C. M., Llyod, R. S., and Stone, M. P. 2004. Mispairing of a site specific major (2S,3S)-N^6-(2,3,4-trihydroxybutyl)-2′-deoxyadenosyl DNA adduct of butadiene diol epoxidewith deoxyguanosine: formation of a dA(anti) dG(anti) paring interaction. Chem. Res. Toxicol. 18:145–153.

Selzer, R. R., and Elfarra, A. A. 1996a. Characterization of N1- and N^6-adenosine adducts and N1-inosine adducts formed by the reaction of butadiene monoxide with adenosine: evidence for the N1-adenosine adducts as major initial products. Chem. Res. Toxicol. 9:875–881.

Selzer, R. R., and Elfarra, A. A. 1996b. Synthesis and biochemical characterization of N1-, N^2-, and N7-guanosine adducts of butadiene monoxide. Chem. Res. Toxicol. 9:126–132.

Selzer, R. R., and Elfarra, A. A. 1997a. Characterization of four N-3-thymidine adducts formed in vitro by the reaction of thymidine and butadiene monoxide. Carcinogenesis 18:1993–1998.

Selzer, R. R., and Elfarra, A. A. 1997b. Chemical modification of deoxycytidine at different sites yields adducts of different stabilities: characterization of N3- and O^2-deoxycytidine and N3-deoxyuridine adducts of butadiene monoxide. Arch. Biochem. Biophys. 343:63–72.

Selzer, R. R., and Elfarra, A. A. 1999. In vitro reactions of butadiene monoxide with single- and double-stranded DNA: characterization and quantitation of several purine and pyrimidine adducts. Carcinogenesis 20:285–292.

Sisk, S. C., Pluta, L. J., Bond, J. A., and Recio, L. 1994. Molecular analysis of lacI mutants from bone marrow of B6C3F1 transgenic mice following inhalation exposure to 1,3-butadiene. Carcinogenesis 15:471–477.

Steen, A. M., Meyer, K. G., and Recio, L. 1997a. Analysis of hprt mutations occurring in human TK6 lymphoblastoid cells following exposure to 1,2,3,4-diepoxybutane. Mutagenesis 12:61–67.

Steen, A. M., Meyer, K. G., and Recio, L. 1997b. Characterization of hprt mutations following 1,2-epoxy-3-butene exposure of human TK6 cells. Mutagenesis 12:359–364.

Tates, A. D., van Dam, F. J., de Zwart, F. A., van Teylingen, C. M., and Natarajan, A. T. 1994. Development of a cloning assay with high cloning efficiency to detect induction of 6-thioguanine-resistant lymphocytes in spleen of adult mice following in vivo inhalation exposure to 1,3-butadiene. Mutat. Res. 309:299–306.

Tretyakova, N., Chiang, S. Y., Walker, V. E., and Swenberg, J. A. 1998. Quantitative analysis of 1,3-butadiene-induced DNA adducts in vivo and in vitro using liquid chromatography electrospray ionization tandem mass spectrometry. J. Mass Spectrom. 33:363–376.

Tretyakova, N., Lin, Y. P., Upton, P. B., Sangaiah, R., and Swenberg, J. A. 1996. Macromolecular adducts of butadiene. Toxicology 113:70–76.

Tretyakova, N., Lin, Y., Sangaiah, R., Upton, P. B., and Swenberg, J. A. 1997a. Identification and quantitation of DNA adducts from calf thymus DNA exposed to 3,4-epoxy-1-butene. Carcinogenesis 18:137–147.

Tretyakova, N., Sangaiah, R., Yen, T. Y., and Swenberg, J. A. 1997c. Synthesis, characterization, and in vitro quantitation of N-7-guanine adducts of diepoxybutane. Chem. Res. Toxicol. 10:779–785.

Tretyakova, N., Sangaiah, R., Yen, T. Y., Gold, A., and Swenberg, J. A. 1997b. Adenine adducts with diepoxybutane: isolation and analysis in exposed calf thymus DNA. Chem. Res. Toxicol. 10:1171–1179.

Valadez, J. G., Liu, L., Loktionova, N. A., Pegg, A. E., and Guengerich, F. P. 2004. Activation of *bis*-electrophiles to mutagenic conjugates by human O^6-alkylguanine-DNA alkyltransferase. Chem. Res. Toxicol. 17:972–982.

Ward, J. B., Jr., Abdel-Rahman, S. Z., Henderson, R. F., Stock, T. H., Morandi, M., Rosenblatt, J. I., and Ammenheuser, M. M. 2001. Assessment of butadiene exposure in synthetic rubber manufacturing workers in Texas using frequencies of hprt mutant lymphocytes as a biomarker. Chem. Biol. Interact. 135–136:465–483.

Ward, J. B., Jr., Ammenheuser, M. M., Bechtold, W. E., Whorton, E. B., Jr., and Legator, M. S. 1994. hprt Mutant lymphocyte frequencies in workers at a 1,3-butadiene production plant. Environ. Health Perspect. 102 Suppl 9:79–85.

Ward, J. B., Jr., Ammenheuser, M. M., Whorton, E. B., Jr., Bechtold, W. E., Kelsey, K. T., and Legator, M. S. 1996. Biological monitoring for mutagenic effects of occupational exposure to butadiene. Toxicology 113:84–90.

Wickliffe, J. K., Ammenheuser, M. M., Salazar, J. J., Abdel-Rahman, S. Z., Hastings-Smith, D. A., Postlethwait, E. M., Lloyd, R. S., and Ward, J. B., Jr. 2003. A model of sensitivity: 1,3-butadiene increases mutant frequencies and genomic damage in mice lacking a functional microsomal epoxide hydrolase gene. Environ. Mol. Mutagen. 42:106–110.

Wickliffe, J. K., Galbert, L. A., Ammenheuser, M. M., Herring, S. M., Xie, J., Masters, O. E., 3rd, Friedberg, E. C., Lloyd, R. S., and Ward, J. B., Jr. 2006. 3,4-Epoxy-1-butene, a reactive metabolite of 1,3-butadiene, induces somatic mutations in Xpc-null mice. Environ. Mol. Mutagen. 47:67–70.

Wickliffe, J. K., Herring, S. M., Hallberg, L. M., Galbert, L. A., Masters, O. E., 3rd, Ammenheuser, M. M., Xie, J., Friedberg, E. C., Lloyd, R. S., Abdel-Rahman, S. Z., and Ward, J. B., Jr. 2007. Detoxification of olefinic epoxides and nucleotide excision repair of epoxide-mediated DNA damage: insights from animal models examining human sensitivity to 1,3-butadiene. Chem. Biol. Interact. 166:226–231.

Xu, W., Merritt, W. K., Nechev, L. V., Harris, T. M., Harris, C. M., Lloyd, R. S., and Stone, M. P. 2007. Structure of the 1,4-bis(2′-deoxyadenosin-N(6)-yl)-2*S*,3*S*-butanediol intrastrand DNA cross-link arising from butadiene diepoxide in the human N-ras codon 61 sequence. Chem. Res. Toxicol. 20:187–198.

Yunes, M. J., Charnecki, S. E., Marden, J. J., and Millard, J. T. 1996. 1,2,5,6-Diepoxyhexane and 1,2,7,8-diepoxyoctane cross-link duplex DNA at 5′-GNC sequences. Chem. Res. Toxicol. 9:994–1000.

Zhang, X. Y., and Elfarra, A. A. 2003. Identification and characterization of a series of nucleoside adducts formed by the reaction of 2′-deoxyguanosine and 1,2,3,4-diepoxybutane under physiological conditions. Chem. Res. Toxicol. 16:1606–1615.

Zhang, X. Y., and Elfarra, A. A. 2004. Characterization of the reaction products of 2′-deoxyguanosine and 1,2,3,4-diepoxybutane after acid hydrolysis: formation of novel guanine and pyrimidine adducts. Chem. Res. Toxicol. 17:521–528.

Zhang, X. Y., and Elfarra, A. A. 2005. Reaction of 1,2,3,4-diepoxybutane with 2′-deoxyguanosine: initial products and their stabilities and decomposition patterns under physiological conditions. Chem. Res. Toxicol. 18:1316–1323.

Zhang, X. Y., and Elfarra, A. A. 2006. Characterization of 1,2,3,4-diepoxybutane-2′-deoxyguanosine cross-linking products formed at physiological and nonphysiological conditions. Chem. Res. Toxicol. 19:547–555.

Zhang, Y., Wu, X., Guo, D., Rechkoblit, O., and Wang, Z. 2002. Activities of human DNA polymerase kappa in response to the major benzo[a]pyrene DNA adduct: error-free lesion bypass and extension synthesis from opposite the lesion. DNA Repair (Amst) 1:559–569.

Zhao, C., Koskinen, M., and Hemminki, K. 1998. ^{32}P-Postlabelling of N^{6}-adenine adducts of epoxybutanediol in vivo after 1,3-butadiene exposure. Toxicol. Lett. 102–103:591–594.

Zhao, C., Vodicka, P., Sram, R. J., and Hemminki, K. 2000. Human DNA adducts of 1,3-butadiene, an important environmental carcinogen. Carcinogenesis 21:107–111.

16

Pharmacogenetics of Drug Bioactivation Pathways

Lauren A. Trepanier
Department of Medical Sciences, School of Veterinary Medicine, University of Wisconsin-Madison, 2015 Linden Drive, Madison, WI 53706-1102, USA
e-mail: latrepanier@svm.vetmed.wisc.edu

Keywords: Polymorphism · Genotype · Phenotype · Cytochrome P450 · Flavin-containing Monooxygenases · Peroxidases · *N*-acetyltransferase · Sulfotransferase · Epoxide Hydrolases

16.1. Introduction

Pharmacogenetics is the study of variation in xenobiotic response that is caused by genetic polymorphisms in drug disposition or drug response genes. These genes may encode receptors, transporters, or biotransformation enzymes. Polymorphisms in biotransformation enzymes, particularly cytochrome P450 s (CYPs), have been most extensively studied. While biotransformation pathways are thought to have evolved to inactivate and allow the elimination of foreign compounds, these pathways can less commonly lead to the bioactivation and increased toxicity of xenobiotics (Figure 16.1). Oxidation of xenobiotics is a common bioactivation reaction, and can be catalyzed by CYPs, flavin-containing monooxygenases (FMOs), peroxidases, or cyclooxygenases (COXs). Less commonly, bioactivation can be mediated by conjugation or hydrolysis reactions. This chapter will review what is known about pharmacogenetic differences in important xenobiotic bioactivation pathways, with an emphasis on the association between functional polymorphisms and clinical and toxicologic outcomes in humans. There are considerable data to support a role for bioactivation polymorphisms in occupational chemical toxicity and in the carcinogenicity of environmental pollutants. In contrast, most idiosyncratic drug toxicities have not been associated to date with genetic variability in bioactivation pathways; however, studies have been limited (Pirmohamed 2006).

A.A. Elfarra (ed.), *Advances in Bioactivation Research*, DOI: 10.1007/978-0-387-77300-1_16,

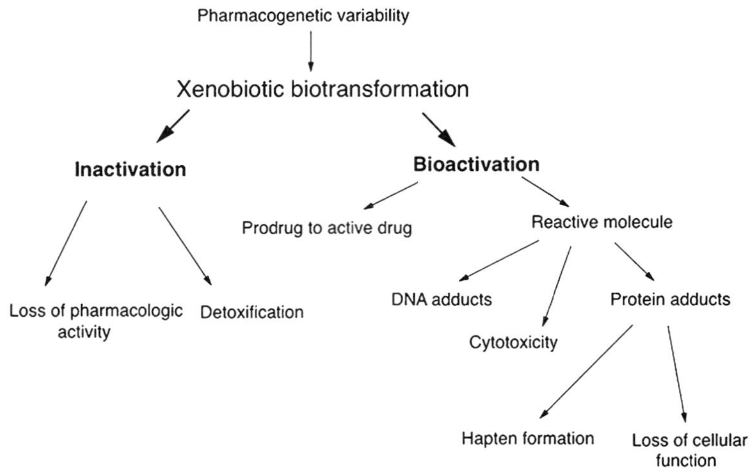

Figure 16.1 Variable potential outcomes due to pharmacogenetic variability in xenobiotic biotransformation pathways.

16.2. Cytochrome P450s

Cytochrome P450s are heme-containing monooxygenases that are expressed in the endoplasmic reticulum (microsomal fraction) of many tissues, including liver, kidney, gut, lung, endocrine glands, and brain. While CYP action most commonly renders xenobiotics less active or more polar, CYPs can also bioactivate compounds via the formation of hydroxylamines, epoxides, and hydroquinones, which can lead to unstable electrophilic by-products (Ioannides and Lewis 2004).

16.2.1. Bioactivation by the CYP1 Family

The CYP1 family is the predominant group of CYPs involved in xenobiotic bioactivation, primarily by CYP1A1, CYP1A2, and CYP1B1. Typical substrates of CYP1 enzymes are lipophilic and planar molecules (Ioannides and Lewis 2004), a number of which are important pro-carcinogens. CYP1A enzymes are inducible by chemicals such as benzo[*a*]pyrene and 2-aminobiphenyl, via the cytosolic aryl hydrocarbon (Ah) receptor. The mutagenicity of CYP1A substrates has been shown to correlate with the degree of induction of these enzymes (Cheung et al. 1994).

16.2.1.1. CYP1A1

CYP1A1 is expressed in extrahepatic tissues such as the lung, skin, and breast, and is highly conserved among species. CYP1A1 bioactivates aromatic amines, polycyclic aromatic hydrocarbons, and heterocyclic amines. CYP1A1 also catalyzes the first step in the bioactivation 17β-estradiol to its genotoxic quinone derivative (Crooke et al. 2006).

CYP1A1 activates the tobacco carcinogen benzo[*a*]pyrene, which is necessary for the formation of genotoxic DNA adducts. High pulmonary CYP1A1 expression has been associated with lung cancer in smokers (Anttila et al. 1992). A high-inducibility polymorphism in *CYP1A1*

(*CYP1A1*2A*) has been characterized, and is identified by an *Msp*I restriction fragment length polymorphism (RFLP) in the 3′-untranslated region (UTR) of the gene (6235 T >C) (Petersen et al. 1991). The *MspI* allele has been associated with an increased risk of lung cancer in Japanese patients (Kawajiri et al. 1990; Nakachi et al. 1991), but not in Caucasians, in which the *MspI* allele is rare (Raunio et al. 1995).

The heterocyclic amine 2-amino-3-methylimidazo[4,5-*f*]quinolone (IQ) is a mammary carcinogen in rodents, and is bioactivated by CYP1A1 in human breast (Williams et al. 1998). The inducible *MspI* allele has been associated with breast cancer risk in Chinese women (Shen et al. 2006), and may interact with antioxidant deficiencies to increase the risk of breast cancer in African-American women (Zhu et al. 2006). However, in other populations of women, the association between *CYP1A1* genotype and breast cancer outcome has been weak or nonsignificant (Boyapati et al. 2005; Le Marchand et al. 2005; Okobia et al. 2005; Singh et al. 2007).

For colorectal cancer, for which dietary heterocyclic amine exposure is a likely risk factor, the relationship between *CYP1A1* genotype and tumor outcome appears to be complex, with varied interactions among this CYP and gender, meat intake, and other polymorphisms (Murtaugh et al. 2005). However, another high-inducibility polymorphism (*CYP1A1*2C*; 462 Ile > Val) (Crofts et al. 1994) was significantly associated with colorectal cancer in a study of patients in Scotland (Sachse et al. 2002).

16.2.1.2. CYP1A2

CYP1A2 is expressed primarily in liver, where it varies more than 50-fold in activity among individuals (Butler et al. 1989; Turesky et al. 1998). CYP1A2 bioactivates heterocyclic aromatic amines such as 2-amino-1-methyl-6-phenylimidazo[4,5-*b*]pyridine (PhIP) and 2-amino-3,8-dimethylimidazo[4,5-*f*]quinoxaline (MeIQX) to reactive hydroxylamine metabolites (Turesky et al. 2002; Figure 16.2). These hydroxylamines are further bioactivated by *O*-acetylation, followed by heterolytic cleavage to form a

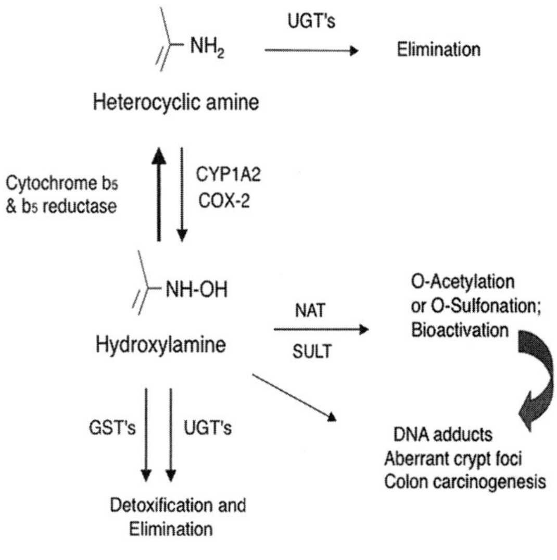

Figure 16.2 Oxidative metabolism of heterocyclic amines such as PhIP, and resulting mutagenic outcome. UDP-glucuronosyltransferases (UGTs) act to enhance elimination of the parent compound. Bioactivation by cytochrome P450 1A2 or cyclooxygenases (COX) 2 leads to an unstable hydroxylamine, which can be eliminated as glutathione or glucuronide conjugates via the action of glutathione-S-transferases (GSTs) or UGTs. Alternatively, the hydroxylamine may be further bioactivated by *N*-acetyltransferases (NAT) or sulfotransferases (SULT) to ultimately form a nitrenium ion, which can form DNA adducts that are thought to initiate colon carcinogenesis.

nitrenium ion, which forms DNA adducts (Turesky and Vouros 2004). CYP1A2 activity is therefore important for the carcinogenicity of these compounds.

The *CYP1A2*1D* allele (-2467delT) has been associated with both increased CYP1A2 activity in vivo (as measured by urinary caffeine metabolites) and increased urine mutagenicity in smokers (Pavanello et al. 2005). Rapid CYP1A2 activity has also been linked to colorectal carcinoma, particularly in association with smoking or red meat intake (Badawi et al. 1996; Bae et al. 2006; Le Marchand et al. 2002). High CYP1A2 activity phenotype has been associated with lung cancer in one study in Chinese women, but only when modulation by *N*-acetyltransferase status was considered (Seow et al. 2001).

CYP1A2 also bioactivates aflatoxin, with low K_m values comparable to concentrations expected from dietary exposure (Gallagher et al. 1996; Gallagher et al. 1994). Aflatoxin is associated with hepatocellular carcinoma in humans, and is the second leading cause of this tumor type, after hepatitis B infection, in high-exposure populations in Africa and Asia (Yu and Yuan 2004). Accordingly, impaired CYP1A2 activity (*CYP1A2*1C* allele) appears to have a protective effect on the outcome of hepatocellular carcinoma among hepatitis B seronegative patients (Chen et al. 2006).

The antihypertensive agent dihydralazine leads to an autoimmune hepatitis in a small subset of patients. Dihydralazine is both bioactivated by CYP1A2 and leads to its induction (Bourdi et al. 1992), and autoantibodies in patients with dihydralazine hepatitis have been shown to target hepatic CYP1A2 (Bourdi et al. 1990). Reactive metabolites generated by CYP1A2 are thought to both inactivate and haptenize this enzyme and lead to autoantibody formation (Bourdi et al. 1994). Given the functional variability in CYP1A2 in humans (http://www.cypalleles.ki.se/cyp1a2.htm), polymorphisms in this enzyme are likely to be a risk factor for this adverse drug reaction; however, this has not yet been evaluated.

16.2.1.3. CYP1B1

CYP1B1 is also involved in the bioactivation and mutagenicity of polycyclic aromatic hydrocarbons such as benzo[*a*]pyrene, and is inducible by dioxin (TCDD). CYP1B1 is found in extrahepatic tissues such as breast (Hellmold et al. 1998), and like CYP1A1, can bioactivate estradiol (Crooke et al. 2006; Jefcoate et al. 2000).

A polymorphism in *CYP1B1* at codon 432 (Val > Leu) has been evaluated in risk analyses of cancer outcome. The wild-type allele (*432 Val*), which is found in approximately 40% of Caucasian women and 70% of African-American women (Bailey et al. 1998), has higher activity in vitro for estradiol activation than *432Leu* (Li et al. 2000; Shimada et al. 1999). Studies have been conflicting, with the *432Val* allele found to be overrepresented among women with estrogen receptor-positive breast tumors (Bailey et al. 1998; De Vivo et al. 2002) or breast cancer patients who smoke (Sillanpaa et al. 2006), while the variant *432 Leu* allele was found to be associated with breast cancer risk in women who take hormone replacement therapy (Rylander-Rudqvist et al. 2003).

16.2.2. Bioactivation by the CYP2 Family

Of the CYP2 family of CYPs, CYP2E1 has the most prominent role in clinically and toxicologically important bioactivation pathways.

16.2.2.1. CYP2E1

CYP2E1 plays a key role in the bioactivation of low-molecular-weight environmental and industrial chemicals, to include tobacco *N*-nitrosamines, styrene, benzene, butadiene, urethane, and vinyl chloride (Ioannides and Lewis 2004). In addition, CYP2E1 bioactivates several clinically important drugs, such as acetaminophen, isoniazid, and halothane. CYP2E1 substrates also include ethanol and other short-chain alcohols. Ethanol induces CYP2E1 expression via stabilization of the protein against proteasomal degradation (Roberts et al. 1995); this acquired increase in CYP2E1 protein expression can lead to discordance between genotype and phenotype among individuals.

The coding sequence of *CYP2E1* is well conserved among humans, likely due to an as yet undefined but important role for this CYP in endogenous metabolism (Hu et al. 1997). Despite relatively low functional variability in the coding region among individuals, *CYP2E1* has several potentially important polymorphisms with toxicological significance. An important high-prevalence allele (*CYP2E1*5B*) comprised of two 5′ flanking region polymorphisms (*Pst*I/*Rsa*I, found at -1293 and -1053, respectively) appears to involve a binding site for the transcription factor HNF1, and leads to increased transcriptional activity in vitro (Hayashi, Watanabe and Kawajiri 1991). This allele has a higher prevalence in Asian populations (approximately 40% are homozygotes or heterozygotes) compared to Caucasian populations (less than 8%) (Bolt, Roos and Their 2003). The *Pst*I/*Rsa*I polymorphism is thought to lead to enhanced bioactivation of 2E1 substrates, such as carcinogenic *N*-nitrosamines (Yu and Yuan 2004). However an in vivo study of CYP2E1 activity (as measured by chlorzoxazone metabolism) found that the *Rsa*I polymorphism was associated with decreased enzyme activity (Le Marchand, Wilkinson and Wilkens 1999), which is discordant with in vitro transcriptional data.

Overall, however, the *Pst*I/*Rsa*I CYP2E1 polymorphism appears to be associated with increased risk of certain cancers. In a meta-analysis of more than 2000 cases of gastric carcinoma in an Asian population, *Pst*I/*Rsa*I homozygotes were significantly overrepresented (Boccia et al. 2007). In addition, this allele was overrepresented among patients with pulmonary adenocarcinoma. (El-Zein et al. 1997), and colorectal cancer (Yu and Yuan 2004).

High CYP2E1 activity appears to be a risk factor for several chemical toxicities. CYP2E1 metabolizes vinyl chloride to the electrophiles chloroethylene oxide and chloroacetaldehyde. Consistent with this, the high-expression *Pst*I polymorphism was overrepresented among workers who developed evidence of liver toxicity following occupational exposure to vinyl chloride (Zhu et al. 2005). This same polymorphism has also been associated with increased expression of mutant p53 protein in the plasma of industrial vinyl chloride workers (Wong et al. 2002). In addition, Chinese smokers who developed signs of bone marrow toxicity after benzene exposure were more likely to harbor the *Pst*I polymorphism (Wan et al. 2002). This apparent effect was particularly pronounced in subjects with loss-of-function polymorphisms in the glutathione-*S*-transferase and NAD(P)H:quinone oxidoreductase 1 (NQO1) detoxification pathways.

The chemical 1,3-butadiene is used in the synthesis of rubber and latex, and is also found in tobacco smoke and automobile exhaust. Butadiene is oxidized to ultimately genotoxic epoxide metabolites in part by CYP2E1 (Duescher and Elfarra 1994, Elfarra, Krause and Selzer 1996), and the response to butadiene may be modulated by *CYP2E1* genotype. Paradoxically, one 5-flanking polymorphism (*CYP2E1*7B*), which leads to enhanced enzyme expression in vitro (Fairbrother et al. 1998), was associated with a trend toward decreased levels of hemoglobin adducts in butadiene-exposed workers (Fustinoni et al. 2002).

CYP2E1 also bioactivates the inhalant anesthetic halothane, generating a reactive trifluoroacetyl chloride metabolite (Bourdi et al. 1996; Kenna et al. 1988). This metabolite leads to protein binding, neohapten formation, and an autoimmune response that is associated with hepatic necrosis (Spracklin et al. 1997). Induction of CYP2E1 leads to enhanced metabolite–protein binding from halothane in vivo in rodents (Eliasson et al. 1998), as well as increased hepatotoxicity (Takagi et al. 1983); however, the role of CYP2E1 polymorphisms in halothane hepatitis in humans has not been evaluated.

16.2.2.2. Other CYP2 Bioactivation Pathways

CYP2A6, like CYP1A2, can also activate aflatoxin and aromatic amines, as well as tobacco nitrosamines. Rapid CYP2A6 phenotype has been associated with an increased risk for colorectal cancer (Nowell et al. 2002), and the *CYP2A6*4C* genotype, in which the entire gene is deleted, has been associated with reduced lung cancer risk in smokers (Kamataki et al. 2005). The relationship between CYP2A6 and lung cancer risk is compounded by the role of this enzyme in inactivating nicotine, which appears to modulate smoking behavior in humans (Malaiyandi, Sellers and Tyndale 2005). Specifically, rapid CYP2A6 activity is associated with an increased risk of habitual smoking, and higher cigarette consumption (Tyndale and Sellers 2002).

CYP2D6 has important polymorphic variability, with approximately 30% of Caucasians expressing low-activity alleles (Bradford 2002), and about 3% of African-Americans showing very high activity due to gene duplication (Gaedigk et al. 2007). CYP2D6 also contributes to the bioactivation of nitrosamines in tobacco (Raunio et al. 1995). In some studies, extensive CYP2D6 activity has been associated with an increased risk of smoking-related lung cancer (Agundez et al. 1994; Hirvonen et al. 1993).

16.2.3. Bioactivation by the CYP3 Family

CYP3A4 has a broad substrate range for therapeutics drugs, and is the most highly expressed CYP in human liver. CYP3A4 bioactivates a number of drugs to reactive metabolites that have been associated with organ toxicity, to include the anticonvulsant carbamazepine, the anti-infective agents dapsone and isoniazid, the estrogen receptor antagonist tamoxifen, and the oral hypoglycemic agent troglitazone (Vignati et al. 2005). CYP3A4 can also bioactivate the genotoxins aflatoxin B1 and ochratoxin (Guengerich 2006; Vignati et al. 2005). Although CYP3A4 expression varies widely in human liver (Guengerich 2006; Vignati et al. 2005), the role of genetic variability in this CYP and xenobiotic toxicity remains to be established.

CYP3A5 shares some substrate specificity with CYP3A4, and also bioactivates aflatoxin, via oxidation to its genotoxic exo-8,9-epoxide. Several CYP3A5 alleles encode proteins with markedly decreased or no activity (for summary, see http://www.cypalleles.ki.se/cyp3a5.htm); accordingly, only about 20% of human livers express stable CYP3A5 protein (Daly 2006). High-activity haplotypes for CYP3A5 alleles *3, *6, and *7 have been found to correlate with higher levels of aflatoxin–albumin adducts among people in Gambia, a region with both high dietary exposure to aflatoxin and a high prevalence of hepatocellular carcinoma (Wojnowski et al. 2004).

CYP3A5, but not CYP3A4, is expressed in human esophagus (Lechevrel et al. 1999). The CYP3A5*3 allele, which leads to markedly decreased activity, is associated with a reduced risk of esophageal cancer, suggesting a role for local bioactivation of esophageal carcinogens by this enzyme (Dandara, Ballo and Parker 2005).

16.3. Other Oxidative Pathways

16.3.1. Flavin-Containing Monooxygenases

Flavin-containing monooxygenases bioactivate drugs by oxidizing a "soft" (i.e., readily oxidized) nucleophilic group (Krueger and Williams 2005), such as those containing nitrogen, sulfur, or phosphorous. FMO2, which is variably expressed in human lung, bioactivates thiourea (used in fertilizer manufacturing and other industries), and related pulmonary toxins (Henderson et al. 2004). Reactive sulfenic acids generated by FMOs lead to redox stress, and may contribute to lung damage from these compounds. No Caucasian or Asian subjects evaluated to date have been found to express functional FMO2. The absence of functional protein in the face of normal mRNA levels is explained by a premature stop codon in the coding sequence, leading to a truncated protein (Krueger et al. 2002). However, one in four African-Americans and one in 20 Hispanics do express functional FMO2 in lung, which could make these populations more susceptible to thiourea lung toxicity. This area requires further study.

FMO3, expressed primarily in liver, bioactivates the antithyroid drug methimazole (Overby, Carver and Philpot 1997), which has been associated with idiosyncratic hepatotoxicity (Woeber 2002), and contributes to the N-oxidation of the antipsychotic drug clozapine (Tugnait et al. 1997), which can lead to agranulocytosis (Iqbal et al. 2003). Pharmacogenetic variability in FMO3 has been documented in human subjects, with at least three lower-activity alleles recognized (Zhou and Shephard 2006), and a nearly 10-fold range in FMO3 expression in human liver (Overby, Carver and Philpot 1997). The relationship between this variability and drug toxicity remains to be established.

16.3.2. Peroxidases

Peroxidases, including myeloperoxidase (MPO), lactoperoxidase, and COXs, have strong oxidizing activity toward drugs and environmental chemicals. Myeloperoxidase has been the most studied, and generates reactive metabolites from many compounds. MPO oxidizes arylamine carcinogens such as 4-aminobiphenyl and PhIP to reactive hydroxylamine metabolites; lactoperoxidase can bioactivate these same carcinogens locally in breast tissue (Gorlewska-Roberts et al. 2004). While MPO polymorphisms are not yet well characterized, a promoter polymorphism (–463 G >A), which leads to decreased transcription of MPO (Piedrafita et al. 1996), has been associated with decreased risk of both breast cancer (Ahn et al. 2004) and lung cancer (Lee et al. 2002).

Myeloperoxidase appears to play a role in benzene toxicity as well. Bone marrow MPO bioactivates benzene hydroquinonone to its reactive 1,4 benzoquinone metabolite. This leads to hematologic toxicity ranging from anemia or leukopenia, to acute myelogenous leukemia (Ross et al. 1996). Accordingly, wild-type MPO (*463GG*) has been associated with depressed leukocyte cell counts in workers exposed to benzene (Lan et al. 2004). In addition, MPO bioactivates many therapeutic drugs (Rubin and Kretz-Rommel 2001; Uetrecht 1995), including the antimicrobials sulfamethoxazole, trimethoprim, and dapsone, the anticonvulsant carbamazepine, the antiarrhythmic drug procainamide, and the antithyroid agent propylthiouracil. However, the relationship between MPO polymorphisms and idiosyncratic toxicity from these drugs has not yet been evaluated.

Cyclooxygenase enzymes have both COX and hydroperoxidase catalytic sites. Both sites can bioactivate xenobiotics and lead to DNA binding (Wiese, Thompson and Kadlubar 2001). COX1 isoforms are present in most tissues, while COX2 is expressed constituitively in sites such as kidney and brain, and is inducible in other tissues during inflammation. A number of carcinogens are COX substrates, including benzidine (Zenser et al. 1983), the industrial chemical 4,4′-methylene-*bis*(2-chloroaniline (MOCA), 4-aminobiphenyl, benzo[*a*]pyrene, MeIQx, and PhIP (Wiese, Thompson and Kadlubar 2001). A high-frequency allele in the promoter region of COX-2, -1195 G > A, leads to increased gene expression, and is overrepresented among Chinese patients with esophageal cancer (Zhang et al. 2005). A 8473 T > C polymorphism in the 3′-UTR of COX2 has been associated with a decreased risk of cancer of the lung (Park et al. 2006) and prostate (Shahedi et al. 2006), but increased risk of breast (Langsenlehner et al. 2006) and lung cancer (Campa et al. 2004) in other studies. The functional consequences of this polymorphism have not yet been established. More work is needed to determine the implications of COX polymorphisms and their relationship to xenobiotic toxicity.

16.4. Conjugation Reactions

In contrast to oxidation reactions mediated by CYP and other oxidative enzymes, biotransformation by conjugation reactions more commonly leads to nontoxic metabolites. However, conjugates formed by both

N-acetyltransferases and sulfotransferases (SULTs) can in some instances undergo heterolytic cleavage to release electrophilic products such as nitrenium ions. These electrophiles can then react with DNA to form genotoxic adducts.

16.4.1. *N*-Acetyltransferases

N*N*-acetyltransferases (NAT1 and NAT2) catalyze the *N*- and *O*-acetylation of aromatic amines, aromatic hydroxylamines, and heterocyclic arylhydroxylamines. These enzymes, in particular NAT2, are polymorphically expressed, (http://www.louisville.edu/medschool/pharmacology/NAT.html) and approximately 50% of Caucasians and African-Americans have low activity for the NAT2 isozyme (Blum et al. 1991).

Both NAT1 and NAT2 can bioactivate, via *O*-acetylation, the *N*-hydroxy derivatives of 2-aminofluorene, MeIQx, and PhIP, leading to the formation of DNA adducts (Hein 1988; Hein et al. 1994; Figure 16.2). Both MeIQx and PhIP are found in meat cooked at high temperatures, and are colon carcinogens in rodents (Nishikawa et al. 2005). Rapid NAT2 phenotype or genotype is overrepresented among patients with colorectal cancer, with modulation by high CYP1A2 activity, smoking, and consumption of well-done meat (Chen, Jiang and He 2005; Hein et al. 2002; Lang et al. 1994; Le Marchand et al. 2002).

The relationship between NAT2 status and breast cancer is less well defined, with both slow and rapid NAT2 associated with breast cancer in different studies (Deitz et al. 2000; Sillanpaa et al. 2005). However, rapid NAT2 has been associated with PhIP breast adducts in women who consume well-done meat (Zhu et al. 2003). For bladder cancer, the NAT2 pathway appears to be detoxifying overall, with rapid NAT2 status associated with a lower risk of bladder tumors (reviewed in Hein 2002). This same relationship was recently found for lung cancer in European patients (Gemignani et al. 2007), although a meta-analysis found no relationship between NAT status and lung cancer (Borlak and Reamon-Buettner 2006).

As for NAT1, a high-activity allele (*NAT1*10*) leads to increased enzyme activity in human tissues (Bell et al.1995). *NAT1*10* appears to contribute to the risk of colorectal cancer (Lilla et al. 2006), and in some studies, cancers of the lung (Abdel-Rahman et al. 1998; Wikman et al. 2001), stomach (Boissy et al. 2000; Katoh et al. 2000), lymphatic system (Morton et al. 2006), and prostate (Fukutome et al. 1999; Hein et al. 2002).

16.4.2. Sulfotransferases

Cytosolic sulfotransferases mediate the sulfonation of a diverse array of xenobiotics and endogenous sterols. This most commonly leads to more polar, readily excreted molecules, but can also lead to reactive by-products, since the sulfate group can undergo cleavage to form an electrophilic cation (Glatt 2000). SULT1A1 (a phenol SULT) bioactivates arylhydroxylamines such as those generated from the tobacco carcinogen 4-aminobiphenyl,

(Chou, Lang and Kadlubar 1995) and the dietary carcinogen PhIP (Muckel, Frandsen and Glatt 2002). Despite the demonstrated role of SULT1A1 in carcinogen mutagenicity (Glatt et al. 2000), epidemiologic studies of colorectal cancer have found either no association of SULT with tumor outcome (Moreno et al. 2005; Peng et al. 2003; Tiemersma et al. 2004), or significantly decreased risk of cancer or colorectal polyps with active SULT1A1 (Bamber et al. 2001; Goode et al. 2007; Lilla et al. 2007; Nowell et al. 2002). This apparent paradox can be attributed to the dual roles of SULTs in both bioactivation and detoxification, as well as their complex roles in the modulation of sterol hormones that can contribute to carcinogenesis (Glatt and Meinl 2004).

16.5. Hydrolysis

16.5.1. Epoxide Hydrolases

Epoxide hydrolases are microsomal enzymes that mediate hydrolysis of epoxides to less-reactive dihydrodiols (Morisseau and Hammock 2005). Overall, these enzymes have a detoxifying role for most substrates. However, epoxide hydrolases can also contribute to the bioactivation of polycyclic aromatic hydrocarbons, such as benzo[*a*]pyrene and 7,12-dimethylbenz[a]anthracene (DMBA; Miyata et al. 1999; Wood et al. 1976) via the formation of unstable diol-epoxides (Morisseau and Hammock 2005). One polymorphism in exon 3 of microsomal epoxide hydrolase, 113Tyr>His, which decreases enzyme activity (Hassett et al. 1994), has been associated with a decreased risk of lung cancer (Gsur et al. 2003; Kiyohara et al. 2006; Lee et al. 2002) and colorectal cancer (Huang et al. 2005; Sachse et al. 2002). Consistent with these findings, a high-activity polymorphism in exon 4 (139 His>Arg) was associated with a possible increase risk of lung cancer (Kiyohara et al. 2006).

16.6. Summary

Xenobiotic bioactivation pathways are well characterized for many environmental carcinogens, industrial chemicals, and therapeutic drugs. Evidence for a significant relationship between altered bioactivation and toxicologic outcome is strongest for the enzymes CYP1A1, CYP1A2, CYP2E1, and the *N*-acetyltransferases (Summary: Table 16.1). The most common outcome evaluated is cancer development, although occupational chemical toxicity and its metabolic risk factors are receiving more attention. It is likely that many idiosyncratic drug reactions are due to drug bioactivation; however, there is little evidence to date to link specific polymorphisms in bioactivation pathways with these relatively rare adverse drug reactions.

Table 16.1 Examples of oxidative biotransformation pathways associated with xenobiotic bioactivation.

Enzyme	Substrates	Outcomes associated with pharmacogenetic variability
CYP1A1	Aromatic amines PAHs HCAAs 17β-estradiol	Cancers of breast, lung, and colon
CYP1A2	HCAAs	Lung and colon cancer
	Aflatoxin	Hepatocellular carcinoma
	Dihydralazine	Drug-induced hepatitis: not evaluated
CYP1B1	PAHs Estradiol	Breast cancer
CYP2E1	Tobacco *N*-nitrosamines	Breast and gastric cancer
	Industrial chemicals (styrene, benzene, butadiene, urethane, vinyl chloride)	Hepatotoxicity (vinyl chloride) Hemoglobin adducts (butadiene) Bone marrow toxicity (benzene)
	Acetaminophen, halothane, isoniazid	Drug-induced hepatopathies: not evaluated
CYP2A6	Aflatoxin	Colorectal and lung cancer
	Aromatic amines Tobacco *N*-nitrosamines	Nicotine addiction
CYP2D6	Tobacco *N*-nitrosamines	Lung cancer
CYP3A4	Carbamazepine, dapsone, isoniazid, tamoxifen, troglitazone	Drug-induced toxicities: not evaluated
	Aflatoxin, ochratoxin	Aflatoxin–albumin adducts Esophageal cancer
CYP3A5	Aflatoxin	
FMO2	Thiourea	Pulmonary toxicity: not evaluated
FMO3	Clozapine, methimazole	Liver and bone marrow toxicities: not evaluated
MPO	Aromatic amines HCAAs	Breast and lung cancer
	Benzene	Hematologic toxicity
	Sulfamethoxazole, trimethoprim, dapsone, carbamazepine, procainamide, propylthiouracil.	Drug-induced toxicities: not evaluated
COX	MCOA Aromatic amines HCAAs Benzidine	Cancers of lung, prostate, breast, and esophagus

Abbreviations: HCAAs, heterocyclic aromatic amines; PAH, polycyclic aromatic hydrocarbons

References

Abdel-Rahman, S. Z., El-Zein, R. A., Zwischenberger, J. B., and Au, W. W. 1998. Association of the NAT1*10 genotype with increased chromosome aberrations and higher lung cancer risk in cigarette smokers. Mutat.Res. 398:43–54.

Agundez, J. A., Martinez, C., Ladero, J. M., Ledesma, M. C., Ramos, J. M., Martin, R., Rodriguez, A., Jara, C., and Benítez, J. 1994. Debrisoquin oxidation genotype and susceptibility to lung cancer. Clin. Pharmacol. Ther. 55:10–14.

Ahn J., Gammon M. D., Santella R. M., Gaudet, M. M., Britton, J. A., Teitelbaum, S. L., Neugut, A. I., Josephy P. D., and Ambrosone, C. B. 2004. Myeloperoxidase genotype, fruit and vegetable consumption, and breast cancer risk. Cancer Res 64:7634–7639.

Anttila, S., Vainio, H., Hietanen, E., Camus, A.-M., Malaveille, C., Brun, G., Husgafvel-Pursiainen, K., Heikkilä, L., Karjalainen, A., and Bartsch, H. 1992. Immunohistochemical detection of pulmonary cytochrome P450IA and metabolic activities associated with P450IA1 and P450IA2 isozymes in lung cancer patients. Environ. Health. Perspect. 98:179–182.

Badawi, A. F., Stern, S. J., Lang, N. P., and Kadlubar, F. F. 1996. Cytochrome P-450 and acetyltransferase expression as biomarkers of carcinogen–DNA adduct levels and human cancer susceptibility. Prog. Clin. Biol. Res. 395:109–140.

Bae, S. Y., Choi, S. K., Kim, K. R., Park, C.-S., Lee, S.-K., Roh, H.-K., Shin, D.-W., Pie, J.-E., Woo, Z.-H., and Kang, J.-H. 2006. Effects of genetic polymorphisms of MDR1, FMO3 and CYP1A2 on susceptibility to colorectal cancer in Koreans. Cancer Sci 97:774–779.

Bailey, L. R., Roodi, N., Dupont, W. D., and Parl, F. F. 1998. Association of cytochrome P450 1B1 (CYP1B1) polymorphism with steroid receptor status in breast cancer. Cancer Res 58:5038–5041.

Bamber, D. E., Fryer, A. A., Strange, R. C., Elder, J. B., Deukin, M., Rajagopal, R., Fawole, A., Gilissen, R. A., Campbell, F. C., and Coughtrie, M. W. 2001. Phenol sulphotransferase SULT1A1*1 genotype is associated with reduced risk of colorectal cancer. 2001. Pharmacogenetics 11:679–685.

Bell, D. A., Badawi, A. F., Lang, N. P., Ilett, K. F., Kadlubar, F. F., and Hirvonen, A. 1995. Polymorphism in the *N*-acetyltransferase 1 (NAT1) polyadenylation signal: association of NAT1*10 allele with higher N-acetylation activity in bladder and colon tissue. Cancer Res 55:5226–5229.

Blum, M., Demierre, A., Grant, D. M., Heim, M., and Meyer, U. A. 1991. Molecular mechanism of slow acetylation of drugs and carcinogens in humans. Proc. Natl. Acad. Sci. USA 88:5237–5241.

Boccia, S., De Lauretis, A., Gianfagna, F., van Duijn, C. M., and Ricciardi G. 2007. CYP2E1*PstI*/*RsaI* polymorphism and interaction with tobacco, alcohol and GSTs in gastric cancer susceptibility: A meta-analysis of the literature. Carcinogenesis 28:101–106.

Boissy R. J., Watson M. A., Umbach D. M., Deakin M., Elder, J., Strange, R. C., and Bell, D. A. 2000. A pilot study investigating the role of NAT1 and NAT2 polymorphisms in gastric adenocarcinoma. Int. J. Cancer 87:507–511.

Bolt, H. M., Roos, P. H., and Their, R. 2003. The cytochrome P-450 isoenzyme CYP2E1 in the biological processing of industrial chemicals: consequences for occupational and environmental medicine. Int Arch Occup Environ Health 76:174–185.

Borlak, J., and Reamon-Buettner, S. M. 2006. *N*-acetyltransferase 2 (NAT2) gene polymorphisms in colon and lung cancer patients. BMC Med. Genet. 7:58.

Bourdi, M., Chen, W., Peter, R. M., Martin, J. L., Buters, J. T. M., Nelson, S. D., and Pohl, L. R. 1996. Human cytochrome P450 2E1 is a major autoantigen associated with halothane hepatitis. Chem. Res. Toxicol. 9:1159–1166.

Bourdi, M., Gautier, J. C., Mircheva, J., Larrey, D., Guillouzo, A., Andre, C., Belloc, C., and Beaune, P. H. 1992. Anti-liver microsomes autoantibodies and dihydralazine-induced hepatitis: specificity of autoantibodies and inductive capacity of the drug. Mol. Pharmacol. 42:280–285.

Bourdi, M., Larrey, D., Nataf, J., Bernuau, J., Pessayre, D., Iwasaki, M., Guengerich, F. P., and Beaune, P. H. 1990. Anti-liver endoplasmic reticulum

autoantibodies are directed against human cytochrome P-450IA2. A specific marker of dihydralazine-induced hepatitis. J. Clin. Invest. 85:1967–1973.
Bourdi, M., Tinel, M., Beaune, P. H., and Pessayre, D. 1994. Interactions of dihydralazine with cytochromes P4501A: a possible explanation for the appearance of anti-cytochrome P4501A2 autoantibodies. Mol. Pharmacol. 45: 1287–1295.
Boyapati, S. M., Shu, X. O., Gao, Y. T., Cai, Q., Jin, F., and Zheng, W. 2005. Polymorphisms in CYP1A1 and breast carcinoma risk in a population-based case–control study of Chinese women. Cancer 103:2228–2235.
Bradford L. D. 2002. CYP2D6 allele frequency in European Caucasians, Asians, Africans and their descendants. Pharmacogenomics 3:229–243.
Butler M. A., Iwasaki M., Guengerich F. P., and Kadlubar F. F. 1989. Human cytochrome P-450 PA (P-450IA2),·the phenacetin *O*-deethylase, is primarily responsible for the hepatic 3-demethylation of caffeine and N-oxidation of carcinogenic arylamines. Proc Natl Acad Sci USA 86:7696–7700.
Campa D., Zienolddiny S., Maggini V., Skaug, V., Haugen, A., and Canzian, F. 2004. Association of a common polymorphism in the cyclooxygenase 2 gene with risk of non-small cell lung cancer. Carcinogenesis 25:229–235.
Chen, K., Jiang, Q. T.and He, H. Q. 2005. Relationship between metabolic enzyme polymorphism and colorectal cancer. World J. Gastroenterol. 11:331–335.
Chen, X., Wang, H., Xie, W., Liang R., Wei, Z., Zhi, L., Zhang, X., Hao, B., Zhong, S., Zhou, G., Zhang, L., Gao, X., Zhu, Y., He, F. 2006. Association of CYP1A2 genetic polymorphisms with hepatocellular carcinoma susceptibility: a case–control study in a high-risk region of China. Pharmacogenet Genomics 16:219–227.
Cheung, Y. L., Puddicombe, S. M., Gray, T. J., and Ioannides, C. 1994. Mutagenicity and CYP1A induction by azobenzenes correlates with their carcinogenicity. Carcinogenesis 15:1257–1263.
Chou, H. C., Lang, N. P., and Kadlubar, F. F. 1995. Metabolic activation of the *N*-hydroxy derivative of the carcinogen 4-aminobiphenyl by human tissue sulfotransferases. Carcinogenesis 16:413–417.
Crofts, F., Taioli, E., Trachman, J., Cosma, G. N., Currie, D., Toriolo, P., and Garte, S. J. 1994. Functional significance of different human CYP1A1 genotypes. Carcinogenesis 15:2961–2963.
Crooke, P. S., Ritchie, M. D., Hachey, D. L., Dawling, S., Roodi, N., and Parl, F. F. 2006. Estrogens, enzyme variants, and breast cancer: a risk model. Cancer Epidemiol. Biomarkers Prev. 15:1620–1629.
Daly, A. K. 2006. Significance of the minor cytochrome P450 3A isoforms. Clin. Pharmacokinet. 45:13–31.
Dandara, C., Ballo, R., and Parker, M. I. 2005. CYP3A5 genotypes and risk of oesophageal cancer in two South African populations. Cancer Lett. 225:275–282.
De Vivo, I., Hankinson, S. E., Li, L., Colditz, G. A., and Hunter, D. J. 2002. Association of CYP1B1 polymorphisms and breast cancer risk. Cancer Epidemiol. Biomarkers Prev. 11:489–492.
Deitz, A. C., Zheng, W., Leff, M. A., Gross, M., Wen, W.-Q., Doll, M. A., Xiao, G. H., Folson, A. R., and Hein, D. W. 2000. *N*-Acetyltransferase-2 genetic polymorphism, well-done meat intake, and breast cancer risk among postmenopausal women. Cancer Epidemiol. Biomarkers Prev. 9:905–910.
Duescher, R. J., and Elfarra, A. A. 1994. Human liver microsomes are efficient catalysts of 1,3-butadiene oxidation: evidence for major roles by cytochromes P450 2A6 and 2E1. Arch. Biochem. Biophys. 311:342–349.
El-Zein, R. A., Zwischenberger, J. B., Abdel-Rahman, S. Z., Sankar, A. B., and Au, W. W. 1997. Polymorphism of metabolizing genes and lung cancer histology: prevalence of CYP2E1 in adenocarcinoma. Cancer Lett. 112:71–78.

Elfarra, A. A., Krause, R. J., and Selzer, R. R. 1996. Biochemistry of 1,3-butadiene metabolism and its relevance to 1,3-butadiene-induced carcinogenicity. Toxicology 113:23–30.

Eliasson, E., Gardner, I., Hume-Smith, H., de Waziers, I., Beaune, P., Kenna, J. G. 1998. Interindividual variability in P450-dependent generation of neoantigens in halothane hepatitis. Chem. Biol. Interact. 116:123–141.

Fairbrother, K. S., Grove, J., de Waziers, I., Steimel, D. T., Day, C. P., Crespi, C. L., and Daly, A. K. 1998. Detection and characterization of novel polymorphisms in the CYP2E1 gene. Pharmacogenetics 8:543–552.

Fukutome, K., Watanabe, M., Shiraishi, T., Murata, M., Uemura, H., Kubota, Y., Kawamura, J., Ho, H., Yatani, R. 1999. *N*-acetyltransferase 1 genetic polymorphism influences the risk of prostate cancer development. Cancer Lett. 136:83–87.

Fustinoni, S., Soleo, L., Warholm, M., Begemann, P., Rannug, A., Neumann H.-G., Swenberg, J. A., Vimercati, L., Foà, V., and Colombi, A. 2002. Influence of metabolic genotypes on biomarkers of exposure to 1,3-butadiene in humans. Cancer Epidemiol. Biomarkers Prev. 11:1082–1090.

Gaedigk, A., Ndjountche, L., Divakaran, K., Bradford, D., Zineh, I., Oberlander, T. F., Brousseau, D. C., McCarver, D. G., Johnson, J. A., Alander, S. W., Wayne Riggs, K., and Seven Leeder J. 2007. Cytochrome P4502D6 (CYP2D6) gene locus heterogeneity: characterization of gene duplication events. Clin. Pharmacol. Ther. 81:242–251.

Gallagher, E. P., Kunze, K. L., Stapleton, P. L., and Eaton, D. L. 1996. The kinetics of aflatoxin B1 oxidation by human cDNA-expressed and human liver microsomal cytochromes P450 1A2 and 3A4. Toxicol. Appl. Pharmacol. 141:595–606.

Gallagher, E. P., Wienkers, L. C., Stapleton, P. L., Kunze, K. L., and Eaton, D. L. 1994. Role of human microsomal and human complementary DNA-expressed cytochromes P4501A2 and P4503A4 in the bioactivation of aflatoxin B1. Cancer Res 54:101–108.

Gemignani, F., Landi, S., Szeszenia-Dabrowska, N., Zaridze, D., Lissowska J., Rudnai, P., Fabianova E., Mates, D., Foretova, L., Janout, V., Bencko, V., Gaborieau, V., Gioia-Patricola, L., Bellini, I., Barale, R., Canzian, F., Hall, J., Boffetta, P., Hung, R. J., and Brennan, P. 2007. Development of lung cancer before the age of 50: the role of xenobiotic metabolism genes. Carcinogenesis 28:1287–1293.

Glatt, H. 2000. Sulfotransferases in the bioactivation of xenobiotics. Chem. Biol. Interact. 129:141–170.

Glatt, H., Engelke, C. E., Pabel, U., Teubner, W., Jones, A. L., Coughtrie, M. W., Andrae, U., Falanay, C. N., and Meinl, W. 2000. Sulfotransferases: genetics and role in toxicology. Toxicol. Lett. 112–113:341–348.

Glatt, H., and Meinl, W. 2004. Pharmacogenetics of soluble sulfotransferases (SULTs). Naunyn Schmiedebergs Arch. Pharmacol. 369:55–68.

Goode, E. L., Potter, J. D., Bamlet, W. R., Rider, D. N., and Bigler, J. 2007. Inherited variation in carcinogen-metabolizing enzymes and risk of colorectal polyps. Carcinogenesis 28:328–341.

Gorlewska-Roberts, K. M., Teitel, C. H., Lay, J. O., Jr.,Roberts, D. W., and Kadlubar, F. F. 2004. Lactoperoxidase-catalyzed activation of carcinogenic aromatic and heterocyclic amines. Chem. Res. Toxicol. 17:1659–1666.

Gsur, A., Zidek, T., Schnattinger, K., Feik, E., Haidinger, G., Hollaus, P., Mohn-Staudner, A., Armbruster, C., Madersbacher, S., Schatzl, G., Trieb, K., Vutuc, C., and Micksche, M. 2003. Association of microsomal epoxide hydrolase polymorphisms and lung cancer risk. Br. J. Cancer 89:702–706.

Guengerich F. P. 2006. Cytochrome P450 s and other enzymes in drug metabolism and toxicity. 2 AAPS J. 8:E101–111.

Hassett, C., Aicher, L., Sidhu, J. S., and Omieclnskl, C. J. 1994. Human microsomal epoxide hydrolase: genetic polymorphism and functional expression in vitro of amino acid variants. Hum. Mol. Genet. 3:421–428.
Hayashi, S., Watanabe, J., and Kawajiri, K. 1991. Genetic polymorphisms in the 5'-flanking region change transcriptional regulation of the human cytochrome P450IIE1 gene. J. Biochem. (Tokyo) 110:559–565.
Hein, D. W. 1988. Acetylator genotype and arylamine-induced carcinogenesis. Biochim. Biophys. Acta 948:37–66.
Hein, D. W. 2002. Molecular genetics and function of NAT1 and NAT2: role in aromatic amine metabolism and carcinogenesis. Mutat. Res. 506–507:65–77.
Hein, D. W., Leff, M. A., Ishibe, N., Sinha, R., Frazier, H. A., Doll, M. A., Xiao, G. H., Weinrich, M. C., Caporaso, N. E. 2002. Association of prostate cancer with rapid *N*-acetyltransferase 1 (NAT1*10) in combination with slow *N*-acetyltransferase 2 acetylator genotypes in a pilot case–control study. Environ. Mol. Mutagen. 40:161–167.
Hein, D. W., Rustan, T. D., Ferguson, R. J., Doll, M. A., and Gray, K. 1994. Metabolic activation of aromatic and heterocyclic *N*-hydroxyarylamines by wild-type and mutant recombinant human NAT1 and NAT2 acetyltransferases. Arch. Toxicol. 68:129–133.
Hellmold, H., Rylander, T., Magnusson, M., Reihnér, E., Warner, M., and Gustafsson, J.-A. 1998. Characterization of cytochrome P450 enzymes in human breast tissue from reduction mammaplasties. J. Clin. Endocrinol. Metab. 83:886–895.
Henderson, M. C., Krueger, S. K., Stevens, J. F., and Williams, D. E. 2004. Human flavin-containing monooxygenase form 2 S-oxygenation: sulfenic acid formation from thioureas and oxidation of glutathione. Chem. Res. Toxicol. 17:633–640.
Hirvonen, A., Husgafvel-Pursiainen, K., Anttila, S., Karjalainen, A., and Vainio, H. 1993. Polymorphism in CYP1A1 and CYP2D6 genes: possible association with susceptibility to lung cancer. Environ. Health Perspect. 101 Suppl 3:109–112.
Hu, Y., Oscarson, M., Johansson, I., Yue, Q.-Y., Dahl, M.-L., Tabone, M., Arincò, S., Albano, E., and Ingelman-Sundberg, M. 1997. Genetic polymorphism of human CYP2E1: characterization of two variant alleles. Mol. Pharmacol. 51:370–376.
Huang, W. Y., Chatterjee, N., Chanock, S., Dean, M., Yeager, M., Schoen, R. E., Hou, L. F., Berndt, S. I., Yadavalli, S., Johnson, C. C., and Hayes, R. B. 2005. Microsomal epoxide hydrolase polymorphisms and risk for advanced colorectal adenoma. Cancer Epidemiol. Biomarkers Prev. 14:152–157.
Ioannides, C., and Lewis, D. F. 2004. Cytochromes P450 in the bioactivation of chemicals. Curr. Top. Med. Chem. 4:1767–1788.
Iqbal, M. M., Rahman, A., Husain, Z., Mahmud, S. Z., Ryan, W. G., and Feldman, J. M. 2003. Clozapine: a clinical review of adverse effects and management. Ann. Clin. Psychiatry 15:33–48.
Jefcoate, C. R., Liehr, J. G., Santen, R. J., Sutter, T. R., Yager, J. D., Yue, W., Santer, S. J., Tekmal, R., Demers, L., Pauley, R., Naftolin, F., Mor, G., and Berstein, L. 2000. Tissue-specific synthesis and oxidative metabolism of estrogens. J. Natl. Cancer Inst. Monogr. 27:95–112.
Kamataki, T., Fujieda, M., Kiyotani, K., Iwano S., and Kunitoh, H. 2005. Genetic polymorphism of CYP2A6 as one of the potential determinants of tobacco-related cancer risk. Biochem. Biophys. Res. Commun. 338:306–310.
Katoh, T., Boissy, R., Nagata, N., Kitagawa, K., Kuroda, Y., Itoh, H., Kawamoto, T., and Bell, D. A. 2000. Inherited polymorphism in the *N*-acetyltransferase 1 (NAT1) and 2 (NAT2) genes and susceptibility to gastric and colorectal adenocarcinoma. Int. J. Cancer 85:46–49.

Kawajiri, K., Nakachi, K., Imai, K., Hayashi, S., and Watanabe, J. 1990. Individual differences in lung cancer susceptibility in relation to polymorphisms of P-450IA1 gene and cigarette dose. Princess Takamatsu Symp 21:55–61.
Kenna, J. G., Satoh, H., Christ, D. D., and Pohl, L. R. 1988. Metabolic basis for a drug hypersensitivity: antibodies in sera from patients with halothane hepatitis recognize liver neoantigens that contain the trifluoroacetyl group derived from halothane. J. Pharmacol. Exp. Ther. 245:1103–1109.
Kiyohara, C., Yoshimasu, K., Takayama, K., Nakanishi, Y. 2006. EPHX1 polymorphisms and the risk of lung cancer: a HuGE review. Epidemiology 17:89–99.
Krueger, S. K., Martin, S. R., Yueh, M. F., Pereira, C. B., and Williams, D. E. 2002. Identification of active flavin-containing monooxygenase isoform 2 in human lung and characterization of expressed protein. Drug Metab. Dispos. 30:34–41.
Krueger, S. K.,and Williams, D. E. 2005. Mammalian flavin-containing monooxygenases: structure/function, genetic polymorphisms and role in drug metabolism. Pharmacol. Ther. 106:357–387.
Lan, Q., Zhang, L., Li, G., Vermeulen, R., Weinberg, R. S., Dosemeci, M., Rappaport, S. M., Shen, M., Alter, B. P., Wu, Y., Koop, W., Waidyanatha, S., Rabkin, C., Guo, W., Chanock, S., Hayes, R. B., Linet, M., Kim, S., Yin, S., Rothman, N., and Smith, M. T. 2004. Hematotoxicity in workers exposed to low levels of benzene. Science 306:1774–1776.
Lang, N. P., Butler, M. A., Massengill, J., Lawson, M., Stotts, R. C., Hauer-Jensen, M., and Kadlubar, F. F. 1994. Rapid metabolic phenotypes for acetyltransferase and cytochrome P4501A2 and putative exposure to food-borne heterocyclic amines increase the risk for colorectal cancer or polyps. Cancer Epidemiol. Biomarkers Prev. 3:675–682.
Langsenlehner, U., Yazdani-Biuki, B., Eder, T., Renner, W., Wascher, T. C., Paulweber, B., Weitzer, W., Samonigg, H., and Krippl, P. 2006. The cyclooxygenase-2 (PTGS2) 8473T>C polymorphism is associated with breast cancer risk. Clin. Cancer Res. 12:1392–1394.
Le Marchand, L., Donlon, T., Kolonel, L. N., Henderson, B. E., and Wilkens, L. R. 2005. Estrogen metabolism-related genes and breast cancer risk: the multiethnic cohort study. Cancer Epidemiol. Biomarkers Prev. 14:1998–2003.
Le Marchand, L., Hankin, J. H., Pierce, L. M., Sinha, R., Nerurkar, P. V., Franke, A. A., Wilkens, L. R., Kolonel, L. N., Donlon, T., Seifried, A., Custer, L. J., Lum-Jones, A., and Chang, W. 2002. Well-done red meat, metabolic phenotypes and colorectal cancer in Hawaii. Mutat. Res. 506–507:205–214.
Le Marchand, L., Wilkinson, G. R., and Wilkens L. R. 1999. Genetic and dietary predictors of CYP2E1 activity: a phenotyping study in Hawaii Japanese using chlorzoxazone. Cancer Epidemiol. Biomarkers Prev. 8:495–500.
Lechevrel, M., Casson, A. G., Wolf, C. R., Hardie, L. J., Flinterman, M. B., Montesano, R., and Wild, C. R. 1999. Characterization of cytochrome P450 expression in human oesophageal mucosa. Carcinogenesis 20:243–248.
Lee, W. J., Brennan, P., Boffetta, P., London, S. J., Benhamous, S., Rannug, A., To-Figueras, J., Ingelman-Sundberg, M., Shields, P., Gaspari, L., and Taioli, E. 2002. Microsomal epoxide hydrolase polymorphisms and lung cancer risk: a quantitative review. Biomarkers 7:230–241.
Li, D. N., Seidel, A., Pritchard, M. P., Wolf, C. R., and Friedberg, T. 2000. Polymorphisms in P450 CYP1B1 affect the conversion of estradiol to the potentially carcinogenic metabolite 4-hydroxyestradiol. Pharmacogenetics 10:343–353.
Lilla, C., Risch, A., Verla-Tebit, E., Hoffmeister, M., Brenner, H., and Chang-Claude, J. 2007. SULT1A1 genotype and susceptibility to colorectal cancer. Int. J. Cancer 120:201–206.
Lilla, C., Verla-Tebit, E., Risch, A., Jäger, B., Hoffmeister, M., Brenner, H., Chang-Claude, J. 2006. Effect of NAT1 and NAT2 genetic polymorphisms on

colorectal cancer risk associated with exposure to tobacco smoke and meat consumption. Cancer Epidemiol. Biomarkers Prev. 15:99–107.
Malaiyandi, V., Sellers, E. M., and Tyndale, R. F. 2005. Implications of CYP2A6 genetic variation for smoking behaviors and nicotine dependence. Clin. Pharmacol. Ther. 77:145–158.
Miyata, M., Kudo, G., Lee, Y. H., Yang, T. J., Gelboin, H. V., Fernandez-Salguero, P., Kimura, S., and Gonzalez, F. J. 1999. Targeted disruption of the microsomal epoxide hydrolase gene. Microsomal epoxide hydrolase is required for the carcinogenic activity of 7,12-dimethylbenz[a]anthracene. J. Biol. Chem. 274:23963–23968.
Moreno, V., Glatt, H., Guino, E., Fisher E., Meinl, W., Navarro, M., Badosa, J. M., Boeing, H., Bellvitge Colorectal Cancer Study Group. 2005. Polymorphisms in sulfotransferases SULT1A1 and SULT1A2 are not related to colorectal cancer. Int. J. Cancer 113:683–686.
Morisseau, C., and Hammock, B. D. 2005. Epoxide hydrolases: mechanisms, inhibitor designs, and biological roles. Annu. Rev. Pharmacol. Toxicol. 45:311–333.
Morton, L. M., Schenk, M., Hein, D. W., Davis, S., Zahm, S. H., Cozen, W., Cerhan, J. R., Hartge, P., Welch, R., Chanock, S. J., Rothman, N, and Wang, S. S. 2006. Genetic variation in *N*-acetyltransferase 1 (NAT1) and 2 (NAT2) and risk of non-Hodgkin lymphoma. Pharmacogenet. Genomics 16:537–545.
Muckel E., Frandsen H., and Glatt H. R. 2002. Heterologous expression of human *N*-acetyltransferases 1 and 2 and sulfotransferase 1A1 in *Salmonella typhimurium* for mutagenicity testing of heterocyclic amines. Food Chem. Toxicol. 40:1063–1068.
Murtaugh, M. A., Sweeney, C., Ma, K. N., Caan, B. J., and Slattery, M. L. 2005. The CYP1A1 genotype may alter the association of meat consumption patterns and preparation with the risk of colorectal cancer in men and women. J. Nutr. 135:179–186.
Nakachi, K., Imai, K., Hayashi, S., Watanabe, J., and Kawajiri, K. 1991. Genetic susceptibility to squamous cell carcinoma of the lung in relation to cigarette smoking dose. Cancer Res. 51:5177–5180.
Nishikawa, A., Imazawa, T., Kuroiwa, Y., Kitamura, Y., Kannki, K., Ishii, Y., Umemura, T., and Hirose, M. 2005. Induction of colon tumors in C57BL/6 J mice fed MeIQx, IQ, or PhIP followed by dextran sulfate sodium treatment. Toxicol. Sci. 84:243–248.
Nowell, S., Coles, B., Sinha, R., MacLeod, S., Ratnasinghe, D. L., Stotts, C., Kadlubar, F. F., Ambrosone, C. B., and Lang, N. P. 2002. Analysis of total meat intake and exposure to individual heterocyclic amines in a case–control study of colorectal cancer: contribution of metabolic variation to risk. Mutat. Res.506–507:175–185.
Okobia, M., Bunker, C., Zmuda, J., Kammerer, C., Vogel, V., Uche, E., Anyanwu, S., Ezeome, E., Ferrell, R., and Kuller, L. 2005. Cytochrome P4501A1 genetic polymorphisms and breast cancer risk in Nigerian women. Breast Cancer Res. Treat. 94:285–293.
Overby, L. H., Carver, G. C., and Philpot, R. M. 1997. Quantitation and kinetic properties of hepatic microsomal and recombinant flavin-containing monooxygenases 3 and 5 from humans. Chem. Biol. Interact. 106:29–45.
Park, J. M., Choi, J. E., Chae, M. H., Lee W. K., Cha, S. I., Son, J.-W., Kim, C. H., Kam, S., Kang, Y. M., Jung, T. H., and Park, J. Y. 2006. Relationship between cyclooxygenase 8473T>C polymorphism and the risk of lung cancer: a case–control study. BMC Cancer 6:70.
Pavanello, S., Pulliero, A., Lupi, S., and Gregorio, P. 2005. Influence of the genetic polymorphism in the 5'-noncoding region of the CYP1A2 gene on CYP1A2 phenotype and urinary mutagenicity in smokers. Mutat. Res. 587:59–66.
Peng, C. T., Chen, J. C., Yeh, K. T., Wang, Y. F., Hou, M. F., Lee, T. P., Shih, M. C., and Chang, J. Y., and Chang, J. G. 2003. The relationship among the

polymorphisms of SULT1A1, 1A2 and different types of cancers in Taiwanese. Int. J. Mol. Med. 11:85–89.

Petersen, D. D., McKinney, C. E., Ikeya, K., Smith, H. H., Bale, A. E., McBride, O. W., Nebert, D. W. 1991. Human CYP1A1 gene: cosegregation of the enzyme inducibility phenotype and an RFLP. Am. J. Hum. Genet. 48:720–725.

Piedrafita, F. J., Molander, R. B., Vansant, G., Orlova, E. A., Pfahl, M., and Reynolds, W. F. 1996. An Alu element in the myeloperoxidase promoter contains a composite SP1-thyroid hormone-retinoic acid response element. J Biol Chem 271:14412–14420.

Pirmohamed, M. 2006. Genetic factors in the predisposition to drug-induced hypersensitivity reactions. AAPS J. 8:E20–26.

Raunio, H., Husgafvel-Pursiainen, K., Anttila, S., Hietanen, E., Hirvonen, A., and Pelkonen, O. 1995. Diagnosis of polymorphisms in carcinogen-activating and -inactivating enzymes and cancer susceptibility–a review. Gene 159:113–121.

Roberts, B. J., Song, B. J., Soh, Y., Park, S. S., and Shoaf, S. E. 1995. Ethanol induces CYP2E1 by protein stabilization. Role of ubiquitin conjugation in the rapid degradation of CYP2E1. J. Biol. Chem. 270:29632–29635.

Ross, D., Siegel, D., Schattenberg, D. G., Sun, X.-M., and Moran, J. L. 1996. Cell-specific activation and detoxification of benzene metabolites in mouse and human bone marrow: identification of target cells and a potential role for modulation of apoptosis in benzene toxicity. Environ. Health. Perspect. 104 Suppl 6:1177–1182.

Rubin, R. L., and Kretz-Rommel, A. 2001. Phagocyte-mediated oxidation in idiosyncratic adverse drug reactions. Curr. Opin. Hematol. 8:34–40.

Rylander-Rudqvist, T., Wedren, S., Granath, F., Humphreys K., Ahlberg, S., Weiderpass, E., Oscarson, M., Ingelman-Sundberg, M., and Persson, I. 2003. Cytochrome P450 1B1 gene polymorphisms and postmenopausal breast cancer risk. Carcinogenesis 24:1533–1539.

Sachse, C., Smith, G., Wilkie, M. J., Barrett, J. H., Waxman, R., Sullivan F., Forman, D., Bishop, D. T., Wolf, C. R., and the Colorectal Cancer Study Group. 2002. A pharmacogenetic study to investigate the role of dietary carcinogens in the etiology of colorectal cancer. Carcinogenesis 23:1839–1849.

Seow, A., Zhao, B., Lee, E. J., Poh, W.-T., Teh, M., Eng, P., Wang, Y.-T., Tan, W.-C., and Lee, H.-P. 2001. Cytochrome P4501A2 (CYP1A2) activity and lung cancer risk: a preliminary study among Chinese women in Singapore. Carcinogenesis 22:673–677.

Shahedi K., Lindstrom S., Zheng S. L., Wiklund, F., Adolfsson, J., Sun, J., Augustsson-Bälter, K., Chang, B. L., Adami, H. O., Liu, W., Grönberg, H., and Xu, J. 2006. Genetic variation in the COX-2 gene and the association with prostate cancer risk. Int. J. Cancer 119:668–672.

Shen, Y., Li, D. K., Wu, J., Zhang, Z., and Gao, E. 2006. Joint effects of the CYP1A1 MspI, ERalpha PvuII, and ERalpha XbaI polymorphisms on the risk of breast cancer: results from a population-based case–control study in Shanghai, China. Cancer Epidemiol. Biomarkers Prev. 15:342–347.

Shimada, T., Watanabe, J., Kawajiri, K., Sutter, T. R., Guengeruch, F. P., Gillam, E. M. J., and Inoue, K. 1999. Catalytic properties of polymorphic human cytochrome P450 1B1 variants. Carcinogenesis 20:1607–1613.

Sillanpaa, P., Heikinheimo, L., Kataja, V., Eskelinen, M., Kosma, V. M., Uusitupa, M., Vainio, H., Metsola, K., Hirvonen, A. 2006. CYP1A1 and CYP1B1 genetic polymorphisms, smoking and breast cancer risk in a Finnish Caucasian population. Breast Cancer Res. Treat. 104:287–297.

Sillanpaa, P., Hirvonen, A., Kataja, V., Eskelinen, M., Kosma, V. M., Uusitupa, M., Vainio, H., Mitrunen, K. 2005. NAT2 slow acetylator genotype as an important modifier of breast cancer risk. Int. J. Cancer 114:579–584.

Singh, V., Rastogi, N., Sinha, A., Kumar, A., Mathur, N., and Singh, M. P. 2007. A study on the association of cytochrome-P450 1A1 polymorphism and breast cancer risk in North Indian women. 2007. Breast Cancer Res. Treat. 101:73–81.

Spracklin, D. K., Hankins, D. C., Fisher, J. M., Kumar, A., Mathur, N., and Singh, M. P. 1997. Cytochrome P450 2E1 is the principal catalyst of human oxidative halothane metabolism in vitro. J. Pharmacol. Exp. Ther. 281:400–411.

Takagi, T., Ishii, H., Takahashi, H., Kato, S., Okuno, F., Ebihara, Y., Yamauchi, H., Nagata, S., Tashiro, M., Tsuchiya, M. 1983. Potentiation of halothane hepatotoxicity by chronic ethanol administration in rat: an animal model of halothane hepatitis. Pharmacol. Biochem. Behav. 18 Suppl 1:461–465.

Tiemersma, E. W., Voskuil, D. W., Bunschoten, A., Hogendoorn, E. A., Witteman, B. J. M., Nagengast, F. M., Glatt, H., Kok, F. J., and Kampman, E. 2004. Risk of colorectal adenomas in relation to meat consumption, meat preparation, and genetic susceptibility in a Dutch population. Cancer Causes Control 15:225–236.

Tugnait, M., Hawes, E. M., McKay, G., Rettie, A. E., Haining, R. L., and Midha, K. K. 1997. N-oxygenation of clozapine by flavin-containing monooxygenase. Drug Metab. Dispos. 25:524–527.

Turesky, R., Guengerich, F., Guillouzo, A., and Langouet, S. 2002. Metabolism of heterocyclic aromatic amines by human hepatocytes and cytochrome P4501A2. Mutat. Res. 506–507:187–195.

Turesky, R. J., Constable, A., Richoz, J., Varga, N., Markovic, J., Martin, M. V., and Guengerich, F. P. 1998. Activation of heterocyclic aromatic amines by rat and human liver microsomes and by purified rat and human cytochrome P450 1A2. Chem. Res. Toxicol. 11:925–936.

Turesky, R. J., and Vouros, P. 2004. Formation and analysis of heterocyclic aromatic amine–DNA adducts in vitro and in vivo. J. Chromatogr. B Analyt. Technol. Biomed. Life Sci. 802:155–166.

Tyndale, R. F., and Sellers, E. M. 2002. Genetic variation in CYP2A6-mediated nicotine metabolism alters smoking behavior. Ther. Drug Monit. 24:163–171.

Uetrecht, J. P. 1995. Myeloperoxidase as a generator of drug free radicals. Biochem. Soc. Symp. 61:163–170.

Vignati, L., Turlizzi, E., Monaci, S., Grossi, P., de Kanter, R., and Monshouwer, M. 2005. An in vitro approach to detect metabolite toxicity due to CYP3A4-dependent bioactivation of xenobiotics. Toxicology 216:154–167.

Wan, J., Shi, J., Hui, L., Wu, D., Jin, X., Zhao, N., Huang, W., Xia, Z., and Hu, G. 2002. Association of genetic polymorphisms in CYP2E1, MPO, NQO1, GSTM1, and GSTT1 genes with benzene poisoning. Environ. Health Perspect. 110:1213–1218.

Wiese, F. W., Thompson, P. A., and Kadlubar, F. F. 2001. Carcinogen substrate specificity of human COX-1 and COX-2. Carcinogenesis 22:5–10.

Wikman, H., Thiel, S., Jager, B., Schmezer, P., Spiegelhalder, B., Edler, L., Dienemann, H., Kayser, K., Schulz V., Drings, P., Bartsch, H., and Risch, A. 2001. Relevance of *N*-acetyltransferase 1 and 2 (NAT1, NAT2) genetic polymorphisms in non-small cell lung cancer susceptibility. Pharmacogenetics 11:157–168.

Williams, J. A., Stone, E. M., Millar, B. C., Gusterson, B. A., Grover, P. L., and Phillips, D. H. 1998. Determination of the enzymes responsible for activation of the heterocyclic amine 2-amino-3-methylimidazo[4,5-f]quinoline in the human breast. Pharmacogenetics 8:519–528.

Woeber, K. A. 2002. Methimazole-induced hepatotoxicity. Endocr. Pract. 8:222–224.

Wojnowski, L. Turner, P. C., Pedersen B., Hustert, E., Bruckmöller, J., Mendy, M., Whittle, H. C., Kirk, G., Wild, C. P. 2004. Increased levels of aflatoxin–albumin adducts are associated with CYP3A5 polymorphisms in The Gambia, West Africa. Pharmacogenetics 14:691–700.

Wong, R. H., Du, C. L., Wang, J. D., Chan, C.-C., Luo, J.-C. J., and Cheng, T.-J. 2002. XRCC1 and CYP2E1 polymorphisms as susceptibility factors of plasma mutant p53 protein and anti-p53 antibody expression in vinyl chloride monomer-exposed polyvinyl chloride workers. Cancer Epidemiol. Biomarkers Prev. 11:475–482.

Wood, A. W., Levin, W., Lu, A. Y., Yagi, H., Hernandez, O., Jerina, D. M., Conney, A. H. 1976. Metabolism of benzo(a)pyrene and benzo (a)pyrene derivatives to mutagenic products by highly purified hepatic microsomal enzymes. J. Biol. Chem. 251:4882–4890.

Yu, M. C., and Yuan, J. M. 2004. Environmental factors and risk for hepatocellular carcinoma. Gastroenterology 127:S72–78.

Zenser, T. V., Mattammal, M. B., Wise, R. W., Rice, J. R., and Davis, B. B. 1983. Prostaglandin H synthase-catalyzed activation of benzidine: a model to assess pharmacologic intervention of the initiation of chemical carcinogenesis. J. Pharmacol. Exp. Ther. 227:545–550.

Zhang, X., Miao, X., Tan, W., Ning, B., Liu, Z., Hong, Y., Song, W., Guo, Y., Zhang, X., and Shen, Y. 2005. Identification of functional genetic variants in cyclooxygenase-2 and their association with risk of esophageal cancer. Gastroenterology 129:565–576.

Zhou, J., and Shephard, E. A. 2006. Mutation, polymorphism and perspectives for the future of human flavin-containing monooxygenase 3. Mutat. Res. 612:165–171.

Zhu, J., Chang, P., Bondy, M. L., Sahin, A. A., Singletary, S. E., Takahashi, S., Shirai, T., Li, D. 2003. Detection of 2-amino-1-methyl-6-phenylimidazo[4,5-b]-pyridine-DNA adducts in normal breast tissues and risk of breast cancer. Cancer Epidemiol. Biomarkers Prev. 12:830–837.

Zhu, K., Hunter, S., Payne-Wilks, K., Sutclife, C., Bentley, C., Roland, C. L., and Williams, S. M. 2006. Potential differences in breast cancer risk factors based on CYP1A1 *Msp*I and African-American-specific genotypes. Ethn. Dis. 16:207–215.

Zhu S.-M., Ren X.-F., Wan J.-X., and Xia, Z.-L. 2005. Evaluation in vinyl chloride monomer-exposed workers and the relationship between liver lesions and gene polymorphisms of metabolic enzymes. World J. Gastroenterol. 11:5821–5827.

17

Human Phenanthrene Metabolites as Probes for the Metabolic Activation and Detoxification of Carcinogenic Polycyclic Aromatic Hydrocarbons

Stephen S. Hecht

The Cancer Center, University of Minnesota, 420 Delaware Street SE – MMC 806, Minneapolis, MN 55455, USA

e-mail: hecht002@umn.edu

Keywords: Lung Cancer Risk · Individual Differences in PAH Metabolism · Genetic Polymorphism

17.1. Introduction

In 1915, Yamagiwa and Ichikawa demonstrated that repeated application of coal tar to the ears of rabbits produced tumors, providing experimental support for observations in the nineteenth century and earlier that occupational exposure to coal tar and related materials was associated with skin cancer. The classic fractionation studies of Kennaway, Cook, and others in London then established that polycyclic aromatic hydrocarbons (PAHs), fluorescent products of incomplete combustion, were the responsible agents. This led to the synthesis and characterization of a number of these compounds and, in 1930, dibenz[*a,h*]anthracene was shown to induce tumors locally by repeated application to mouse skin, the first example of tumor induction by a pure chemical. Following this, many PAHs were synthesized and tested for carcinogenicity. The structures of some PAHs and their carcinogenic activities are summarized in Figure 17.1.

Considerable evidence supports a major role for PAHs as causes of lung cancer in smokers (Hecht 1999; Hecht 2003; Pfeifer et al. 2002). Carcinogenic PAH in cigarette smoke include BaP, benz[*a*]anthracene, methylchrysenes, benzofluoranthenes, indeno[1,2,3-*cd*]pyrene, dibenz[*a,h*]anthracene, and others, with concentrations in mainstream smoke totaling about 100–200 ng per cigarette (International Agency for Research on Cancer 2004a). Certain PAHs, including some of those in cigarette smoke, are potent locally acting carcinogens which induce lung tumors in rodents (Hecht 1999). Fractions of cigarette smoke condensate enriched in PAHs

A.A. Elfarra (ed.), *Advances in Bioactivation Research*, DOI: 10.1007/978-0-387-77300-1_17,

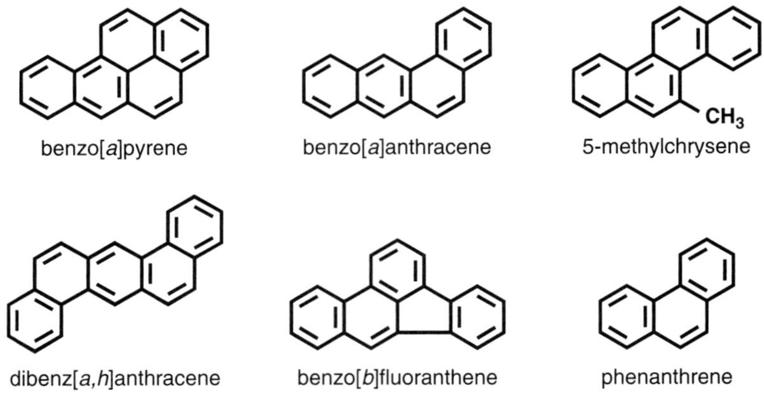

Figure 17.1 Structures of some PAHs in cigarette smoke.

are carcinogenic on mouse skin (Hecht 1999). The uptake of PAHs in smokers has been clearly demonstrated and there is solid evidence for the presence of benzo[*a*]pyrene diol epoxide–DNA (BPDE–DNA) adducts in lung tissue from some smokers (Beland et al. 2005; Boysen and Hecht 2003; Hecht 2002). The pattern of mutations in the *p53* gene in lung tumors from smokers is similar to the pattern of DNA damage caused in vitro by PAH diol epoxides and by BaP in cell culture (Denissenko et al. 1996; Pfeifer et al. 2002; Smith et al. 2000; Tretyakova et al. 2002), although similar results are obtained with acrolein (Feng et al. 2006). The pattern of *KRAS* mutations observed in lung tumors from smokers is also similar to that found in lung tumors of animals treated with PAH such as BaP (Ahrendt et al. 2001; Mills et al. 1995; Nesnow et al. 1998; Westra et al. 1993). Collectively, these observations strongly support the role of PAHs as major causes of lung cancer in smokers. There is also extensive evidence that other cigarette smoke carcinogens such as the tobacco-specific nitrosamine 4-(methylnitrosamino)-1-(3-pyridyl)-1-butanone (NNK) are involved (Hecht 1999; Hecht 2003).

Polycyclic aromatic hydrocarbons are also regarded as causes of cancers of the lung and skin due to occupational exposures to coke oven emissions, soots, coal tars, and related combustion products (International Agency for Research on Cancer 1983, 1984, 1985). PAH are considered as "reasonably anticipated to be human carcinogens" by the U.S. Dept. of Health and Human Services (U.S.Department of Health and Human Services 2004). BaP has recently been evaluated as "carcinogenic to humans" by the International Agency for Research on Cancer (Straif et al. 2005).

17.2. Metabolic Activation and Detoxification of PAH

Polycyclic aromatic hydrocarbons themselves are quite unreactive and require metabolic activation to be converted to electrophiles that react with DNA. Reaction with DNA to form adducts with miscoding potential is firmly established as the key step in the carcinogenic process. Without conversion to electrophilic metabolites, PAH are not mutagenic and will not be carcinogenic. PAH–DNA adducts cause miscoding events in the DNA of human cells, and if these events occur in critical regions of critical genes such as the tumor suppressor gene *p53* or the oncogene *KRAS*, the result can be loss of normal cellular growth control mechanisms, genomic instability, and ultimately cancer. The role of DNA adducts and the consequent mutations in cancer induction is firmly established through studies of DNA repair deficiency syndromes that lead to extraordinarily high cancer risks.

The major established route of metabolic activation of BaP and a number of other PAH to DNA adducts is formation of diol epoxides with one carbon terminus of the epoxide ring in the "bay region" of the PAH molecule (Figure 17.2). The first step in the metabolic activation of BaP by this pathway is formation of BaP-7,8-epoxide, catalyzed by cytochromes P450 1A1, 1B1, and several others. This metabolite then undergoes epoxide hydrolase (EH)-catalyzed hydration to produce BaP-7,8-diol. This product is stable and nonreactive, but has an isolated double bond in its terminal ring. This bond is readily oxidized, with catalysis by cytochromes P450 and other enzymes, yielding BaP-7,8-diol-9,10-epoxide (BPDE). Four stereoisomers are possible, but the major one formed in human cells and the most reactive with DNA is the "*trans, anti*" isomer (from *trans*- ring opening of the epoxide ring that is *anti*- to the 7-hydroxyl group) illustrated in Figure 17.2. BPDE is a "bay-region diol epoxide" and such compounds are reactive with DNA (depending on stereochemistry). In the case of BPDE, the major DNA reaction product results from *trans*- addition of the exocyclic amino group of deoxyguanosine to the 10-position of the epoxide ring. This adduct has miscoding properties and is considered to play a major role in cancer induction by BaP. While BPDE is more DNA-reactive than other BaP metabolites, its major reaction is with H_2O, producing *trans*-, *anti*-BaP-tetraol, a nonreactive metabolite that is the major detoxification product of BPDE.

There are other pathways of BaP metabolic activation. One involves the generation of electrophiles via one-electron oxidation, yielding a variety of DNA adducts which spontaneously depurinate leaving apurinic sites (Devanesan et al. 1996). A second involves oxidation of BaP-7,8-diol to a catechol and subsequent cycling of this metabolite with BaP-7,8-quinone, producing oxidative damage to DNA (Jiang et al. 2005; Yu et al. 2002). These pathways have been definitively elucidated in vitro and in some animal studies, but there is presently limited evidence that they occur in humans, in contrast to the BPDE pathway. In addition, the bay-region diol epoxide metabolic activation pathway is generalizable to many other PAHs.

Competing with the metabolic activation of BaP are a variety of detoxification reactions. BaP is initially oxidized to several simple epoxides, and these undergo spontaneous rearrangements to phenols (Figure 17.2). The epoxides can also be detoxified by reaction with glutathione, catalyzed by glutathione-*S*-transferases, a pathway that also detoxifies diol epoxides. Diols that are formed by hydration of the epoxides can be detoxified by conversion to glucuronides. The 1,3-, 1,6-, and 6,12-quinones are also common BaP metabolites that are generally regarded as detoxification products.

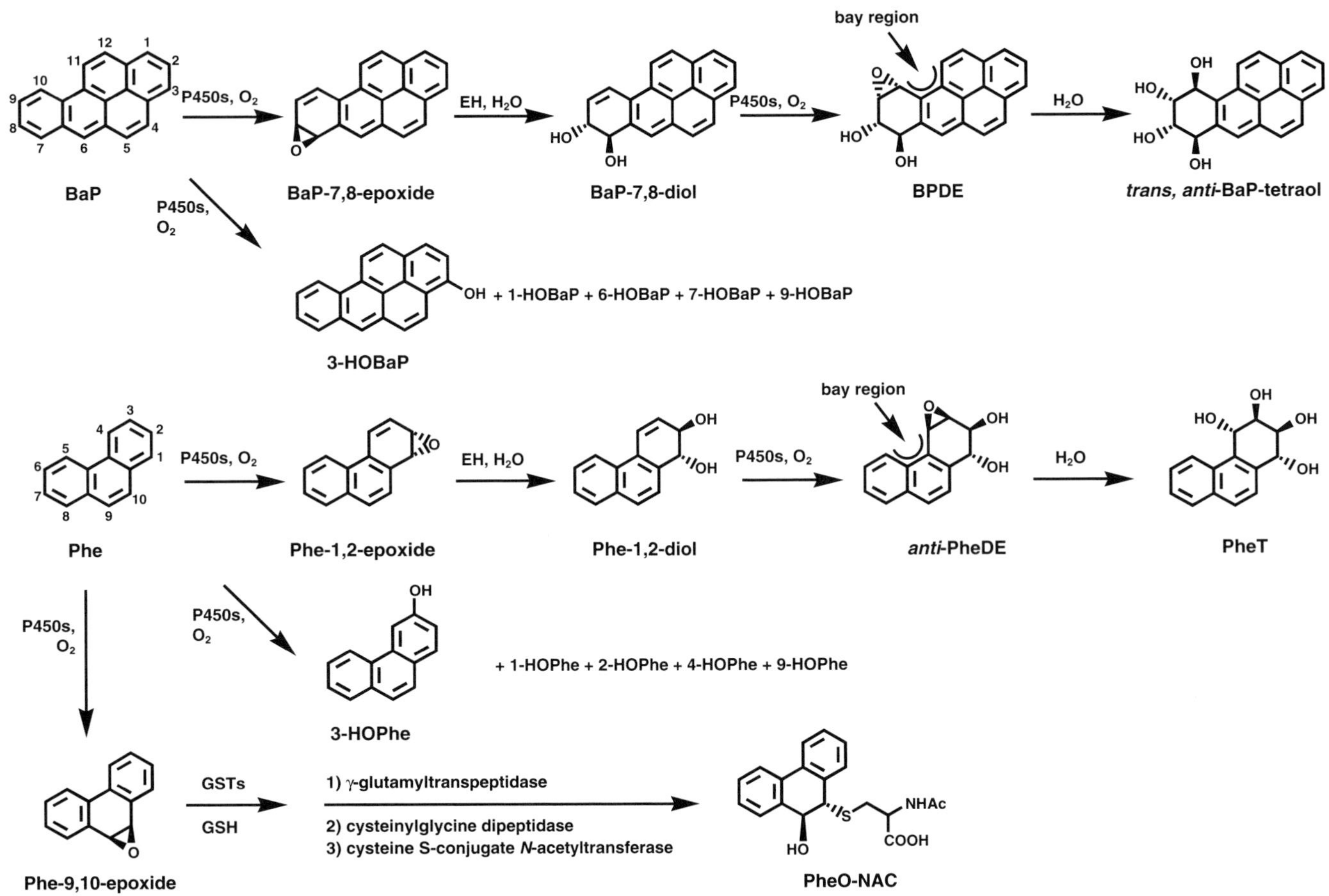

Figure 17.2 Metabolism of BaP to *trans, anti*-BaP-tetraol via BPDE (metabolic activation pathway) and to phenols, such as 3-HOBaP (metabolic detoxification pathway), and corresponding metabolism of phenanthrene (Phe) to PheT, phenanthrols, such as 3-HOPhe, and PheO-NAC.

The picture that emerges from this brief overview of BaP metabolism is a complex one. There is one firmly established metabolic activation pathway and a multitude of detoxification pathways including the formation of phenols, quinones, and glutathione or glucuronide conjugates. Similar pathways of metabolic activation and detoxification have been established for other PAHs.

Numerous studies have demonstrated that there are large interindividual differences in the human metabolism of PAH (Alexandrov et al. 2002; Harris et al. 1976; Kiyohara et al. 1998; McLemore et al. 1990; Nebert 2000; Nowak et al. 1988; Sabadie et al. 1981), giving rise to the hypothesis that individuals who efficiently metabolically activate PAH are at a higher risk for cancer. Interindividual differences in PAH metabolism and their relationship to cancer have been investigated extensively.

Beginning with the work of Conney and co-workers in the 1960s and continuing to the present, these studies have employed a variety of approaches. Some have investigated the inducibility of PAH metabolism. The aryl hydrocarbon receptor (AhR) regulates the *CYP1A1*, *1A2*, and *1B1* genes (which code for cytochromes P450 1A1, 1A2, and 1B1). Various dietary and environmental substances bind to the AhR and induce these enzymes (known in the older literature as aryl hydrocarbon hydroxylase or AHH) (Nebert, McKinnon and Puga 1996; Nebert et al. 2004; Tang, Lin and Lu 2005). About 10% of the Caucasian population has a high-inducibility phenotype for AHH, which co-segregates with *CYP1A1*2A* (Petersen et al. 1991). It is well established that cigarette smoking induces CYP1A and CYP1B enzymes, most likely through the binding of PAH and other smoke constituents to the AhR (International Agency for Research on Cancer 1986, 2004b; Kim et al. 2004; Nebert, McKinnon and Puga 1996; Nebert et al. 2004; Port et al. 2004; Tang, Lin and Lu 2005). The relationship between AHH inducibility and lung cancer risk in smokers has been examined with conflicting results (International Agency for Research on Cancer 1986, 2004b; Kiyohara et al. 1998; Nebert, McKinnon and Puga 1996; Nebert et al. 2004), possibly because AHH inducibility affects both the metabolic activation and detoxification of PAH.

Many studies have used genotyping methods to assess the relationship between polymorphisms in particular genes or combinations of genes involved in PAH metabolism and lung cancer risk. Some recent reviews and pooled analyses are illustrative (Bartsch et al. 2000; Smith et al. 2001). Two *CYP1A1* polymorphisms, the *Msp*I polymorphism due to a T-to-C substitution within the 3′ noncoding region of the gene (*CYP1A1Msp*I or *CYP1A1*2A*), and an A-to-G substitution in exon 7 resulting in the substitution of valine for isoleucine (*CYP1A1*I462V or *CYP1A1*2C*) have been extensively studied, and relationships to lung cancer have been found, particularly in Asian populations where these polymorphisms are more common than in Caucasians (Bartsch et al. 2000). A meta-analysis published in 2000 found little support for the role of these variants in lung cancer risk (Houlston 2000). However, a pooled analysis found a clear association between the homozygous *CYP1A1*2A* variant and lung cancer risk in smokers (Vineis et al. 2003). Another pooled analysis found a gene dosage effect for the *CYP1A1*2C* variant and lung cancer, particularly in never-smokers and women (Le Marchand et al. 2003). A pooled analysis in nonsmokers showed a significant effect of the heterozygous *CYP1A1*2C* variant on lung cancer risk, but not *CYP1A1*2A*. There was also a significant effect of the combined *CYP1A1*2C* and *GSTM1*-null genotype (Hung et al. 2003), but no effect of *GSTM1*-null genotype alone (Benhamou et al. 2002). A further pooled analysis replicated the effect of *CYP1A1*2A* on lung cancer risk in smokers and indicated an interaction between this genotype and *GSTM1* (Vineis et al. 2004). A meta-analysis and pooled analysis did not find consistent effects of EH polymorphisms on lung cancer risk (Lee et al. 2002). Collectively, these results indicate that there may be some effect of polymorphisms in *CYP1A1* and *GST* genes on lung cancer risk, presumably due to alterations in PAH metabolism, but the effects reported in these studies are small. It is likely that PAH metabolism is simply too complex to assess individual differences by polymorphisms in one or two genes, especially since some of the resultant enzymes catalyze both metabolic activation and detoxification.

17.3. Carcinogen Metabolite Phenotyping to Assess Individual Differences in PAH Metabolism

We propose to use carcinogen metabolite phenotyping, for example, actual measurement of PAH metabolites in urine, to assess individual differences in PAH metabolism and their possible relationship to cancer risk. We initiated our studies in this area by developing a method for analysis of *trans-,anti*-BaP-tetrol in urine. As mentioned above, this metabolite is the major end product of the BPDE metabolic activation pathway and its levels would represent the flux of BaP metabolism through this critical pathway in humans. A highly sensitive method was developed but the levels of *trans, anti*-BaP-tetraol were so low (1–100 fmol ml^{-1} urine, even in some highly exposed individuals) that multiple purification steps were needed prior to gas chromatography-mass spectrometry (GC-MS) analysis, and the method would not be practical for even modest-size clinical and epidemiologic studies.

Therefore, we turned our attention to phenanthrene (Phe). Phe is the simplest PAH with a bay region, but is not carcinogenic. Several studies have clearly demonstrated similarities in metabolism between Phe and other PAHs containing a bay region, such as BaP, chrysene, and benz[*a*]anthracene (Figure 17.1; Feng et al. 2006; Nordquist et al. 1981; Shou et al. 1994b; Thakker et al. 1985). These studies show that common P450 enzymes, particularly P450 s 1A1 and 1A2, are involved in the formation of Phe-1,2-diol and *anti*-PheDE as well as the corresponding dihydrodiols and diol epoxides of BaP, chrysene, and benz[*a*]anthracene, and that the stereochemistry of these transformations is similar for different PAHs, leading to the formation of bay-region diol epoxides with *R,S,S,R*- absolute configuration from dihydrodiols with *R,R*- configuration (as shown in Figure 17.2). Nevertheless, neither Phe nor its dihydrodiol metabolites exhibits significant tumorigenicity on mouse skin, and its diol epoxide metabolites, including *anti*-PheDE, while having some mutagenic activity in *Salmonella typhimurium* and Chinese hamster V79 cells, show no tumorigenic activity in newborn mice, a test system highly sensitive to the tumorigenic activities of BPDE and other PAH diol epoxides (Buening et al. 1979; Chaturapit and Holder 1978). To quote from Nordqvist et al, "the lack of tumorigenicity for phenanthrene lies solely in the fact that its bay-region diol epoxides have extremely weak biological activity, since metabolism of phenanthrene to bay-region diol epoxides closely parallels that of tumorigenic hydrocarbons". (Nordquist et al. 1981) Consistent with these observations, the binding of PheDE to DNA was only 1/250th as great as that of BPDE (unpublished data).

We propose that the measurement of Phe metabolites in human urine is an effective surrogate for those of carcinogenic PAH, and that Phe metabolite ratios can provide an accurate assessment of individual differences in PAH metabolism. This would ultimately allow us to test the hypothesis that individual differences in PAH metabolism are related to cancer susceptibility. An advantage of this carcinogen metabolite phenotyping approach is that it integrates all enzymatic, genetic, and environmental factors that impact on carcinogen metabolism.

17.4. Development of Methods for Analysis of Phe Metabolites in Human Urine

As shown in Figure 17.2, the metabolism of Phe by the diol epoxide metabolic activation pathway results in the formation of *anti*-PheDE, which reacts with H_2O to produce PheT. We developed a gas chromatography (GC)-negative ion chemical ionization-mass spectrometry method for analysis of PheT in human urine (Hecht et al. 2003). A typical chromatogram obtained from a PheT analysis in a nonsmoker's urine is illustrated in Figure 17.3. In contrast to *trans, anti*-BaP-tetraol, this metabolite was readily detected. PheT is present in all human urine samples. The other isomers of Phe tetraol are also observed but their levels are considerably lower than those of PheT. Amounts of PheT in smokers' urine are about 4.5 pmol mg^{-1} creatinine while in nonsmokers levels are about 1.5 pmol mg^{-1} creatinine. Levels of PheT in the urine of individuals exposed to high levels of PAH, such as coke oven workers, were about 26 pmol mg^{-1} creatinine, more than 10 000 times the amounts of *trans, anti*-BaP-tetraol in the same samples. This method provides a practical way to monitor the metabolic activation of Phe, as a surrogate for carcinogenic PAH, and can be applied in large studies. A similar method for analysis of PheT in human plasma has also been developed (Carmella, Yoder and Hecht 2006).

Levels of PheT will be influenced by both exposure and metabolic activation. While both are important in determining the ultimate outcome, our main focus in this work is to explore metabolic differences in individuals with a given PAH exposure. Therefore, we need to correct for exposure. In order to do this, we propose creating a metabolic activation: detoxification ratio. PheT would be in the numerator of this ratio, while phenanthrols (HOPhe), products of detoxification (Figure 17.2), would be in the denominator.

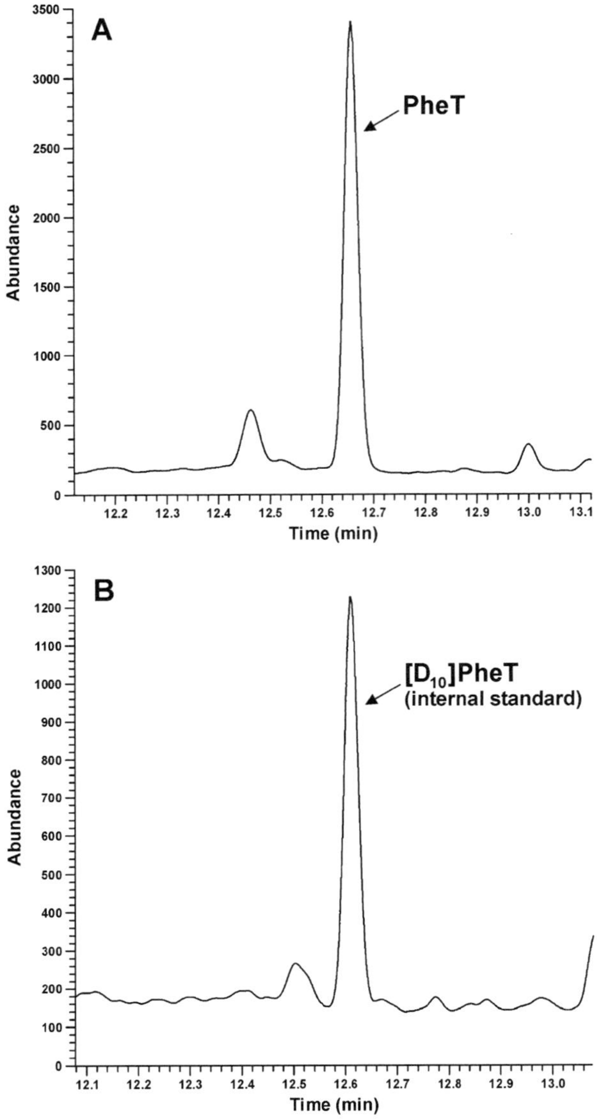

Figure 17.3 GC-MS analysis of phenanthrene-tetraol in human urine: (**a**) analyte, and (**b**) internal standard.

Five HOPhe- 1-HOPhe, 2-HOPhe, 3-HOPhe, 4-HOPhe, and 9-HOPhe- can be formed from Phe (Figure 17.2), and all have been previously identified in human urine (Angerer, Mannschreck and Gundel 1997; Jacob and Seidel 2002). Several methods have been published for quantitation of HOPhe in human urine. These used either high-performance liquid chromatography (HPLC) (Bentsen-Farmen et al. 1999; Gundel et al. 1996; Heudorf and Angerer 2001; Kuusimaki et al. 2003; Lintelmann et al. 1994; Mannschreck, Gundel and Angerer 1996), GC (Grimmer, Dettbarn and Jacob 1993; Hoepfner et al. 1987), or GC-MS (Gmeiner et al. 1998; Grimmer et al. 1997; Jacob, Grimmer and Dettbarn 1999; Serdar et al. 2003; Smith et al. 2002a, 2002b) for detection and quantitation. We developed a GC-positive ion chemical ionization-MS method for quantitation of HOPhe in human urine (Carmella et al. 2004). Our method quantified the HOPhe, except 9-HOPhe. Levels of total HOPhe measured by our method in smokers and nonsmokers were similar, about 2–3 pmol mg^{-1} creatinine. Our data were generally similar to those reported in previous studies (Carmella et al. 2004).

We then developed a method for quantitation of a mercapturic acid, *N*-acetyl-*S*-(9,10-dihydro-9-hydroxy-10-phenanthryl)-L-cysteine (PheO-NAC, Figure 17.2), the end product of reaction of Phe-9,10-epoxide with glutathione (Upadhyaya et al. 2006). This would provide an indicator of the glutathione detoxification pathway. PheO-NAC was quantified by liquid chromatography-electrospray ionization-tandem mass spectrometry with selected reaction monitoring. PheO-NAC was detected in the urine of 46 of 104 smokers, with an average amount of approximately 0.06 pmol ml^{-1} urine, considerably lower than the amounts of PheT or HOPhe. PheO-NAC was detected significantly more frequently in subjects who were *GSTM1*-positive than in those who were *GSTM1*-null, and the levels of PheO-NAC were significantly higher in the *GSTM1*-positive subjects, consistent with a role for *GSTM1* in the detoxification of phenanthrene-9,10-epoxide. There were no significant relationships between PheO-NAC levels and the occurrence of two *GSTP1* polymorphisms. These results provided the first evidence for a PAH-derived mercapturic acid in human urine, but the levels were fairly low, so would not contribute markedly to the PheT:HOPhe ratios.

17.4.1. Longitudinal Study of Urinary Phe Metabolite Ratios

As described above, we propose that a ratio of PheT (as a marker of metabolic activation) to HOPhe (as a marker of detoxification) would be characteristic of a given individual's ability to metabolically activate or detoxify PAH. One major goal was to determine the longitudinal consistency of this ratio in a person (Hecht et al. 2005). This would provide essential information with respect to the design of epidemiologic studies using this biomarker. A second goal was to compare the ratio in smokers and nonsmokers. Twelve smokers and 10 nonsmokers were enrolled in the study. First morning urine samples were collected daily on days 1–7, then weekly on days 14, 21, 28, 35, 42, and 49 of the study.

As a measure of longitudinal stability, coefficients of variation (C.V.) for PheT, 3-HOPhe, total HOPhe, and the ratios PheT:3-HOPhe and PheT:total HOPhe over the 49-day period for smokers and nonsmokers are summarized in Table 17.1. PheT:3-HOPhe ratios were included because the internal standard in our HOPhe analysis is [^{13}C]3-HOPhe. Therefore, results for this particular HOPhe isomer should be the most reliable. Variation in PheT levels was greater than that in 3-HOPhe or total HOPhe. Coefficient of variation for PheT:3-HOPhe and PheT:total HOPhe ratios were 37.3 ± 17.1% and 36.3 ± 18.4% in smokers, respectively, while the corresponding figures in nonsmokers for these two ratios were 44.0 ± 20.8% and 45.7 ± 20.3%. Overall, there were no significant variations in PheT, 3-HOPhe, total HOPhe, or either ratio with continuous time. The results were the same in both smokers and nonsmokers.

Data for the ratio PheT:total HOPhe in smokers and nonsmokers are illustrated in Figure 17.4. This ratio was significantly higher in smokers

Table 17.1 Geometric means of PheT, phenanthrols, and PheT: phenanthrol ratios over a 49-day period in smokers and nonsmokers.

		PheT			3-HOPhe			Total HOPhe			PheT: 3-HOPhe			PheT Total HOPhe		
Smokers	**CPD**[a]	**Mean**[b]	**S.D.**	**C.V.**[c]	**Mean**[b]	**S.D.**	**C.V.**	**Mean**[b]	**S.D.**	**C.V.**	**Mean**	**S.D.**	**C.V.**	**Mean**	**S.D.**	**C.V.**
1	30	0.76	0.21	27.0	0.99	0.22	22.5	2.58	0.70	26.9	0.76	0.24	31.6	0.29	0.11	38.9
2	20	2.50	0.62	24.9	0.42	0.12	27.8	1.62	0.42	25.8	5.92	1.50	25.4	1.54	0.36	23.1
3	15	4.84	3.35	69.3	0.73	0.44	59.8	2.51	1.61	64.2	6.59	1.88	28.5	1.93	0.50	26.1
4	40	3.02	0.81	27.0	0.70	0.36	51.2	2.20	1.18	53.5	4.32	1.56	37.0	1.37	0.51	36.9
5	30	3.34	0.42	12.5	1.07	0.16	14.9	3.77	0.41	10.9	3.13	0.60	19.2	0.88	0.13	14.5
6	20	1.49	0.29	19.3	0.64	0.15	23.4	2.16	0.47	21.7	2.33	0.62	26.8	0.69	0.17	24.3
7	25	5.59	3.28	58.8	0.91	0.31	34.0	2.29	1.39	60.4	6.12	3.28	53.7	2.44	1.39	56.9
8	15	4.24	2.42	57.2	0.60	0.16	26.3	1.88	0.48	25.3	7.02	4.57	65.1	2.26	1.49	65.9
9	20	3.68	0.76	20.6	0.89	0.29	32.5	2.79	0.66	23.7	4.15	1.17	28.1	1.32	0.25	18.6
10	5	2.37	1.68	70.7	0.63	0.23	36.7	1.93	0.68	35.1	3.75	2.66	70.9	1.23	0.84	67.9
11	10	6.24	4.90	78.5	0.96	0.50	52.4	2.93	1.45	49.6	6.51	2.57	39.5	2.13	0.87	41.0
12	10	42.3	8.37	19.8	4.35	0.83	19.1	10.1	2.24	22.2	9.72	2.09	21.5	4.20	0.92	22.0
overall[d]				40.5 ± 24.2			33.4 ± 14.3			34.9 ± 17.4			37.3 ± 17.1			36.3 ± 18.4
Non-smokers																
1		1.44	0.63	43.9	0.76	0.27	35.8	2.04	0.89	43.4	1.91	0.35	18.2	0.71	0.16	22.2
2		1.65	0.62	37.6	0.56	0.098	17.7	1.50	0.26	17.0	2.96	1.11	37.6	1.10	0.44	39.8
3		0.80	0.32	39.3	0.37	0.086	23.3	1.22	0.29	23.5	2.16	0.76	35.1	0.66	0.24	36.7
4		0.63	0.26	41.2	0.48	0.25	50.9	1.45	0.65	44.6	1.31	0.45	34.4	0.44	0.13	30.4
5		0.89	0.24	26.5	0.39	0.12	29.9	1.33	0.48	36.3	2.30	0.47	20.3	0.67	0.14	21.4
6		2.73	1.33	48.9	0.70	0.20	28.9	4.05	0.93	22.9	3.89	2.06	53.1	0.67	0.39	57.9
7		1.42	0.53	37.1	0.49	0.066	13.6	1.40	0.29	20.6	3.04	1.31	42.9	1.05	0.52	49.0
8		3.94	2.19	55.4	1.18	0.23	19.0	4.28	1.76	41.1	3.29	1.50	45.6	0.91	0.44	48.1
9		1.47	0.99	67.1	0.24	0.069	29.3	0.98	0.28	28.3	6.22	5.47	87.9	1.51	1.32	87.4
10		1.56	0.52	33.1	0.55	0.24	44.3	2.23	0.91	40.6	2.85	1.85	64.7	0.70	0.45	63.7
overall[d]				43.0 ± 11.6			29.3 ± 11.8			31.8 ± 10.5			44.0 ± 20.8			45.7 ± 20.3

[a] CPD, cigarettes per day.
[b] pmol/mg creatinine.
[c] C.V., coefficient of variation.
[d] Arithmetic means ± S.D.

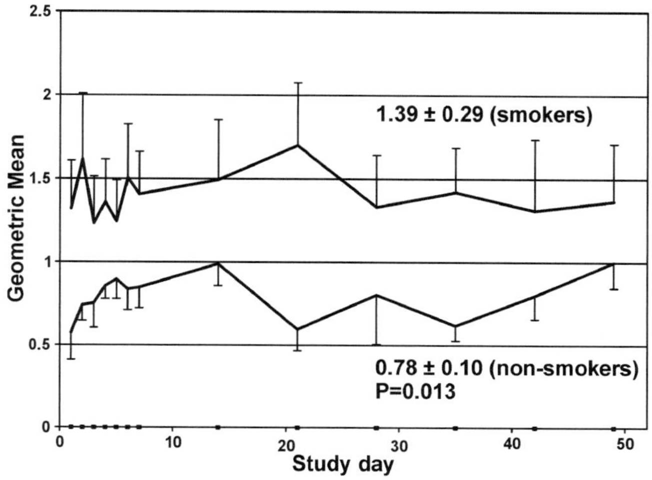

Figure 17.4 PheT:total HOPhe ratios in smokers and nonsmokers over a 49-day period.

than in nonsmokers. The ratio PheT:3-HOPhe was also higher in smokers than in nonsmokers, but the difference barely missed significance. Total HOPhe was not different in smokers and nonsmokers. The results of this study indicated that, when comparing Phe metabolites or their ratios between groups such as smokers and nonsmokers, a single sampling would probably be sufficient. Sampling in both groups should be done at about the same time. When comparing individual levels, multiple sampling would be advisable if feasible.

A potentially important finding of this study was the significantly higher PheT:total HOPhe ratio in smokers than in nonsmokers (Figure 17.4). Although it is known that smoking induces P450 1A1, 1A2, and 1B1 through binding of smoke constituents to the AhR, there are no previous studies that have examined the consequences of this induction with respect to metabolic activation versus detoxification of PAH in humans. These results demonstrated that the diol epoxide metabolic activation pathway of Phe was induced to a greater extent than the HOPhe detoxification pathway in smokers (Figure 17.4). The greater induction of the diol epoxide than the HOPhe metabolism pathway is logical because P450 1A1, 1A2 and 1B1 are involved in two steps in diol epoxide formation but only one step in HOPhe formation (Figure 17.2).

17.4.2. Relationship of PheT: HOPhe Ratios to Genotyping Data

In this study, our goal was to investigate the relationship of polymorphisms in PAH-metabolizing genes to PheT:HOPhe ratios in smokers (Hecht et al. 2006). This was designed to be a genotype:phenotype comparison study. We explored the association of urinary PheT:HOPhe ratios with particular polymorphisms in these genes to determine whether these polymorphisms, individually or in combination, could predict high PheT:HOPhe ratios. We recruited 346 smokers and collected a blood sample for genotyping and a first morning urine sample for analysis of PheT and HOPhe. Genotyping was carried out for 11 polymorphisms in genes involved in PAH metabolism: *CYP1A1Msp*I; *CYP1A1*I462 V; *CYP1B1*R48G; *CYP1B1*A119S; *CYP1B1*L432 V; *CYP1B1*N453S; *EPHX1*Y113H; *EPHX1*H139R; *GSTP1*I105 V; *GSTP1*A114 V; and *GSTM1*- null. *CYP1A1* and *CYP1B1* code for cytochromes P450 1A1 and 1B1, which, as discussed above, catalyze both the metabolic activation of PAH by the diol epoxide pathway, and their detoxification by phenol formation (Figure 17.1; Bauer et al. 1995; Kim et al. 1999; Shimada et al. 1996, 1999; Shou et al. 1994a, 1994b). *EPHX1* codes for microsomal EH which is involved in the metabolic activation of PAH through the diol epoxide pathway (Cooper, Grover and Sims 1983; Guenthner and Oesch 1981). *GSTM1* and *GSTP1* code for glutathione S-transferases which catalyze the detoxification of PAH diol epoxides (Robertson et al. 1986; Sundberg et al. 1997, 1998, 2002).

The distribution of PheT:3-HOPhe ratios is illustrated in Figure 17.5. The geometric mean PheT:3-HOPhe ratio was 4.08. Ten percent of the smokers had PheT:3-HOPhe ratios of 9.90 and higher, and we would predict that these smokers should be at higher risk for lung cancer.

The relationship of PheT:3-HOPhe ratios to polymorphisms is summarized in Table 17.2. There was no significant effect of the *CYP1A1Msp*I polymorphism (also known as *CYP1A1*2A*). The PheT:3-HOPhe ratio was significantly higher in individuals heterozygous or homozygous for *CYP1A1*I462 V (also known as *CYP1A1*2C*) [5.68 (95% CI 4.20, 7.68)] than in normals [3.99 (3.70,4.31)], $P = 0.02$. A gene dosage effect was not observed, as the ratio for heterozygotes was greater than for homozygotes. However, there were only four homozygotes (1.18%). Individuals heterozygous in *CYP1A1* I462 V were significantly overrepresented in the top 10% and underrepresented in the bottom 10% of PheT:3-HOPhe ratios ($P = 0.03$). With one exception, all subjects heterozygous or homozygous for *CYP1A1*I462 V were also either

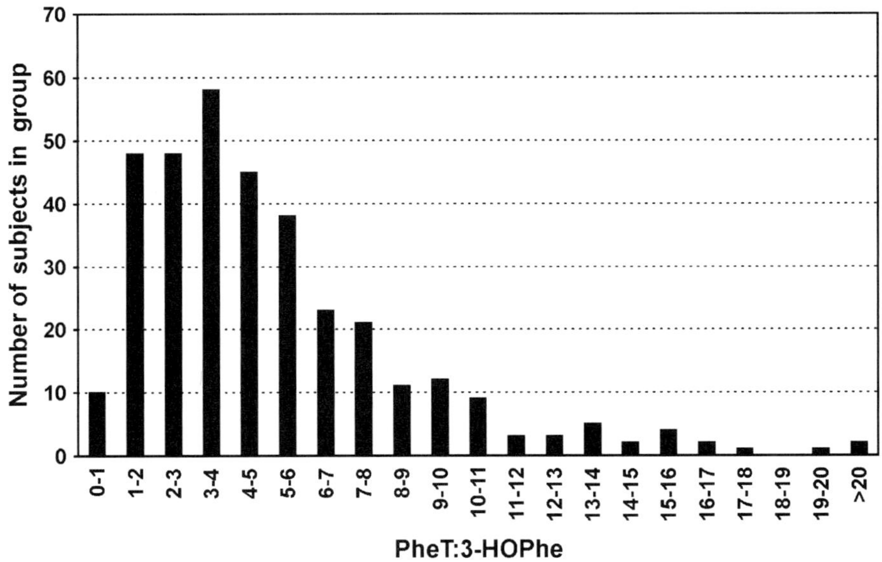

Figure 17.5 Frequency plot of PheT:3-HOPhe ratios in 346 smokers.

Table 17.2 Effects of polymorphisms on PheT:3-HOPhe ratios in 346 smokers.

		Percent occurrence			Geometric mean PheT:3-HOPhe (95% C.I.)				
Gene polymorphism	rs Number	Heterozygotes	Homozygotes	Combined	Normal	Heterozygotes	Homozygotes	Combined	P^a
*CYP1A1Msp*I	4646903	26.1	1.55	27.6	4.26 (3.91, 4.65)	3.93 (3.38, 4.57)	4.81 (2.11, 10.97)	3.98 (3.44, 4.60)	0.42
*CYP1A1*I462 V	1048943	5.59	1.18	6.77	3.99 (3.70, 4.31)	6.02 (4.22, 8.59)	4.31 (2.16, 8.60)	5.68 (4.20, 7.68)	0.02
*CYP1B1*R48G	10012	39.4	12.7	52.1	4.88 (4.39, 5.41)	3.76 (3.33, 4.23)	3.11 (2.50, 3.88)	3.59 (3.23, 3.98)	<0.0001
*CYP1B1*A119S	1056827	40.9	12.8	53.7	4.98 (4.49, 5.52)	3.61 (3.23, 4.05)	3.09 (2.50, 3.82)	3.48 (3.15, 3.85)	<0.0001
*CYP1B1*L432 V	1056836	43.7	25.2	68.9	4.18 (3.61, 4.85)	3.83 (3.45, 4.24)	4.59 (3.91, 5.38)	4.09 (3.75, 4.47)	0.79
*CYP1B1*N453S	1800440	21.5	2.65	24.2	4.04 (3.71, 4.40)	4.26 (3.66, 4.96)	8.49 (5.34, 13.48)	4.59 (3.96, 5.34)	0.14
*EPHX1*Y113H	1051740	36.5	10.5	47.0	4.12 (3.70, 4.58)	4.14 (3.68, 4.66)	4.46 (3.68, 5.40)	4.21 (3.81, 4.66)	0.78
*EPHX1*H139R	2234922	34.4	5.21	39.6	4.14 (3.78, 4.55)	4.03 (3.48, 4.67)	4.25 (3.10, 5.84)	4.06 (3.56, 4.64)	0.80
*GSTP1*I105 V	947894	45.8	14.0	59.8	4.31 (3.84, 4.84)	4.00 (3.57, 4.49)	4.23 (3.40, 5.25)	4.05 (3.67, 4.48)	0.43
*GSTP1*A114 V	1799811	12.7	0	12.7	4.11 (3.80, 4.45)	3.99 (3.19, 5.00)	—	3.99 (3.19, 5.00)	0.80
GSTM1 null	none	—[b]	64.6	64.6	3.80 (3.37, 4.29)	—[b]	4.42 (4.00, 4.90)	4.42 (4.00, 4.90)	0.07

[a] Normal vs. Combined; [b] Not done

heterozygous or homozygous for *CYP1A1MspI*. Therefore, the effects on PheT:3-HOPhe ratios in individuals with both polymorphisms (also known as *CYP1A1*2B*) were virtually identical to those with only a *CYP1A1*I462 V polymorphism.

The PheT:3-HOPhe ratio was significantly lower in individuals heterozygous or homozygous for *CYP1B1*R48G (3.59 (3.23, 3.98)), than in normals (4.88 (4.39, 5.41)), $P<0.0001$. It was also significantly lower in individuals heterozygous or homozygous for *CYP1B1*A119S (3.48 (3.15, 3.85)) than in normals (4.98 (4.49, 5.52)), $P < 0.0001$. A gene dosage effect was observed for both of these *CYP1B1* variants.

There were no significant effects of *EPHX1* or *GSTP1* polymorphisms on the PheT:3-HOPhe ratio (Table 17.3). The ratio was higher (4.42 (4.00, 4.90)) in *GSTM1*-null individuals than in those with *GSTM1* present (3.80 (3.37, 4.29)), but this difference was not significant, $P = 0.07$.

When the data were stratified by gender, a strong relationship was observed between the *CYP1A1*I462 V polymorphism and PheT:3-HOPhe ratio in females. The ratio was significantly higher in females heterozygous or homozygous for this polymorphism (6.49 (4.28, 9.85)) than normals (3.80 (3.43, 4.21)), $P< 0.01$. A gene dosage effect was not observed, but there were only four homozygotes. No significant effect of *CYP1A1*I462 V on PheT:3-HOPhe ratio was observed in males.

The data were further stratified, forming groups of ≤15, 16–25, and ≥26 cigarettes per day. The strongest relationships between PheT:3-HOPhe or PheT:total HOPhe ratios and *CYP1A1*I462 V polymorphism were seen in females in the 16–25 cigarettes per day group. The PheT:3-HOPhe ratio was 7.74 (4.38, 13.7) in females heterozygous or homozygous for this polymorphism compared to normals 3.74 (3.12, 4.47), $P= 0.04$. PheT itself was also significantly higher in this group in heterozygous or homozygous females (9.73 (4.42, 21.45)) than in normals (3.30 (2.76, 3.93)) $P= 0.002$, but no effects were observed on 3-HOPhe or total HOPhe.

The combination of *CYP1A1*I462 V and *GSTM1*-null was investigated. In individuals who were either homozygous or heterozygous for *CYP1A1*I462 V and also had the *GSTM1*-null genotype ($N = 15$), the PheT:3-HOPhe ratio (6.85 (4.50, 10.4)) was significantly higher than in normals ($N = 102$) (3.78 (3.33, 4.29)), $P < 0.01$. Stratifying by gender, this combined effect was restricted to females, and was significant for PheT:3-HOPhe ($P = 0.003$), PheT:total HOPhe ($P < 0.001$), and PheT ($P = 0.013$). Smokers with the combination of *CYP1A1*I462 Val homozygous or heterozygous and *GSTM1*-null were significantly overrepresented in the top 10% and underrepresented in the bottom 10% of PheT:3-HOPhe ratios ($P = 0.02$). There were no consistent significant effects on PheT:3-HOPhe ratios of the combination of *CYP1A1*I462 V and *GSTP1* polymorphisms or of the combination of *CYP1A1MspI* and *GSTM1*-null or *GSTP1* polymorphisms.

The strongest relationship between a combination of polymorphisms and PheT:3-HOPhe ratios in the top 10% of our subjects was found for *CYP1A1*I462 V and *GSTM1*-null. Nevertheless, only four of these individuals had both polymorphisms and about 25% did not have either one. We investigated whether the highest 10% of PheT:3-HOPhe ratios could be predicted by any of the 11 polymorphisms individually or by certain combinations. The combinations were *CYP1A1*I462 V and *GSTM1*-null; *CYP1A1MspI* and

GSTM1-null; and each of the four *CYP1B1* polymorphisms individually with *GSTM1*-null. The model could not accurately predict high PheT:3-HOPhe ratios.

Some interesting effects of polymorphisms in *CYP* genes were observed in this study. The *CYP1A1*I462 V polymorphism was associated with a significant increase in Phe metabolic activation, as determined by PheT:HOPhe ratios, and this effect was particularly strong in female smokers, and in combination with *GSTM1*-null. We also observed a consistent modifying effect of the *CYP1B1*R48G and *CYP1B1*A119S polymorphisms, in which the metabolic activation of Phe was decreased. An important result of this study was that the polymorphisms alone or in logical combinations could not predict elevated PheT:HOPhe ratios, indicating that genotyping alone is not sufficient for evaluating individual differences in PAH metabolism.

It is interesting to compare the results to those of previous studies in which polymorphisms have been studied with respect to lung cancer. The *CYP1A1*I462 V polymorphism was not associated overall with lung cancer risk in a cohort of men in Shanghai, China, although there was some suggestion that having at least one valine allele might be related to increased risk of lung cancer among smokers of less than 20 cigarettes per day, particularly among *GSTM1*-null individuals (London et al. 2000). Quite similar results were obtained in two other studies in China (Chen et al. 2001; Song et al. 2001). A study among Chinese women demonstrated that the *CYP1A1*I462 V genotype was associated with a significantly elevated risk of lung cancer in both smokers and nonsmokers, with the risk being greater in the latter (Yang et al. 2004). Another study showed a higher risk of lung cancer in nonsmoking Chinese women with the *CYP1A1*I462 V genotype than in those with the normal genotype (Ng et al. 2005). A pooled analysis of the Genetic Susceptibility to Environmental Carcinogens database found that there was a significant gene dosage effect for the *CYP1A1*I462 V polymorphism with respect to lung cancer in the US, and that the effect appeared to be stronger in Caucasians than Asians. The effect of the polymorphism was strongest in never-smoking females (Le Marchand et al. 2003). Collectively, the results of these studies were quite consistent with our data, if one assumes that higher PheT:3-HOPhe ratios are associated with higher risk for lung cancer, as predicted based on metabolic considerations.

The results of this study also showed that polymorphisms in PAH-metabolizing genes cannot accurately predict Phe metabolism, and likely the metabolism of other PAH, in smokers. This calls into question the strategy of genotyping for identification of individuals who might be particularly susceptible or resistant to PAH carcinogenesis. This conclusion is logical because enzyme activities are not dictated by genotype alone. Differences in enzyme expression, induction, and inhibition, among others, will affect PAH metabolic activation and detoxification. Although metabolic phenotyping is presently more technically demanding than genotyping, current advances in analytical chemistry should lead to rapid phenotyping methods suitable for application in epidemiologic studies.

17.5. Future Directions in Phe Metabolite Phenotyping

It is apparent from the studies described above that genotyping cannot predict the balance of Phe metabolism by the diol epoxide metabolic activation pathway versus the phenol-forming detoxification pathway. Although the extent to which Phe metabolism correlates with the metabolism of carcinogenic PAH is unknown, available data indicate that there are strong similarities. Therefore, it is plausible that Phe metabolite phenotyping may be an approach to rigorously test the hypothesis that individual differences in PAH metabolism are related to cancer risk.

How would such studies actually be performed? Presently, there are stored urine and plasma samples in a number of very large screening or epidemiologic studies in which cancer outcomes are known. These samples were obtained when healthy subjects entered the studies, long before disease developed. Comparing PheT:HOPhe ratios in samples from subjects who developed cancer versus appropriately matched controls who did not, provides an attractive approach to testing the hypothesis. Since the longitudinal study described above did show considerable variation in this ratio in some individuals, it would probably be advisable to study the factors related to the variation and to carry out further longitudinal studies to assess ratio consistency. The present methodology for determining PheT:HOPhe ratios is somewhat complex but still applicable to fairly large studies. This methodology can most likely be streamlined to allow more rapid analysis.

If the results of such molecular epidemiology studies do support the hypothesis that differences in PAH metabolism are related to cancer risk, it would be important to develop a predictive model which included such information. There is presently no such model for lung cancer, and we still do not know which smoker will be affected. It is conceivable that a PAH metabolism term would be an important part of such a model. The phenotyping method could be applied at a relatively young age and might be helpful in encouraging susceptible individuals in particular to quit smoking.

References

Ahrendt, S. A, Decker, P. A, Alawi, E. A, Zhu Yr, Y. R, Sanchez-Cespedes, M, Yang, S. C, Haasler, G. B, Kajdacsy-Balla, A, Demeure, M. J., and Sidransky, D. 2001. Cigarette smoking is strongly associated with mutation of the K-*ras* gene in patients with primary adenocarcinoma of the lung. Cancer 92: 1525–1530.

Alexandrov, K, Cascorbi, I, Rojas, M, Bouvier, G, Kriek, E., and Bartsch, H. 2002. CYP1A1 and GSTM1 genotypes affect benzo[*a*]pyrene DNA adducts in smokers' lung: comparison with aromatic/hydrophobic adduct formation. Carcinogenesis 23:1969–1977.

Angerer, J, Mannschreck, C., and Gundel, J. 1997. Biological monitoring and biochemical effect monitoring of exposure to polycyclic aromatic hydrocarbons. Int. Arch. Occup. Environ. Health 70:365–377.

Bartsch, H, Nair, U, Risch, A, Rojas, M, Wikman, H., and Alexandrov, K. 2000. Genetic polymorphism of CYP genes, alone or in combination, as a risk modifier of tobacco-related cancers. Cancer Epidemiol. Biomarkers & Prev. 9:3–28.

Bauer, E, Guo, Z, Ueng, Y. F, Bell, L. C, Zeldin, D., and Guengerich, F. P. 1995. Oxidation of benzo[*a*]pyrene by recombinant human cytochrome P450 enzymes. Chem. Res. Toxicol. 8:136–142.

Beland, F. A, Churchwell, M. I, Von Tungeln, L. S, Chen, S, Fu, P. P, Culp, S. J, Schoket, B, Gyorffy, E, Minarovits, J, Poirier, M. C, Bowman, E. D, Weston, A., and Doerge, D. R. 2005. High-performance liquid chromatography electrospray ionization tandem mass spectrometry for the detection and quantitation of benzo[*a*]pyrene–DNA adducts. Chem. Res. Toxicol. 18:1306–1315.

Benhamou, S, Lee, W. J, Alexandrie, A. K, Boffetta, P, Bouchardy, C, Butkiewicz, D, Brockmoller, J, Clapper, M. L, Daly, A, Dolzan, V, Ford, J, Gaspari, L, Haugen, A, Hirvonen, A, Husgafvel-Pursiainen, K, Ingelman-Sundberg, M, Kalina, I, Kihara, M, Kremers, P, Le Marchand, L, London, S. J, Nazar-Stewart, V, Onon-Kihara, M, Rannug, A, Romkes, M, Ryberg, D, Seidegard, J, Shields, P, Strange, R. C, Stucker, I, To-Figueras, J, Brennan, P., and Taioli, E. 2002. Meta- and pooled analyses of the effects of glutathione S-transferase M1 polymorphisms and smoking on lung cancer risk. Carcinogenesis 23:1343–1350.

Bentsen-Farmen, R. K, Botnen, I. V, Noto, H, Jacob, J., and Ovrebo, S. 1999. Detection of polycyclic aromatic hydrocarbon metabolites by high-pressure liquid chromatography after purification on immunoaffinity columns in urine from occupationally exposed workers. Int. Arch. Occup. Environ. Health 72:161–168.

Boysen, G. and Hecht, S. S. 2003. Analysis of DNA and protein adducts of benzo[*a*]pyrene in human tissues using structure-specific methods. Mutation Res. 543:17–30.

Buening, M. K, Levin, W, Karle, J. M, Yagi, H, Jerina, D. M., and Conney, A. H. 1979. Tumorigenicity of bay-region epoxides and other derivatives of chrysene and phenanthrene in newborn mice. Cancer Res. 39:5063–5068.

Carmella, S. G, Chen, M, Yagi, H, Jerina, D. M., and Hecht, S. S. 2004. Analysis of phenanthrols in human urine by gas chromatography-mass spectrometry: potential use in carcinogen metabolite phenotyping. Cancer Epidemiol. Biomarkers & Prev. 13:2167–2174.

Carmella, S. G, Yoder, A., and Hecht, S. S. 2006. Combined analysis of *r*-1,*t*-2,3,*c*-4-tetrahydroxy-1,2,3,4-tetrahydrophenanthrene and 4-(methylnitrosamino)-1-(3-pyridyl)-1-butanol in smokers' plasma. Cancer Epidemiol. Biomarkers & Prev. 15:1490–1494.

Chaturapit, S. and Holder, G. M. 1978. Studies on the hepatic microsomal metabolism of [^{14}C]phenanthrene. Biochem. Pharmacol. 27:1865–1871.

Chen, S, Xue, K, Xu, L, Ma, G., and Wu, J. 2001. Polymorphisms of the CYP1A1 and GSTM1 genes in relation to individual susceptibility to lung carcinoma in Chinese population. Mutat. Res. 458:41–47.

Cooper, C. S, Grover, P. L., and Sims, P. 1983. The metabolism and activation of benzo[*a*]pyrene. Prog. Drug Metab. 7:295–396.

Denissenko, M. F, Pao, A, Tang, M., and Pfeifer, G. P. 1996. Preferential formation of benzo[*a*]pyrene adducts at lung cancer mutational hot spots in P53. Science 274:430–432.

Devanesan, P. D, Higginbotham, S, Ariese, F, Jankowiak, R, Suh, M, Small, G. J, Cavalieri, E. L., and Rogan, E. G. 1996. Depurinating and stable benzo[a]pyrene–DNA adducts formed in isolated rat liver nuclei. Chem. Res. Toxicol. 9:1113–1116.

Feng, Z, Hu, W, Hu, Y., and Tang, M. S. 2006. Acrolein is a major cigarette-related lung cancer agent: Preferential binding at p53 mutational hotspots and inhibition of DNA repair. Proc. Natl. Acad. Sci. USA. 103:15404–15409.

Gmeiner, G, Krassnig, C, Schmid, E., and Tausch, H. 1998. Fast screening method for the profile analysis of polycyclic aromatic hydrocarbon metabolites in urine using derivatization–solid-phase microextraction. J. Chromatogr. B Biomed. Sci. Appl. 705:132–138.

Grimmer, G, Dettbarn, G., and Jacob, J. 1993. Biomonitoring of polycyclic aromatic hydrocarbons in highly exposed coke plant workers by measurement of urinary phenanthrene and pyrene metabolites (phenols and dihydrodiols). Int. Arch. Occup. Environ. Health 65:189–199.

Grimmer, G, Jacob, J, Dettbarn, G., and Naujack, K. W. 1997. Determination of urinary metabolites of polycyclic aromatic hydrocarbons (PAH) for the risk assessment of PAH-exposed workers. Int. Arch. Occup. Environ. Health 69:231–239.

Guenthner, T. M. and Oesch, F. 1981. Microsomal epoxide hydrolase and its role in polycyclic aromatic hydrocarbon biotransformation. In Polycyclic Hydrocarbons and Cancer, Vol. 3, eds. H. V. Gelboin, and P. O. P. Ts'o, pp. 183–212. New York: Academic Press

Gundel, J, Mannschreck, C, Buttner, K, Ewers, U., and Angerer, J. 1996. Urinary levels of 1-hydroxypyrene, 1-, 2-, 3-, and 4- hydroxyphenanthrene in females living in an industrial area of Germany. Arch. Environ. Contam. Toxicol. 31:585–590.

Harris, C. C, Autrup, H, Connor, R, Barrett, L. A, McDowell, E. M., and Trump, B. F. 1976. Interindividual variation in binding of benzo[*a*]pyrene to DNA in cultured human bronchi. Science 194:1067–1069.

Hecht, S. S. 1999. Tobacco smoke carcinogens and lung cancer. J. Natl. Cancer Inst. 91:1194–1210.

Hecht, S. S. 2002. Human urinary carcinogen metabolites: biomarkers for investigating tobacco and cancer. Carcinogenesi*s* 23:907–922.

Hecht, S. S. 2003. Tobacco carcinogens, their biomarkers, and tobacco-induced cancer. Nature Rev. Cancer 3:733–744.

Hecht, S. S, Carmella, S. G, Yoder, A, Chen, M, Li, Z, Le, C, Jensen, J., and Hatsukami, D. K. 2006. Comparison of polymorphisms in genes involved in polycyclic aromatic hydrocarbon metabolism with urinary phenanthrene metabolite ratios in smokers. Cancer Epidemiol. Biomarkers & Prev. 15:1805–1811.

Hecht, S. S, Chen, M, Yagi, H, Jerina, D. M., and Carmella, S. G. 2003. *r*-1,*t*-2,3,*c*-4-Tetrahydroxy-1,2,3,4-tetrahydrophenanthrene in human urine: a potential biomarker for assessing polycyclic aromatic hydrocarbon metabolic activation. Cancer Epidemiol. Biomarkers & Prev. 12:1501–1508.

Hecht, S. S, Chen, M, Yoder, A, Jensen, J, Hatsukami, D, Le, C., and Carmella, S. G. 2005. Longitudinal study of urinary phenanthrene metabolite ratios: effect of smoking on the diol epoxide pathway. Cancer Epidemiol. Biomarkers & Prev. 14:2969–2974.

Heudorf, U. and Angerer, J. 2001. Urinary monohydroxylated phenanthrenes and hydroxypyrene – the effects of smoking habits and changes induced by smoking on monooxygenase-mediated metabolism. Int. Arch. Occup. Environ. Health 74:177–183.

Hoepfner, I, Dettbarn, G, Scherer, G, Grimmer, G., and Adlkofer, F. 1987. Hydroxy-phenanthrenes in the urine of nonsmokers and smokers. Toxicol. Lett. 35:67–71.

Houlston, R. S. 2000. *CYP1A1* polymorphisms and lung cancer risk: a meta-analysis. Pharmacogenetics 10:105–114.

Hung, R. J, Boffetta, P, Brockmoller, J, Butkiewicz, D, Cascorbi, I, Clapper, M. L, Garte, S, Haugen, A, Hirvonen, A, Anttila, S, Kalina, I, Le Marchand, L, London, S. J, Rannug, A, Romkes, M, Salagovic, J, Schoket, B, Gaspari, L., and Taioli, E. 2003. CYP1A1 and GSTM1 genetic polymorphisms and lung cancer risk in Caucasian nonsmokers: a pooled analysis. Carcinogenesis 24:875–882.

International Agency for Research on Cancer. 1983. Polynuclear Aromatic Compounds, Part 1, Chemical, Environmental, and Experimental Data. In IARC Monographs on the Evaluation of the Carcinogenic Risk of Chemicals to Humans, Vol. 32, pp. 33–91. Lyon, FR: IARC.

International Agency for Research on Cancer. 1984. Polynuclear Aromatic Compounds, Part 3. Industrial Exposures in Aluminum Production, Coal Gasification, Coke Production, and Iron and Steel Founding. In IARC Monographs on the Evaluation of the Carcinogenic Risk of Chemicals to Humans, Vol. 34, pp. 65–131. Lyon, FR: IARC.

International Agency for Research on Cancer. 1985. Polynuclear Aromatic Compounds, Part 4. Bitumens, Coal-Tars and Derived Products, Shale Oils and Soots. In IARC Monographs on the Evaluation of the Carcinogenic Risk of Chemicals to Humans, Vol. 35, pp. 83–241. Lyon, FR: IARC

International Agency for Research on Cancer. 1986. Tobacco Smoking. In IARC Monographs on the Evaluation of the Carcinogenic Risk of Chemicals to Humans, Vol. 38, pp. 186–188. Lyon, FR: IARC

International Agency for Research on Cancer. 2004b. Tobacco Smoke and Involuntary Smoking. In IARC Monographs on the Evaluation of Carcinogenic Risks to Humans, Vol. 83, p. 1009. Lyon, FR: IARC

International Agency for Research on Cancer. 2004a. Tobacco Smoke and Involuntary Smoking. In IARC Monographs on the Evaluation of Carcinogenic Risks to Humans, Vol. 83, pp. 53–119. Lyon, FR: IARC

Jacob, J, Grimmer, G., and Dettbarn, G. 1999. Profile of urinary phenanthrene metabolites in smokers and non-smokers. Biomarkers 4:319–327.

Jacob, J. and Seidel, A. 2002. Biomonitoring of polycyclic aromatic hydrocarbons in human urine. J. Chromatog. B 778:31–47.

Jiang, H, Shen, Y. M, Quinn, A. M., and Penning, T. M. 2005. Competing roles of cytochrome P450 1A1/1B1 and aldo–keto reductase 1A1 in the metabolic activation of (+/–)-7,8-dihydroxy-7,8-dihydro-benzo[*a*]pyrene in human bronchoalveolar cell extracts. Chem. Res. Toxicol. 18:365–374.

Kim, J. H, Sherman, M. E, Curriero, F. C, Guengerich, F. P, Strickland, P. T., and Sutter, T. R. 2004. Expression of cytochromes P450 1A1 and 1B1 in human lung from smokers, non-smokers, and ex-smokers. Toxicol. Appl. Pharmacol. 199:210–219.

Kim, J. H, Stansbury, K. H, Walker, N. J, Trush, M. A, Strickland, P. T., and Sutter, T. R. 1999. Metabolism of benzo[*a*]pyrene and benzo[*a*]pyrene-7,8-diol by human cytochrome P450 1B1. Carcinogenesis 19:1847–1853.

Kiyohara, C, Nakanishi, Y, Inutsuka, S, Takayama, K, Hara, N, Motohiro, A, Tanaka, K, Kono, S., and Hirohata, T. 1998. The relationship between CYP1A1 aryl hydrocarbon hydroxylase activity and lung cancer in a Japanese population. Pharmacogenetics 8:315–323.

Kuusimaki, L, Peltonen, Y, Mutanen, P, Peltonen, K., and Savela, K. 2003. Urinary hydroxy-metabolites of naphthalene, phenanthrene and pyrene as markers of exposure to diesel exhaust. Int. Arch. Occup. Environ. Health 77:23–30.

Le Marchand, L, Guo, C, Benhamou, S, Bouchardy, C, Cascorbi, I, Clapper, M. L, Garte, S, Haugen, A, Ingelman-Sundberg, M, Kihara, M, Rannug, A, Ryberg, D, Stucker, I, Sugimura, H., and Taioli, E. 2003. Pooled analysis of the CYP1A1 exon 7 polymorphism and lung cancer (United States). Cancer Causes Control 14:339–346.

Lee, W. J, Brennan, P, Boffetta, P, London, S. J, Benhamou, S, Rannug, A, To-Figueras, J, Ingelman-Sundberg, M, Shields, P, Gaspari, L., and Taioli, E. 2002. Microsomal epoxide hydrolase polymorphisms and lung cancer risk: a quantitative review. Biomarkers 7:230–241.

Lintelmann, J, Hellemann, C., and Kettrup, A. 1994. Coupled-column high-performance liquid chromatographic method for the determination of four metabolites of polycyclic aromatic hydrocarbons, 1-, 4- and 9-hydroxyphenanthrene and 1-hydroxypyrene, in urine. J. Chromatog. B 660:67–73.

London, S. J, Yuan, J. M, Coetzee, G. A, Gao, Y. T, Ross, R. K., and Yu, M. C. 2000. CYP1A1 I462 V genetic polymorphism and lung cancer risk in a cohort of men in Shanghai, China. Cancer Epidemiol. Biomarkers & Prev. 9:987–991.

Mannschreck, C, Gundel, J., and Angerer, J. 1996. Occupational exposure to PAHs – biological monitoring of hydroxylated metabolites. Polycycl. Aromat. Comp. 11:11–18.

McLemore, T. L, Adelberg, S, Liu, M. C, McMahon, N. A, Yu, S. J, Hubbard, W. C, Czerwinski, M, Wood, T. G, Storeng, R, Lubet, R. A, Eggleston J. C, Boyd M. R., and Hines, R. N. 1990. Expression of CYP1A1 gene in patients with lung cancer: evidence for cigarette smoke-induced gene expression in normal lung tissue and for altered gene regulation in primary pulmonary carcinomas. J. Natl. Cancer Inst. 82:1333–1339.

Mills, X. E, Fishman, C. L, Rom, W. N, Dubin, N., and Jacobson, D. R. 1995. Increased prevalence of K-*ras* oncogene mutations in lung adenocarcinma. Cancer Res. 55:1444–1447.

Nebert, D. W. 2000. Drug-metabolizing enzymes, polymorphisms and interindividual response to environmental toxicants. Clin. Chem. Lab. Med. 38:857–861.

Nebert, D. W, Dalton, T. P, Okey, A. B., and Gonzalez, F. J. 2004. Role of aryl hydrocarbon receptor-mediated induction of the CYP1 enzymes in environmental toxicity and cancer. J Biol. Chem. 279:23847–23850.

Nebert, D. W, McKinnon, R. A., and Puga, A. 1996. Human drug-metabolizing enzyme polymorphisms: effects on risk of toxicity and cancer. DNA Cell Biol. 15:273–280.

Nesnow, S, Ross, J. A, Mass, M. J., and Stoner, G. D. 1998. Mechanistic relationships between DNA adducts, oncogene mutations, and lung tumorigenesis in Strain A mice. Exp. Lung Res. 24:395–405.

Ng, D. P, Tan, K. W, Zhao, B., and Seow, A. 2005. CYP1A1 polymorphisms and risk of lung cancer in non-smoking Chinese women: influence of environmental tobacco smoke exposure and GSTM1/T1 genetic variation. Cancer Causes Control 16:399–405.

Nordquist, M, Thakker, D. R, Vyas, K. P, Yagi, H, Levin, W, Ryan, D. E., and Thomas, P. E. 1981. Metabolism of chrysene and phenanthrene to bay-region diol epoxides by rat liver enzymes. Mol. Pharmacol. 19:168–178.

Nowak, D, Schmidt-Preuss, U, Jorres, R, Liebke, F., and Rudiger, H. W. 1988. Formation of DNA adducts and water-soluble metabolites of benzo[*a*]pyrene in human monocytes is genetically controlled. Int. J. Cancer 41:169–173.

Petersen, D. D, McKinney, C. E, Ikeya, K, Smith, H. H, Bale, A. E, McBride, O. W., and Nebert, D. W. 1991. Human CYP1A1 gene: cosegregation of the enzyme inducibility phenotype and an RFLP. Am. J. Hum. Genet. 48:720–725.

Pfeifer, G. P, Denissenko, M. F, Olivier, M, Tretyakova, N, Hecht, S. S., and Hainaut, P. 2002. Tobacco smoke carcinogens, DNA damage and p53 mutations in smoking-associated cancers. Oncogene 21:7435–7451.

Port, J. L, Yamaguchi, K, Du, B, De Lorenzo, M, Chang, M, Heerdt, P. M, Kopelovich, L, Marcus, C. B, Altorki, N. K, Subbaramaiah, K., and Dannenberg, A. J. 2004. Tobacco smoke induces CYP1B1 in the aerodigestive tract. Carcinogenesis 25:2275–2281.

Robertson, I. G. C, Guthenberg, C, Mannervik, B., and Jernström, B. 1986. Differences in stereoselectivity and catalytic efficiency of three human glutathione transferases in the conjugation of glutathione with 7β,8α-dihyroxy-9α,10α-oxy-7,8,9,10-tetrahydrobenzo(a)pyrene. Cancer Res. 46:2220–2224.

Sabadie, N, Richter-Reichhelm, H. B, Saracci, R, Mohr, U., and Bartsch, H. 1981. Inter-individual differences in oxidative benzo(*a*)pyrene metabolism by normal and tumorous surgical lung specimens from 105 lung cancer patients. Int. J. Cancer 27:417–425.

Serdar, B, Waidyanatha, S, Zheng, Y., and Rappaport, S. M. 2003. Simultaneous determination of urinary 1- and 2-naphthols, 3- and 9-phenanthrols, and 1-pyrenol in coke oven workers. Biomarkers 8:93–109.

Shimada, T, Gillam, E. M. J, Oda, Y, Tsumara, F, Sutter, T. R, Guengerich, F. P., and Inoue, K. 1999. Metabolism of benzo[*a*]pyrene to *trans*-7,8-dihydroxy-7,8-dihydrobenzo[*a*]pyrene by recombinant human cytochrome P450 1B1 and purified liver epoxide hydrolase. Chem. Res. Toxicol. 12:623–629.

Shimada, T, Hayse, C. L, Yamazaki, H, Amin, S, Hecht, S. S, Guengerich, F. P., and Sutter, T. R. 1996. Activation of chemically diverse procarcinogens by human cytochrome P450 1B1. *Cancer Res.* 56:2979–2984.

Shou, M, Korzekwa, K. R, Crespi, C. L, Gonzalez, F. J., and Gelboin, H. V. 1994a. The role of 12 *c*DNA-expressed human, rodent, and rabbit cytochromes P450 in the metabolism of benzo[*a*]pyrene and benzo[*a*]pyrene *trans*-7,8-dihydrodiol. Mol. Carcinogenesis 10:159–168.

Shou, M, Korzekwa, K. R, Krausz, K. W, Crespi, C. L, Gonzalez, F. J., and Gelboin, H. V. 1994b. Regio- and stereo-selective metabolism of phenanthrene by twelve cDNA-expressed human, rodent, and rabbit cytochromes P-450. Cancer Lett. 83:305–313.

Smith, C. J, Huang, W, Walcott, C. J, Turner, W, Grainger, J., and Patterson, D. G, Jr. 2002a. Quantification of monohydroxy-PAH metabolites in urine by solid-phase extraction with isotope dilution-GC-MS. Anal. Bioanal. Chem. 372:216–220.

Smith, C. J, Walcott, C. J, Huang, W, Maggio, V, Grainger, J., and Patterson Jr., D. G. 2002b. Determination of selected monohydroxy metabolites of 2-, 3- and 4-ring polycyclic aromatic hydrocarbons in urine by solid-phase microextraction and isotope dilution gas chromatography-mass spectrometry. J. Chromatogr. B 778:157–164.

Smith, G. B, Harper, P. A, Wong, J. M, Lam, M. S, Reid, K. R, Petsikas, D., and Massey, T. E. 2001. Human lung microsomal cytochrome P4501A1 (CYP1A1) activities: impact of smoking status and CYP1A1, aryl hydrocarbon receptor, and glutathione S-transferase M1 genetic polymorphisms. Cancer Epidemiol. Biomarkers & Prev. 10:839–853.

Smith, L. E, Denissenko, M. F, Bennett, W. P, Li, H, Amin, S, Tang, M., and Pfeifer, G. P. 2000. Targeting of lung cancer mutational hotspots by polycyclic aromatic hydrocarbons. J. Natl. Cancer Inst. 92:803–811.

Song, N, Tan, W, Xing, D., and Lin, D. 2001. CYP 1A1 polymorphism and risk of lung cancer in relation to tobacco smoking: a case–control study in China. Carcinogenesis 22:11–16.

Straif, K, Baan, R, Grosse, Y, Secretan, B, El Ghissassi, F., and Cogliano, V. 2005. Carcinogenicity of polycyclic aromatic hydrocarbons. Lancet Oncol. 6:931–932.

Sundberg, K, Dreij, K, Seidel, A., and Jernstrom, B. 2002. Glutathione conjugation and DNA adduct formation of dibenzo[*a*,l]pyrene and benzo[*a*]pyrene diol epoxides in V79 cells stably expressing different human glutathione transferases. Chem. Res. Toxicol. 15:170–179.

Sundberg, K, Johansson, A. S, Stenberg, G, Widersten, M, Seidel, A, Mannervik, B., and Jernstrom, B. 1998. Differences in the catalytic efficiencies of allelic variants of glutathione transferase P1-1 towards carcinogenic diol epoxides of polycyclic aromatic hydrocarbons. Carcinogenesis 19:433–436.

Sundberg, K, Widersten, M, Seidel, A, Mannervik, B., and Jernstrom, B. 1997. Glutathione conjugation of bay- and fjord-region diol epoxides of polycyclic aromatic hydrocarbons by glutathione transferase M1-1 and P1-1. Chem. Res. Toxicol. 10:1221–1227.

Tang, C, Lin, J. H., and Lu, A. Y. 2005. Metabolism-based drug–drug interactions: what determines individual variability in cytochrome P450 induction? Drug Metab. Dispos. 33:603–613.

Thakker, D. R, Yagi, H, Levin, W, Wood, A. W, Conney, A. H., and Jerina, D. M. 1985. Polycyclic aromatic hydrocarbons: metabolic activation to ultimate carcinogens. In Bioactivation of Foreign Compounds, ed. M. W. Anders, pp. 177–242. New York: Academic Press, Inc.

Tretyakova, N. T, Matter, B, Jones, R., and Shallop, A. 2002. Formation of benzo[*a*]pyrene diol epoxide–DNA adducts at specific guanines within K-ras and p53 gene sequences: stable isotope-labeling mass spectrometry approach. Biochemistry 41:9535–9544.

U.S.Department of Health and Human Services. 2004. Report on Carcinogens, 11th Edition. p. III-220-III-222 Research Triangle Park, N.C.

Upadhyaya, P, Rao, P, Hochalter, J. B, Li, Z. Z, Villalta, P. W., and Hecht, S. S. 2006. Quantitation of *N*-Acetyl-*S*-(9,10-dihydro-9-hydroxy-10-phenanthryl)-L-cysteine in human urine: comparison with glutathione-S-transferase genotypes in smokers. Chem. Res. Toxicol. 19:1234–1240.

Vineis, P, Veglia, F, Anttila, S, Benhamou, S, Clapper, M. L, Dolzan, V, Ryberg, D, Hirvonen, A, Kremers, P, Le Marchand, L, Pastorelli, R, Rannug, A, Romkes, M, Schoket, B, Strange, R. C, Garte, S., and Taioli, E. 2004. CYP1A1, GSTM1 and GSTT1 polymorphisms and lung cancer: a pooled analysis of gene–gene interactions. Biomarkers 9:298–305.

Vineis, P, Veglia, F, Benhamou, S, Butkiewicz, D, Cascorbi, I, Clapper, M. L, Dolzan, V, Haugen, A, Hirvonen, A, Ingelman-Sundberg, M, Kihara, M, Kiyohara, C, Kremers, P, Le Marchand, L, Ohshima, S, Pastorelli, R, Rannug, A, Romkes, M, Schoket, B, Shields, P, Strange, R. C, Stucker, I, Sugimura, H, Garte, S, Gaspari, L., and Taioli, E. 2003. CYP1A1 T3801 C polymorphism and lung cancer: a pooled analysis of 2451 cases and 3358 controls. Int. J. Cancer 104:650–657.

Westra, W. H, Slebos, R. J, Offerhaus, G. J. A, Goodman, S. N, Evers, S. G, Kensler, T. W, Askin, F. B, Rodenhuis, S., and Hruban, R. H. 1993. K-ras oncogene activation in lung adenocarcinomas from former smokers. Cancer 72:432–438.

Yang, X. R, Wacholder, S, Xu, Z, Dean, M, Clark, V, Gold, B, Brown, L. M, Stone, B. J, Fraumeni, J. F, Jr., and Caporaso, N. E. 2004. CYP1A1 and GSTM1 polymorphisms in relation to lung cancer risk in Chinese women. Cancer Lett. 214:197–204.

Yu, D, Berlin, J. A, Penning, T. M., and Field, J. 2002. Reactive oxygen species generated by PAH *o*-quinones cause change-in-function mutations in p53. Chem. Res. Toxicol. 15:832–842.

Index

Printed in the United States of America